Interdisciplinary Approaches to Overlap Disorders in Dermatology & Rheumatology

Amit Garg • Joseph F. Merola
Laura Fitzpatrick
Editors

Interdisciplinary Approaches to Overlap Disorders in Dermatology & Rheumatology

Springer

Editors
Amit Garg
Department of Dermatology
Donald and Barbara Zucker School of Medicine at Hofstra Northwell
Hempstead, NY
USA

Laura Fitzpatrick
Department of Dermatology
Donald and Barbara Zucker School of Medicine at Hofstra Northwell
Hempstead, NY
USA

Joseph F. Merola
Department of Dermatology
Department of Medicine
Division of Rheumatology
Inflammation and Immunity
Brigham and Women's Hospital
Harvard Medical School
Boston, MA
USA

ISBN 978-3-319-18445-6 ISBN 978-3-319-18446-3 (eBook)
https://doi.org/10.1007/978-3-319-18446-3

This Springer imprint is published by the registered company Springer Nature Switzerland AG
The registered company address is: Gewerbestrasse 11, 6330 Cham, Switzerland

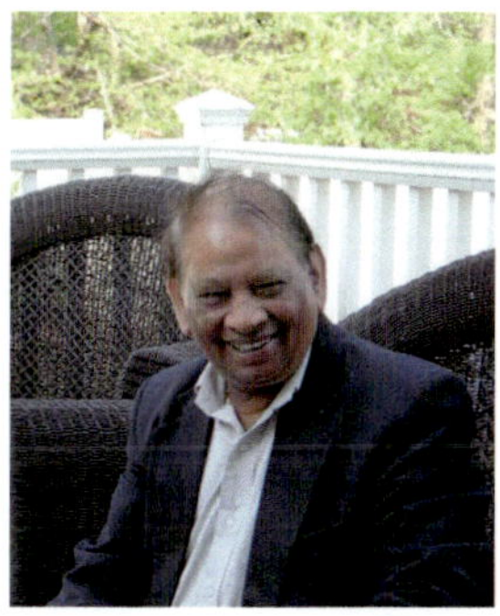

This book was inspired by my late father, Dr. Shankar Lal Garg, who loved rheumatology. He had the great fortune of training with his mentor Dr. John J. Calabro. Thereafter, my father practiced rheumatology for over 45 years in central Massachusetts. What I appreciated most while spending time in his office after school was that his patients adored him, even at a time when health outcomes in rheumatology, in the absence of truly disease modifying treatments, were modest. It was his compassion, kindness, skills, and knowledge which drove this sentiment. My observations in his practice and our dinner table conversations ultimately inspired me to pursue an inter-related focus with the specialty about which he was so passionate.

My father was the youngest of nine siblings and grew up in a village on the outskirts of old Delhi. He was accepted into the prestigious All India Institute of Medical Sciences and graduated as one of their Gold Medalists. His elder brother Baghat, the only other sibling with any sort of higher education, sold his scooter to pay for my father's flight to the United States so that he could pursue their shared dream of him practicing medicine abroad. And Boy, did he!

My father practiced rheumatology until he passed in late 2016. One of my most beloved life moments was reacquainting with one of his patients, someone I had first met in his office when I was just 12 years of age. He dropped in while I was cleaning out my father's office to share stories about his care with my father. I'm certain there were hundreds of patients who had the same cherished experiences, ones I try and build with my own patients each week as a medical dermatologist.

A quote by Nelson Mandela resonated with my father, because it aligned with his own personal philosophy in life, and he inspired me to live by it as well. If I can be half as inspiring to my own kids as my father was to me, they will be just fine.

There's no passion to be found in playing small – in settling for a life that is less than the one you are capable of living – Nelson Mandela.

Foreword

Rheumatic skin diseases are at the core of complex medical dermatology. Drs. Garg, Merola and Fitzpatrick have assembled a group of nationally known dermatologists, rheumatologists and one pulmonologist to deal with these systemic diseases with prominent cutaneous manifestations.

Cutaneous manifestations are important clues to rapid and accurate diagnosis. In addition, cutaneous diseases may complicate therapies directed at control of systemic disease. The approach that is taken in this book is to first approach diagnosis. Over a century ago, Louis A. Duhring stated that "*The power of making a correct diagnosis is the key to all success in the treatment of skin diseases; without this faculty, the physician can never be a thorough dermatologist, and therapeutics at once cease to hold their proper position, and become empirical.*" The first two chapters speak directly to this issue by first laying out the findings in order to make a correct diagnosis and then detailing the evaluation that is necessary. Subsequently the authors deal with traditional diseases in chapters on lupus, dermatomyositis, scleroderma, psoriasis and psoriatic arthritis, vasculitis, and sarcoidosis before ending with two chapters on the complications of therapy.

The editors and authors have provided the reader with information that will improve diagnostic acumen and should result in improved patient care.

Jeffrey P. Callen
Professor of Medicine (Dermatology)
Chief, Division of Dermatology
University of Louisville School of Medicine
Louisville, KY, USA

Preface

To my colleagues and all learners of overlap diseases involving the integument:

I very much hope you enjoy reading the first edition of our textbook *Interdisciplinary Approaches to Overlap Disorders in Dermatology & Rheumatology*. While there are a number of available sources on this subject area, there are few which exist as consolidated evidence-based inter-disciplinary summaries. This book was in part inspired by a magnificent predecessor of sorts, titled *Cutaneous Manifestations of Rheumatic Diseases*, by Sontheimer and Provost, with the acknowledgment that our knowledge in this field has evolved significantly over the past two decades. My own personal inspiration was also drawn from experiences with my father, a rheumatologist, about whom I have written in the Dedication.

The dynamic nature of new information made it a challenge for us to stay current, even through the initial drafting of content and the editorial process, especially with respect to approval of new treatments (i.e., biologic therapies) and observations of mucocutaneous reactions to novel chemotherapies, for example. We also gave our authors the freedom to write in their own styles as well as some flexibilities in format, with the intent of allowing the experts the ability to relate and emphasize content which flowed naturally for the subject area. This has resulted in some variation in the way the chapters read, something that will likely be better harmonized in a second edition.

Despite some of the challenges common to first edition textbooks, this project was a joy to pursue. Joe and Laura were terrific partners in this endeavor. It was a privilege to have one of my mentors and accomplished medical dermatologist, Dr. Jeffrey Callen, write the foreword. For the content, we recruited the very best experts, many of whom are responsible for the primary evidence described in the chapters. I want to extend my deepest gratitude to all of my aforementioned colleagues for skillfully engaging this project.

Nearly all chapters provide an interdisciplinary perspective, one from dermatology, and the other from rheumatology or another related subspecialty, based on the topic. We felt this was a unique and critical value addition to the resource which would facilitate an expanded scope of perspective and practice. The value to dermatologists is derived from knowledge and pearls related to multi-system examinations, workup, and assessments. The value to rheumatologists and other subspecialists originates from detailed morphologic descriptions or eruptions and dermatologic assessments that will support, and often specify, diagnosis. We are also certain that students of medicine and trainees across medical specialties will find value in the comprehensive multidisciplinary perspectives that will support disease recognition and early referral or management.

Hempstead, NY, USA Amit Garg

Contents

Contributors

Allireza Alloo, MD Department of Dermatology, Donald and Barbara Zucker School of Medicine at Hofstra Northwell, Hempstead, NY, USA

Robert P. Baughman, MD University of Cincinnati Medical Center, Department of Internal Medicine, Cincinnati, OH, USA

Lorinda Chung, MD, MS Division of Immunology and Rheumatology, Stanford University School of Medicine, Palo Alto, CA, USA

VA Palo Alto Health Care System, Palo Alto, CA, USA

M. Kari Connolly, MD University of California San Francisco, Dermatology and Medicine, San Francisco, CA, USA

Alisa N. Femia, MD Ronald O. Perelman Department of Dermatology, NYU Grossman School of Medicine, New York, NY, USA

Laura Ferris, MD University of Pittsburgh, Pittsburgh, PA, USA

David Fiorentino, MD, PhD Department of Dermatology, Stanford University School of Medicine, Redwood City, CA, USA

Amit Garg, MD Department of Dermatology, Donald and Barbara Zucker School of Medicine at Hofstra Northwell, Hempstead, NY, USA

Tania C. González-Rivera, MD University of Pennsylvania, Internal Medicine, Division of Rheumatology, Philadelphia, PA, USA

Anna Helena Jonsson, MD, PhD Brigham and Women's Hospital, Division of Rheumatology, Inflammation, and Immunity, Department of Medicine, Boston, MA, USA

Harvard Medical School, Boston, MA, USA

Matt Lewis, MD, MPH Department of Dermatology, Stanford University School of Medicine, Redwood City, CA, USA

Ada Man, MD University of Manitoba, Winnipeg, MB, Canada

Daniel R. Mazori, MD Ronald O. Perelman Department of Dermatology, NYU Grossman School of Medicine, New York, NY, USA

Peter A. Merkel, MD, MPH Division of Rheumatology, University of Pennsylvania, Philadelphia, PA, USA

Joseph F. Merola, MD, MMSc Department of Dermatology, Department of Medicine, Division of Rheumatology, Inflammation and Immunity, Brigham and Women's Hospital, Boston, MA, USA

Harvard Medical School, Boston, MA, USA

Robert G. Micheletti, MD Department of Dermatology, University of Pennsylvania, Philadelphia, PA, USA

Lisa Pappas-Taffer Corporal Michael J. Crescenz VAMC, Philadelphia, PA, USA

Department of Dermatology, University of Pennsylvania, Philadelphia, PA, USA

Mital Patel-Cohen, MD Summit Health, Florham Park, NJ, USA

Soumya Reddy, MD NYU Langone School of Medicine, New York, NY, USA

Shelly Rivas, MD Department of Dermatology, Donald and Barbara Zucker School of Medicine at Hofstra Northwell, Hempstead, NY, USA

Misha Rosenbach, MD Dermatology & Internal Medicine, Cutaneous Sarcoidosis Clinic, University of Pennsylvania, Philadelphia, PA, USA

Jordan Taylor Said, BA Harvard Medical School, Boston, MA, USA

Peter H. Schur, BS, MD Brigham and Women's Hospital, Division of Rheumatology, Inflammation, and Immunity, Department of Medicine, Boston, MA, USA

Harvard Medical School, Boston, MA, USA

Robert W. Simms, MD Boston University School of Medicine, Boston, MA, USA

Marleigh Stern, MD New York University School of Medicine, New York, NY, USA

Victoria P. Werth, MD, MS Corporal Michael J. Crescenz VAMC, Philadelphia, PA, USA

Department of Dermatology, University of Pennsylvania, Philadelphia, PA, USA

1 Evaluation of the Integumentary and Musculokeletal Systems: An Approach to the Interdisciplinary Examination for Overlap Diseases

Mital Patel-Cohen, Amit Garg, Jordan Taylor Said, and Joseph F. Merola

Introduction

A comprehensive skin examination is an integral component to the evaluation of patients with, or suspected to have, an inflammatory or autoimmune musculoskeletal disease. Integumentary findings, inclusive of the skin, nails and hair, often provide specificity when clinical features otherwise yield an indeterminate diagnosis. These findings, although sometimes subtle (i.e., periungual swelling and erythema), may be detected through an attentive awareness of these signs and proper approach. While a full description of the dermatological lexicon and the comprehensive examination of the integument is beyond the scope of this chapter, the most important aspects of the examination that will support the evaluation and management of patients with connective tissue conditions are described herein. We conclude with a summary of elements of the musculoskeletal and joint exam that we recommend synthesizing with skin examination findings, particularly in the case of evaluating patients with rheumatologic skin disease.

M. Patel-Cohen (✉)
Summit Health, Florham Park, NJ, USA
e-mail: mpatelcohen@smgnj.com

A. Garg
Department of Dermatology, Donald and Barbara Zucker School of Medicine at Hofstra Northwell, Hempstead, NY, USA

J. T. Said
Harvard Medical School, Boston, MA, USA

J. F. Merola
Department of Dermatology, Department of Medicine, Division of Rheumatology, Inflammation and Immunity, Brigham and Women's Hospital, Boston, MA, USA

Harvard Medical School, Boston, MA, USA

General Recommendations

The examination of the integument should be performed in a well-lit room, ideally with natural sunlight, as this type of light is least likely to alter the perception of erythema color. A penlight is helpful in examining areas such as the mouth or the ears in which there is less natural light exposure. The dermatoscope, a hand-held magnifier and specialized light source, may be helpful in visualizing small structures such as capillary loops in the nailfolds. Dermoscopy is particularly helpful in examining the nailfolds of patients with systemic sclerosis, dermatomyositis, systemic lupus erythematosus, mixed connective tissue disease, and Raynaud's phenomenon. Several studies suggest that the use of dermoscopy can replace the need for nailfold capillaroscopy in many instances (Bergman, JAMA Derm 2003).

A. Garg et al. (eds.), *Interdisciplinary Approaches to Overlap Disorders in Dermatology & Rheumatology*,
https://doi.org/10.1007/978-3-319-18446-3_1

The patient should be undressed at least to undergarments and donning a proper hospital gown. The patient should remove eyeglasses, dentures when feasible, jewelry including the watch, as well as make-up and nail polish, so that relevant findings are not hidden. It is important to be mindful of respecting the patient's modesty when undressed. Asking the patient's permission to move the gown or undergarments to expose the skin during the examination and informing the patient when examining sensitive areas helps to alleviate any unease.

A systematic approach that is used for every patient's examination will help ensure all relevant areas of integument are thoroughly evaluated. In patients with connective tissue disease, take note of several commonly affected areas, including the scalp, conchal bowls of the ears, face including the eyelids, oral mucosa, neck, upper chest, upper back, dorsal hands, nails and nail folds. It is important to examine all affected areas to determine the exact distribution of an eruption. In addition, making note of the eruption's color, shape, configuration, secondary changes such as scale, and palpability complete the morphologic assessment.

In addition, a complete and appropriately tailored rheumatologic/musculoskeletal examination can complement a thorough skin exam, informing the diagnosis and management for patients with rheumatologic-dermatologic overlap conditions. We focus here on the overview of assessing joint pathology; a thorough examination of neuromuscular disease is outside the scope of this introduction.

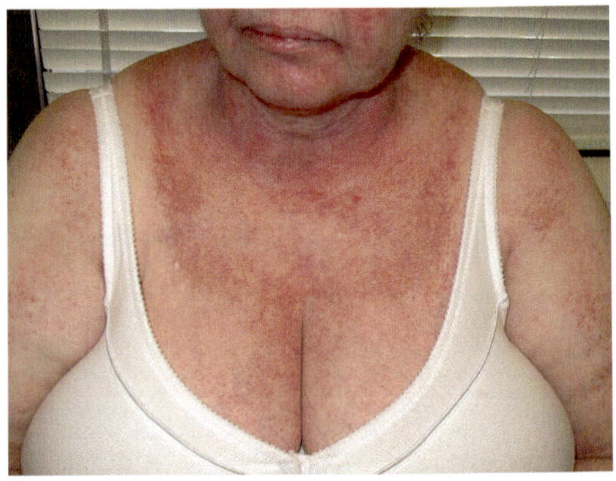

Fig. 1.1 Photodistributed. Erythema and poikiloderma most prominent over the cheeks, neck, and upper chest in a patient with dermatomyositis

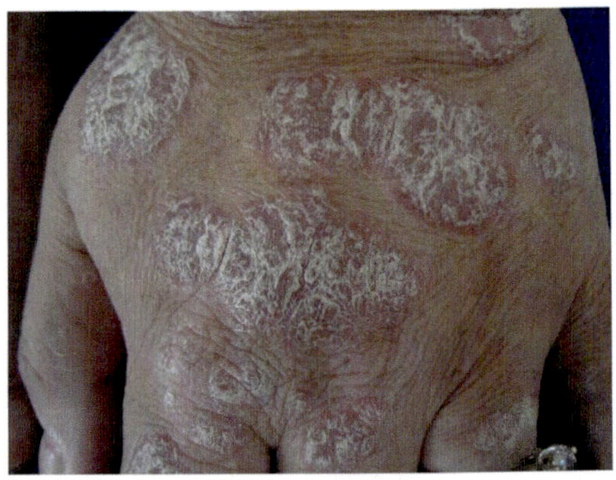

Fig. 1.2 Extensor. Well demarcated red erythematous plaque of psoriasis with white to silver colored scale on the dorsum of the hand

Distribution

The most important distribution pattern to recognize among patients with autoimmune and connective tissue diseases is the **photodistributed** eruption (Fig. 1.1). Photodistributed eruptions occur in areas usually not covered by clothing, which thereby receive the most direct ultraviolet exposure. These areas namely include the forehead, bilateral cheeks, nose, lower chin, lateral neck, a triangular area corresponding to the opening of a V-neck shirt on the anterior upper chest, the upper back, flexor forearms, and dorsal hands including the phalanges. Typically, there is also relative sparing of skin fully protected from the sun. Photosensitive eruptions occur in systemic and cutaneous lupus erythematous, Sjogren's syndrome, and dermatomyositis.

Plaques of psoriasis among patients with psoriatic arthritis are classically **extensor** (Fig. 1.2) in their distribution pattern. These plaques occur over the scalp, buttocks and extensor surfaces of all four extremities, including the elbows and knees. This is in contrast to atopic dermatitis (eczema) which is most often apparent on flexural surfaces. Psoriasis plaques are also commonly **bilateral and symmetric**, particularly on extensor surfaces. In some cases, psoriasis

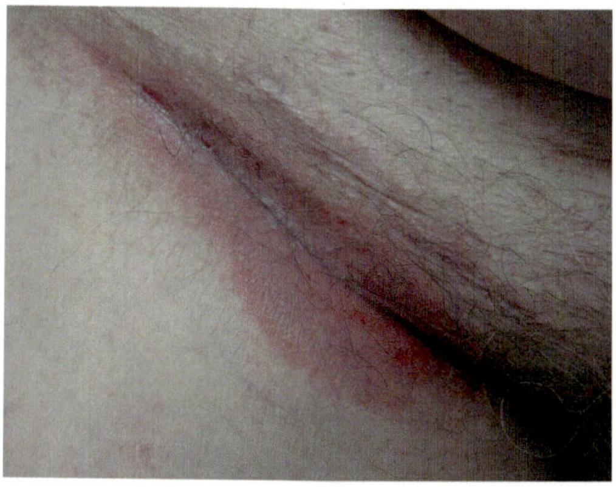

Fig. 1.3 Inverse. Well demarcated red erythematous plaque of psoriasis without scale in the inguinal crease

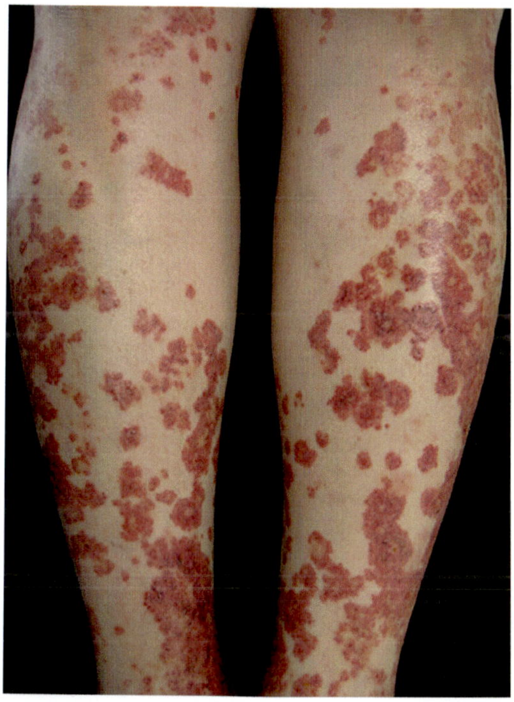

Fig. 1.4 Dependent. Purpuric (non-blanching) red to purple patches, papules and plaques over the lower extremities and more prominent distal to the knees

patients may present with an **inverse** distribution (Fig. 1.3), in which well-demarcated pink erythematous non-scaly plaques will appear in intertriginous folds such as the axillae, inframammary folds, and inguinal creases.

In leukocytoclastic vasculitis, palpable purpura is noted on **dependent** areas of the body (Fig. 1.4), such as the ankles and lower legs, and occasionally the buttocks and back in bedridden patients.

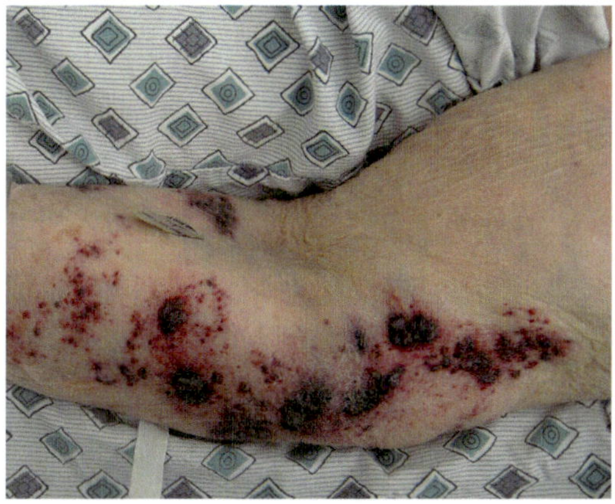

Fig. 1.5 Dermatomal. Grouped hemorrhagic vesicles and plaques following the C6 dermatome in this patient with herpes zoster

A **dermatomal or zosteriform** (Fig. 1.5) distributed eruption is in the distribution of a single spinal afferent nerve root (dermatome). It is unilateral and does not cross the midline of the body. The classic dermatomal eruption is herpes zoster, which commonly afflicts patients with chronic disease, immunotherapies, or advanced age.

Color

Perhaps the most important additional feature of an eruption, other than its distribution, is color. Color, which is often the first visual assessment made, is reliably reproducible with particular types of pathologics, including connective tissue diseases. As such, color provides meaningful insight into pathologic processes of the skin and facilitates clinical diagnosis.

Erythema represents the blanchable pink to red color of skin or mucous membrane. It exists in different colors, and to call a primary lesion *erythematous* alone is incomplete. Describing erythema with the color it most closely resembles provides a meaningful clue to diagnosis. For example, violaceous erythema of the periorbital area (heliotrope, Fig. 1.6), and in particular the lid margin, is highly suggestive of dermatomyositis. We note the same color of erythema in other dermatoses of connective tissue disease which also involve an interface dermatitis and dermal-epidermal junction. As another example, lilac colored erythema surrounding a slightly whitish and firm plaque is suggestive of morphea.

Red blood cells that extravasate from cutaneous vessels into skin or mucous membranes result in reddish-purple patches referred to as purpura. The application of pressure with two glass slides or an unbreakable clear lens (diascopy) on a reddish-purple lesion is a simple and reliable method for differentiating redness due to vascular dilatation (erythema) from redness due to extravasated erythrocytes or erythrocyte products (purpura). If the redness is non-blanching under the pressure of the slides, the lesion is purpuric. As extravasated red blood cells decompose over time, the color of purpuric lesions changes from bluish-red to yellowish-brown or green. Petechiae are tiny, pinpoint purpuric macules. Ecchymoses are larger, bruise-like purpuric patches. These lesions correspond to a non-inflammatory extravasation of blood. If a lesion is purpuric and palpable ("palpable purpura"), the suggestion of an inflammatory insult to the vessel wall as a cause of extravasation of blood and inflammatory cells exists. The classic histopathological correlate to palpable purpura is leukocytoclastic vasculitis (Fig. 1.4).

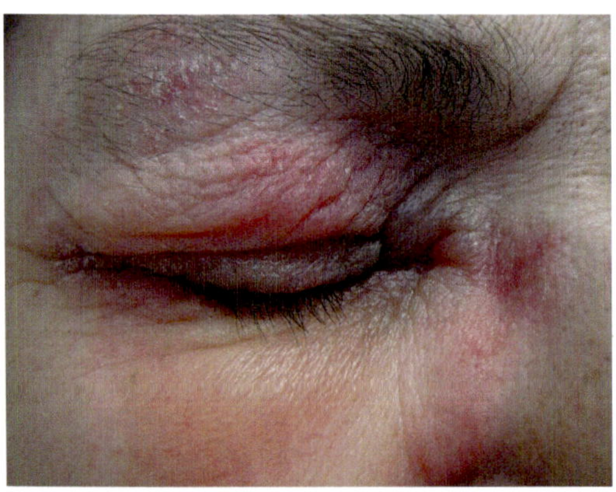

Fig. 1.6 Violaceous color. Intensely pink to purplish erythema, swelling and scale in the periorbital region representing the heliotrope in this patient with dermatomyositis

Erythema of any type is difficult to detect in darker skinned patients. Erythema in these instances may appear subtle or may appear more violaceous in color even when the true color is red or pink.

Shape or Configuration

Accurate appreciation of the shape or configuration of lesion(s) will facilitate narrowing of the differential diagnosis and specificity in diagnosis. There are several shapes and configurations of relevance to patients with inflammatory and autoimmune connective tissue diseases.

A linear configuration describes a lesion which resembles a straight line. This configuration may apply to a single lesion or to the arrangement of multiple lesions. Its appearance may suggest that the Koebner phenomenon (Fig. 1.7), defined as the appearance of the same lesion on previously normal appearing skin, has occurred in response to scratching or trauma. Psoriasis and Behcet's are two examples of conditions that exhibit koebnerization.

Round to oval, or coined-shaped, lesions that are uniform from the edges to the center of the lesion may be termed discoid (Fig. 1.8). Discoid lupus erythematous typically presents with coin-shaped plaques involving the scalp, face, and conchal bowls of the ears.

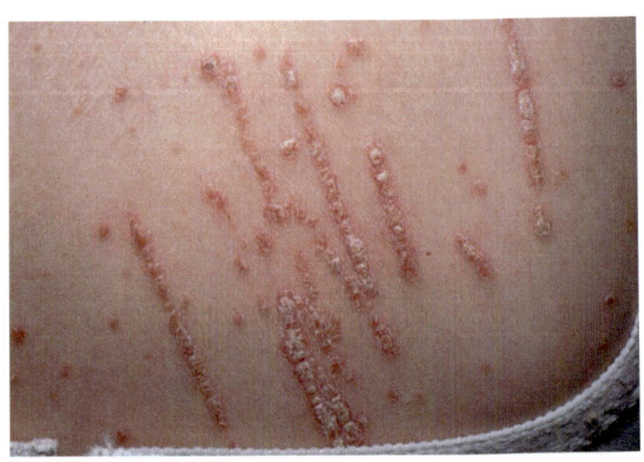

Fig. 1.7 Linear configuration. Well demarcated red erythematous linearized plaques on the back over areas that have been stimulated by scratching in a psoriasis patient

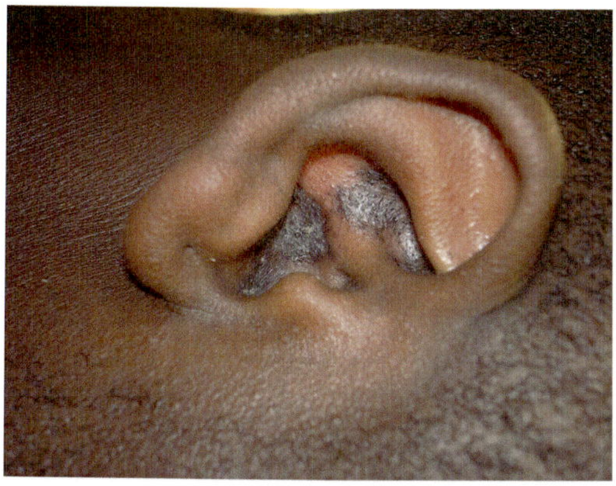

Fig. 1.8 Discoid shape. Rounded brown and slightly erythematous think plaques with follicular plugging in the conchal bowl of this patient with discoid lupus

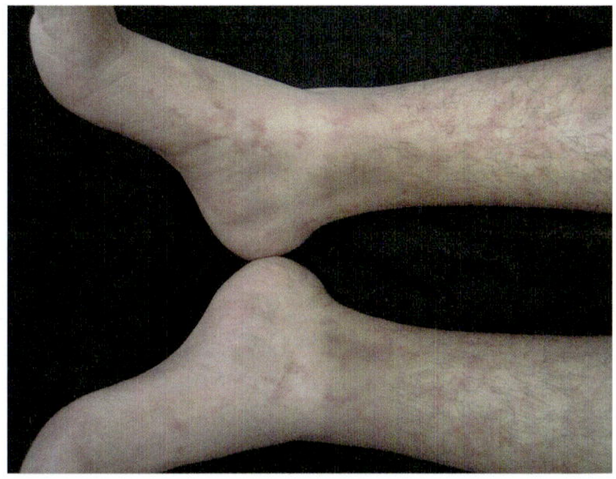

Fig. 1.10 Reticular. Light purple patches forming irregular, broken networks on the lower extremities and feet of this patient with cutaneous polyarteritis nodosa

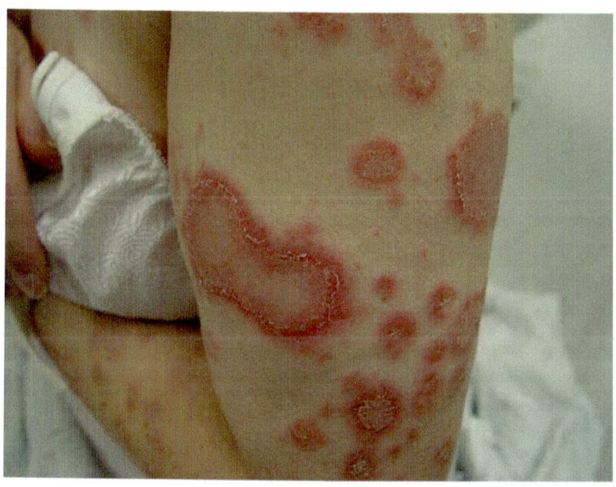

Fig. 1.9 Annular. Red erythematous annular plaques with peripherally located scale on the upper arms in this patient with terbinafine-induced subacute cutaneous lupus

In annular or ring-shaped lesions, the edge differs from the center, either by being flatter, more raised, scaly, or differing in color. Annular lesions that are incomplete form an arcuate shape. Annular lesions may coalesce to form circles or rings, in a polycyclic configuration. The annular, arcuate, and polycyclic patterns represent one form of subacute cutaneous lupus erythematosus (SCLE) (Fig. 1.9). Urticaria also commonly presents with the same shapes and configurations.

The reticular configuration is represented by net-like or lacy patches with somewhat regularly spaced rings or partial rings and sparing of intervening skin. The netlike pattern is more regular in livedo reticularis, whereas the rings in livedo racemosa tend to be more broken up and jagged (i.e., cutaneous polyarteritis nodosa, Fig. 1.10).

Scaling

When epidermal differentiation is disordered, accumulation and casting of stratum corneum become apparent as scale, which ranges in size from fine dust-like particles to extensive parchment-like sheets. Not all scales are similar, and the expert dermatologist with a well-trained eye can obtain diagnostically useful information from close examinations of the type of scale present.

Scale may be fine or thick, dry or greasy, loose or adherent, and may range in color from silvery-white to yellow or brown. In some instances, the diagnosis is based on specifying the type of scale present. For example, SCLE and psoriasis may both present with rounded well demarcated red erythematous plaques with scale. However, the scale in SCLE may be finer and more prominent around the periphery, whereas the silver-white colored scale in psoriasis will cover the plaque. Although layered, the scale in psoriasis is adherent and leads to pinpoint hemorrhage when peeled away. Scale in SCLE easily flakes off without bleeding. Plaques in discoid lupus erythematous also have an adherent scale which extends into the orifices of dilate hair follicles.

When the scale on these plaques is lifted, keratotic spikes formed with hair follicles under the surface of the scale may be visualized. These spikes are said to resemble carpet tacks, and hence this finding specific to Discoid lupus erythematosus (DLE) is known as the as "carpet tack" sign. Complete absence of scale is also helpful in differentiating eruptions. For example, urticaria and urticarial vasculitis may present as erythematous annular and polycyclic plaques, similar to SCLE. However, the former eruptions have no scale.

Consistency

Palpation of lesions is an important part of the physical examination. Plaques that are thick or firm may suggest fibroses of the skin, such as in morphea or systemic sclerosis. When the pannus of the skin in inflamed, as with erythema nodosum, the presentation typically includes rubbery to firm nodules on the lower extremities.

A similar, more diffuse firmness along with tiny dimples in the skin can be appreciated with deep fascial inflammation noted in eosinophilic fasciitis. "Rock" hard whitish plaques or nodules may represent calcinosis, seen in patients with dermatomyositis who have had an aggressive course, delay in treatment, or undertreatment, or in juvenile patients with the disease. Similar nodules can be seen in patients with limited scleroderma.

Scalp/Hair/Nails/Oral Mucosa

In addition to the skin examination, evaluation of the hair, nails, and oral mucosa offers important clues in the diagnosis of connective tissue disorders. Patients with Sjogren's syndrome have decreased salivary pools in the mouth, and in longstanding cases, the dorsum of the tongue may appear lobulated. In systemic lupus erythematosus, patients may have painful oral ulcers, most frequently observed on the roof of the mouth at the junction of hard and soft palates. In Behcet's disease, patients may present with multiple, painful, large aphthous ulcers on the mucosal lips, buccal mucosa and tongue.

The nail unit is comprised of the nail plate, nail bed, nail matrix, lunula, eponychium (cuticle), proximal nail folds (skin at base of nail plate), perionychium (skin at sides of nail plate), and the hyponychium (skin under free edge of nail plate). In connective tissue disorders, one or several of these structures may be altered. In psoriasis, for example, involvement of the nail matrix results in pitting of the nail plate. This finding, however, is not specific to psoriasis and can be seen in several other conditions, including alopecia areata and eczemas, and may also be present in otherwise healthy individuals. In psoriasis, patients will typically have multiple pits (>10) involving several fingernails. Psoriasis patients also commonly have yellow colored "oil spots" at the distal portions of the nail (Fig. 1.11). The discoloration occurs when the nail plate separates from the involved nailbed. The cuticles in patients with dermatomyositis become hypertrophic and appear ragged, a finding known as Samitz sign (Fig. 1.12). The proximal nailfold is also typically erythematous and edematous with dilatations in capillary loops, as it is in patients with systemic lupus erythematosus (Fig. 1.13). Capillary loops are also altered in patients with lupus erythematous and systemic sclerosis. In patients with systemic sclerosis, capillary loss ("dropout") often alternates with dilated capillary loops, forming a distinc-

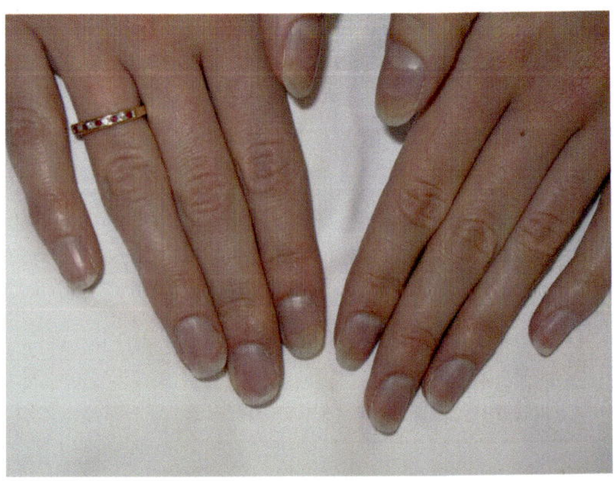

Fig. 1.11 Oil spot. Yellowish discoloration of the distal fingernails due to separation of the nail plate from the nail bed (onycholysis) in psoriasis

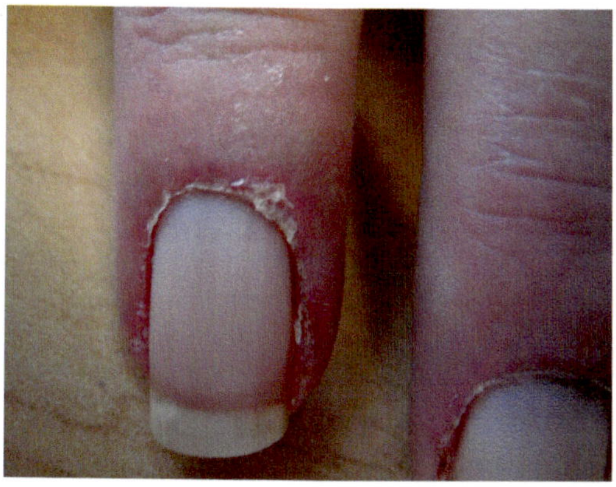

Fig. 1.12 Ragged cuticles. Periungual erythema and hyperkeratosis of the proximal and lateral nail folds (Samitz sign) in this patient with dermatomyositis

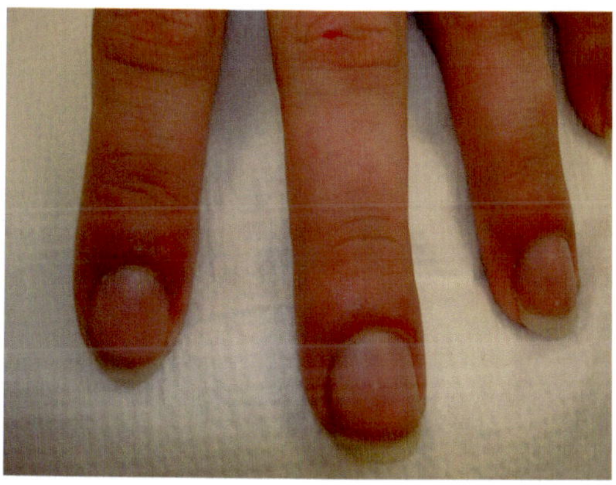

Fig. 1.13 Periungual erythema. Edema and periungual erythema in patients with systemic lupus erythematosus

tive pattern. The capillary abnormalities in systemic lupus erythematosus are more subtle and less specific but can include capillary dropout, alterations in capillary length (either sorter or longer) and alterations in capillary morphology (including tortuous or meandering capillaries); capillary microhemorrhages may also be present. (Fig. 1.14).

The scalp examination is particularly important in patients suspected of having psoriasis or dermatomyositis. Not infrequently, the only manifestation of psoriasis among patients with psoriatic arthritis is scalp involvement. Psoriasis plaques in the scalp tend to be well marginated, often involving the hairline of the scalp, and have a characteristic silver-colored scale. Patients with dermatomyositis frequently demonstrate diffuse scalp erythema of a similar color to the heliotrope sign involving the periorbital area.

Alopecia involving the scalp is a frequent finding in patients with lupus erythematosus. Patients with systemic disease commonly have non-scarring alopecia, i.e., hair loss without damage or destruction of the follicle. They may experience excessive diffuse shedding of scalp hairs, with the potential for hair to regrow. In discoid lupus erythematosus, however, inflammatory injury of the follicular epithelium leads to scarring alopecia. Once lost, these hairs do not regrow, even when the inflammatory process has regressed with or without treatment. Along with

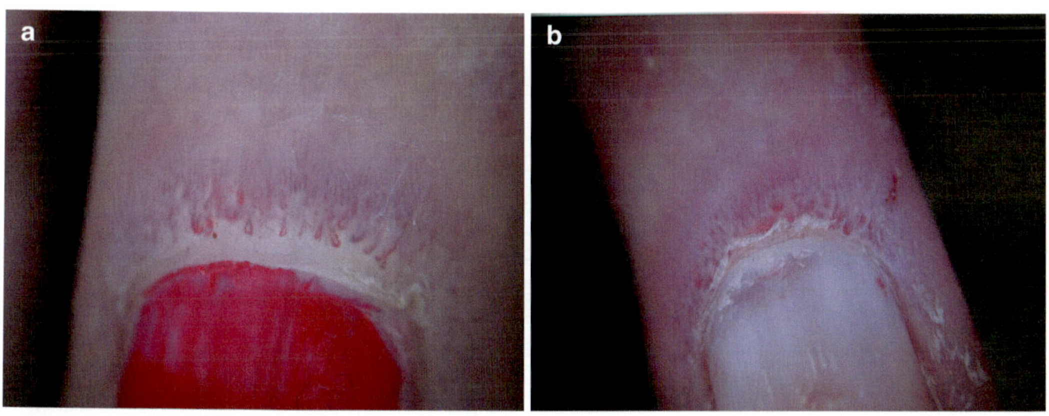

Fig. 1.14 Altered capillary loops. (**a**) sclerosis of proximal nail fold and dilatation of capillary loops in a patient with systemic sclerosis. (**b**) Advanced sclerosis of proximal nail fold with dilatation and further obliteration of capillary loops in a patient with systemic sclerosis

atrophy and discoloration of the skin, scarring alopecia results in significant morbidity. As such, this condition should be managed early and appropriately to minimize the occurrence of permanent hair loss.

Rheumatologic Musculoskeletal Examination

A targeted joint and musculoskeletal examination should be synthesized with the findings of a skin examination, particularly for patients with psoriasis who are at-risk for psoriatic arthritis, hidradenitis suppurativa (where increased prevalence of peripheral and/or axial spondyloarthritis occurs), connective tissue disorders, and other overlap conditions. Herein, we will review the hallmarks of the joint and muscle examinations that are most relevant for overlap diseases.

Joint Examination

Just as for the skin examination, a high-quality joint examination begins with establishing the optimal setting. Lighting should allow for visualization of the joint and any gross changes such as swelling, protrusions, overlying skin changes. The patient should be comfortable and in a gown or other non-restrictive clothing; this is important for both observation of the joints and the range of motion. Socks and shoes must be removed to properly assess all lower extremity joints.

A systematic and consistent approach to the examination will ensure a comprehensive and efficient evaluation. One commonly employed order includes evaluation of distal interphalangeal finger joints, proximal interphalangeal finger joints, metacarpal joints, wrist joints, elbow joints, shoulder joints, hip joints, knee joints, ankle joints, midtarsal joints, subtalar joints, metatarsal joints, proximal interphalangeal toe joints, distal interphalangeal toe joints, and spine (cervical to sacral), in succession.

Examination should begin with observation of each joint while the joint is at rest in order to assess for overlying skin changes [i.e., erythema, scale, papules, plaques, nodules), swelling, or gross deformities. Joint swelling is soft tissue swelling surrounding the joint, which is detectable along the joint margins. When a synovial effusion is present, it invariably means the joint has swelling.

After a joint is observed, it should be palpated. The objective of joint palpation is to assess for *warmth*, which may suggest inflammatory, infectious or crystal-induced arthritis; *tenderness,* and *swelling*. While the specific technique for joint palpation varies with each joint, the examiner should press into the fluid-filled bursa between the overlying muscle and bone. Sufficiently deep palpation of the joint bursa ensures that the examination is assessing the underlying joint, rather than the overlying muscle. Palpation is also necessary to confirm suspected swelling and to rule out bony swelling or deformity. Fluctuation is a characteristic feature of swollen joints.

Joint tenderness is pain in a joint under defined circumstances. Tenderness may occur at rest with pressure (i.e., MCPs and wrist joints); on movement of a joint (i.e., shoulder and tarsal joints); or may be assessed through questioning about joint pain (i.e., hips and cervical spine). Pain with physical manipulation of the bursa cushioning a specific joint may also suggest bursitis. When assessing for tenderness through palpation, pressure should be exerted by the examiner's thumb and index fingers to a sufficient degree to cause "whitening" of the examiner's nail bed, blanching about one-third to half-way down on the thumb to achieve adequate standard pressure.

Of particular utility is the assessment of 'entheseal' points; that is, points of tendon or ligament insertion into bone. Tenderness at these sites may suggest enthesitis, inflammation at the enthesis insertion, which is of particular relevance to the seronegative inflammatory arthritides such as psoriatic arthritis and other spondylo-athritis variants. Typical sites of examination include those noted in the Leeds Enthesitis Index, at the lateral epicondyles of the humerus, medial femoral condyles, and bilateral Achilles tendon insertions. The additional presence of widespread soft tissue tenderness might suggest a central sensitization syndrome such as fibromyalgia with referral to differentiating from inflammatory entheseal disease. To elicit diffuse soft tissue pain, palpation with similar pressure as noted above, to soft tissue areas of the upper back, upper arms and forearms, away from tendon insertion points or joints is applied. The finding of diffuse and often severe pain as experienced by the patient might suggest a concurrent or isolated pain syndrome such as central sensitization / fibromyalgia; it is worth noting that there is a relatively high co-prevalence of fibromyalgia with other inflammatory arthritides which means they may not be mutually exclusive in nature.

Finally, range of motion testing should be assessed for each joint. The patient's joints may be moved as tolerated to assess passive range of motion, or the patient can be observed performing active range of motion. Range of motion testing is important to assess restriction of movement, particularly in active range of motion testing. Range of motion testing can also be useful in determining presence of underlying swelling. For example, decreased dorsiflexion of the wrist and decreased elbow extension may suggest swelling of the involved joints.

The number of involved joints and overall distribution of joint tenderness and/or swelling is important for an examiner to synthesize. Joint diseases can be divided into monoarticular (one joint), oligoarticular (2–5), or polyarticular (>5) disease. The number of affected joints can inform the differential diagnosis of a patient's joint pain. For example, a monoarticular joint pain may be caused by crystal-induced disease (gout, calcium pyrophosphate deposition), septic arthritis, or a traumatic hemarthrosis; whereas, oligo- or polyarticular disease raises the possibility of rheumatoid arthritis, psoriatic arthritis, systemic lupus erythematosus (SLE), and viral infection (i.e., parvovirus B19), psoriatic arthritis, for example.

Distributions of disease may be described as symmetrical or asymmetrical, or may be small joint-predominant (MCPs, PIPs, DIPs) or large joint-predominant (knees, hips, shoulders, spine). Absence of disease in key joints may help to distinguish inflammatory joint diseases. For example, rheumatoid arthritis and osteoarthritis both involve joints of the upper and lower extremities. Rheumatoid arthritis tends to involve the MCPs and PIPs symmetrically while sparing the DIPs, while osteoarthritis involves the DIPs and can spare the MCPs. Involvement of the base of the thumb would be most typical of osteoarthritis.

Finally, an examination of the joints should include an assessment of the spine and chest. As with other joints, examination should begin with observation of overlying skin and any present deformities or swelling, and then proceed to palpation of the joint spaces of the cervical to sacral spine. A wide variety of specialized techniques exist that may be used to assess for presence of joint disease involving the spine, the details of which are beyond the scope of this chapter. However, a brief look at cervical neck range of motion and consideration of maneuvers such as the modified Schober test are useful in considering axial involvement of disease and can be successfully performed by the non-rheumatologist. The FABER (leg flexed, thigh abducted, externally rotated) test can also be helpful in eliciting hip, lumbar spine or sacroiliac pathology.

Other specialized assessments may be applied when specific conditions are uspected. For example, dactylitis of the fingers and toes is a common feature in psoriatic arthritis, and other peripheral / axial spondyloarthritides. A simple count of affected digits is relevant. For a more comprehensive entheseal evaluation, the Leeds dactylitis instrument can be utilized.

Muscle Examination

The muscular examination is comprised of both palpation and strength testing. Deep palpation of the muscle is unnecessary, in contrast to when joint palpation is performed. Tenderness upon palpation of muscle may suggestan underlying inflammatory myositis, such as dermatomyositis, polymyositis, or anti-synthetase syndrome.

Finally, a full-strength examination should be completed by assessing the force of each of the joint movements under resistance. Procedures for the strength examination vary with the muscle group being assessed, but it should always be conducted with resistance. For example, abduction of the elbow may be assessed with the examiner applying an adducting force to the forearm. Similarly, extension at the knee may be assessed against force applied to the anterior shin. Of note, the finding of reduced strength on examination is a non-specific sign, and may point to disease processes at the level of the bone, muscle, joint, or the nervous supply.

Conclusion

This chapter has reviewed the fundamentals of the skin and musculoskeletal examinations relevant for overlap diseases. The astute clinician, attentive to the myriad of integumentary disorders that may afflict patients with these diseases, will have an opportunity to add specificity to the overall evaluation with the goal of early and accurate diagnosis.

Serologic Evaluation in the Rheumatology-Dermatology Overlap Patient

2

Anna Helena Jonsson, Marleigh Stern, Alisa N. Femia, and Peter H. Schur

Key Points

- A functional appreciation of the application and limitations of serologic and other laboratory tests is essential for the evaluation and management of patients with inflammatory and autoimmune skin and musculoskeletal diseases.
- Serologic tests are utilized to support diagnosis, and in some cases, they may be useful in predicting prognosis or monitoring disease activity.
- Presence of antibodies in asymptomatic patients does not equate to development of disease. Diagnosis should never be based on the presence or absence of antibodies alone. Diagnosis requires clinical context.
- An understanding of the relative sensitivities and specificities of serologic tests will facilitate an accurate interpretation of results in the diagnosis of patients with inflammatory and autoimmune diseases.

Interdisciplinary Introduction

Laboratory testing has an important role in the diagnostic work-up of most rheumatology-dermatology overlap conditions, as well as in monitoring of disease activity in some cases. This chapter discusses the most useful serologic and other laboratory tests available to clinicians. Radiologic imaging and other selected diagnostic studies will also be addressed. A practical understanding of these tests and studies is important, as integrating laboratory and radiologic data with the clinical impression is vital to making an accurate diagnosis in patients with overlap diseases.

Erythrocyte Sedimentation Rate and C-reactive Protein

The erythrocyte sedimentation rate (ESR) and C-reactive protein (CRP) level are acute phase reactants which serve as markers of inflammation which can support diagnosis and assessment of disease activity. Patients with an ESR of 100, or in the case of CRP, 100 times the upper limit of normal warrant a more aggressive and faster-paced work-up than someone with an ESR and/or CRP that is just over the normal range. Normal

A. H. Jonsson · P. H. Schur (✉)
Brigham and Women's Hospital, Division of Rheumatology, Inflammation, and Immunity, Department of Medicine, Boston, MA, USA

Harvard Medical School, Boston, MA, USA
e-mail: pschur@partners.org

M. Stern
New York University School of Medicine, New York, NY, USA

A. N. Femia
Ronald O. Perelman Department of Dermatology, NYU Grossman School of Medicine, New York, NY, USA

A. Garg et al. (eds.), *Interdisciplinary Approaches to Overlap Disorders in Dermatology & Rheumatology*,
https://doi.org/10.1007/978-3-319-18446-3_2

Table 2.1 Age correction for upper limit of normal for ESR and CRP

	Men	Women
ESR	Age	Age + 10
CRP	Age	Age + 30

values of ESR and CRP do not rule out an autoimmune or inflammatory condition. However, in cases of low clinical pre-test probability of overlap disease, such values may further support the clinician's impression of disease absence.

ESR and CRP generally tend to track together, i.e. when one is elevated, the other is also usually elevated. CRP levels tend to respond more rapidly to progression and regression of inflammatory states than does ESR. As such, CRP is more likely to be elevated when onset of inflammatory disease is acute (e.g. within several days). Likewise, CRP tends to decrease toward the normal range more quickly than ESR with disease control. Overall, we find it useful to monitor both values.

It is important to remember that both ESR and CRP are non-specific markers and typically do not suggest the underlying cause of inflammation. Elevations in ESR and CRP occur in various types of inflammatory conditions, including rheumatologic, dermatologic, infectious, cardiovascular, and malignant diseases. Aging, obesity, tobacco smoking, and uremia have also been shown to increase baseline ESR and CRP levels. While ESR and CRP may be corrected for age, (Table 2.1) validated equations that quantify the influence of obesity, tobacco smoking, or renal function have not yet been developed. Clinical judgment and other ancillary data should be applied to support clinical decision making when ESR and CRP levels twice the upper limit of normal are observed in an overweight tobacco smoker with renal insufficiency, for example, who may not have a baseline measure.

Antibodies in Rheumatologic Disease – General Principles

In most instances, serologic tests for rheumatologic conditions are utilized to support diagnosis. However, in some cases, they may be useful in predicting prognosis or monitoring disease activity. Disease-associated antibodies are often present for years prior to the development of clinical symptoms, and so, it is rarely useful to repeat previously negative serologies unless significant time has passed or new symptoms have developed.

Even with the presence of particular antibodies (ie., antinuclear antibodies, ANA), many patients never develop disease. This is especially true in elderly patients since the prevalence of autoimmune antibodies increases with age. Conversely, not all patients with a particular autoimmune disease (ie., systemic lupus erythematosus, SLE) will have all of the antibodies commonly associated with that disease. In SLE, a meaningfully elevated titer of ANA is essentially required for diagnosis, while a high titer of Smith antibody, seen in only a subset of SLE patients, is highly predictive of disease. As such, one should have a sound clinical basis prior to ordering serologic tests. Furthermore, diagnosis, and certainly treatment decisions, should never be based on the presence or absence of antibodies alone. Having a functional understanding of sensitivity and specificity for serologic tests will also aid interpretation of results and application to the clinical context.

Sensitivity of a test refers to the percentage of patients with a particular disease in whom a particular antibody is present. For example, the sensitivity of the ANA test for SLE is over 99%, meaning that more than 99% of patients with true SLE will have an elevated ANA titer. Anti-Smith antibodies, on the other hand, have a sensitivity in the 10–40% range, meaning that only 10–40% of patients with SLE have anti-Smith antibodies. Specificity, on the other hand, refers to the percentage of patients with a positive value for a particular blood test who have a particular associated disease. For example, the specificity of the ANA test for SLE is 15%, meaning that only 15% of patients with an elevated ANA titer truly have SLE. The other 85% are healthy or have some other disease associated with ANA. Anti-Smith antibodies; however, have a specificity of 97%, meaning that nearly all patients with elevated titers of Smith antibodies have true SLE. It is rare for a serologic test to have both high specificity and high sensitivity. As such, the diagnostic work-up for a given patient will likely include both high-sensitivity/low-specificity tests as well as low-sensitivity/high-specificity tests. The high-sensitivity/low-specificity antibodies are most useful for ruling out associated diseases. For example, if the ANA titer is normal, then it is extremely unlikely the patient has SLE. An elevated titer of a low-sensitivity/high-specificity antibody may strengthen clinical suspicion of the associated disease. For example, the suspicion for SLE is high when Smith antibody titers are elevated.

Numerous studies have evaluated prognostic utility for serologic antibodies. In some conditions, such as scleroderma and dermatomyositis, the associations between antibody and disease manifestations are well-documented. For other conditions, including SLE, the available data are conflicting. Herein, we will discuss antibody associations which we feel are strong and dependable.

Anti-nuclear Antibody

The ANA is arguably the most well-known serology test, one that every medical student learns is connected to SLE. In practice, the association of ANA to disease is more complex, as the ANA is also observed in those having a number of other rheumatologic and non-rheumatologic diseases, as well as in healthy patients (Table 2.2).

Many healthy people without autoimmune disease also have a positive ANA. In fact, among people with a positive ANA, only 15% will have SLE. The number of false positive ANAs decreases with increasing titers. Approximately 13% of healthy controls have an ANA with a titer of 1:80 or higher, while only about 3% of the general population has an ANA titer of 1:320 or higher [17]. In other words, the higher the ANA titer, the more likely it is that a patient has an autoimmune disease.

ANA is the prototype for a low specificity test, although the sensitivities and specificities vary significantly among the different methods by which the ANA is measured. The current gold standard method to determining the presence of ANA is by indirect immunofluorescence on HEp-2 cells (IF-ANA). In this method, HEp-2 cells (a human epidermoid cancer cell line) are incubated with patient serum at serial dilutions. Antibodies in the sera that bind to the HEp-2 cells are then detected with fluorescence-conjugated anti-human Ig antibodies. This is a labor-intensive and costly method that requires subjective analysis of immunofluorescence staining by lab technicians. Less costly alternatives have been developed over the years, including ELISA or flow cytometry assays which use a mixture of nuclear contents as the antigen. However, the sensitivity of these assays is significantly lower. The gold-standard IF-ANA has a sensitivity for SLE of >99%, whereas flow cytometry-based ANA assays have a sensitivity approximating 50% [2, 14]. Similarly, in a side-by-side comparison of IF-ANA with ELISA-based assays, the ELISA was positive in only 56% of patients with a positive IF-ANA, and the ELISA-based assay had a sensitivity of only 75% for SLE [5]. These lower sensitivities alter the way that the ANA is interpreted in the diagnostic work-up, and so the American College of

Table 2.2 Sensitivity of the ANA test

Condition	Sensitivity of ANA
Systemic lupus erythematosus	99–100% by IF-ANA (lower for ELISA- or flow cytometry-based assays)
Drug-induced lupus	100%
Mixed connective tissue disease	100%
Discoid lupus	15%
Scleroderma	60–80%
Polymyositis/dermatomyositis	60%
Sjogren syndrome	40–70%
Pauciarticular juvenile idiopathic arthritis	70%
Raynaud's phenomenon	60%
Anti-phospholipid antibody syndrome	50%
Rheumatoid arthritis	50%
Graves' disease	50%
Autoimmune thyroid disease (Hashimoto's thyroiditis, Grave's disease)	35–50%
Autoimmune liver disease (autoimmune hepatitis, autoimmune cholangitis, primary biliary cirrhosis)	Varies, but positive ANA is common

Rheumatology supports the use of IF-ANA over these alternative methods. However, many commercial labs continue to use ELISA or other methods to detect ANA, and we recommend that clinicians take note of the method being used to perform the ANA assay when interpreting the result.

In terms of cutaneous lupus, the malar ("butterfly") rash of cutaneous lupus signifies acute cutaneous lupus, and it is frequently associated with SLE. In this case, an IF-ANA will essentially always be positive. In contrast, ANA is only present in about 10–20% of patients with discoid lupus erythematosus (DLE, a form of chronic cutaneous lupus). In subacute cutaneous lupus, ANA is present in roughly 60–80% of patients, while anti-Ro/SSA is present in approximately 80% and anti-La/SSB in 30–50% of patients.

A number of other autoimmune diseases are also associated with an elevated ANA titer (Table 2.2); however, caution must be used with regard to using ANA as criterion to diagnose autoimmune conditions. For example, positive ANA is a diagnostic criterion for drug-induced lupus (DIL) and mixed connective tissue disease (MCTD), so the sensitivity in these diseases is 100%. In contrast, since only a minority of patients with DLE have a positive ANA, this test is not helpful for diagnosis. Similarly, patients with dermatomyositis may have a positive ANA; however, ANA is often negative in this patient population, and therefore this test is not useful for diagnosis. Furthermore, up to 50% of patients with RA have a positive ANA, which may make establishing a diagnosis in these patients more challenging. In such cases, one must carefully review clinical symptoms in the context of additional lab testing, such as rheumatoid factor, anti-CCP antibodies, anti-dsDNA antibodies, and anti-extractible nuclear antigens (ENAs) including the Sm, RNP, Ro (SS-A) and La (SS-B) antigens. As a general rule, clinical symptoms and examination in the context of complete laboratory work-up is more helpful in establishing a diagnosis than ANA alone.

The pattern of ANA staining (e.g. speckled or diffuse) may be used to guide diagnosis, though we find that testing for anti-ENA antibodies is more helpful. The exception is the anti-centromere pattern, which has sensitivity of 25–50% for systemic sclerosis with clinical manifestations of limited systemic sclerosis (CREST) syndrome. ENA antibodies are discussed further in this chapter.

A negative ANA (as determined by immunofluorescence testing) strongly argues against a diagnosis of SLE, MCTD, and DIL. It also makes a diagnosis of scleroderma somewhat less likely. In patients with SLE, it is not useful to follow ANA titers over time since titers are not predictive of disease activity.

SLE-Associated Serologies

ANA antibodies are diverse in their antigen specificity, targeting any of the hundreds of proteins, nucleic acids, and other components of cellular nuclei. Different conditions tend to feature antibodies that target particular nuclear components, such as double-stranded DNA (dsDNA) or histones. A number of commercially available tests that evaluate antibodies targeting these individual nuclear antigens (Table 2.3) are useful in the diagnostic work-up of SLE and several other autoimmune diagnoses.

Anti-dsDNA antibodies have higher specificity for SLE (97%) than the ANA test and should be evaluated in all cases of suspected SLE. The sensitivity is relatively poor (70%), so it is not adequate as the sole test for suspected SLE. Anti-dsDNA antibodies may also be found in some asymptomatic patients taking minocycline, TNF blockers, and procainamide, drugs which are known to cause DIL. These medications, in other words, may cause anti-dsDNA antibodies even in the absence of clinical lupus or DIL symptoms.

Importantly, anti-dsDNA antibodies are useful in monitoring disease activity in some (but not all) patients with SLE. While there is some controversy on this matter in the literature, we have observed that in patients with detectable anti-dsDNA antibodies at baseline, levels tend to increase just prior to and during flares, and

Table 2.3 Sensitivity and specificity of selected extractable nuclear antigens

	dsDNA	ssDNA	Histone	Smith	RNP	SSA (Ro)	SSB (La)
SLE Sen Spec	70% 95%	80% –	30-80% 50%	25-30% Mod	45% 99%	40% 87-94%	15% –
Drug LE Sen Spec	1-5% –	80% 50%	95% High	50% Mod	– –	Low –	Low –
RA Sen Spec	1% –	Mod Mod	Low –	25% Low	47% –	Low –	Low –
Sjogren Sen Spec	1-5% –	Mod Mod	Low Low	1-5% –	5-60% –	8-70% 87%	14-60% 94%
SSc Sen Spec	<1% –	– –	<1% –	<1% –	20% –	– –	– –
PM/DM Sen Spec	<1% –	– –	<1% –	<1% –	– –	Low –	– –

SLE systemic lupus erythematosus, *Drug LE* drug induced lupus erythematosus, *RA* rheumatoid arthritis, *SSc* systemic sclerosis, *PM/DM* polymyositis or dermatomyositis

they tend to decrease during periods of relative remission. This is especially true in patients with lupus nephritis. In contrast, elevated anti-dsDNA titers are not associated with neuropsychiatric lupus, suggesting that this form of SLE may also have a different pathophysiologic mechanism.

Like anti-dsDNA antibodies, anti-Smith antibodies have high specificity (97%) for SLE. However, the sensitivity (10–40%) is significantly lower for patients with SLE. Anti-Smith antibodies appear to be more common among African-Americans and Asians with SLE than among Caucasians with SLE. Unlike with anti-dsDNA antibodies, titers of anti-Smith antibodies do not correlate with disease activity. However, the presence of anti-Smith antibodies may be associated with other findings. For example, one large cross-sectional study found that patients with SLE and DLE are more likely to have anti-Smith antibodies. In this study, patients with SLE and DLE were also more likely to have photosensitivity and leukopenia and less likely to experience pleuritis and arthritis as compared to patients with SLE but without DLE [11]. Interestingly, prior data supports that the presence of DLE in SLE is associated with a lower risk of SLE nephritis [10].

Antibodies against Ro (SS-A) and La (SS-B) may occur together, although anti-Ro antibodies are also observed in the absence of anti-La antibodies. With only 0.1–0.5% of healthy controls testing positive for these antibodies, they are rare in the general population. Ro and La antibodies are observed in 30–50% of patients with SLE. These antibodies are present in 75% of patients with primary Sjogren's syndrome (SS) and impart a greater risk of SS-associated vasculitis. Anti-Ro and -La antibodies are less common in secondary SS (e.g. Sjogren's in the context of SLE or rheumatoid arthritis). In patients with SLE, anti-Ro and anti-La antibodies have been associated with interstitial lung disease.

One form of cutaneous lupus, known as subacute cutaneous lupus erythematosus (SCLE), is particularly associated with anti-Ro and anti-La antibodies, irrespective of whether concomitant SLE is present. Some patients with SCLE have anti-Ro antibodies even in the absence of a positive ANA, and hence the presence of these antibodies could potentially aid in the diagnosis of SCLE [15]. Roughly 80% of patients with SCLE have detectable anti-Ro antibodies. At least 1/3 of cases of SCLE are thought to be drug-induced; in these cases anti-Ro antibodies are also usually positive, and may become undetectable in serum several weeks after withdrawal of the offending drug. However, the persistence of SCLE as well as of anti-Ro or anti-La antibodies after drug withdrawal is also possible. Anti-Ro and anti-La may also be present in patients with DLE in the absence of systemic disease. Ro and La antibodies are important to assess in all women with SLE of childbearing age, as they are also associated with increased risk of neonatal lupus and congenital heart block in the newborn. In a patient with suspected neonatal lupus, anti-Ro and anti-La antibodies, and rarely, anti-U1RNP antibodies, can be detected in serum of the neonate at up to 6 months of age due to transplacental passage from the mother. Finally, anti-Ro and -La antibodies may be observed in patients with MCTD and JIA, among other autoimmune diseases.

Antibodies to collagen VII are associated with bullous cutaneous lupus, in which vesicles and bullae form on an inflammatory base, typically within areas of acute cutaneous lupus. This eruption tends to occur in patients with severe SLE, particularly in those with renal involvement. Around 69% of patients with bullous SLE have detectable anti-collagen VII antibodies in serum. In one report, antibodies to collagen VII rose prior to presentation with bullous SLE and then fell after its resolution, suggesting that antibody presence may correlate with disease activity [4]. In a cutaneous bullous disorder known as epidermolysis bullosa acquisita, antibodies to collagen VII are also characteristic; this disorder may occur in the setting of SLE, although it is more commonly associated with inflammatory bowel disease.

The presence of high titers of anti-RNP antibodies is characteristic of MCTD, a syndrome with clinical features of lupus, scleroderma, myositis, and rheumatoid arthritis. However, anti-RNP antibodies are also observed among patients having symptoms of only one of these diseases, as opposed to the combination of symptoms seem in patients with overlap disorders.

The presence of anti-histone antibodies is the serologic hallmark of DIL, though the sensitivity of this test varies widely based on the inducing medication. Anti-histone antibodies are frequently found in cases of DIL associated with procainamide, hydralazine, and chlorpromazine. However, this antibody is infrequently observed in DIL induced by TNF inhibitors or minocycline. Additional laboratory testing is useful when distinguishing DIL from SLE without rash. For example, elevated titers of anti-dsDNA or anti-Smith antibodies favor a diagnosis of SLE, as these antibodies are rare in DIL. Anti-neutrophil cytoplasmic antibodies (ANCAs) to myeloperoxidase (MPO) or proteinase 3 (PR3) may be seen with DIL but are uncommonly observed among patients with SLE.

Work-up for patients with established SLE or with suspected SLE who demonstrate features of anti-phospholipid antibody syndrome (APS) should include a complete panel of anti-phospholipid (APL) antibodies. Testing for APL antibodies should also be considered in patients with persistent livedo racemosa, retiform purpura, or unexplained cutaneous ulcerations, even if there is no pre-existing suspicion of an autoimmune process. APL antibodies include anti-cardiolipin antibodies (IgM and IgG), lupus anticoagulant [which often also includes a dilute Russell viper venom test (DRVVT)], anti-beta-2-glycoprotein-1 antibodies (IgM and IgG), and anti-phosphotidylserine antibodies. Positive testing for APL antibodies should be repeated 12 weeks later to confirm persistence of these antibodies over time. It is important to remember that positive APL antibodies do not by themselves confer the diagnosis of APS.

Testing of complement levels or function is also helpful in evaluating patients with suspected SLE. Levels of the C3 and C4 components are preferentially depleted in active SLE. CH50, which tests the function of many different complement components, also decreases with flares. As such, these complements tests may be supportive in establishing diagnosis and more so in monitoring disease activity. In contrast, infections or other inflammatory conditions typically increase complement levels, which also serve as acute phase reactants. In cases of severe sepsis however, CH50 and C3, but not C4, may be depleted due to activation of the alternative pathway of complement activation. Complement levels may increase during pregnancy in healthy women, and this may complicate interpretation of complement levels in pregnant patients who develop SLE.

Further SLE associations with autoantibodies are being investigated in the hopes of finding clinical phenotypes that match an autoantibody profile. One study of Chinese patients with SLE found that patients could be divided into three clusters characterized by autoantibodies and clinical manifestations; one end of the spectrum includes patients with anti-dsDNA antibodies who have higher rates of renal disorder, and the other includes patients with anti-Ro, anti-La, anti-Smith, anti-RNP, and APL antibodies who were more likely to have malar rash, photosensitivity, and arthritis, amongst other findings [9]. This analysis also showed an association between anti-dsDNA antibodies and hematological involvement. These findings warrant further consideration, and investigation regarding serologies in SLE are ongoing.

Systemic Sclerosis (Scleroderma)

Approximately 85% of patients with systemic sclerosis have an elevated ANA titer. While there are other more specific antibodies associated with scleroderma, the sensitivities of these antibodies are generally low. It is therefore important to consider that many patients with scleroderma have an absence of disease-specific antibodies.

Anti-Scl70 antibodies, also known as anti-topoisomerase antibodies, are found in approximately 15–20% of patients. When present, these antibodies indicate higher risk of diffuse scleroderma (i.e. skin involvement proximal to the forearms) and interstitial lung disease. Anti-Scl70 is also a marker for renal involvement and greater overall mortality in scleroderma.

Anti-RNA polymerase I, II, or III antibodies are found in approximately 20% of patients with systemic sclerosis. The most frequently observed subtype is the RNA polymerase III antibody, found in 7–12% of patients. This antibody has high specificity for systemic sclerosis, and it tends to be associated with rapid onset disease characterized by severe skin involvement, calcinosis, scleroderma renal crisis, and gastric antral vascular ectasia (GAVE, also known as watermelon stomach). Anti-RNA polymerase III antibodies are associated with a higher modified Rodnan score as compared with anti-centromere antibodies. This skin score indicates both more diffuse cutaneous involvement and increased skin thickness. Anti-RNA polymerase III antibodies have also been associated with a higher risk of malignancy (most commonly breast cancer) occurring in close temporal association to SSc when compared with other systemic sclerosis-associated antibodies [13].

The anti-centromere antibody does not represent a distinct serologic test per se, but rather it is a pattern of immunofluorescence for the ANA test. It has a sensitivity of approximately 25–50% in scleroderma. The anti-centromere antibody is associated with a form of limited systemic sclerosis known as the CREST syndrome (calcinosis, Raynaud's phenomenon, esophageal dysmotility, scleroderma, telangiectasia). In CREST syndrome, cutaneous disease is mostly limited to distal areas, such as the hands, forearms, face, and neck. In addition, anti-centromere antibodies are associated with an elevated risk of pulmonary arterial hypertension but a lower likelihood of developing interstitial lung disease and scleroderma renal crisis.

Several other antibodies have been connected to scleroderma, including U1-RNP, U3-RNP, PM-Scl, Th/To, and RPC1. However, these antibodies have lower sensitivities, and their prognostic utility is not clear. For these reasons, we do not routinely check these antibodies in the work-up of scleroderma patients.

Dermatomyositis

Creatinine kinase (CK) and aldolase levels help to differentiate inflammatory myositis (and non-inflammatory myopathies) from deconditioning and steroid myopathy, which are often on the differential diagnosis for patients with classic dermatomyositis. Most patients with inflammatory myositis will have elevations of one or both muscle enzymes, whereas patients with deconditioning or steroid myopathy typically have normal levels of both enzymes. Because some patients with inflammatory myositis may have elevations in only one of these enzymes, we recommend evaluating both enzymes initially. It is well-documented that "normal" CK levels vary by gender and ethnicity, although any measurement above the normal range, or above a patient's prior baseline, should trigger further exploration, especially in the context of cutaneous and other features that prompt suspicion for dermatomyositis. The differential diagnosis for an elevated CK level is quite broad and includes trauma (including from vigorous exercise), toxins (including from statins), endocrine dyscrasias, malignancy, and genetic diseases (e.g. glycogen storage disorders, some muscular dystrophies). Statins may cause a mild increase in CK levels, and in approximately 1 in 10,000 patients, statins may cause a more severe necrotizing myopathy. It should be noted that approximately one-fifth of all patients with dermatomyositis have clinically amyopathic disease, meaning that they have no clinical evidence of muscle involvement, and may lack serum muscle enzyme level elevations.

Obtaining mysotitis-specific antibodies should be considered in patients with dermatomyositis as the may correlate with phenotype and prognosis. (Table 2.4) Each of these antibodies is found only in a small percentage of patients with dermatomyositis, and thus these antibodies are not helpful for diagnosis. However, when present, these antibodies may provide important prognostic information related to risk for other organ involvement, such as interstitial lung disease. Additionally, autoantibodies in dermatomyositis may help stratify cancer risk. Most myositis panels include the anti-synthetase antibodies, which help to define a subset of patients with anti-synthetase syndrome - an entity that manifests with a combination of dermatomyositis (or polymyositis), interstitial lung disease, fevers, arthritis, and mechanic's hands (hyperkeratosis on the lateral and palmar surfaces of the fingers). Jo-1, an antibody against histidyl-tRNA synthetase, is the most common anti-synthetase antibody and is observed in approximately 10% of patients with dermatomyositis and 20% of patients with polymyositis [7]. Other anti-synthetase antibodies include anti-PL7, anti-PL12, anti-OJ, anti-EJ, anti-KS, anti-SC, anti-JS, anti-Ha, anti-tryptophanyl, and anti-Zo.

Table 2.4 Myositis-associated antibodies

Antibody	Target antigen	Frequency	Clinical phenotype
Jo-1	Histidyl-tRNA	15–30%	PM/DM, ILD, Raynaud, mechanic's hands
PL-7	Threonyl-tRNA	5–10%	ILD, mild myositis
PL-EJ	Glycyl-tRNA	5–10%	
PL12			90% have ILD
OJ			ILD
KS			ILD
Zo, YRS, PMS			
SRP	Signal recognition particle		Necrotizing myopathy
Mi-2	218/240kDA		DM>PM, classic dermatomyositis, favorable prognosis
MDA5 (CADM140)	140kDa, melanoma differentiation- associated protein 5	50%	Amyopathic DM, rapidly progressive interstitial lung disease
TIF1ϒ (p140/p155)	Transcriptional intermediary factor	20%	DM, especially cancer-associated
U1RNP	U1 small nuclear RNP	10%	Overlap myositis
Ku	DNA-PK	20–30%	PM-SSc (Japanese), overlap syndromes
PM-Scl	Nucleolar proteins	8–10%	PM-SSc (Caucasian)
NXP-2	Nuclear matrix protein	20–25% juvenile DM, 1–30% adult DM	Calcinosis, malignancy, dysphagia, myalgia, peripheral edema

The presence of certain antibodies suggests an increased risk for serious complications of dermatomyositis. The anti-melanoma differentiation-associated protein 5 (MDA5) antibody (previously known as CADM-140) has been associated with interstitial lung disease, which is often rapidly progressive, and is associated with a high mortality rate [8]. This antibody is more often seen in clinically amyopathic dermatomyositis than in classic dermatomyositis. Asian populations, in particular Japanese patients, seem to be at particular risk for this complication of MDA5+ dermatomyositis, but recent data from the United States suggests that this complication is not limited to the Japanese population, as it has been observed in Caucasian, Latino, Pacific Islander, and African American patients. Physical features associated with anti-MDA5 antibodies include skin ulcers, which tend to occur on the extensor surfaces of the dorsal hand (often within Gottron papules), elbows, or lateral nailfolds. Tender palmar papules, oral pain or ulceration, hand swelling, alopecia, and arthritis are also associated with MDA5 antibodies. Recently, the presence of anti-MDA5 was also shown to be associated with a lower likelihood of achieving clinical remission of cutaneous dermatomyositis. Given the prognostic value of the MDA5 antibody, testing for this antibody should be considered in patients with dermatomyositis, particularly in those with clinically amyopathic disease or in those who exhibit the aforementioned cutaneous features. In such patients, pulmonary status must be closely monitored.

Searching for the presence of additional antibodies can be useful in characterizing patients with dermatomyositis. For example, anti-TIF-1γ antibodies are associated with a significantly increased risk of malignancy, significantly above the baseline cancer risk of the total population of dermatomyositis. Patients with the anti-transcriptional intermediary factor -1γ (anti-TIF-1γ) antibody are more likely to have extensive skin involvement, although their risk of systemic involvement other than associated malignancy appears to be lower than in patients with dermatomyositis without anti-TIF-1γ positivity. Unique features of cutaneous dermatomyositis, namely hyperkeratotic, verrucous palmar papules, psoriasis-like patches, hypopigmented and telangiecatic "red on white" patches, and an ovoid palatal patch have been associated with TIF-1γ positivity in dermatomyositis. The palatal patch is described as erythematous with white macular markings, and its presence has a strong association with both anti-TIF-1γ antibodies and internal malignancy [1]. Patients with TIF-1γ antibodies seem to have a lower prevalence of certain extracutaneous manifestations, including interstitial lung disease, Raynaud phenomenon, and arthritis. Although TIF-1γ is not typically included on initial screening panels for dermatomyositis as testing for this antibody is not widely available, when these clinical findings are present, testing for anti-TIF-1γ antibodies can be helpful in establishing prognosis and assessing malignancy risk.

Additional antibodies in dermatomyositis include nuclear matrix protein 2 (NXP-2) antibodies (formerly known as MJ). This autoantibody has been associated with calcinosis as well as with an increased risk of malignancy, particularly in male patients with dermatomyositis. Anti-NXP2 has also been associated with dysphagia, myalgia, and peripheral edema, as well as with milder cutaneous involvement and a decreased incidence of Gottron's sign.

Anti-Ku antibodies are thought to be a marker of an overlap syndrome that often includes features of polymyositis or dermatomyositis, SLE, and systemic sclerosis [3]. The clinical features of Raynaud phenomenon, arthritis/arthralgia, myositis, sicca symptoms, and interstitial lung disease are often seen in patients with anti-Ku antibodies. Patients with dermatomyositis who also exhibit features of a sclerosing skin disorder may benefit from testing for the presence of anti-Ku antibodies.

Psoriatic Arthritis

There are no blood tests that specify a diagnosis of psoriatic arthritis (PsA), although seronegativity for rheumatoid factor is included in the CASPAR classification criteria. Approximately

8–12% of patients with PsA will be seropositive for rheumatoid factor or cyclic citrullinated peptide antibody, and so serologic testing alone should not be used to include or exclude PsA as a diagnosis. These are in general low titer positive results in the context of PsA. The majority of PsA patients will not have increased levels of acute phase reactants, though there is data to suggest that patients with elevated CRP at diagnosis may have worse prognosis, including increased joint erosion and damage.

Vasculitis

When there is evidence of systemic involvement with vasculitis, either because it is suggested by review of systems or because presentation on skin would suggest larger vessel involvement, laboratory evaluation can confirm systemic involvement and provide clinical data which may specify etiology.

To screen for evidence of systemic involvement, we recommend at minimum a complete blood count, serum creatinine, and urinalysis with microscopic sediment to assess for protein, red blood cells (RBCs), or casts which might suggest the presence of glomerulonephritis. ANCAs have a high sensitivity and relatively high specificity for medium vessel vasculitides including granulomatosis with polyangiitis (GPA) and microscopic polyangiitis (MPA). Eosinophilic granulomatosis with polyangiitis (EGPA) is also considered an ANCA-associated vasculitis, but the sensitivity of ANCA for EGPA is lower than for GPA and MPA. Drug-induced vasculitis and rheumatoid vasculitis (RV) may also feature positive ANCA antibodies. The diagnosis of these ANCA-associated conditions must also include correlation to the clinical presentation, examination, and histopathology. In terms of cutaneous involvement, ANCA-positive vasculitis may manifest with features that include palpable purpura, tender erythematous-violaceous cutaneous nodules that may ulcerate, livedo racemosa, and retiform purpura.

ANCA testing is performed by immunofluorescence, which generally demonstrates either a cytoplasmic or perinuclear pattern. The cytoplasmic pattern (c-ANCA) is strongly associated with antibodies directed to PR3, whereas the perinuclear pattern (p-ANCA) is associated with antibodies to MPO. However, these associations are not absolute, and several other ANCA antibodies have been identified (e.g. antibodies to elastase, lactoferrin, and other cytoplasmic proteins). When an ANCA is ordered in our laboratory, analysis is performed to determine ANCA positivity and immunofluorescence pattern, and to determine presence of antibodies to MPO and PR3. This has been shown to increase the sensitivity and specificity of the ANCA test.

Antibodies to PR3 are detected in over 90% of patient with acute or rapidly progressive multi-organ (in particular renal) GPA. However, only approximately 60% of patients who have "limited" GPA, involving only the sinuses or upper airways, have a positive ANCA. Antibodies to PR3 are also found in 50% of patients with MPA and in 5–10% of patients with polyarteritis nodosa or EGPA.

Antibodies to MPO are seen in 50–70% of patients with MPA, 50–85% of patients with idiopathic necrotizing glomerulonephritis, 70–85% of patients with EGPA, 10–30% of patients with anti-GBM (Goodpasture's disease), and in 5–10% of patients with GPA. These antibodies may also be observed in some patients with SLE, RA, and other rheumatologic disorders.

While testing for antibodies to PR3 and MPO is useful in establishing diagnosis of vasculitis, their utility in monitoring for early signs of relapse is controversial. In general, patients with anti-PR3 antibodies tend to relapse more frequently than patients with anti-MPO antibodies. A number of studies have attempted to address whether an increase in titers PR3 or MPO antibodies predicts relapse. Altogether, the data suggest that while increased titers often predict flares, flares also occur in the context of stable or decreasing titers, and increasing titers are not always associated with subsequent relapse [18]. Overall, the correlation between increasing anti-PR3 or -MPO antibody titers and disease relapse is not strong enough to recommend routine monitoring of asymptomatic patients. It is reasonable, however, to assess anti-PR3 or anti-MPO titers when a relapse of disease is suspected clinically. An increase in titer would modestly support the suspicion of flare, especially when the patient has renal disease [6]. If, on the other hand, a patient has converted to being anti-PR3 and anti-MPO antibody-negative during treatment, his or her risk of relapse is lower than in patients with persistent ANCA, although this risk is not entirely negated.

Drug-induced vasculitis (DIV) occurs in response to a number of medications and illicit drugs, and it may feature the same antibodies as primary vasculitides. Positive ANCA has been observed in patients with DIV triggered by hydralazine, minocycline, and propylthiouracil. In most of these cases, the pattern is perinuclear (i.e. p-ANCA) targeting MPO, though there have also been cases of antibodies to PR3 or other ANCA antigens, such as elastase. These patients often have serologies and symptoms to suggest DIL, and there seems to be significant overlap between these two conditions. Patients with drug-induced small vessel vasculitis (leukocytoclastic vasculitis) do not typically demonstrate serologic antibodies.

RV occurs almost exclusively in patients with longstanding seropositive rheumatoid arthritis who have a history of severe joint disease. Rheumatoid factor is present in essentially all patients with RV, and the occurrence of vasculitis is often heralded by a high spike in the titer. While the prevalence of antibodies to CCP in RV is somewhat lower, the titer is also high when present. ANCA antibodies are not particularly useful in making a diagnosis of RV, as they can be present in patients with rheumatoid arthritis who do not have vasculitis. Complement levels or activity are low in some, but not all, patients with RV, limiting the utility of such testing in this setting.

Mixed cryoglobulinemia is another condition marked by an increase in rheumatoid factor level, but these patients usually do not have a history of rheumatoid arthritis and antibodies to CCP are not likely to be present. Cryoglobulinemia can produce a cutaneous vasculitis that may manifest as palpable purpura, retiform purpura, or necrotic ulcerations.

Urticarial vasculitis may present with mainly cutaneous disease or may involve severe organ-threatening disease. The cutaneous presentation ranges from erythematous plaques similar to plain urticaria, to violaceous and purpuric plaques similar to small vessel cutaneous vasculitis. The more severe cases with systemic involvement are often referred to as hypocomplementemic urticarial vasculitis syndrome, and as the name suggests, this condition is characterized by low complement activity and reduced C3 and C4 levels. Levels of C1q are also often low, and anti-C1q antibodies may be detected. Patients with urticarial vasculitis frequently have high titers of ANA. Taken together, these observations are quite similar in SLE, and it can be challenging to distinguish the two diagnoses. Clinical presentation and the absence of anti-dsDNA antibodies help to distinguish the SLE from urticarial vasculitis. In patients with urticarial vasculitis and normal complement levels, systemic involvement is rarely seen.

Still's Disease

Still's disease is an uncommon but serious form of inflammatory arthritis that may present in children or adults. Symptoms include fever and daily appearance of a characteristic fleeting eruption that is typically described as salmon-colored and may wax and wane with fever, although the clinical appearance may vary. There is no specific test to establish diagnosis for this disease. ESR and CRP are often elevated. Rheumatoid factor and ANA are usually negative. Ferritin levels are often quite elevated (>3000). Some studies have suggested that the proportion of ferritin that is glycosylated is relatively low, and this may be helpful in distinguishing Still's disease from other rheumatologic diseases associated with elevated ferritin levels.

Sarcoidosis

There is no specific serologic test to establish a diagnosis for sarcoidosis. Angiotensin Converting Enzyme (ACE) levels may be elevated in these patients, but this test does not specify sarcoidosis. We recommend relying on plain radiograph, and when necessary, computed tomography scanning to look for hilar adenopathy in the chest. Tissue sampling of skin, lymph node, or other involved tissue are often necessary to make a diagnosis.

Lyme disease

Lyme disease is becoming increasingly common and widespread in North America. Clinicians must have a high index of suspicion for early disease manifestations in order to diagnose and treat patients prior to progression to later stage disease. Testing for Lyme infection is performed by a screening ELISA, which if positive, is followed by either a confirmatory Western blot assay or an ELISA or chemiluminescence assay for antibodies against specific Borrelia proteins. At least five out of a predefined group of 10 immunoglobulin G bands are required for the Western blot to be considered positive. Additional information on laboratory testing for Lyme disease is available from the CDC website.

Three quarters of adults will develop erythema migrans days to a month after the bite of an ixodes tick transmitting the spirochete Borrelia burgdorferi. IgM antibodies emerge 2–4 weeks after the eruption appears and peak 6–8 weeks following the rash. As such, many patients with the eruption may not have yet seroconverted at this early stage, and so the utility of Lyme serologies in establishing a diagnosis of Lyme disease is low. Bell's palsy, heart block, and arthritis are later stage manifestations which develop months to years after the tick bite. At this later stage, serologies are almost always positive. If serologies are negative in the presence of arthritis, a different cause of the arthritis should be considered. Lyme serologies remain positive for years, even after treatment with antibiotics. This poses a problem when there is suspicion of re-infection in a previously infected patient. The quantified levels of antibodies may drop over time, so an increase in the absolute amount of anti-*Borrelia* IgM or IgG antibodies may suggest a new infection. Additionally, the appearance of new bands on the Western blot is strong evidence of a new infection. PCR amplification of bacterial products from blood, skin, or synovial fluid has been performed in several research studies [12, 16], but in our experience, this assay has a relatively low sensitivity in most commercial laboratories and is therefore of limited utility.

Lastly, it should be noted that there are a number of other *Borrelia* strains, such as *B. miyamotoi*, *B. afzelii*, and *B. garinii* that can cause either Lyme disease or other tick-borne illnesses. At this point in time, only *B. burgdorferi* is thought to cause a significant burden of disease in North America, and this is the strain for which North American serological assays are designed. These ELISA and Western blots may not react in cases of infections with other strains of *Borrelia*, for example in cases where patients may have been exposed abroad. However, as already stated, non-*burgdorferi* strains of *Borrelia* remain very rare in North America.

Summary

A functional appreciation of the application and limitations of serologic and other laboratory tests will effectively support the evaluation and management of patients with complex inflammatory and autoimmune skin and musculoskeletal diseases. Table 2.5 provides a summary of high yield evaluative laboratory tests for common overlap diseases.

Table 2.5 Suggested initial work-up for common rheumatologic diseases

Tests to consider if you suspect…	
Systemic lupus erythematosus	ANA, CBC, C3, C4, dsDNA, Cr, urinalysis with sediment
Discoid lupus erythematosus	ANA, dsDNA, anti-histone antibody
Sjogren syndrome	ANA, Ro, La
Dermatomyositis	CK, aldolase, ANA, Jo-1, myositis panel, consider MDA5 and TIF1Υ
Psoriatic arthritis	ESR, CRP, RF, CCP
Rheumatoid arthritis	RF, CCP
Vasculitis	ESR, CRP, ANCA, MPO, PR3, Cr, urinalysis with sediment Also consider ANA, RF, C3, C4, cryoglobulin/cryofibrinogen, hepatitis C serologies, anti-GBM antibodies.

Suggested Reading

Schur PH. Laboratory evaluation of patients with systemic lupus erythematosus. In: Lahita RG, Tsokos G, Buyon J, Koike T, editors. Systemic lupus erythematosus. 5th ed. Amsterdam: Elsevier; 2011. p. 629–54.

References

In addition to the specific references below, we are indebted to the work of many authors of UpToDate (for which Dr. Schur has been a long-time editor), which provided the groundwork for much of the general information in this chapter. We also refer the reader to the following chapter:

1. Bernet LL, Lewis MA, Rieger KE, et al. Ovoid palatal patch; a novel finding in dermatomyositis associated with anti-TIF1-γ (p155) antibodies. JAMA Dermatol. 2016;152(9):1049–51.
2. Bonilla E, Francis L, Allam F, et al. Immunofluorescence microscopy is superior to fluorescent beads for detection of antinuclear antibody reactivity in systemic lupus erythematosus patients. Clin Immunol. 2007;124:18–21.
3. Cavazzana I, Ceribelli A, Quinzanini M, et al. Prevalence and clinical associations of anti-Ku antibodies in systemic autoimmune diseases. Lupus. 2008;17(8):727–32.
4. Grabell DA, Matthews LA, Yancey KB, et al. Detection of Type VII collagen autoantibodies before the onset of bullous systemic lupus erythematosus. JAMA Dermatol. 2015;151(5):539–43.
5. Hira-Kazal R, Shea-Simonds P, Peacock JL, Maher J. How should a district general hospital immunology service screen for anti-nuclear antibodies? An 'in-the-field' audit. Clin Exp Immunol. 2015;180:52–7.
6. Kemna MJ, Damoiseaux J, Austen J, et al. ANCA as a predictor of relapse: useful in patients with renal involvement but not in patients with nonrenal disease. J Am Soc Nephrol. 2015;26:537–42.
7. Lega JC, Fabien N, Reynaud Q, et al. The clinical phenotype associated with myositis-specific and associated autoantibodies: a meta-analysis revisiting the so-called antisynthetase syndrome. Autoimmun Rev. 2014;13:883–91.
8. Li L, Wang Q, Wen X, et al. Assessment of anti-MDA5 antibody as a diagnostic biomarker in patients with dermatomyositis-associated interstitial lung disease or rapidly progressive interstitial lung disease. Oncotarget. 2017;8(44):76129–76,140.
9. Li PH, Wong WH, Lee TL, et al. Relationship between autoantibody clustering and clinical subsets in SLE: cluster and association analyses in Hong Kong Chinese. Rheumatology (Oxford). 2013;52(2):337–45.
10. Merola JF, Chang CA, Sanchez MR, et al. Is chronic cutaneous discoid lupus protective against severe renal disease in patients with systemic lupus erythematosus? J Drugs Dermatol. 2011;10(12):1413–20.
11. Merola JF, Prystowsky SD, Iversen C, et al. Association of discoid lupus erythematosus with other clinical manifestations among patients with systemic lupus erythematosus. J Am Acad Dermatol. 2013;69(1):19–24.
12. Nadelman H. Mukherjee NEJM; 2012.
13. Moinzadeh P, Fonseca C, Hellmich M, et al. Association of anti-RNA polymerase III autoantibodies and cancer in scleroderma. Arthritis Res Ther. 2014;16:R53.
14. Nifli AP, Notas G, Mamoulaki M, et al. Comparison of a multiplex, bead-based fluorescent assay and immunofluorescence methods for the detection of ANA and ANCA autoantibodies in human serum. J Immunol Methods. 2006;311:189–97.
15. Patsinakidis N, Gambichler T, Lahner N, et al. Cutaneous characteristics and association with antinuclear antibodies in 402 patients with different sub-

types of lupus erythematosus. J Eur Acad Dermatol Venereol. 2016;30(12):2097–104.
16. Shin JJ, Glickstein LJ, Steere AC. High levels of inflammatory chemokines and cytokines in joint fluid and synovial tissue throughout the course of antibiotic-refractory lyme arthritis. Arthritis Rheum. 2007;56:1325–35.
17. Tan EM, Feltkamp TE, Smolen JS, et al. Range of antinuclear antibodies in "healthy" individuals. Arthritis Rheum. 1997;40:1601–11.
18. Tomasson G, Grayson PC, Mahr AD. Value of ANCA measurments during remission to predict a relapse of ANCA-associated vasculitis – a meta-analysis. Rheumatology (Oxford). 2012;51:100–9.

Cutaneous Lupus

3

Lisa Pappas-Taffer, Tania C. Gonzalez-Rivera, and Victoria P. Werth

Key Points

- Cutaneous disease in systemic lupus erythematosus (SLE) is common. In contrast, the likelihood of systemic disease in patients with cutaneous lupus is variable and depends on cutaneous lupus subtype.
- Cutaneous lupus subtypes may have significant overlap, both clinically and histologically. Clinicopathologic correlation and careful observation of lesion morphology is essential in establishing subtype.
- In the setting of new onset subacute cutaneous lupus, a thorough evaluation of prescription and over-the-counter medication history is important to rule out iatrogenic disease.
- Patients with cutaneous lupus should be evaluated for the presence of systemic disease through a complete history, review of systems, physical examination, and serologic testing as appropriate.
- The goal of treating cutaneous lupus is to prevent progression of existing lesions and formation of new ones. Aggressive treatment is warranted to prevent disfigurement in scarring subtypes.

Interdisciplinary Introduction

Lupus erythematosus (LE) can affect the skin, the internal organs, or both. In this chapter we review the cutaneous findings specific to LE as well as the nonspecific skin findings that may be associated with systemic LE. Cutaneous disease represents the second most common presentation in systemic lupus erythematosus (SLE), and as such, dermatologists play an important role in the evaluation and diagnosis for these patients by correlating clinical findings with those demonstrated on skin biopsy if needed, and by undertaking initial risk assessment for systemic disease.

In patients with significant systemic disease, including central nervous system (CNS), renal, or other internal organ involvement, co-management in an interdisciplinary fashion is important, and the managing team should include a rheumatologist, nephrologist, neurologist, or other relevant specialists. An interdisciplinary approach may also be beneficial in patients with skin-limited disease who are managed with systemic medications, which can result in multi-

L. Pappas-Taffer · V. P. Werth (✉)
Corporal Michael J. Crescenz VAMC, Philadelphia, PA, USA

Department of Dermatology, University of Pennsylvania, Philadelphia, PA, USA
e-mail: Lisa.Pappas-Taffer@pennmedicine.upenn.edu; werth@pennmedicine.upenn.edu

T. C. Gonzalez-Rivera
University of Pennsylvania, Internal Medicine, Division of Rheumatology, Philadelphia, PA, USA

A. Garg et al. (eds.), *Interdisciplinary Approaches to Overlap Disorders in Dermatology & Rheumatology*,
https://doi.org/10.1007/978-3-319-18446-3_3

system morbidity, including infection, osteoporosis, and metabolic or cardiovascular effects.

Epidemiology & Classification

Epidemiology

The incidence of cutaneous lupus erythematosus (CLE) is similar to that of SLE, but CLE is more common than SLE in males and in older adults [1, 2]. The female to male ratio in CLE is closer to 3 or 4:1, as opposed to the much higher ratio seen in SLE [2]. In CLE, smoking is a risk factor for refractoriness to therapy [3, 4].

Classification of Cutaneous Lupus Erythematosus

Gilliam Classification (Table 3.1)

Classification of lupus erythematosus (LE)-specific skin changes is based on lesion morphology. According to the widely used classification scheme suggested by Gilliam and Sontheimer [5], CLE may be divided as follows: acute cutaneous LE (ACLE); subacute cutaneous LE (SCLE); and chronic cutaneous LE (CCLE), with the last category including discoid LE (DLE), chilblain LE, tumid LE, and lupus profundus [5] (Table 3.1). We review the clinical features of each subtype in detail below.

Table 3.1 Specific skin findings for CLE [5]

Acute cutaneous LE (ACLE)
1. Localized ACLE (malar or butterfly rash)
2. Generalized ACLE (maculopapular rash, SLE rash, photosensitive lupus dermatitis)
Subacute cutaneous LE (SCLE)
1. Annular SCLE
2. Papulosquamous SCLE
Chronic cutaneous LE (CCLE)
1. Classic discoid LE (DLE)
(a). Localized DLE
(b). Generalized DLE
2. Hypertrophic/verrucous DLE
3. Lupus profundus/lupus panniculitis
4. Mucosal DLE
(a). Oral DLE
(b). Conjunctival DLE
5. Lupus tumidus (urticarial plaque of LE)
6. Chilblains LE (chilblains lupus)
7. Lichenoid DLE (LE/lichen planus overlap, lupus planus), nonspecific skin disease

Of note, there can be significant overlap between CLE subtypes, both clinically and histologically, and it is typically not possible to classify subtypes based solely on histology. Clinicopathologic correlation is extremely important, and careful observation of lesion morphology is paramount. It may not always be possible to make a definitive diagnosis of CLE subtype in every patient.

Other Approaches to CLE Subgrouping

Variants of the Gilliam classification have been proposed. There is a lack of international agreement on the proper classification of CLE, and there has been a recent proliferation of the potential ways to group subtypes of CLE [6, 7]. An international effort to develop definitions and groupings for subtypes of CLE is ongoing [8, 9].

LE-Nonspecific Skin Changes (Table 3.2)

There are numerous skin findings that can be seen in patients with LE but are not specific for LE, including vasculitis, vasculopathy, and nonscarring alopecia, among others. These findings, reviewed in detail in Table 3.2, are more frequently associated with SLE than is CLE alone [10]. The presence of these findings in patients with established disease should also prompt evaluation for an underlying flare of SLE.

CLE Association with SLE

The likelihood of SLE in patients with CLE is variable and depends largely on CLE subtype. In localized DLE, extracutaneous involvement is relatively uncommon. Patients with generalized DLE or papulosquamous SCLE are more likely to meet criteria for SLE, although they may have lower likelihood of CNS or renal involvement than other groups with SLE.

Table 3.2 Nonspecific skin findings in LE

Cutaneous vascular disease
1. Vasculitis
(a). Leukocytoclastic vasculitis
(i). Palpable purpura
(ii). Urticarial vasculitis
(b). Polyarteritis nodosa-like cutaneous lesions
2. Vasculopathy
(a). Degos disease-like lesions
(b). Secondary atrophie blanche (livedoid vasculitis, livedo vasculitis)
3. Periungual telangiectasia
4. Livedo reticularis
5. Thrombophlebitis
6. Raynaud phenomenon
7. Erythromelalgia
Nonscarring alopecia
1. "Lupus hair"
2. Telogen effluvium
3. Alopecia areata
Other cutaneous manifestations
1. Sclerodactyly
2. Rheumatoid nodules
3. Calcinosis cutis
4. LE-nonspecific bullous lesions
5. Urticaria
6. Papulonodular mucinosis
7. Cutis laxa/anetoderma
8. Acanthosis nigricans (type B insulin resistance)
9. Erythema multiforme
10. Leg ulcers
11. Lichen planus

By contrast, about 80% of SLE patients have specific skin changes. The commonly used ACR-97 criteria for SLE diagnosis [11, 12] place great importance on skin manifestations, including both LE-specific skin changes (butterfly rash, discoid lesions), and relatively nonspecific skin changes (oral and nasal mucosal ulcers, and photosensitivity). In many patients with isolated cutaneous LE, skin signs and symptoms alone may thus fulfill the required four ACR criteria for SLE [13, 14] (Table 3.3).

New criteria for SLE were developed by the Systemic Lupus International Collaborating Clinics (SLICC) in 2012 [15], including 11 clinical and six immunologic criteria. Fulfillment of four or more criteria (including at least one clinical and one immunologic item) is required for a diagnosis of SLE. Among other changes, the SLICC criteria reduce the relative weighting of skin findings as compared to ACR-97 by consolidating the skin findings in LE into fewer categories, eliminating the redundancy in ACR-97 that allows patients to meet SLE criteria with skin-limited disease. Of note, alopecia is added as a criterion in the SLICC criteria, though this presents challenges, as SLE patients can have alopecia for many different reasons, not all of which are related to SLE. Differentiating alopecia

Table 3.3 The American College of Rheumatology 1982 revised criteria for classification of systemic lupus erythematosus (6). Sm, Smith

Criterion	Definition
1. Malar Rash	Fixed erythema, flat or raised, over the malar eminences, tending to spare the nasolabial folds
2. Discoid rash	Erythematous raised patches with adherent keratotic scaling and follicular plugging; atrophic scarring may occur in older lesions
3. Photosensitivity	Skin rash as a result of unusual reaction to sunlight, by patient history or physician observation
4. Oral ulcers	Oral or nasopharyngeal ulceration, usually painless, observed by physician
5. Nonerosive Arthritis	Involving 2 or more peripheral joints, characterized by tenderness, swelling, or effusion
6. Pleuritis or Pericarditis	1. Pleuritis – convincing history of pleuritic pain or rubbing heard by a physician or evidence of pleural effusion *OR* 2. Pericarditis – documented by electrocardiogram or rub or evidence of pericardial effusion
7. Renal Disorder	1. Persistent proteinuria > 0.5 grams per day or > than 3+ if quantitation not performed *OR* 2. Cellular casts - may be red cell, hemoglobin, granular, tubular, or mixed

(continued)

Table 3.3 (continued)

Criterion	Definition
8. Neurologic Disorder	1. Seizures – in the absence of offending drugs or known metabolic derangements; e.g. uremia, ketoacidosis, or electrolyte imbalance *OR* 2. Psychosis – in the absence of offending drugs or known metabolic derangements, e.g., uremia, ketoacidosis, or electrolyte imbalance
9. Hematologic Disorder	1. Hemolytic anemia: with reticulocytosis *OR* 2. Leukopenia: < 4000 mm^3 on ≥ 2 occasions *OR* 3. Lymphopenia: < 1500 mm^3 on ≥ 2 occasions *OR* 4. Thrombocytopenia: < 100,000 mm^3 in the absence of offending drugs
10. Immunologic Disorder	1. Anti-DNA: antibody to native DNA in abnormal titer *OR* 2. Anti-SM: presence of antibody to Sm nuclear antigen *OR* 3. False-positive serologic test for syphilis known to be positive for at least 6 months confirmed by Treponema pallidum immobilization or fluorescent treponemal antibody absorption test
11. Positive Antinuclear Antibody	An abnormal titer of antinuclear antibody by immunofluorescence or an equivalent assay at any point in time and in the absence of drugs known to be associated with drug-induced lupus

related to SLE from alopecia due to other causes (e.g., medication-related telogen effluvium, androgenic alopecia, and alopecia areata, among others) is frequently challenging. For many patients the etiology of hair loss is multifactorial (Table 3.4).

Not surprisingly based on the changes reviewed, studies suggest greater sensitivity for the SLICC criteria as compared with the ACR-97, but poorer specificity [16]. Further testing and validation will be needed to determine the optimal criteria for SLE [15, 17].

Pathogenesis of Cutaneous Lupus Erythematosus

The pathogenesis of CLE is incompletely understood but involves the interaction of genetic and environmental factors to promote the development of a complex inflammatory cascade. Identified pathogenic factors include ultraviolet irradiation compounded by the accumulation of apoptotic cells due to decreased clearing or impaired macrophage phagocytic capacity, B cell defects, dysregulation of T cells, activation of dendritic cells (DCs), and chemokine and cytokine imbalances, particularly in type 1 interferon (IFN) [18]. Autoantibody-mediated antibody-dependent cellular cytotoxicity (ADCC) is a potential mechanism of tissue injury, particularly as certain autoantibodies are associated with certain phenotypes, as reviewed below [19].

Genetic Factors

Major genetic associations with CLE include the human leukocyte antigen (HLA) A1, B8, DR3, B7 and DR2 haplotypes [20]. In the SCLE subtype in particular, genetic studies have identified HLA types A1, B8, DR3, DQ2, DRw52 and C4null as susceptibility haplotypes [21]. SCLE is closely associated with the HLA haplotype DRB1*0301-B*08.6, which includes the 308A TNFa promoter polymorphism. This polymorphism has been associated with increased UV-induced TNFa production in keratinocytes [20, 22].

Additionally, polymorphisms affecting many genetic regions outside the major histocompatibility complex (MHC) regions increase susceptibility to CLE. These include genes encoding cytokines (IL-1 locus 2q13; IL-10 locus 1q31), cytokine receptors (gamma receptor II Fc RII locus 1q23; T cell receptor TCR locus 7q35),

Table 3.4 SLICC 2012 SLE classification criteria

Clinical criteria	
Acute cutaneous lupus or subacute cutaneous lupus	Acute cutaneous lupus, including lupus malar rash (do not count if malar discoid); bullous lupus; toxic epidermal necrolysis variant of SLE; maculopapular lupus rash; photosensitive lupus rash in the absence of dermatomyositis; *or* Subacute cutaneous lupus (nonindurated psoriasiform and/or annular polycyclic lesions that resolve without scarring, although occasionally with postinflammatory depigmentation or telangiectasia)
Chronic cutaneous lupus	Classic discoid rash (localized or generalized); hypertrophic (verrucous) lupus; lupus panniculitis (profundus); mucosal lupus; lupus erythematous tumidus; chilblains lupus; discoid lupus/lichen planus overlap
Oral ulcers	Palate, buccal, tongue or nasal ulcers in the absence of other causes, such as vasculitis, Behçet disease, infection (herpes), inflammatory bowel disease, reactive arthritis, and acidic foods
Nonscarring alopecia	Diffuse thinning or hair fragility with visible broken hairs in the absence of other causes, such as alopecia areata, drugs, iron deficiency, and androgenic alopecia
Synovitis involving two or more joints	Swelling, or effusion, or tenderness in 2 or more joints, and 30 minutes or more of morning stiffness
Serositis	Typical pleurisy for more than 1 day, or pleural effusions, or pleural rub; *or* Typical pericardial pain (pain with recumbency improved by sitting forward) for more than 1 day, or pericardial effusion, or pericardial rub, or pericarditis by electrocardiography; *and* The absence of other causes, such as infection, uremia, and Dressler's pericarditis
Renal	Urine protein/creatinine (or 24-hour urine protein) representing 500 mg of protein/24 hour; *or* Red blood cell casts
Neurologic	Seizures; psychosis; mononeuritis multiplex (in the absence of other known causes, such as primary vasculitis); myelitis; peripheral or cranial neuropathy (in the absence of other known causes such as primary vasculitis, infection or diabetes mellitus); acute confusional state (in the absence of other causes, including toxic-metabolic, uremia, drugs).
Hemolytic anemia	
Leukopenia or leukopenia	Leukopenia <4000 mm^3 at least once (in the absence of other known causes such as Felty syndrome, drugs and portal hypertension); *or* Lymphopenia (<1000 mm^3 at least once) in the absence of other known causes such as corticosteroids, drugs, and infection
Thrombocytopenia	<100,000/mm^3 at least once in the absence of other known causes, such as drugs, portal hypertension, and TTP
Immunologic criteria	
ANA	Above laboratory reference range
Anti-dsDNA	Above laboratory reference range, except ELISA: twice above laboratory reference range
Anti-Sm	
Antiphospholipid antibody	Any of the following: lupus anticoagulant, false positive RPR, medium or high titer anticardiolipin (IgA, IgG or IgM), anti-β2 glycoproteins I (IgA, IgG or IgM)
Low complement	Low C3, low C4, low CH50
Direct Coombs test	In the absence of hemolytic anemia

adhesion molecules (ICAM-1 locus 19p13.3–p13.2; E-selectin locus 1q23–25), antioxidant enzymes (glutathione-S-transferase M1 GST M1 locus 1p13), and apoptosis genes (Fas locus 10q24.1;TRIM39), ITGAM, TYK2, and CTLA4 [23–27]. Genes in the IFN pathway (e.g. IRF5) are associated with SLE and may also play a role in CLE [28].

Inherited deficiencies of complement components have also been strongly linked to CLE. The likely mechanism is accumulation of DNA and/or RNA inside cells, leading to IRF-3 dependent production and release of IFNa. Patients with C1q deficiency frequently develop LE-like photosensitive skin eruptions. C1q binds apoptotic cells and appears to play a role in the clearance of apoptotic keratinocytes [29]. C1 inhibitor, C1q, C2, and partial C4b deficiencies have been described in CLE.

Certain complement deficiencies have been associated with specific CLE subtypes: C2/C4 deficiencies are associated with SCLE, while C4 deficiency has been associated with LE profundus [30].

Missense mutations in the TREX1 gene, an exonuclease that digests single-stranded or mispaired double-stranded DNA, underlies familial chilblain LE [31].

Ultraviolet Light and Apoptosis

Both Ultraviolet A (UVA) and Ultraviolet B (UVB) exposure can trigger CLE, although irradiation of a large spot size on a normally photo-exposed area is required to see induction of lesions in about half of CLE patients [32–34]. The exact role of UVR in CLE induction is unclear. UVB irradiation induces changes in keratinocyte membrane expression of autoantigens [35, 36]. It also is known that UVR induces DNA damage and that there are increased apoptotic cells in the epidermis in CLE. These increased apoptotic cells are seen in more than half of CLE biopsies after irradiation, and CLE patients may have defects in clearance of these cells [37]. As reviewed, patients deficient in C1q develop a photosensitive form of LE [38].

Innate Immunity

Antimicrobial peptides, including LL-37, are expressed in inflammatory and epithelial cells. These are upregulated in CLE skin [39, 40]. Antimicrobial peptides and other molecules present in CLE skin, including HMGB1, hyaluronic acid, self-nucleic acids, and nucleic acid-containing immune complexes, upregulate DCs through toll-like receptors and pathogen recognition receptors [41, 42]. Type I interferons are upregulated in CLE and activate the JAK/STAT1/2 signaling pathway, causing expression of IFN-stimulated genes that activate the adaptive immune system.

Inflammatory Cells

The interface dermatitis that is the hallmark of most subtypes of CLE, as reviewed below, includes an inflammatory infiltrate of DCs, as well as CCR5+, CD4+ T cells. CD8+ T cells can predominate in long-standing DLE. Th17, CD4+ T cells are important in SLE pathogenesis, but activation of type I IFN and IFN-g are more characteristic of DLE than activation of the IL-17 pathway [43]. Regulatory T cells are locally decreased in CLE, potentially contributing to autoimmunity [44].

Inflammatory Cytokines and Chemokines

A distinctive IFN signature is observed in the skin and blood of certain CLE patients [45, 46]. Specifically, this signature can be found only in subsets of CLE characterized by an interface dermatitis (DLE, SCLE); it correlates with CLE disease activity, but there is no difference in IFN signature in those meeting criteria for SLE relative to CLE alone [46].

The expression pattern of IFN-inducible proteins in CLE reflects the characteristic histological distribution of infiltrating immune cells in each subset [47]. Studies have demonstrated the CXCR3 ligands CXCL9 (interferon-gamma [IFNg]-induced monokine), CXCL10 (IFNg-inducible protein 10), and CXCL11 (IFN-inducible T cell alpha chemoattractant) as the most abundantly expressed chemokine family members in cutaneous LE [48]. In addition, IFN-lambda, recently demonstrated in the epidermis of CLE, is produced by keratinocytes and induces expression of CXCL9 [49]. Within cutaneous LE lesions, plasmacytoid and myeloid DCs accumulate in the dermis and are activated to produce type I IFN, as detected by the expression of IRF7 and MxA [50]. Type I INF induce proinflammatory cytokines and chemokines that support the cellular immune response.

The proinflammatory cytokines TNFa and IL-1 are upregulated by UVR and therefore may be important in CLE [51]. In addition, increased TNFa produced by peripheral blood mononuclear cells (PBMCs) in CLE patients correlates with increased disease activity [52].

Clinical Features

Each subtype of CLE has distinctive clinical features and differing frequency of association with SLE. However, the histology can overlap in some subtypes. Subtypes with scarring (e.g., DLE and lupus panniculitis) have the deepest and most dense inflammatory infiltrate on histology, while clinically transient subtypes (e.g., ACLE) are characterized by the most superficial infiltrate.

Acute Cutaneous Lupus Erythematosus (ACLE)

ACLE is an acute, non-scarring, photosensitive eruption that occurs in patients who frequently meet criteria for SLE. It is transient, and its appearance tends to mirror increased systemic activity. ACLE is associated with a younger age of SLE onset. Co-occurrence with other subtypes of CLE, especially SCLE, can occur.

Classically, ACLE presents as erythematous patches with fine scale and/or edema. Patients may initially mistake this rash for sunburn and only seek medical attention after it persists for several days. There are both localized and generalized forms of ACLE.

Localized ACLE is more common than generalized; it may present as either the classic "butterfly rash," involving the malar cheeks and nasal bridge with sparing of the nasolabial folds, or between joints on the dorsal fingers. Involvement of other photodistributed sites (forehead, periorbital, sides of neck) can occur.

The generalized form of ACLE is less common and can be non-bullous or bullous. Non-bullous ACLE may appear as symmetric, discrete or coalescing macules and/or papules. It can also mimic dermatomyositis. Bullous ACLE can mimic bullous fixed drug or Stevens-Johnson syndrome (SJS)/toxic epidermolytic necrolysis (TEN), presenting with flaccid bullae and epidermal detachment. (See section below entitled " *Vesicobullous disease occurring as severe variants of ACLE, SCLE, and rarely, DLE.*")

Not all patients with SLE develop ACLE, however presence of ACLE is typically a sign of SLE. Malar ACLE was reported in up to 52% of SLE patients at the time of diagnosis in one study [53], and large U.S. lupus cohorts reported malar ACLE in 20–60% of patients. Rosacea can be mistaken for malar ACLE. Persistence of the eruption, involvement past the nasolabial fold onto the lip, presence of papules, and dynamic flushing would go against a diagnosis of ACLE. A biopsy may be needed to confirm the diagnosis.

ACLE tends to wax and wane with systemic activity. It does not scar but can result in post-inflammatory hyper- or hypopigmentation. Treatment of ACLE often requires treatment of underlying SLE.

Subacute Cutaneous Lupus Erythematosus (SCLE)

SCLE is a highly photosensitive, non-scarring CLE subtype. An estimated 35–40% of patients with SCLE meet criteria for SLE, although many patients do so by fulfilling 4 or more of the ACR-97 criteria involving skin lesions, photosensitivity, and serologies [2, 54, 55]. SCLE patients with SLE typically have only mild systemic symptoms, most commonly arthritis and myalgias; in the original series, no SCLE patients had serious CNS or renal disease [56].

SCLE most commonly involves sun exposed areas, including the upper chest and back in a 'V' distribution, the extensor aspect of arms, and, occasionally, the sides of the face. The mid-face, scalp, and skin below the waist are usually spared.

Clinically, there are two forms of SCLE: annular and papulosquamous. Annular SCLE is characterized by scaly, erythematous, thin, coin-shaped plaques with raised red borders and a central clearing. The annular plaques tend to coalesce, producing a polycyclic array. In contrast, papulosquamous SCLE (Fig. 3.1) tends to have a psoriasis or eczema-like appearance in a sun-exposed distribution. Lesions may begin as small erythematous papules or plaques with fine scale. Although most patients are asymptomatic,

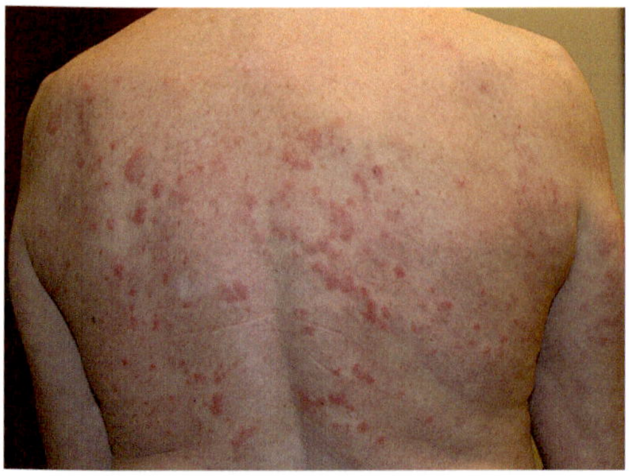

Fig. 3.1 Papulosquamous SCLE. Erythematous scaly patches and plaques on back

mild pruritus may occur. Most patients have chronically active disease with intermittent sun-induced exacerbations, and although SCLE does not scar, it can result in significant hyperpigmentation or hypopigmentation.

Up to 30% of SCLE cases are induced or exacerbated by a medication [54]. Widespread involvement may favor a drug-induced etiology. Presence of eosinophils on histopathology does not appear to reliably distinguish drug-induced from idiopathic disease. A 2012 population-based case-control study found terbinafine, TNF-alpha antagonists, antiepileptics, and proton pump inhibitors to be the most frequent culprits [54]. However, over 100 different agents have been implicated, with additional culprits including anti-hypertensive medications (calcium channel blockers and ACE inhibitors), nonsteroidal anti-inflammatory drugs, other antifungal agents, and chemotherapy agents. There have been reports of radiation therapy-induced SCLE and paraneoplastic SCLE [57].

In suspected cases of SCLE, consider testing for the anti-SSA/Ro antibody, the titers for which may be positive in up to 5% of cases when the ANA test is negative. Women with SCLE and certain autoan tibodies (typically anti-SSA but rarely anti-RNP) have an increased risk of giving birth to infants with neonatal lupus (NL), due to transplacental passage of the autoantibody. Presence of Ro/SSA Antobody is also associated with risk of congenital heart block in the fetus or newborn. Women with anti-SSA/Ro antibody who become pregnant should be evaluated by Maternal-Fetal Medicine.

Discoid Lupus Erythematosus (DLE)

DLE is the most common type of CLE. Active DLE lesions often present as erythematous, scaly plaques. These may cause scarring, alopecia, and dyspigmentation, manifestations that become more pronounced over time. Patients classically develop atrophic plaques with central hypopigmentation and peripheral hyperpigmentation. Vitiligo-like hypopigmentation may also be seen (Fig. 3.2). Although typically asymptomatic, lesions may be tender. Erythema, tenderness, and/or scale are all signs of disease activity that can fluctuate and should be treated. Disfiguring scarring, burning pain and alopecia cause significant morbidity. Interestingly, a recent survey study noted that patients are bothered more by signs of activity (e.g. redness) than damage (scarring and dyspigmentation) [58, 59].

DLE can occur in a localized or a generalized distribution (Fig. 3.3). Localized DLE, which is more common, presents with lesions limited to the head and neck, with a propensity for the scalp and conchal bowl of the ear. Generalized DLE, the less common form, presents with lesions below the neck, typically on the extensor forearms and hands; these patients are at higher risk for developing SLE than those with localized disease [60, 61]. DLE lesions occur most commonly in sun-exposed areas but can also occur in non-sun-exposed regions, including, rarely, the palms and soles (<2%) as well as the mucosa (lips, oral cavity, genitalia) (Fig. 3.4a, b) [62].

Hypertrophic DLE is a variant of DLE in which thick, keratotic plaques occur on the arms, hands, and face. Hypertrophic DLE can be confused clinically and histologically with warts, keratoacanthomas, squamous cell carcinomas, and hypertrophic lichen planus; a skin biopsy is often needed to confirm the diagnosis. Although hypertrophic DLE can mimic squamous cell carcinoma (SCC), SCC can also rarely develop within a DLE lesion, and a high index of suspicion is necessary for diagnosis [63].

Although most patients with DLE have skin-limited disease, recent data suggest that the risk of progression to SLE may be higher than previously thought. In 1975, Prystowsky et al. reported that <5–10% of adults with DLE progress to SLE [64], while in 2011, Grohhagen et al. reported a 16.7% risk of progression within 3 years of diagnosis [54]. Children with DLE are believed to have a greater likelihood of developing SLE than adults, with reported risk ranging from 23.5–26% [60, 65, 66]. In one retrospective study looking at 34 children <16 years old over a nine-year period, an association between DLE and SLE was seen in 23.5% of patients, with disseminated DLE lesions more frequent in those meeting SLE criteria (87.5% *vs.* 34%).

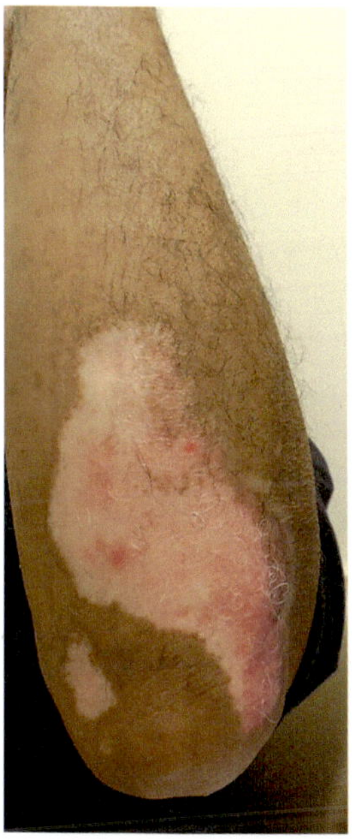

Fig. 3.2 DLE with post-inflammatory hypopigmentation. Note the presence of activity (pink) and damage (hypopigmentation)

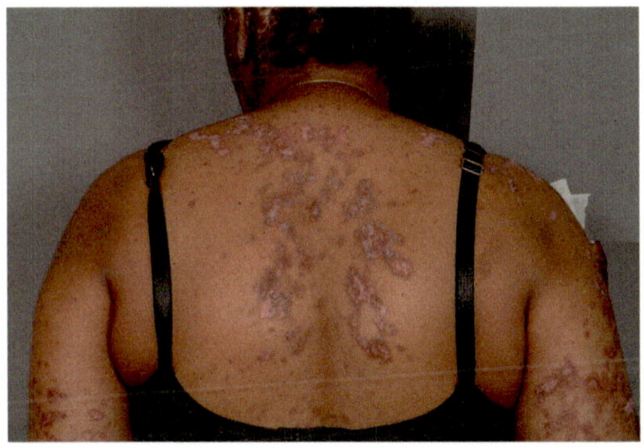

Fig. 3.3 Generalized DLE. Erythematous, scaly atrophic plaques on back and arms, with central hypopigmentation and hyperpigmentation at the periphery

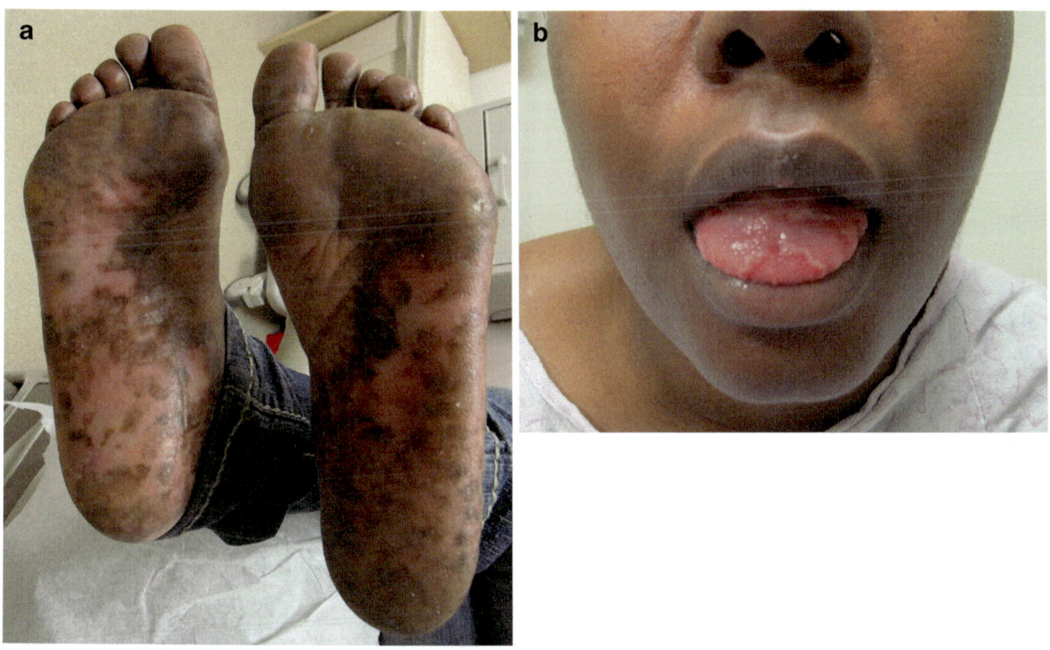

Fig. 3.4 Non-sun-exposed DLE (**a**) DLE affecting soles of feet. (**b**) Intraoral DLE

Cutaneous Lupus: Additional LE-Specific Skin Variants

Lupus Erythematosus Tumidus (Tumid Lupus)

Tumid lupus is a relatively uncommon variant of cutaneous lupus that is generally considered to be a skin-limited condition. Clinically, lesions appear as erythematous, edematous papules or plaques, sometimes annular, without overlying epidermal change or scarring. Tumid LE is characterized by extreme photosensitivity, with lesions occurring most commonly on the face, V of the neckline, upper back, and extensor upper extremities.

Histologically, there is no vacuolar interface dermatitis at the dermal-epidermal junction (DEJ), and direct immunofluorescence (DIF) is negative. Patients are typically ANA negative and do not have underlying SLE.

Lupus Erythematosus Panniculitis/ Lupus Profundus

Lupus erythematous (LE) panniculitis is a scarring subtype of CLE characterized by intense inflammation in the fat lobules. It typically presents with tender, erythematous plaques or subcutaneous nodules without epidermal change. It occurs most commonly on the face, proximal extremities, upper trunk, and buttocks, but also scalp, breasts, and thighs. Lupus panniculitis involving the breast, also known as "lupus mastitis", may present similarly to inflammatory breast cancer, and biopsy should readily rule out a malignancy. Lesions of LE panniculitis frequently occur in sun-protected areas, are often painful, and evolve into disfiguring, depressed areas of focal lipoatrophy (Fig. 3.5a, b). One third of cases of LE panniculitis may present with overlying DLE, in a phenomenon clinically termed "lupus profundus."

Clinically and histologically, lupus panniculitis can closely resemble subcutaneous panniculitis-like T-cell lymphoma [67]. Biopsy specimens should be reviewed by a dermatopathologist, and T-cell markers and gene rearrangement studies may be necessary to help differentiate the two entities.

Chilblain Lupus

Chilblain lupus is a rare form of CLE that resembles frostbite and occurs most commonly in children and young to middle-aged women. In a series of 33 patients with chilblains lasting more than one month, 24% were found to meet classification criteria for SLE at the time of diagnosis [68]. Patients present with single or multiple, erythematous to violaceous, painful and/or pruritic nodules, most commonly located on the dorsolateral aspect of fingers and toes, and rarely on the ears and nose. Lesions arise 12–24 hours after exposure to a cold and wet environment. Unlike classic chilblains, lesions of chilblain lupus often persist beyond cold months.

Neonatal Lupus

Neonatal lupus (NL) is a self-limited syndrome that occurs in infants whose mothers have anti-SSA/Ro antibodies, or less commonly anti-SSB/La or anti-RNP antibodies, due to transplacental passage of these antibodies. The cutaneous eruption in NL occurs in 1–2% of infants born to mothers with SLE or Sjögren Syndrome with positive anti-SSA/Ro but can occur in asymptomatic mothers as well. In one series, 44% of NL mothers were asymptomatic without a history of connective tissue disease, with 50% of these mothers subsequently developing SLE or Sjögren syndrome within 10 years [69].

Unlike most CLE subtypes, NL occurs equally in male and female infants [70]. It can include one or more of the following features: an SCLE-like eruption (15–95%); congenital heart block (10%); hepatobiliary disease (9–25%); cytopenias, including leukopenia, neutropenia, or thrombocytopenia (10–15%); varying neurologic findings, including hydrocephalus, non-specific white matter changes, and calcification of the basal ganglia; vasculopathy; and, rarely, stippling

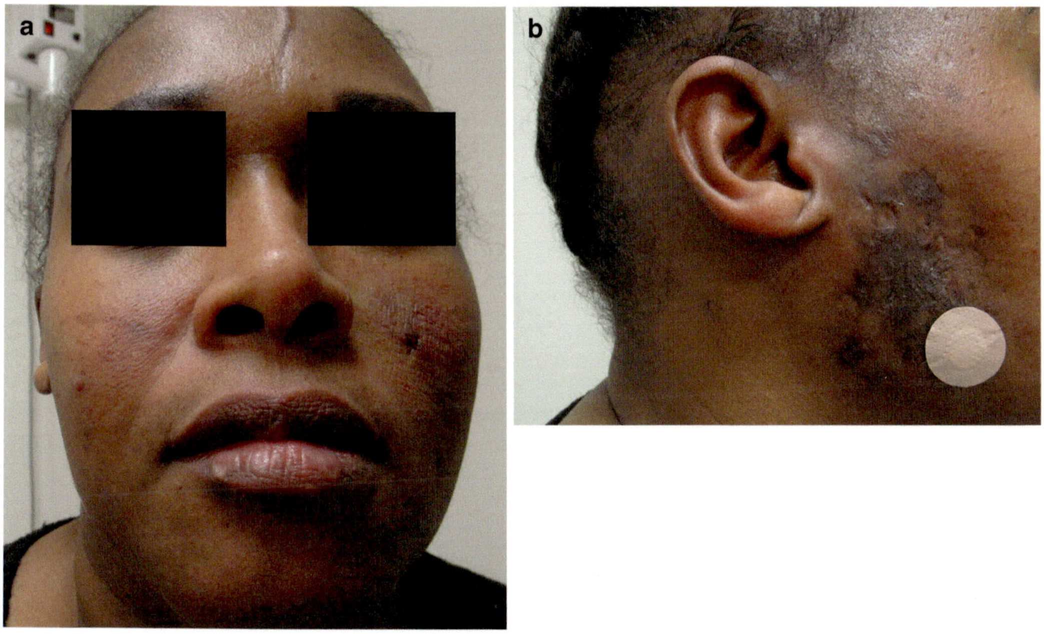

Fig. 3.5 (**a**) Lupus panniculitis of the face in a patient with SLE. Firm, violaceous plaques on the cheeks, rather than patches of erythema seen with ACLE. (**b**) Lupus profundus. Lupus panniculitis with overlying DLE involving the face

of the epiphyses (chondrodysplasia punctata) on x-ray [70, 71]. Complete heart block, which is permanent, is the most feared complication of NL; the other findings are transient and self-limited, typically self-resolving within 6–8 months as the maternal antibodies are cleared.

Skin The skin eruption of NL can be present at birth but is most commonly detected between 4–6 weeks of age, often following the first sun exposure. Skin lesions morphologically resemble the annular lesions of SCLE and have the same histologic findings; further similarities between NL and adult SCLE include photosensitivity and a strong association with anti-SSA/Ro. Unlike SCLE, however, NL has a predilection for the periorbital face (resulting in the finding known as "raccoon eyes") and scalp, though it can also present elsewhere on the body.

The skin lesions of NL typically self-resolve in the first year of life but can result in dyspigmentation and residual telangiectasias in 10–20% of patients. Corticosteroids can hasten resolution of NL, but there is no evidence that sequelae are prevented with treatment. Photoprotection is important, and pulsed dye laser can be used to treat residual telangiectasias.

Cardiac Autoantibody-induced cardiac conduction abnormalities occur in the setting of a normal heart in NL, which is the most common cause of congenital heart block diagnosed in utero or during the neonatal period (*See Disease Assessment section below for screening recommendations*). Of note, anti-SSA/Ro is responsible for cardiac manifestations; NL induced by anti-RNP does not involve the heart. Cardiac NL has a mortality rate of approximately 20%, and approximately two-thirds of affected children require pacemakers [72].

Hematologic Any hematological lineage can be affected in NL, but thrombocytopenia is the most common manifestation, generally occurring within the 1st week of life and self-resolving by age 2–4 weeks. Neutropenia occurs later, at 4–8 weeks (10–15%). Rare cases of hemolytic anemia, pancytopenia, or aplastic anemia have been reported [70].

Hepatobiliary Hepatobiliary disease has been reported in 9–25% of infants with NL. The severity of involvement can vary widely, ranging from asymptomatic elevations in liver function tests, to mild hepatosplenomegaly, cholestasis, and hepatitis, to, rarely, death [70, 71].

Lupus-specific Vesiculobullous Disease

Bullous SLE (BSLE)

BSLE, also referred to as "bullous lupus," is a neutrophilic, subepidermal, antibody-mediated, vesiculobullous condition that occurs as a clinical manifestation of SLE. It is occasionally the presenting sign of SLE. Unlike ACLE, blistering activity does not necessarily correlate with systemic disease activity, although parallel exacerbations, often between BSLE and lupus nephritis, have been described.

Clinically and histologically, BSLE can resemble neutrophil-rich bullous pemphigoid, epidermolysis bullosa acquisita, linear IgA dermatosis, or dermatitis herpetiformis, presenting with tense, fluid filled vesicles or bullae. It often scars and may lead to the development of milia. The bullous eruption has a rapid onset and is typically widespread and symmetric, favoring the upper trunk, proximal upper extremities, neck, and face. However, it can occur on both sun-exposed and unexposed skin, as well as nasal, oral, and genital mucous membranes. Skin lesions are typically pruritic, with symptoms ranging from mild to severe. Mucosal lesions are typically painful.

Elements required for diagnosis of BSLE include (1) meeting criteria for SLE, (2) having an acquired bullous eruption, (3) a skin biopsy showing a neutrophilic subepidermal blister, and (4) direct immunofluorescence (DIF) demonstrating IgG (typically linear deposition at the DEJ), with or without IgM or IgA. Lastly, evidence of antibodies to type VII collagen may be demonstrated by DIF, indirect IF, or ELISA [73, 74]. The cutaneous lesions in BSLE typically respond well to treatment with dapsone.

Vesiculobullous Disease Occurring as Severe Variants of ACLE, SCLE, and Rarely, DLE.

The lupus-specific vesiculobullous eruptions are distinctly different from BSLE in that they present with flaccid rather than tense bullae, typically have a positive Nikolsky sign, often involve the mucosa, can occur in the setting of any CLE subtype, and may occur in patients without SLE. The frequency of these vesiculobullous eruptions is unclear due to the differing presentations and nomenclature reported in the literature.

In TEN-like ACLE, also known as apoptotic pan-epidermolysis (ASAP), patients with SLE present with diffuse or patchy erythema, often photodistributed, that evolves rapidly into flaccid bullae [75]. Unlike drug-induced TEN, there is typically no or limited mucosal involvement, no clear drug culprit, and a better prognosis [76]. TEN-like SCLE, by contrast, is described as widespread, flaccid bullae in the context of pre-existing, photodistributed SCLE lesions and positive anti-SSA/Ro or anti-SSB/La.

Erythema multiforme (EM)-like ACLE, SCLE, or DLE, also known as Rowell syndrome, is characterized by EM-like lesions (targetoid, erythematous plaques with central flaccid bullae and erosions) in the context of lupus erythematosus (Fig. 3.6) [76, 77]. In the original case series from 1963, Rowell et al. described four adult women with longstanding DLE, chilblain LE, and skin lesions resembling EM [78]. Zeitouni et al. redefined the diagnostic criteria in 2000 to require all of three major criteria (including the presence of lupus erythematosus, EM-like lesions, and a speckled pattern of ANA), as well as one of the minor criteria (including chilblains, positive anti-SSA/Ro or anti-SSB/La, or a positive rheumatoid factor) [79].

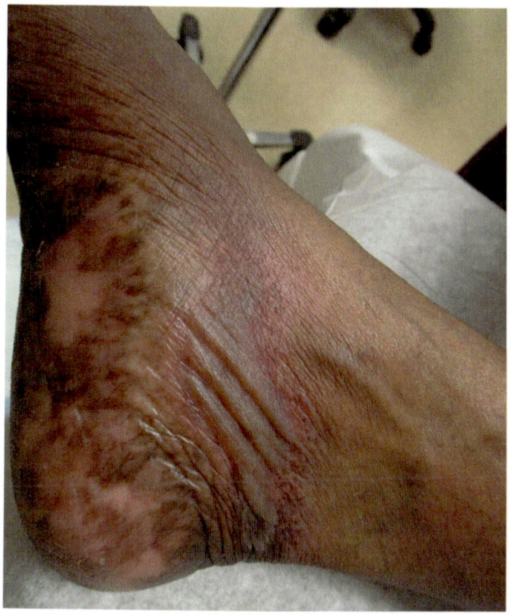

Fig. 3.6 Bullous DLE/EM-like DLE. Bullae with surrounding violaceous erythema on the foot

A review compiling 142 cases from the international literature noted that EM-like CLE differed from classic EM in that it did not preferentially affect the distal extremities, infrequently involved the mucous membranes, and was only rarely associated with an identifiable trigger [76]. It is difficult to differentiate the EM-like lesions of Rowell syndrome from classic EM on routine skin biopsy. However, positive DIF has been reported in more than 50% of cases; this frequency is similar to that seen in classic SCLE/ACLE, suggesting that EM-like lesions represent morphologic variants of CLE [76]. Nonetheless, whether or not Rowell syndrome truly represents a variant of CLE or an entity in its own right is controversial.

Non-specific Cutaneous Lesions of LE

Vascular findings have been reported to occur in approximately 50% of patients with lupus. These include: Raynaud phenomenon, livedo reticularis, palmar erythema, subtle periungual telangiectasias, leukocytoclastic or urticarial vasculitis, antiphospholipid vasculopathy, and atrophy blanche.

Non-scarring alopecia related to SLE may be telogen effluvium (caused by the underlying condition or by medications such as methotrexate or glucocorticoids) or "lupus hair." Lupus hair is characterized by thin, unruly terminal hairs that fracture easily, usually along the frontal hairline, and typically during exacerbations of SLE. The hair grows back when the disease activity subsides [80].

Other nonspecific cutaneous manifestations of LE can include photosensitivity, reticular erythematous mucinosis (REM), erythromelalgia, and anetoderma.

Diagnostic Considerations

A biopsy of lesional skin is the cornerstone of CLE diagnosis. DIF may be a useful adjunct, while lupus serologies are often less helpful. In the setting of new onset SCLE, a careful evaluation of prescription and over-the-counter medication history is important to rule out drug-induced disease.

Diagnosis of Cutaneous Lupus

Histopathology

CLE histology classically shows an interface dermatitis (vacuolar degeneration of the DEJ) with perivascular lymphocytic inflammation and increased dermal mucin (Fig. 3.7). Of note, CLE and dermatomyositis may look histologically identical. However, the two conditions can be differentiated clinically.

The CLE subtypes differ in the amount and depth of inflammation, though there may be overlapping histologic findings between the clinical phenotypes. ACLE, SCLE, and DLE all demonstrate vacuolar interface dermatitis but vary in the degree of dermal inflammation. ACLE has the sparsest and most superficial inflammation of the subtypes, while the superficial lymphocytic infiltrate in SCLE is slightly more robust. DLE dem-

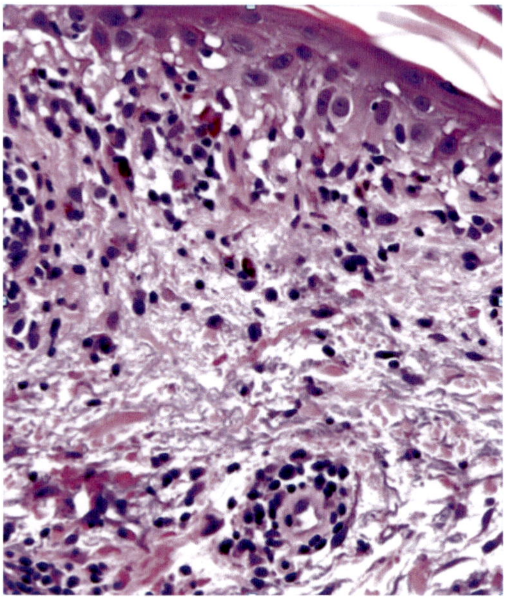

Fig. 3.7 Hematoxylin and eosin stained section of CLE skin lesion. Discoid LE showing focal interface dermatitis and dense perivascular and periadnexal lymphoid infiltrates

onstrates the greatest and deepest dermal inflammation, including periadnexal involvement with follicular plugging and scarring of the epidermis.

Both tumid lupus and lupus panniculitis lack epidermal changes. The findings seen in tumid lupus include prominent dermal mucin and a variable degree of perivascular and periadnexal lymphocytic infiltrate. Lupus panniculitis is characterized by a lobular lymphocytic infiltrate, hyalinizing fat necrosis, periseptal lymphoid follicles, and occasionally calcium deposition or overlying changes of DLE.

NL, if biopsied, looks identical to SCLE, while chilblain LE is characterized by a lymphocytic vasculitis with dermal edema. BSLE demonstrates a subepidermal, neutrophilic-rich blister, and the diagnosis can be confirmed by a positive DIF and ANA. The bullous variants of ACLE, SCLE, and DLE can look identical to drug-related TEN, SJS, or EM on histology, making a thorough history and a high index of suspicion important for accurate diagnosis.

Antibody Deposits in the Skin (DIF)

Skin biopsy to examine immunoreactant deposition by direct immunofluorescent (DIF) testing can be useful in either CLE or SLE. DIF may be performed on lesional skin in active lesions of CLE. When a DIF is performed on nonlesional, non-sun exposed skin, it is referred to as a "lupus band test." Either test is considered positive when a continuous band of immunoreactants along the DEJ is observed. Antibody deposition at the DEJ is the most characteristic immunohistologic finding in lesions of cutaneous lupus and normal skin of patients with SLE. Although the lesional DIF can be helpful in establishing the diagnosis of CLE if the routine biopsy findings are non-specific, it does not replace routine histology as the method of choice for establishing a diagnosis of CLE.

In patients with known SLE, a lupus band test sampled from sun-exposed skin will be positive in 75% [81], and unexposed skin 50% of the time [82]. However 20% of the general population will have a positive lupus band test if sun-exposed skin is biopsied.

Uniquely, SCLE can demonstrate intraepidermal deposits by DIF, thought to be due to anti-Ro/SSA autoantibodies depositing directly in the epidermis rather than at the DEJ.

Autoantibodies

Patients with anti-Smith, anti-RNP, and antiphospholipid antibodies have a greater prevalence of malar rash, while high titer anti-SSA and anti-SSB are associated with SCLE and neonatal LE [19, 83, 84]. The anti-SSA specificity in SCLE is for the SSA/Ro60 antigen.

Evaluation for Systemic Disease

Both the ACR and SLICC criteria for SLE rely heavily on cutaneous manifestations for classification of SLE. Thus, as reviewed, according to the ACR-97 criteria, a patient with a positive ANA, photosensitivity, a malar rash and discoid lesions will fulfill criteria for SLE despite the absence of internal organ involvement. Despite this caveat, CLE can frequently accompany serious systemic involvement. In such cases, the rheumatologist can assist the dermatologist in co-management.

To date, there is no definitive way to predict if a lupus patient with solely cutaneous disease will develop involvement of other organs (Fig. 3.8). Once the diagnosis of CLE is confirmed by histology, a review of systems and a physical examination should be performed to evaluate for mucosal ulcers, fatigue, pleurisy, photosensitivity, joint pain, Raynaud's syndrome, alopecia, history of miscarriages, or thrombotic events.

Initial serology screening should include the ANA measured by the immunofluorescence method. If the patient is being evaluated in the outpatient setting, it is prudent to wait for the results of the ANA test prior to ordering additional serologies. However, if the patient is acutely ill or meets criteria for SLE, additional initial serologies can include anti-dsDNA, anti-Smith, anti-SSA and -SSB antibodies, and C3 and C4 levels. If there is a history of thrombocytopenia, miscarriages, or thrombotic events, evaluation for the antiphospholipid syndrome with dilute Russell viper venom time (DRVVT), anticardiolipin antibodies, and anti-β2-glycoprotein-1 antibodies should be performed.

Principles of Management

The aim of treating CLE is to prevent progression of existing skin lesions and formation of new ones, with aggressive treatment warranted to prevent disfigurement in scarring subtypes. Management strategies include patient education and behavior modification, topical, and systemic therapies, often in combination (Table 3.5). Many systemic therapies have a delayed onset of action in CLE, and initial treatment with topical and intralesional corticosteroids can be important.

Prevention/Patient Education

Sun Protection

UVA and UVB exposure have been shown to induce CLE lesions [85], non-specific cutaneous eruptions, and even systemic symptoms in patients with and without SLE. A vehicle-controlled, randomized, double-blind trial demonstrated that the use of a broad-spectrum sunscreen by those with photosensitive CLE can prevent development of skin lesions [86]. Thus, minimizing UV exposure is a critical component of therapy, even in patients who do not report photosensitivity or worsening of skin lesions following sun exposure.

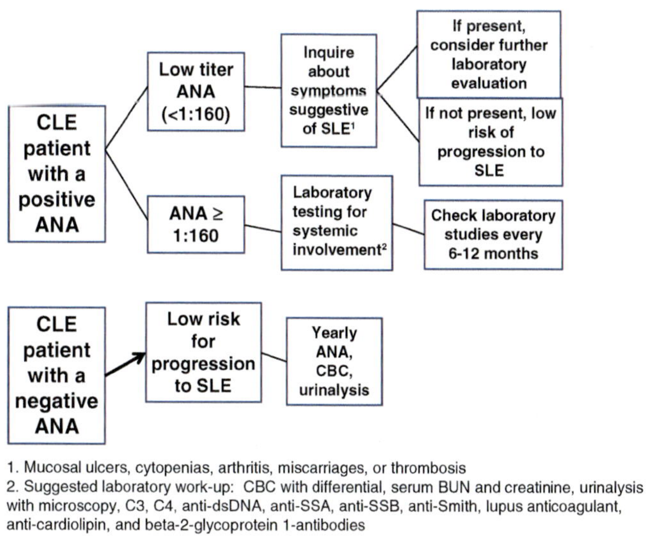

Fig. 3.8 Evaluation/Management. 1. Mucosal ulcers, cytopenias, arthritis, miscarriages, or thrombosis. 2. Suggested laboratory work-up: CBC with differential, serum BUN and creatinine, urinalysis with microscopy, C3, C4, anti-dsDNA, anti-SSA, anti-SSB, anti-Smith, lupus anticoagulant, anti-cardiolipin, and beta-2-glycoprotein 1-antibodies

Table 3.5 Treatment Summary

Prevention	Local Therapy	Systemic Therapy
Sun protection Smoking cessation	Topical or intralesional corticosteroids Calcineurin inhibitors Pulsed dye laser	1st LINE: Antimalarials HCQ CQ +/− addition of Quinacrine 2nd LINE: Immunosuppressants Methotrexate Mycophenolate mofetil Azathioprine Systemic corticosteroids Immunomodulators Dapsone Thalidomide/Lenalidamide Oral retinoids IVIG

Strict sunscreen use is recommended. It should be applied 20–30 minutes prior to expected exposure in sufficient amount (approximately one ounce is required to cover the body of most adults), and with reapplication every 2 hours if sun exposure continues. The sunscreen should be labeled "broad spectrum" (indicating that it provides protection against both UVA and UVB), with a sun protection factor (SPF) of at least 50. Sun-protective clothing is important, including tight-weave fabrics, dark garments and wide-brimmed hats. Sunscreen-impregnated clothing can also be helpful.

UVB-specific protection techniques include avoiding extended outdoor exposure during peak UVB times (10 A.M. to 2 P.M.). Consideration may also be given to using fluorescent light bulbs with the lowest irradiance and/or applying UV-blocking shields to indoor lighting [87, 88], as indoor fluorescent lighting can emit UVB and exacerbate CLE.

UVA is harder to block, as it varies minimally by time of day or by season and can penetrate window glass. However, UV-blocking films can be applied to glass windows in cars, offices, and homes. Sunscreens providing UVA protection (such as those containing titanium dioxide, zinc oxide, mexoryl XL, and others) can also be helpful.

Evaluation for vitamin D deficiency is important in sun-avoiding patients, as sunlight is required for vitamin synthesis. Daily supplementation with at least 400 IU of vitamin D3 and periodic monitoring of 25-hydroxyvitamin D levels for deficiency are recommended.

Smoking Cessation

Multiple studies have reported that cigarette smokers with CLE have more severe disease than nonsmokers and that a subset of these patients are more refractory to therapies [3, 4, 89, 90]. Based on this, and the increased risk of cardiovascular disease in SLE, patients should therefore be counseled on smoking cessation [3].

Camouflage

Makeup products such as Dermablend, Covermark, or Bare Minerals can be helpful in improving cosmesis for patients with active CLE disease or residual pigmentary alterations.

Local Therapy

Topical corticosteroids, calcineurin inhibitors, and intralesional corticosteroids are first-line therapies for CLE.

Topical Steroids

High-potency topical corticosteroids have long been the mainstay for treatment of CLE, including for scarring subtypes of CLE on the face.

However, there is only one randomized, controlled trial examining the efficacy of high-potency topical steroids in CLE. In a 12-week cross-over study of 78 DLE patients, excellent improvement or resolution of lesions was seen in 27% of patients treated with fluocinonide 0.05% cream at 6 weeks, as compared to 10% of patients treated with hydrocortisone 1% cream [91, 92].

Calcineurin Inhibitors

Topical calcineurin inhibitors are a good alternative for patients with persistent facial lesions despite therapy with topical corticosteroids, in whom the risk of continued potent topical steroid use outweighs the benefit. In a randomized, vehicle-controlled, multicenter trial, 20 patients with CLE treated with tacrolimus 0.1% ointment showed significantly more improvement after 28 and 56 days as compared to those treated with vehicle, though the difference was not significant at 84 days [93]. A double-blind, randomized, controlled trial compared tacrolimus 0.1% ointment to clobetasol propionate 0.05% ointment in 20 patients, using a split-face design. The two ointments showed equal efficacy, however, 61% of patients developed telangiectasias on the clobetasol side, as early as 3 weeks into therapy [94]. Although calcineurin inhibitors do not carry a risk of skin thinning, telangiectasias, cataracts, or glaucoma, patients may develop lentigines localized to the treatment site. In addition, calcineurin inhibitors carry a black box warning for a heightened risk of malignancy, specifically lymphoma, although there is no evidence to suggest a causal relationship [95].

Intralesional corticosteroids

Intralesional triamcinolone, given in concentrations ranging from 2.5–20 mg/cc depending on the thickness and location of the lesion being treated, can be effective in DLE. The injections may be repeated monthly while the lesions are active.

Laser

Although typically not used as first line therapy, pulsed-dye laser (PDL) has been demonstrated in several case reports and series to be a safe and effective treatment for DLE. An open prospective study of 12 DLE patients treated with PDL demonstrated efficacy after 6 weeks of treatment [96].

Systemic Therapy

Presently, there are no FDA-approved medications approved specifically for the treatment of CLE. Systemic therapies are indicated for CLE when disease is widespread, when a scarring subtype such as DLE or LE panniculitis affects a cosmetically disfiguring location, or in cases that are refractory to topical or intralesional therapy.

Many of the same systemic medications used to treat SLE are frequently employed in CLE. Exceptions include systemic corticosteroids, which are frequently used in SLE but reserved for severe, rapid-onset CLE; leflutamide, which is used in SLE but not CLE, and thalidomide, which is used for CLE but typically not for SLE.

Antimalarials

Oral antimalarials are considered first-line systemic therapy for all CLE subtypes that are not completely responsive to topical modalities. In addition, it has been suggested that the initiation of hydroxychloroquine (HCQ) for CLE may prevent development of SLE. Specifically, James et al. reported the treatment of HCQ resulted in a significant delay in the time from onset of the first symptom to SLE classification [97].

Antimalarials are immunomodulatory drugs with a mechanism of action that is incompletely understood but thought to involve inhibition of TLR signaling and subsequent inhibition of pro-inflammatory cytokines, as well as antithrombotic properties. It takes 2–3 months to obtain steady-state concentrations, which may account for the slow onset of therapeutic benefit. Because antimalarials can take up to 3–6 months to reach maximum efficacy, bridging with topical and intralesional therapy is important in CLE.

The three antimalarials currently used include HCQ (200–400 mg/day, ≤6.5 mg/kg/day), chloroquine (125–250 mg/day, ≤3.5–4 mg/kg/day), and quinacrine (100 mg/day). Quinacrine is currently only available at compounding companies and may not be covered by insurance.

In practice, HCQ is the antimalarial of choice due to the lower risk for retinopathy as compared to chloroquine (CQ). If there is no response or an incomplete response to HCQ therapy after 2 months, quinacrine may be added. Chang et al. demonstrated a 67% improvement rate of cutaneous disease with the addition of quinacrine to HCQ in patients who had previously failed HCQ monotherapy [98]. Interestingly, Frances et al. recently reported an association between complete remission and higher blood concentrations of HCQ, suggesting that it may be useful to consider checking serum HCQ concentrations in patients with refractory CLE [99]. Finally, if no response is seen, switching from HCQ to CQ can be therapeutically beneficial. Due to weight-based CQ dosing recommendations, patients may be advised not to take the medication on a certain number of days per week.

Antimalarials most commonly cause ocular and cutaneous side effects, most of which are reversible. All ocular side effects are more common with CQ than HCQ, and combined CQ and HCQ use is contraindicated because of additive eye toxicity. Quinacrine does not appear to cause eye toxicity. Corneal drug deposition may cause reversible ocular side effects that are not a contraindication to continued antimalarial therapy, including halos, blurred vision, photophobia, and reduction in accommodation.

True, irreversible retinopathy is uncommon with HCQ and preventable with screening. Premaculopathy (retinal pigment deposition resulting in paracentral and pericentral scotoma, usually without vision change), is reversible with cessation of antimalarials. However, continued administration can result in true retinopathy ("bull's eye" pigment deposition, central scotoma, and visual acuity changes). In a 10-year retrospective study, eye toxicity was shown to be quite rare below 6.5 mg/kg ideal body weight per day of HCQ [100]. Recent CQ/HCQ retinopathy screening guidelines published by the American Academy of Ophthalmology suggest that the risk for retinopathy for patients treated with HCQ at 400 mg/day and CQ at 250 mg/day in the first 5 years of therapy is negligible; at 5 years, the risk increases to 1% [101]. However, the authors' current practice is to monitor yearly with HCQ and at least twice a year with CQ. There has been a movement in the ophthalmology community to decrease HCQ dosing to 5 mg/kg/day. Our observation however is that many cutaneous lupus patients require higher dosing to control skin disease. When necessary, dosing options may be reviewed collaboratively with a retina specialist.

Cutaneous side effects of antimalarials include reversible blue-grey hyperpigmentation (10–30% of patients), progressive bleaching of skin or hair roots (10% of CQ), and yellow discoloration (quinacrine), among others.

Other side effects of antimalarials include gastrointestinal effects (CQ > HCQ, up to 10% intolerable), infrequent CNS effects (restlessness, headache, seizures, toxic psychosis), and rare hematologic effects (aplastic anemia caused by quinacrine and agranulocytosis caused by CQ) [102, 103]. There are also rare reports of ototoxicity, neuromyotoxicity, cardiomyopathy, and rhabdomyolysis [104, 105].

It is well known that HCQ has a positive effect on glucose and lipid levels [106–109]. Thus, CLE patients treated with HCQ benefit from decreased disease activity but possibly also improved glycemic and lipid control.

Antimalarial-resistant Disease

In patients with CLE who fail antimalarial therapy, a wide range of therapeutic options are available. Medication choice should be guided by comorbidities and the presence or absence of systemic involvement. Unfortunately, patients who fail antimalarial combination therapy are often also refractory to other systemic treatments.

Antimalarials are typically continued while additional agents are added, specifically either immunosuppressants or immunomodulators.

Immunosuppressant Agents

Only about 50% of patient with CLE refractory to antimalarials respond to immunosuppressant therapy [58, 110]. Agents utilized include systemic corticosteroids, methotrexate, mycophenolate mofetil (MMF), and azathioprine (AZA). Choice of systemic agent for CLE should include consideration of other systemic manifestations of disease. For example, patients with concurrent arthritis may benefit from methotrexate, while presence of some types of nephritis may improve with MMF or AZA. Collaborative decision making for patients with active integumentary and systemic disease is necessary. It should be noted that all immunosuppressant medications confer increased risk of malignancy, particularly lymphoproliferative and skin cancers, in the group of patients with systemic disease.

Methotrexate

In patients who fail antimalarials, methotrexate at doses of 7.5–25 mg orally or subcutaneously once weekly has been noted to be effective in in retrospective studies and case reports [111–115]. A retrospective analysis of 43 treatment-refractory CLE patients who were started on oral or subcutaneous methotrexate found improvement in 98% of cases. Seven out of 43 patients developed severe side effects necessitating discontinuation of therapy [114].

Potential side effects of methotrexate include gastrointestinal toxicity, bone marrow suppression, supratherapeutic dosing in the setting of renal insufficiency, hepatotoxicity, pulmonary interstitial pneumonitis or fibrosis, and phototoxicity [111]. Co-administration of folic acid 1–5 mg daily, as well as rigorous evaluation for drug interactions prior to prescription, can be helpful in preventing bone marrow suppression. Folic acid is helpful for treating oral ulcerations and preventing or treating gastrointestinal upset. Switching to subcutaneous administration can also be helpful to prevent or ameliorate GI upset, and to avoid absorptive limitations at higher doses. Dividing the weekly methotrexate dose and administering 12 hours apart may increase bioavailability and therefore efficacy. Importantly, methotrexate is teratogenic (pregnancy class X), and pregnancy should be prevented during treatment and for 3 months after discontinuation.

Mycophenolate Mofetil (MMF) or Mycophenolate Sodium

Mycophenolate mofetil (MMF, 1–3 g/day) and mycophenolate sodium (720–2160 mg/day) have been shown to be effective in treating SCLE, DLE, and chilblain lupus in multiple case reports and small studies [116–122]. In some of these cases, patients were also being treated with HCQ. In an open pilot study, 10 patients with SCLE resistant to antimalarials and topical steroids achieved statistically significant reductions in the Cutaneous Lupus Erythematosus Disease Area and Severity Index (CLASI) (from 10.8 ± 6 to 2.9 ± 2.6) following 3-month treatment with MMF (1440 mg/day) [119]. A large multicenter trial of 370 patients compared MMF to cyclophosphamide for treatment of the non-renal aspects of lupus, including skin lesions. At 24 weeks, mucocutaneous LE had improved to mild or non-detectable disease in 84% of patients on MMF *vs.* 93% of patients on cyclophosphamide [123]. One small study demonstrated failure to MMF in 5 of 7 patients [124].

Gastrointestinal toxicity is common with MMF and can occur in up to 50% of patients. This can be prevented by taking the medication on a full stomach or changing to enteric-coated mycophenolate sodium. Hematologic abnormalities due to bone marrow suppression can occur in 2–11% of patients, including agranulocytosis, neutropenia, anemia, and thrombocytopenia.

The malignancy risk conferred by MMF is controversial. In the transplant population, <1% of patients treated with 2–3 g daily of MMF in combined immunosuppressive regimens develop lymphoma or lymphoproliferative disorders. In the dermatologic literature, there have been case reports of lymphoma, solid tumors, and Kaposi sarcoma developing in patients treated with MMF. The literature also includes conflicting data regarding the risk of non-melanoma skin cancer, with some studies reporting an increased risk of basal cell carcinomas in MMF, and some showing no association. MMF is teratogenic (pregnancy class D), and measures to prevent pregnancy are needed during treatment and 6 weeks following discontinuation of medication.

Azathioprine

Azathioprine (AZA) is used more commonly to treat SLE than CLE [125]. However, several small case series from the 1980s demonstrated successful treatment of DLE with AZA, dosed up to 2–2.5 mg/kg/day [126–128]. As with MMF, GI intolerance is the most common adverse effect of AZA, though dividing the dose to three times daily and taking the medication with meals can help.

AZA may carry an increased risk of lymphoproliferative malignancies and cutaneous SCC. However, one retrospective study (n = 358) comparing the incidence of lymphoma and other malignancies in patients with SLE treated with AZA versus those who had not received the drug found no significant difference between the two groups [129].

Other side effects of AZA include bone marrow suppression, with excess risk found in patients (up to 10%) who are deficient in thiopurine methyltransferase (TPMT); screening is important if planning to start at higher doses. Rarely, hepatitis (<1%) or a systemic hypersensitivity reaction such as drug reaction with systemic symptoms/drug-induced hypersensitivity syndrome (DRESS/DIHS) can occur. AZA is pregnancy category D, although some authors have suggested it is relatively safe in pregnancy.

Systemic Corticosteroids

Systemic corticosteroids are generally avoided as therapy for CLE due to the well-known side effects with chronic use; LE patients are at increased risk for developing avascular necrosis (AVN) at baseline. Systemic corticosteroids may, however, be beneficial for short courses in patients with severe or disfiguring CLE, when quick onset of action is needed. In such instances, prednisone may be initiated at 0.5–1 mg/kg/day and tapered over 2–4 weeks.

Important adverse effects of systemic corticosteroids include AVN and osteoporosis [130], particularly with long-term use. To date, there are no specific guidelines to assess and manage osteoporosis in lupus patients. In 2010, the American College of Rheumatology published recommendations for the prevention and treatment of glucocorticoid-induced osteoporosis [131], which were updated in 2017, providing a risk stratification scheme to determine which patients would benefit from bone mineral density testing and bisphosphonate therapy, among other interventions. It is important to encourage bone health and minimize fracture risk by encouraging patients to take vitamin D and calcium supplementation, engage in weight-bearing activities, stop smoking, and reduce alcohol intake. Fall risk assessment is also important.

AVN results from compromise of the bone vasculature with resultant death of the bone marrow and trabecular bone. Several pathologic processes may cause ischemia to bone, and in some instances the cause is not easily identifiable. The most common clinical presentation is pain, most commonly in the anterolateral femoral head. Plain film radiography may be helpful in the initial assessment of AVN, but the plain radiograph can remain normal for months after symptoms appear. Magnetic resonance imaging (MRI) is the most sensitive imaging modality to assess for AVN.

Immunomodulators

Dapsone

Dapsone (25–150 mg/day) has been employed in the treatment of BSLE, lupus panniculitis, SCLE, and DLE. The combined results of three case series including 55 CLE patients treated with dapsone showed a 55% improvement rate [132, 133]. Despite this report, dapsone is widely viewed as less effective in the treatment of CLE, with the exception of BSLE. Because dapsone targets neutrophils, it has been found to be exceptionally useful in treating this subtype, with dramatic response to doses as low as 50 mg/day [73].

Anticipated, dose-related side effects of dapsone include hemolytic anemia (presenting with fatigue and dark urine) and methemoglobinemia (shortness of breath, fatigue, headache, and blue lips). Although hemolytic anemia is expected, with an anticipated average decrease in hemoglobin by 2 g/dL, screening for G6PD deficiency is necessary to avoid severe hemolysis. Patients with diabetes should be counseled that dapsone-induced hemolysis can result in falsely low levels of HgbA1c. In addition, pulse oximetry readings can be spuriously low in all patients and should not necessarily be interpreted as a sign of respiratory decompensation in the absence of other findings. Methemoglobinemia can potentially be prevented with vitamin E (800 IU daily) or cimetidine (400 mg 3 times a day) [134, 135].

Idiosyncratic adverse effects of dapsone therapy include agranulocytosis (rare, presenting with fevers and signs of infection within the first 12 weeks of therapy), reversible peripheral neuropathy (predominantly motor, +/− sensory), GI upset, dapsone hypersensitivity syndrome (typically 3–6 weeks into therapy, and equivalent to DRESS/DIHS).

Thalidomide

Thalidomide (50–100 mg/day) has been shown to be highly efficacious in the treatment of DLE, SCLE, and tumid lupus [136–138], with studies showing 60–80% of patients achieving complete response. CLE typically responds quickly, beginning at 2–4 weeks, and doses can often be tapered after improvement [136, 139]. Hence, thalidomide works well as a rescue medication or for maintenance at low or intermittent dosing (e.g. 25 mg every 2–3 days) in an effort to minimize toxicity.

Common adverse effects of thalidomide include drowsiness, constipation, peripheral edema, and irregular menses. Use of thalidomide is limited by its more serious adverse effects, which include teratogenicity, idiosyncratic peripheral sensory neuropathy, venous thrombosis, and rare leukopenia. Only clinicians registered with the Risk Evaluation and Management Strategy (REMS) program can prescribe thalidomide. Pregnancy prevention is critical, and pregnancy tests are monitored via REMS. CBC should be done at baseline and after starting the drug. Neurologic examinations with sensory nerve action potential (SNAP) amplitudes should be done every 6 months.

Lenalidomide

Lenalidomide is a thalidomide derivative with a better side effect profile. It is a potential alternative to thalidomide in CLE, given promising results in a case series and two small open-label trials [46, 136, 140]. Like thalidomide, lenalidomide is helpful in treating refractory CLE; however, it carries less risk of sedation, constipation, peripheral neuropathy, and thrombophilic effects. Monitoring should include CBC (to evaluate for thrombocytopenia, neutropenia, leukopenia, or anemia), thyroid function tests (TFTs, as patients can develop hypothyroidism), and nerve conduction tests (for peripheral neuropathy). Of note, studies in transplant patients on lenalidamide have noted an increased risk for NMSC, and thus patients should have full body skin exams every 6–12 months.

Oral Retinoids

Oral retinoids are another option for CLE patients who fail antimalarial therapy. Multiple case reports support the efficacy of isotretinoin in this condition, while a randomized, controlled trial found acitretin to be effective in 50% of CLE patients [141–143]. Systemic retinoids are also strongly linked with teratogenicity, and pregnancy prevention is essential. Patients should also be monitored for leukopenia, pseudotumor cerebri, triglyceridemia, and rare hepatitis. Increased myalgias and muscle breakdown with elevated CPK are noted with isotretinoin in the absence of rhabdomyolysis, and bexarotene can be associated with central hypothyroidism.

Other Therapies

Other agents reported in the literature as treatments for CLE include clofazamine, rituximab, intravenous immunoglobulin (IVIG) and belimumab. Rituximab has recently been shown to have limited efficacy [144]. IVIG tends have a short-lived response in CLE, with mixed efficacy reported [145–147]. In general, IVIG can be used as a bridge while waiting for another systemic medication to take effect. Belimumab is a B-cell activating factor inhibitor that is FDA-approved for treatment of SLE; further evaluation for efficacy in treating CLE is warranted [148].

Disease and Comorbidity Assessment (Table 3.6)

Systemic Screening

For patients with CLE only, yearly screening with a CBC with differential, serum albumin, serum creatinine, urinalysis with microscopy, and spot urine for protein/creatinine ratio when significant proteinuria is detected on urinalysis is recommended and is the current practice of the authors. In addition to laboratory evaluation, careful review of systems and physical exam are needed at each visit to evaluate for signs or symptoms such as mucosal ulcers, pleurisy, and joint pain.

Malignancy Risk

The most significant systemic comorbidities seen in CLE affect patients with SLE. However, there is literature to suggest that SCLE in particular is associated with malignancy. There are about 15 reported cases associating SCLE with cancers, including adenocarcinoma of the breast, uterus, esophagus, lung and stomach, Hodgkin's lymphoma, and hepatocellular carcinoma [57, 149–151]. The emergence of new SCLE in an older individual with otherwise negative serologic work-up for systemic or drug-induced lupus should prompt consideration for an underlying malignancy [149]. All patients with CLE should remain up to date with age-appropriate cancer screening.

Pregnancy

Pregnant women with CLE should be checked for ANA, anti-SSA/Ro, anti-SSB/La, and anti-U1-RNP if status is unknown, in order to risk stratify for development of NL in the infant. If maternal positivity of these autoantibodies is found, in utero frequent pulsed Doppler fetal echocardiography starting at 18 weeks gestational age is recommended. If second degree heart block is detected, treatment with fluorinated corticosteroids is recommended.

Table 3.6 Approach to co-morbid conditions in a CLE or SLE patient

Comorbidity	Intervention
Malignancy	Follow age-appropriate malignancy screening guidelines Discuss family history of cancer and screen accordingly Advise smoking cessation
Avascular necrosis (AVN)	Minimize glucocorticoid exposure Consider radiographic evaluation with x-ray and/or MRI if there is clinical suspicion Refer to orthopedic surgery if diagnosis of AVN is made
Osteoporosis	Minimize glucocorticoid exposure Recommend engaging in weight-bearing and muscle strengthening exercises to improve agility, strength, posture and balance Assess fall risk Screen for osteoporosis with DEXA scan Counsel on smoking cessation and minimizing alcohol intake
Neonatal lupus	Check SSA and SSB status in all women of childbearing age Refer to maternal fetal medicine/high risk obstetrician if patient with positive SSA and/or SSB becomes pregnant Serial fetal echocardiography and fluorinated glucocorticoids may be indicated

Infants born to mothers with positive ANA, anti-SSA/Ro, anti-SSB/La, or anti-U1-RNP should be evaluated at birth for hematologic and hepatic involvement (via CBC-D and liver function tests [LFTs]), regardless of whether they have rash. Neonates should also undergo electrocardiogram and possibly echocardiogram, in order to identify first-degree heart block, which may be clinically silent but puts them at risk for cardiac progression.

Neonates with no heart block at birth and a normal electrocardiogram typically do not develop heart block at a later date. It is reasonable to check CBC and LFTs periodically during the first year of life, although there is no universally accepted frequency of screening.

For women who give birth to an infant with NL, the risk for NL in subsequent pregnancies is approximately 25%. Subsequent pregnancies should be considered high risk and monitored closely. In addition, preemptive HCQ can be considered.

Summary

Patients with skin manifestations of lupus erythematosus must be systematically evaluated for SLE, as well as associated comorbidities, such as malignancy. Treatment is guided by the organ systems involved and the severity of the cutaneous disease. All patients should be counseled on sun avoidance, sunscreens, and sun protective clothing; those with vitamin D deficiency should receive replacement therapy.

Steroids and steroid-sparing agents can both be employed as topical therapies. There are few rigorous studies on the efficacy of systemic therapy in CLE, but antimalarials play an important role in the management of many patients with cutaneous lupus and may prevent progression to systemic disease. If HCQ alone is ineffective, combination therapy with HCQ and quinacrine is recommended. For aggressive or unresponsive skin disease, the addition of immunosuppressive agents or thalidomide (or its derivatives), often with oral steroids as bridge treatment, may be required.

Ongoing surveillance for flares or progression to systemic disease is required, but recommendations should be tailored to the severity of the underlying systemic disease. At least yearly systemic monitoring of urinalysis and CBC is recommended for patients with stable skin disease.

Patients with significant systemic disease or medication complications are often best managed through an interdisciplinary approach, with specialists including dermatologists, rheumatologists, and potentially nephrologists and neurologists, depending on the manifestations of the disease. In addition, patients should be monitored for co-existent autoimmune diseases and co-morbidities related to disease and therapies.

References

1. Jarukitsopa S, Hoganson DD, Crowson CS. Epidemiology of systemic lupus erythematosus and cutaneous lupus in a predominantly white population in the United States. Arthritis Care Res Hoboken; 2015.
2. Durosaro O, et al. Incidence of cutaneous lupus erythematosus, : a population-based study. Arch Dermatol. 2009;145:249–53.
3. Piette EW, Foering KP, Chang AY. Impact of smoking in cutaneous lupus erythematosus. Arch Dermatol. 2012;148:317–22.
4. Moghadam-Kia S, Chilek K, Gaines E. Cross-sectional analysis of a collaborative Web-based database for lupus erythematosus-associated skin lesions: prospective enrollment of 114 patients. Arch Dermatol. 2009;145:255–60.
5. Gilliam JN, Sontheimer RD. Distinctive cutaneous subsets in the spectrum of lupus erythematosus. J Am Acad Dermatol. 1981;4(4):471–5.
6. Kuhn A, et al. Clinical manifestations of cutaneous lupus erythematosus. Dermatol Ges. 2007;5:1124–37.
7. Lipsker D. The need to revisit the nosology of cutaneous lupus erythematosus: the current terminology and morphologic classification of cutaneous LE: difficult, incomplete and not always applicable. Lupus. 2010;19:1047–9.
8. Schultz HY, et al. From pathogenesis, epidemiology, and genetics to definitions, diagnosis, and treatments of cutaneous lupus erythematosus and dermatomyositis: a report from the 3rd International Conference on Cutaneous Lupus Erythematosus (ICCLE). Dermatology. 2015;135:7–12.
9. Merola JF, Nyberg F, Furukawa F. Redefining cutaneous lupus erythematosus: a proposed international consensus approach and results of a preliminary questionnaire. Lupus Sci Med. 2015;2:e000085.

10. Zecevic RD, et al. Skin lesions-an indicator of disease activity in systemic lupus erythematosus? Lupus. 2001;10:364.
11. Tan EM, Cohen AS, Fries JF. The revised criteria for the classification of systemic lupus erythematosus. Arthritis Rheum. 1982;25:1271.
12. Hochberg MC. Updating the American College of Rheumatology revised criteria for the classification of systemic lupus erythematosus. Arthritis Rheum. 1997;40:1725.
13. Tan EM. Criteria for the classification of systemic lupus erythematosus. Arthritis Rheum. 1984;25:53.
14. Albrecht JA, Braverman IM, Callen JP. Dermatology position paper on the revision of the ACR criteria for SLE. Lupus. 2004;13:839.
15. Petri M, Orbai AM, Alarcon GS. Derivation and validation of systemic lupus international collaborating clinics classification criteria for systemic lupus erythematosus. Arthritis Rheum. 2012;64(8):2677–86.
16. Ighe A, et al. Application of the systemic lupus interna tional collaborating clinics classification criteria on a Regional Swedish systemic lupus erythematosus register. Arthritis Res Ther. 2015;17:3.
17. Ines L, Silva C, Galindo M. Classification of systemic lupus erythematosus: systemic lupus international collaborating clinics versus american college of rheumatology criteria. Arthritis Care Res Hoboken; 2015.
18. Dey-Rao R, Sinha AA. Genome-wide transcriptional profiling of chronic cutaneous lupus erythematosus (CCLE) peripheral blood identifies systemic alterations relevant to the skin manifestation. Genomics. 2015;105:90–100.
19. Lee LA, et al. Autoantibodies of neonatal lupus erythematosus. Dermatol Antibodydependent cellular cytotoxicity and skin disease. J Invest Dermatol. 1985;85(suppl 165):963–6.
20. Millard TP, Kondeatis E, Cox A. A candidate gene analysis of three related photosensitivity disorders: cutaneous lupus erythematosus, polymorphic light eruption and actinic prurigo. Br J Dermatol. 2001;145:229.
21. Fischer GF, et al. Association between chronic cutaneous lupus erythematosus and HLA class II alleles. Hum Immunol. 1994;41:280–4.
22. Werth VP, et al. Association of a promoter polymorphism of TNFalpha with subacute cutaneous lupus erythematosus and distinct photoregulation of transcription. J Invest Dermatol. 2000;115:726–30.
23. Osmola A, et al. Genetic background of cutaneous forms of lupus erythematosus: update on current evidence. J Appl Genet. 2004;45:77–86.
24. Jarvinen TM, et al. Polymorphisms of the ITGAM gene confer higher risk of discoid cutaneous than of systemic lupus erythematosus. PLoS One. 2010;5:14212.
25. Kim-Howard X, Maiti AK, Anaya JM. ITGAM coding variant (rs1143679) influences the risk of renal disease, discoid rash and immunological manifestations in patients with systemic lupus erythematosus with European ancestry. Ann Rheum Dis. 2010;69:1329–32.
26. Sanchez E, Nadig A, Richardson BC. Phenotypic associations of genetic susceptibility loci in systemic lupus erythematosus. Ann Rheum Dis. 2011;70:1752–7.
27. Kunz M, Konig IR, Schillert A. Genome-wide association study identifies new susceptibility loci for cutaneous lupus erythematosus. Exp Dermatol. 2015;24(7):510–5.
28. Jarvinen TM, Hellquist A, Koskenmies S. Tyrosine kinase 2 and interferon regulatory factor 5 polymorphisms are associated with discoid and subacute cutaneous lupus erythematosus. Exp Dermatol. 2010;19:123–31.
29. Pickering MC, et al. Ultraviolet-radiation-induced keratinocyte apoptosis in C1q-deficient mice. J Invest Dermatol. 2001;117:52.
30. Nousari HC, et al. Generalized lupus panniculitis and antiphospholipid syndrome in a patient without complement deficiency. Ped Dermatol. 1999;16:273.
31. Lee-Kirsch MA, Gong M, Schulz H. Familial chilblain lupus, a monogenic form of cutaneous lupus erythematosus, maps to chromosome 3p. Am J Hum Genet. 2006;79:731.
32. Sanders CJ, et al. Photosensitivity in patients with lupus erythematosus:a clinical and photobiological study of 100 patients using a prolonged phototest protocol. Br J Dermatol. 2003;149:131–7.
33. Kuhn A, et al. Photoprovocation in cutaneous lupus erythematosus: study evaluating a standardized protocol. J Invest Dermatol. 2011;131:1622–30.
34. Rosenbaum M, Billet S, Patel P. Failure of physiologic doses of pure UVB or UVA to induce lesions in photosensitive lupus erythematosus: implications for phototesting and sunblocking strategies. Photodermatol Photoimmunol Photomed. 2006;22:290.
35. Furukawa F, et al. Binding of antibodies to the extractable nuclear antigens SS-A/Ro and SS-B/La is induced on the surface of human keratinocytes by ultraviolet light (UVL): implications for the pathogenesis of photosensitive cutaneous lupus. J Invest Dermatol. 1990;94:77.
36. Casciola-Rosen LA, Anhalt G, Rosen A. Autoantigens targets in systemic lupus erythematosus are clustered in two populations of surface structures on apoptotic keratinocytes. J Exp Med. 1994;179:1317.
37. Kuhn A, Herrmann M, Kleber S. Accumulation of apoptotic cells in the epidermis of patients with cutaneous lupus erythematosus after ultraviolet irradiation. see comment. Arthritis Rheum. 2007;54:939.
38. Botto M, Walport MJ. C1q, autoimmunity and apoptosis. Immunobiology. 2002;205:395–406.
39. Kreuter A, et al. Expression of antimicrobial peptides in different subtypes of cutaneous lupus erythematosus. Acad Dermatol. 2011;65:125–33.
40. Villanueva E, et al. Netting neutrophils induce endothelial damage, infiltrate tissues, and expose

immunostimulatory molecules in systemic lupus erythematosus; 2011. p. 538–52.
41. Popovic K, Ek M, Espinosa A. Increased expression of the novel proinflammatory cytokine high mobility group box chromosomal protein 1 in skin lesions of patients with lupus erthematosus. Arthritis Rheum. 2005;52:3639.
42. Chang LM, Maheshwari P, Werth S. Identification and molecular analysis of glycosaminoglycans in cutaneous lupus erythematosus and dermatomyositis. J Histochem Cytochem. 2011;59:336–45.
43. Jabbari A, et al. Dominant Th1 and minimal Th17 skewing in discoid lupus revealed by transcriptomic comparison with psoriasis. J Invest Dermatol. 2014;134:87–95.
44. Franz B, Fritzsching B, Riehl A. Low number of regulatory T cells in skin lesions of patients with cutaneous lupus erythematosus. Arthritis Rheum. 2007;56:1910–20.
45. Wong D, et al. Interferon and biologic signatures in dermatomyositis skin: specificity and heterogeneity across diseases. PLoS One. 2012;7:29161.
46. Braunstein I, et al. The interferon-regulated gene signature is elevated in SCLE and DLE and correlates with CLASI score. Br J Dermatol. 2012;166:971–5.
47. Wenzel J, et al. The expression pattern of interferon-inducible proteins reflects the characteristic histological distribution of infiltrating immune cells in different cutaneous lupus erythematosus subsets. Br J Dermatol. 2007;157:752–7.
48. Gambichler T, et al. Cytokine and chemokine ligand expression in cutaneous lupus erythematosus. Eur J Dermatol. 2012;22:319–23.
49. Zahn S, et al. Evidence for a pathophysiological role of keratinocyte-derived type III interferon (IFNlambda) in cutaneous lupus erythematosus. J Invest Dermatol. 2011;131:133–40.
50. Meller S, Winterberg F, Gilliet M. Ultraviolet radiation-induced injury, chemokines, and leukocyte recruitment: an amplification cycle triggering cutaneous lupus erythematosus. Arthritis Rheum. 2005;52:1504–16.
51. Werth VP, Zhang W. Wavelength-specific synergy between ultraviolet radiation and interleukin-1 alpha in the regulation of matrix-related genes: mechanistic role for tumor necrosis factor-alpha. J Invest Dermatol. 1999;113:196–201.
52. Nabatian AS, et al. TNFα release in peripheral blood mononuclear cells of cutaneous lupus & dermatomyositis patients. Arthritis Res Ther. 2012;4:R1.
53. Rothfield N, Sontheimer RD, Bernstein M. Lupus erythematosus: systemic and cutaneous manifestations. Clin Dermatol. 2006;24:348–62.
54. Gronhagen CM, et al. Cutaneous lupus erythematosus and the association with systemic lupus erythematosus: a population-based cohort of 1088 patients in Sweden. Br J Dermatol. 2011;164:1335–41.
55. Cohen MR, Crosby D. Systemic disease in subacute cutaneous lupus erythematosus: a controlled comparison with systemic lupus erythematosus. J Rheumatol. 1994;21:1665–9.
56. Sontheimer RD, Thomas JR, Gilliam JN. Subacute cutaneous lupus erythematosus: a cutaneous marker for a distinct lupus erythematosus subset. Arch Dermatol. 1979;115(12):1409–15.
57. Evans KG, Heymann WR. Paraneoplastic subacute cutaneous lupus erythematosus: an underrecognized entity. Cutis. 2013;91:25–9.
58. Chang AY, et al. Quality of life differences between responders and nonresponders in the treatment of cutaneous lupus erythematosus. JAMA Dermatol. 2013;149:104–6.
59. Verma SM, et al. The impact of skin damage due to cutaneous lupus on quality of life. Br J Dermatol. 2014;170:315–21.
60. Sampaio MC, et al. dos Discoid lupus erythematosus in children-a retrospective study of 34 patients. Pediatr Dermatol. 2008;25:163–7.
61. Vera-Recabarren MA, et al. Comparative analysis of subacute cutaneous lupus erythematosus and chronic cutaneous lupus erythematosus: clinical and immunological study of 270 patients. Br J Dermatol. 2010;162:91–101.
62. Parish LC, Kennedy RJ, Hurley J. Palmar lesions in lupus erythematosus. Arch Dermatol. 1967;96:273–6.
63. Tao J, et al. Squamous cell carcinoma complicating discoid lupus erythematosus in Chinese patients: review of the literature. Acad Dermatol. 2012;66:695.
64. Prystowsky SD, Gilliam JN. Discoid lupus erythematosus as part of a larger disease spectrum. Correlation of clinical features with laboratory findings in lupus erythematosus. Arch Dermatol. 1975;111:1448–52.
65. Gysel D, et al. Van de Waard- Childhood discoid lupus erythematosus: report of five new cases and review of the literature. Acad Dermatol Venereol. 2002;16:143–7.
66. Moises-Alfaro C, et al. Discoid lupus erythematosus in children: clinical, histopathologic, and follow-up features in 27 cases. Pediatr Dermatol. 2003;20:103–7.
67. Magro CM, et al. Atypical lymphocytic lobular panniculitis: a clonal subcutaneous T-cell dyscrasia. J Cutan Pathol. 2008;35:947–54.
68. Viguier M, Pinquier L, Cavelier-Balloy B. Clinical and histopathologic features and immunologic variables in patients with severe chilblains. A study of the relationship to lupus erythematosus. Medicine (Baltimore). 2001;80:180–8.
69. Rivera TL, Izmirly PM, Birnbaum BK. Disease progression in mothers of children enrolled in the Research Registry for Neonatal Lupus. Ann Rheum Dis. 2009;68:828–35.
70. Buyon JP, et al. Neonatal lupus: basic research and clinical perspectives. Rheum Dis Clin North Am. 2010;31:299–313.

71. Lee LA, Sokol RJ, Buyon JP. Hepatobiliary disease in neonatal lupus: prevalence and clinical characteristics in cases enrolled in a national registry. Pediatrics. 2002;109:E11.
72. Buyon JP. Neonatal lupus and autoantibodies reactive with SSA/Ro-SSB/La. Scand J Rheumatol Suppl. 1998;107:23–30.
73. Hall RP, et al. Bullous eruption of systemic lupus erythematosus. Dramatic response to dapsone therapy. Ann Intern Med. 1982;97:165–70.
74. Gammon WR, et al. Bullous SLE: a phenotypically distinctive but immunologically heterogeneous bullous disorder. J Invest Dermatol. 1993;100:28S–34.
75. Ting W, et al. Toxic epidermal necrolysis-like acute cutaneous lupus erythematosus and the spectrum of the acute syndrome of apoptotic pan-epidermolysis (ASAP): a case report, concept review and proposal for new classification of lupus erythematosus vesiculobullous skin lesions. Lupus. 2004;13:941–50.
76. Torchia D, et al. Erythema multiforme and Stevens-Johnson syndrome/toxic epidermal necrolysis associated with lupus erythematosus. J Am Acad Dermatol. 2012;67:417–21.
77. Ziemer M, et al. Stevens-Johnson syndrome and toxic epidermal necrolysis in patients with lupus erythematosus: a descriptive study of 17 cases from a national registry and review of the literature. Br J Dermatol. 2012;166:575–600.
78. Rowell NR, et al. Lupus erythematosus and erythema multiforme-like lesions. A syndrome with characteristic immunological abnormalities. Arch Dermatol. 1963;83:176–80.
79. Zeitouni NC, et al. Redefining Rowell's syndrome. Br J Dermatol. 2000;142:343–6.
80. Alarcon-Segovia D, Cetina JA. Lupus hair. Am J Med Sci. 1974;267:241–2.
81. Fabre VC, et al. Twenty percent of biopsy specimens from sun-exposed skin of normal young adults demonstrate positive immunofluorescence. Arch Dermatol. 1991;127:1006–11.
82. David-Bajar KM, Davis BM. Pathology, immunopathology, and immunohistochemistry in cutaneous lupus erythematosus. Lupus. 1997;6:145–57.
83. Li PH, Wong WH, Lee TL. Relationship between autoantibody clustering and clinical subsets in SLE: cluster and association analyses in Hong Kong Chinese. Rheumatology (Oxford). 2013;52:337–45.
84. Lee LA, et al. The autoantibody response to Ro/SSA in cutaneous lupus erythematosus. Arch Dermatol. 1994;130:1262.
85. Kuhn A, et al. Phototesting in lupus erythematosus: a 15-year experience. J Am Acad Dermatol. 2001;45:86–95.
86. Kuhn A, et al. Photoprotective effects of a broad-spectrum sunscreen in ultraviolet-induced cutaneous lupus erythematosus: a randomized, vehicle-controlled, double-blind study. J Am Acad Dermatol. 2010;64:37–48.
87. Klein RS, et al. Analysis of compact fluorescent lights for use by patients with photosensitive conditions. Photochem Photobiol. 2009;85(4):1004–10.
88. Sayre RM, Dowdy JC, Poh-Fitzpatrick M. Dermatological risk of indoor ultraviolet exposure from contemporary lighting sources. Photochem Photobiol. 2004;80:47–51.
89. Jewell ML, McCauliffe DP. Patients with cutaneous lupus erythematosus who smoke are less responsive to antimalarial treatment. J Am Acad Dermatol. 2000;42:983–7.
90. Wahie S, et al. Clinical and pharmacogenetic influences on response to hydroxychloroquine in discoid lupus erythematosus: a retrospective cohort study. J Invest Dermatol. 2011;131:1981–6.
91. Jessop S, Whitelaw DA, Delamere FM. Drugs for discoid lupus erythematosus. Cochrane Database Syst Rev. 2009;5:CD002954.
92. Roenigk HH, et al. Discoid lupus erythematosus. Diagnostic features and evaluation of topical corticosteroid therapy. Cutis. 1980;25:281–5.
93. Kuhn A, et al. Efficacy of tacrolimus 0.1 ointment in cutaneous lupus erythematosus a multicenter randomized doubleblind vehiclecontrolled trial. Acad Dermatol. 2011;65:54–64.
94. Tzung TY, et al. Tacrolimus vs. clobetasol propionate in the treatment of facial cutaneous lupus erythematosus a randomized doubleblind bilateral comparison study. Br J Dermatol. 2007;156: 191–2.
95. Thaci D, Salgo R. Malignancy concerns of topical calcineurin inhibitors for atopic dermatitis: facts and controversies. Clin Dermatol. 2010;28:52–6.
96. Erceg A, et al. Efficacy and safety of pulsed dye laser treatment for cutaneous discoid lupus erythematosus. J Am Acad Dermatol. A randomized study of the effect of withdrawing hydroxychloroquine sulfate in systemic lupus erythematosus The Canadian Hydroxychloroquine Study Group 3241504. 1991;60:626–32.
97. James JA, Kim-Howard XR, Bruner BF. Hydroxychloroquine sulfate treatment is associated with later onset of systemic lupus erythematosus. Lupus. 2007;16:401–9.
98. Chang AY, et al. Response to antimalarial agents in cutaneous lupus erythematosus: a prospective analysis. Arch Dermatol. 2011;147:1261–7.
99. Frances C, Cosnes A, Duhaut P. Low blood concentration of hydroxychloroquine in patients with refractory cutaneous lupus erythematosus: a French multicenter prospective study. Arch Dermatol. 2012;148:479–84.
100. Levy GD, et al. Incidence of hydroxychloroquine retinopathy in 1,207 patients in a large multicenter outpatient practice. Arthritis Rheum. 1997;40:1482–6.
101. Marmor MF, et al. Revised recommendations on screening for chloroquine and hydroxychloroquine retinopathy. Ophthalmology. 2011;118:415–22.
102. Ward WQ, et al. Toxic psychosis: a complication of antimalarial therapy. J Am Acad Dermatol. 1985;12:863–5.
103. Schmid I, et al. Marrow transplantation for severe aplastic anemia associated with exposure to quinacrine. Blut. 1990;61:52–4.

104. Siddiqui AK, et al. Hydroxychloroquine-induced toxic myopathy causing respiratory failure. Chest. 2007;131:588–90.
105. Creel N, Werth VP. Rhabdomyolysis associated with quinacrine therapy in a patient with chronic cutaneous lupus erythematosus. J Drugs Dermatol. 2005;4:225.
106. Bili A, et al. Hydroxychloroquine use and decreased risk of diabetes in rheumatoid arthritis patients. J Clin Rheumatol. 2011;17(3):115–20.
107. Wasko MC, et al. Hydroxychloroquine and risk of diabetes in patients with rheumatoid arthritis. JAMA. 2007;298(2):187–93.
108. Chen YM, et al. Hydroxychloroquine reduces risk of incident diabetes mellitus in lupus patients in a dose-dependent manner: a population-based cohort study. Rheumatology (Oxford). 2015;54(7):1244–9.
109. Mercer E, et al. Hydroxychloroquine improves insulin sensitivity in obese non-diabetic individuals. Arthritis Res Ther. 2012;14(3):R135.
110. Wahie S, Meggitt SJ. Long-term response to hydroxychloroquine in patients with discoid lupus erythematosus. Br J Dermatol. 2013;169:653–9.
111. Kuhn A, et al. Methotrexate treatment for refractory subacute cutaneous lupus erythematosus. J Am Acad Dermatol. 2002;46:600–3.
112. Bohm L, Uerlich M, Bauer R. Rapid improvement of subacute cutaneous lupus erythematosus with low-dose methotrexate. Dermatology. 1997;194:307–8.
113. Malcangi G, et al. Bullous SLE: response to methotrexate and relationship with disease activity. Lupus. 2003;12:63–6.
114. Wenzel J, et al. Efficacy and safety of methotrexate in recalcitrant cutaneous lupus erythematosus: results of a retrospective study in 43 patients. Br J Dermatol. 2005;153:157–62.
115. Boehm IB, Boehm GA, Bauer R. Management of cutaneous lupus erythematosus with low-dose methotrexate: indication for modulation of inflammatory mechanisms. Rheumatol Int. 1998;18:59–62.
116. Cetkovska P, Pizinger K. Coexisting subacute and systemic lupus erythematosus after terbinafine administration: successful treatment with mycophenolate mofetil. Int J Dermatol. 2006;45:320–2.
117. Hanjani NM, Nousari CH. Mycophenolate mofetil for the treatment of cutaneous lupus erythematosus with smoldering systemic involvement. Arch Dermatol. 2002;138:1616–8.
118. Boehm I, Bieber T. Chilblain lupus erythematosus Hutchinson: successful treatment with mycophenolate mofetil. Arch Dermatol. 2001;137:235–6.
119. Kreuter A, et al. Mycophenolate sodium for subacute cutaneous lupus erythematosus resistant to standard therapy. Br J Dermatol. 2007;156:1321–7.
120. Goyal S, Nousari HC. Treatment of resistant discoid lupus erythematosus of the palms and soles with mycophenolate mofetil. J Am Acad Dermatol. 2001;45:142–4.
121. Schanz S, et al. Successful treatment of subacute cutaneous lupus erythematosus with mycophenolate mofetil. Br J Dermatol. 2002;147:174–8.
122. Gammon B, et al. Efficacy of mycophenolate mofetil in antimalarial-resistant cutaneous lupus erythematosus. Acad Dermatol. 2011;65:717–21.
123. Ginzler EM, et al. Nonrenal disease activity following mycophenolate mofetil or intravenous cyclophosphamide as induction treatment for lupus nephritis: findings in a multicenter, prospective, randomized, open-label, parallel-group clinical trial. Arthritis Rheum. 2010;62:211–21.
124. Pisoni CN, Obermoser G, Cuadrado MJ. Skin manifestations of systemic lupus erythematosus refractory to multiple treatment modalities: poor results with mycophenolate mofetil. Clin Exp Rheumatol. 2005;23:393–6.
125. Swaak AJ, et al. Statius Azathioprine in the treatment of systemic lupus erythematosus. A threeyear prospective study. Clin Rheumatol. 1984;3:285–91.
126. Ashinoff R, et al. Resistant discoid lupus erythematosus of palms and soles: successful treatment with azathioprine. J Am Acad Dermatol. 1988;19:961–5.
127. Tsokos GC, Caughman SW, Klippel JH. Successful treatment of generalized discoid skin lesions with azathioprine. Its use in a patient with systemic lupus erythematosus. Arch Dermatol. 1985;121:1323–5.
128. Shehade S. Successful treatment of generalized discoid skin lesions with azathioprine. Arch Dermatol. 1986;122:376–7.
129. Nero P, Rahman A, Isenberg DA. Does long term treatment with azathioprine predispose to malignancy and death in patients with systemic lupus erythematosus? Ann Rheum Dis. 2004;63:325–6.
130. Lakshminarayanan S, et al. Factors associated with low bone mineral density in female patients with systemic lupus erythematosus. J Rheumatol. 2001;28(1):102–8.
131. Cohen-Cline H, et al. Use of interactive voice response to improve colorectal cancer screening. Med Care. 2014;52(6):496–9.
132. Coburn PR, Shuster S. Dapsone and discoid lupus erythematosus. Br J Dermatol. 1982;106(1):105–6.
133. Lindskov R, Reymann F. Dapsone in the treatment of cutaneous lupus erythematosus. Dermatologica. 1986;172(4):214–7.
134. Prussick R, et al. The protective effect of vitamin E on the hemolysis associated with dapsone treatment in patients with dermatitis herpetiformis. Arch Dermatol. 1992;128(2):210–3.
135. Coleman MD, et al. The use of cimetidine to reduce dapsone-dependent methaemoglobinaemia in dermatitis herpetiformis patients. Br J Clin Pharmacol. 1992;34(3):244–9.
136. Cortés-Hernández J, et al. Thalidomide in the treatment of refractory cutaneous lupus erythematosus: prognostic factors of clinical outcome. Br J Dermatol. 2012;166(3):616–23.
137. Stevens RJ, et al. Thalidomide in the treatment of the cutaneous manifestations of lupus erythematosus: experience in sixteen consecutive patients. Br J Rheumatol. 1997;36(3):353–9.

138. Burrows NP, et al. Lupus erythematosus profundus with partial C4 deficiency responding to thalidomide. Br J Dermatol. 1991;125:62–7.
139. Pelle MT, Werth VP. Thalidomide in cutaneous lupus erythematosus. Am J Clin Dermatol. 2003;4(6):379–87.
140. Shah AA, Wigley FM, Hummers LK. Telangiectases in scleroderma: a potential clinical marker of pulmonary arterial hypertension. J Rheumatol. 2010;37(1):98–104.
141. Shornick JK, Formica N, Parke AL. Isotretinoin for refractory lupus erythematosus. J Am Acad Dermatol. 1991;24(1):49–52.
142. Ruzicka T, et al. Treatment of cutaneous lupus erythematosus with acitretin and hydroxychloroquine. Br J Dermatol. 1992;127(5):513–8.
143. Furner BB. Subacute cutaneous lupus erythematosus response to isotretinoin. Int J Dermatol. 1990;29(8):587–90.
144. Man A, et al. Changes in forced vital capacity over time in systemic sclerosis: application of group-based trajectory modelling. Rheumatology (Oxford). 2015;54(8):1464–71.
145. Ky C, et al. Efficacy of intravenous immunoglobulin monotherapy in patients with cutaneous lupus erythematosus: results of proof-of-concept study. Dermatol Reports. 2015;7(1):5804.
146. Strauss RM, et al. Good response of linear scleroderma in a child to ciclosporin. Br J Dermatol. 2004;150(4):790–2.
147. De Pità O, et al. Intravenous immunoglobulin therapy is not able to efficiently control cutaneous manifestations in patients with lupus erythematosus. Lupus. 1997;6(4):415–7.
148. Manzi S, et al. Effects of belimumab, a B lymphocyte stimulator-specific inhibitor, on disease activity across multiple organ domains in patients with systemic lupus erythematosus: combined results from two phase III trials. Ann Rheum Dis. 2012;71(11):1833–8.
149. Chaudhry SI, Murphy LA, White IR. Subacute cutaneous lupus erythematosus: a paraneoplastic dermatosis? Clin Exp Dermatol. 2005;30(6):655–8.
150. Jasim ZF, Walsh MY, Armstrong DK. Subacute lupus erythematosus-like rash associated with oesophageal adenocarcinoma in situ. Clin Exp Dermatol. 2007;32(4):443–5.
151. Shaheen B, Milne G, Shaffrali F. Subacute cutaneous lupus erythematosus associated with breast carcinoma. Clin Exp Dermatol. 2009;34(7):e480–1.

Dermatomyositis

4

Matt Lewis, Lorinda Chung, and David Fiorentino

Key Points

- Dermatomyositis (DM) is a systemic autoimmune disease affecting the skin, muscle, and lungs, and is associated with a malignancy in 10–20% of cases.
- Interstitial lung disease (ILD) is a major source of morbidity and mortality in DM, with increased risk conferred by the presence of anti-synthetase and anti-MDA5 antibodies.
- Malignancy screening with computed tomography scans of the chest, abdomen and pelvis may be of benefit to detect occult cancers in patients with DM that may be missed on routine age-appropriate screening.
- Multidisciplinary collaboration between rheumatology and dermatology, among other specialties, is important to assess all potentially involved organs and select an appropriate treatment plan.
- Treatment of cutaneous DM can be challenging and discordant with treatment for the muscle disease. Multiple agents may be necessary to achieve complete remission; the risks and benefits each agent should be considered carefully given the potentially prolonged treatment course.

Interdisciplinary Introduction

Dermatomyositis (DM) is a systemic autoimmune disease characterized by inflammation of multiple organs, most commonly the skin, muscle and lungs. This disease poses a challenge to clinicians because of its rarity, diverse clinical presentations, and variable organ involvement. Depending on the clinical manifestations, patients with DM can present first to either rheumatologists, dermatologists, or neurologists, among other specialists.

A timely diagnosis is imperative, not only to prevent internal organ damage from the disease itself, but also to initiate appropriate malignancy screening, given the increased risk of cancer around the time of first symptoms [1, 2]. In this chapter we review the manifestations of DM and associated differential diagnosis by organ system. However, making the diagnosis of DM necessitates consideration of the complete clini-

M. Lewis · D. Fiorentino (✉)
Department of Dermatology, Stanford University School of Medicine, Redwood City, CA, USA
e-mail: Fiorentino@stanford.edu

L. Chung
Division of Immunology and Rheumatology, Stanford University School of Medicine, Palo Alto, CA, USA

VA Palo Alto Health Care System, Palo Alto, CA, USA

A. Garg et al. (eds.), *Interdisciplinary Approaches to Overlap Disorders in Dermatology & Rheumatology*, https://doi.org/10.1007/978-3-319-18446-3_4

cal context in which the patient presents, including the history of present illness, contributory past medical history, review of systems, physical examination, laboratory analysis, biopsy results, and imaging or electromyographic studies.

Another important goal in DM is to select therapeutic agents that target manifestations in multiple organs to gain control of the disease while minimizing the risks to the patient. Patients with DM are therefore best served by multidisciplinary collaboration. Rheumatologists and dermatologists approach this disorder with unique perspectives, both of which are often necessary for optimal care of the patient. The purpose of this chapter is to highlight the vital contributions that each specialty can make to patient care in this complex disease.

Epidemiology and Risk Factors

Age of onset in DM has a bimodal distribution, occurring in two peaks, one at 5–14 years and the other at 45–64 years of life. The female to male ratio is 2–3:1. There are insufficient epidemiologic data, however, to determine the true incidence and prevalence of DM. Regional variation and differences in case ascertainment methods have complicated efforts to do so [3, 4].

One study based on data from Olmstead County, Minnesota, estimated population age- and sex-adjusted prevalence at 21.42 per 100,000 persons (95% CI, 13.07–29.77) and incidence at 9.63 per million per decade (95% CI 6.09–13.17) [5]. Another estimate, based on review of hospital discharge diagnosis codes in Spain from 1997–2004, found a lower annual incidence, estimated at 4.9 cases/million/year (95% CI, 4.7–5.2). Lower still, the annual incidence determined in a review of one million records from a health insurance database between 2005–2009 was 0.7 cases per 100,000 person-years (95% CI, 0.5–1.0) [6].

The regional variation noted in DM incidence and prevalence may relate in part to geographic differences in risk factors for the disease. For example, intensity of ultraviolet radiation may influence the development and modulate the expression of DM. In the Northern Hemisphere, the relative incidence of DM as compared to polymyositis displays a latitudinal gradient, with the greatest incidence of DM in Athens, Greece and lowest incidence in Reykjavik, Iceland [7]. This finding was replicated in another study across 14 different countries, which found the highest relative proportion of DM in Guatemala and the lowest in Glasgow, Scotland [8]. These authors concluded that surface ultraviolet radiation was the major geoclimatic factor associated with the relative proportion of DM. Similarly, in the United States, Love et al. found a positive association between the annual ultraviolet index in seven U.S. regions and the proportion of patients with DM, along with the relative frequency of anti-Mi-2 autoantibodies in women [9].

On the other hand, Marcelo Petri et al. found a significant difference in the prevalence of anti-Mi-2 antibodies in Mexico City (26/44 DM patients, or 59%) versus Guadalajara (0/17 DM patients), cities that have comparable surface UV radiation, suggesting that additional genetic or environmental factors determine the autoimmune phenotype [10]. Another study found that the prevalence of juvenile DM patients with anti-NXP2 antibodies was inversely correlated with surface UV exposure, suggesting that, at least for some DM patients, UV is not an epidemiologic risk factor [11].

Classification

DM is currently classified as an idiopathic, inflammatory myopathy. In epidemiologic studies, it is often grouped with other inflammatory myopathies, including polymyositis. In 1975, Bohan and Peter empirically defined diagnostic and classification criteria for DM and polymyositis [12, 13]. They divided DM into four groups: idiopathic DM, juvenile DM, DM associated with cancer, and DM associated with other connective tissue diseases.

Since that time, efforts have been made to subclassify patients. The term "amyopathic dermatomyositis" was coined by Carl Pearson in 1979 to describe patients with the classic cutaneous manifestations of DM but minimal to no evidence of muscle involvement [14]. In 1991, Euwer and Sontheimer proposed the designation of "clinically amyopathic dermatomyositis" (CADM) to describe patients with the hallmark skin findings of DM but no clinical evidence of myopathy on physical examination or muscle enzyme analysis for at least 6 months after disease onset [15].

In 2002, Sontheimer proposed cutaneous criteria for establishing a diagnosis of CADM. These included three major criteria and 14 minor criteria. The major criteria were as follows: the pathognomonic heliotrope sign (violaceous erythema on the upper eyelids), Gottron's papules (papules overlying the metacarpophalangeal and interphalangeal joints) and Gottron's sign (erythema overlying the knees, elbows, or interphalangeal joints) (Table 4.1) [16]. The presence of 2 major criteria, or one 1 major criterion and 2 minor criteria, in addition to skin biopsy showing histopathologic changes consistent with DM, was required to establish a diagnosis [16]. Although these criteria have not been formally validated, they are often cited in studies as inclusion criteria for CADM patients.

Table 4.1 Sontheimer's proposed diagnostic criteria for cutaneous dermatomyositis [16]

Diagnosis of cutaneous dermatomyositis requires:
1. Presence of two major criteria, or one major criterion and two minor criteria
AND
2. Skin biopsy changes consistent with cutaneous dermatomyositis
Major criteria
Heliotrope sign
Gottron's papules
Gottron's sign
Minor criteria
Macular violaceous erythema involving (each area counts as one minor criterion):
Scalp or anterior hairline
Malar eminences of face, forehead, or chin
V-area of neck or upper chest (V-neck sign)
Posterior neck or posterior shoulders (shawl sign)
Extensor surfaces of arms or forearms
Linear streaking overlying extensor tendons of dorsal hands
Periungal skin
Lateral thighs or hips (holster sign)
Medial malleoli
Nailfold capillary telangiectasia, hemorrhage-infarct
Poikiloderma
Mechanic's hands
Cutaneous calcinosis
Cutaneous ulcers
Pruritus

We value the CADM classification criteria for formally recognizing the significant subset of roughly 20% [5] of DM patients who do not have overt muscle disease and would therefore otherwise be excluded from a clinical diagnosis of DM as well as from clinical trials and translational studies for DM patients [17]. However, existing data do not support the concept that CADM patients uniformly differ from classic DM patients in any other clinical or pathologic manner. These CADM patients have similar skin manifestations (both clinically and histologically), as well as an increased risk for interstitial lung disease (ILD) and internal malignancy. Any differences that do exist between these two subgroups may be largely accounted for by differences in autoantibody profile (Table 4.2) and not simply the presence or absence of clinical myositis.

Other subclassification schemes have been proposed based on serologies. In 1991, Love et al. suggested that myositis-specific antibodies may define groups of patients who share certain clinical features [18]. Approximately 80% of DM patients will have a detectable myositis-specific antibody, including transcriptional intermediary factor 1-gamma (TIF1-γ), nuclear matrix protein 2 (NXP2), melanoma differentiation-associated gene 5 (MDA5), small ubiquitin-like modifier activating enzyme (SAE), Mi-2, Jo-1 and the other anti-synthetase antibodies. These myositis-specific autoantibodies have been associated with distinct clinical subsets and appear to be useful in the diagnosis and classification of DM (Table 4.2). Dr. Manabu Fujimoto used results from Japanese studies to create an autoantibody-based classification of DM [19]. With improved phenotyping of the myositis-specific antibodies with respect to disease features and clinical course as well as increasing availability of testing for myositis-specific antibodies, this classification method

Table 4.2 Clinical-serologic autoantibody profiles in dermatomyositis [348, 349]

Autoantibody	Autoantigen	Clinical phenotype	Frequency among DM patients (varies by population)
Anti-tRNA synthetase	Jo-1 – Histidyl PL-7 – Threonyl PL-12 – Alanyl EJ – Glycyl OJ – Isoleucyl KS – Asparaginyl Ha – Tyrosinyl Zo – Phenylalanyl	Increased risk of interstitial lung disease (ILD) for all; PL-7 associated with mild skin and muscle disease; [350] PL-12, KS, OJ associated with isolated ILD; [351–353] All associated with the spectrum of findings in the anti-synthetase syndrome, including ILD, fever, arthritis, myositis, mechanic's hands, Raynaud phenomenon	Jo-1 present in up to 20%. Non-Jo-1 anti-tRNA synthetase antibodies present in 1–5%. [354]
Anti-Mi-2	Mi-2; regulates transcription as a component of nucleosome remodeling and deacetylase (NuRD) complex	Classic cutaneous disease; good prognosis and response to therapy	Ethnogeographic frequency variation: 20%in U.S. [351] and Japan [355] 6.7% in Glasgow 60% in Guatemala [8]
Anti-TIF1-γ	p155; transcriptional intermediary factor; plays role in apoptosis, ubiquitination, and innate immunity	Increased cancer risk; Severe cutaneous disease; Low risk of ILD risk	Present in 21–38% [193, 356]
Anti-MDA5	Melanoma differentiation-associated protein 5; cytosolic receptor for viral dsRNA, mediates type I interferon innate immune response	High ILD risk; RP-ILD in Asians; Vasculopathic phenotype – ulcerated palmar papules, livedo; Arthritis, alopecia, gingival pain	Ethnogeographic frequency variation: 7–10% in U.S. [124, 168] 20–35% in Asia [357, 358]
Anti-NXP2	Nuclear matrix protein; transcription	Increased cancer risk in adults; Increased risk of calcinosis	Present in 1.6–30% [30, 191, 193, 359]
Anti-SAE	Small ubiquitin-like modifier activating enzyme; post-translational modification	Skin disease onset before myositis; May have severe disease; Dysphagia	Present in 1.5–10% [360–364]

may add value to existing definitions by facilitating improved prognostication, targeted screening and potentially tailored therapy.

Clinical Presentation

Skin Disease

Classic Features

A careful history will elicit common features of skin disease in DM. In some patients, onset of disease is associated with a recent history of significant UV exposure. Patients may also describe sensitivity to sunlight. Pruritus is typical and further questioning often reveals a subjective dysesthetic component to the itch, often described as a sensation of skin tightness, burning, or crawling. This sensation is especially common on the scalp. Patients complain of swelling of the eyelids, which is frequently misdiagnosed as allergic contact dermatitis or angioedema. Additionally, patients will describe the eruption to be chronic, relapsing, and progressive.

On physical examination, skin changes in DM are distributed on archetypal regions on the body (Table 4.1). Of note, many of these are not necessarily in areas of UV exposure (so-called "photodistributed"). In order to improve the sensitivity of the examination, proper patient positioning and exam room lighting are critical. Overhead lighting tends to cast shadows over the brow, nose, and chin, which may conceal faint erythema or telangiectasias on the body surfaces inferiorly. Also, we find that bright direct lighting often obscures the subtle color changes seen in DM skin. Examination with natural lighting is recommended whenever possible.

The distinction between disease activity and damage in DM skin is critical for clinical decision-making, so that immunosuppressive treatments are not erroneously utilized for skin damage. In addition to itch, cutaneous disease activity is characterized by violaceous erythema, induration (papules or plaques), scale, or ulceration. Epidermal and vascular damage, by contrast, may be evident on examination as telangiectasias, atrophy, and dyspigmentation.

Although erythema is often an important sign of activity, it may also represent damage, and thus care must be taken not to escalate therapy based solely on the presence of erythema. Telangiectasias, for example, cause erythema but are a sign of damage. Livedo reticularis, a vascular phenomenon associated with DM, may likewise be confused with active erythema in DM. Careful identification of the netlike pattern of livedo and presence on photoprotected surfaces may help avoid this confusion. Skin damage due to DM may also be reflected in reticulated patches, but these are more brown, post-inflammatory hyperpigmented patches in areas of prior disease activity.

When substantial inflammation has been present, patients may present with a distinctive and pathognomonic pattern comprised of reticulated, sometimes atrophic, white macules, adjacent to erythema and/or telangiectasias, which we call "red on white" (Fig. 4.1a–c). The scalp and the skin along the bitemporal hairline (Fig. 4.2) are frequent sites of involvement, though this pattern does not necessarily occur only in sun-exposed areas. It is becoming increasingly clear that many of these red on white patches do not necessarily represent permanent damage, as these lesions may slowly resolve with time, even when atrophy is present. However, this morphology can be a

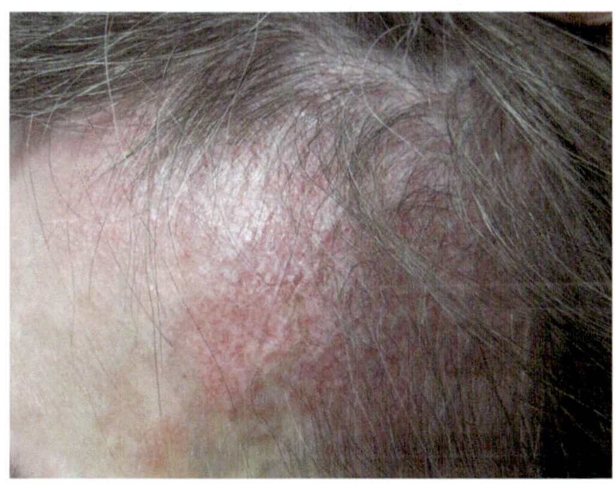

Fig. 4.2 "Red on white" plaques confluent over the frontal hairline and hair-bearing scalp

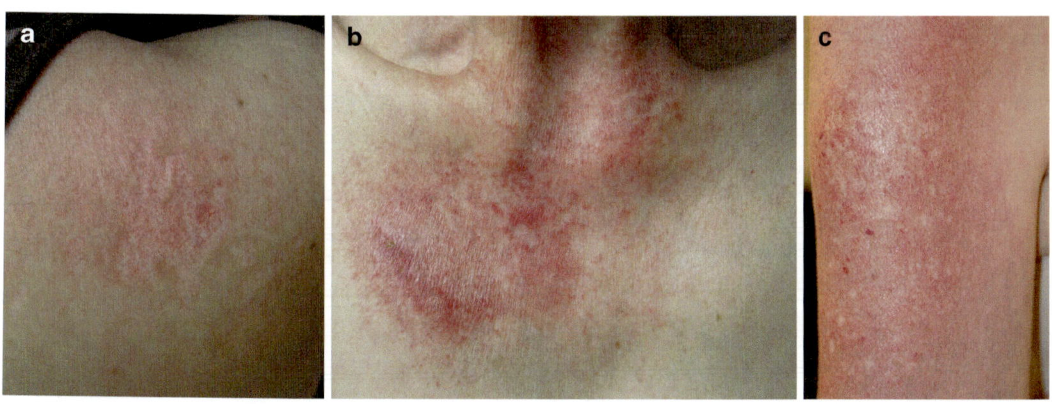

Fig. 4.1 Pathognomonic "red on white" pattern of reticulated, sometimes atrophic, white macules adjacent to erythema and/or telangiectasias, seen on the right upper back (**a**), central chest (**b**) and right lateral upper arm (**c**)

useful diagnostic clue, as it does not seem to be associated with other connective tissue diseases, such as cutaneous lupus, but is more specific to DM.

Longstanding disease activity, typically in sun-exposed areas, results in more significant damage, characterized by atrophy, hypopigmentation, hyperpigmentation and telangiectasias, a constellation of findings that is termed poikiloderma. Poikiloderma is a late manifestation in DM and is not diagnostically specific, as it may result from many other acquired and congenital diseases, including cutaneous lupus, chronic actinic damage (poikiloderma of Civatte), poikilodermatous mycosis fungoides (poikiloderma vasculare atrophicans), borrelia infection (acrodermatitis chronic atrophicans), chronic radiation dermatitis, and graft versus host disease.

Two important signs have been proposed to be pathognomonic for DM. First, violaceous to pink papules over the dorsal proximal interphalangeal and metacarpophalangeal joints are termed Gottron's papules (Fig. 4.3). These may display the same range of features seen elsewhere on DM skin, including poikiloderma, atrophy, hypopigmentation, hyperkeratosis or ulceration. Second, Gottron's sign is characterized by symmetric, macular, violaceous erythema over the interphalangeal joints, olecranon processes (Fig. 4.4), patellas, and medial malleoli.

Other characteristic hand findings in DM include hyperkeratosis and fissuring along the lateral second and third digits (Fig. 4.5), which may be subtle; the rough texture is often evident only with palpation. In patients with antisynthetase antibodies, digital hyperkeratosis and fissuring is often more extensive and usually also affects the palmar fingers and fingertips (so-called "mechanic's hands").

Involvement of the scalp with erythema, fine scale, and pruritus is one of the most ubiquitous cutaneous manifestations in DM. Scalp pruritus may be severe, have a burning or dysesthetic quality and significantly reduce the patient's quality of life. Subtle erythema may be perceptible on the vertex scalp, along the hair part, or on the borders of the hairline, even when the remainder of the cutaneous disease is quiescent.

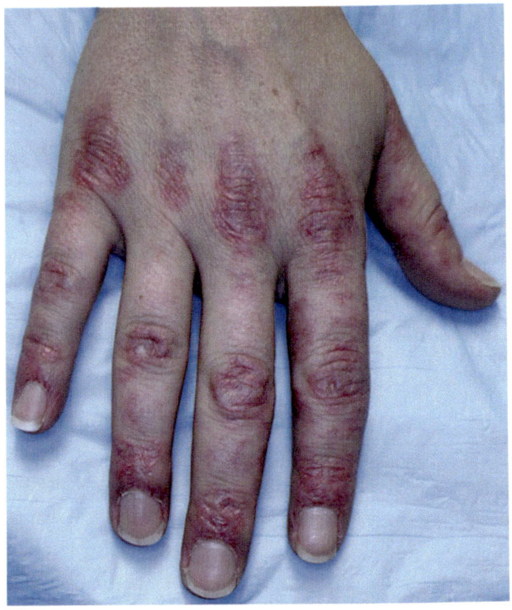

Fig. 4.3 Gottron's papules: violaceous papules overlying the dorsal proximal interphalangeal and metacarpophalangeal joints

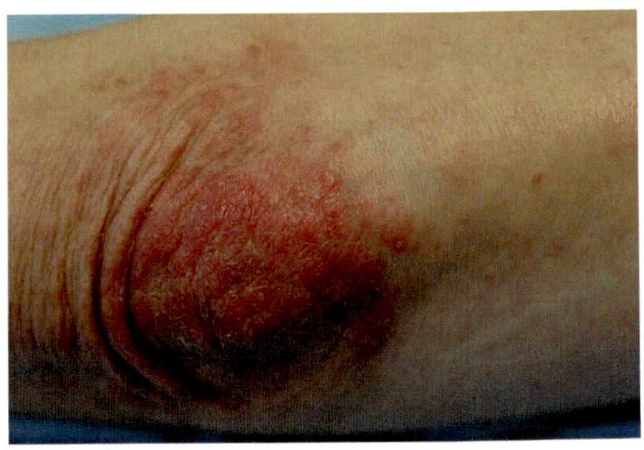

Fig. 4.4 Gottron's sign: symmetric red patches on the elbows

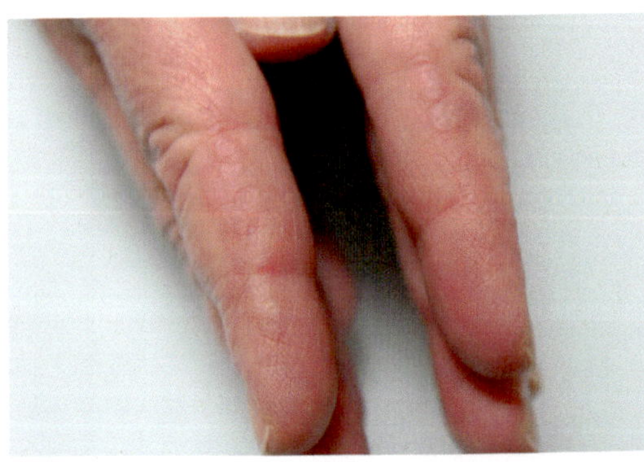

Fig. 4.5 Lateral digit hyperkeratosis: pink papules with rough white scale on the bilateral lateral second digits

The periorbital skin is frequently involved. Patients may present with violaceous patches on the upper eyelids (the heliotrope sign), frequently with associated edema that may be minimal to severe. In addition, erythema of the lateral canthi, medial canthi and adjacent nasal sidewalls is common (Fig. 4.6a, b). The rest of the face may have diffuse erythema or may be uninvolved.

Areas of involvement on the trunk may include the upper back, posterior neck, posterior shoulders (shawl sign), and posterior upper arms. Confluent violaceous erythema on the sun-exposed areas of the lower anterior neck and anterior chest is termed the V-neck sign. In addition, linear patches or urticarial plaques (flagellate erythema), possibly due to excoriation or imprinting from clothing or bed sheets, may be present on the back or upper chest. Biopsy of flagellate erythema shows typical histopathology of DM [20].

We have frequently observed reticulated, violaceous patches on the lateral areas of the flanks and lower back. Violaceous erythema and poikiloderma may also affect the lateral hips and lateral thighs (Holster sign). This finding, consisting of small (1 mm), violaceous, folliculocentric macules or less likely papules, may be confused with the more common condition keratosis pilaris. However, the violaceous color and typically macular nature of the eruption, as well as the distribution typically not involving areas typical for keratosis pilaris (e.g., upper, outer arms) helps to delineate this finding to DM.

The oral mucosa may also be involved in DM. Red on white patches may be observed, particularly on the hard palate and surrounding gingival mucosa. (Fig. 4.7a). When this occurs in a distinctly oval pattern at the junction of the hard and soft palate at the midline, it is termed the "ovoid palatal patch" (Fig. 4.7b). This latter finding appears to occur most frequently in the subset of DM patients with anti-transcriptional intermediary factor 1 gamma (TIF1-γ) antibodies [21]. Biopsies from these lesions demonstrate interface mucositis, consistent with typical findings in DM. In our experience, activity of these mucosal changes seems to mirror the activity of the cutaneous disease: the hard palate changes appear with mild disease activity and fade late in the course as definitive control of the cutaneous disease is achieved. Oral manifestations of DM may be confused with the oral findings seen in discoid lupus or lichen planus, but their consistent localization to the center of the hard palate may aid in the diagnosis of DM when other cutaneous features are non-diagnostic.

The nailfolds are another classic site of involvement for DM. Nailfold capillary changes provide a window into the disease's hallmark microangiopathy. When pronounced and easily visualized with the naked eye, these nailfold capillary changes can be highly suggestive of DM over other connective tissue disorders. The classic findings include, red, edematous, often tender, proximal nailfolds. Capillary loops are ramified and dilated, with intervening pale to white avascular areas characterized by capillary dropout, as

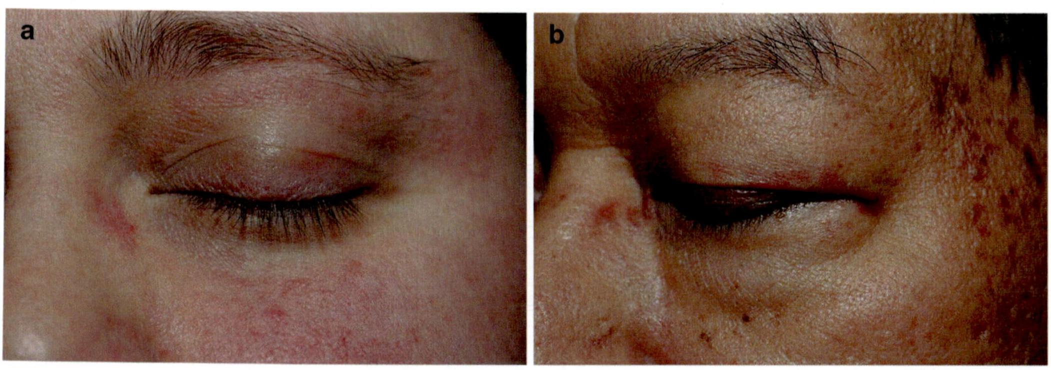

Fig. 4.6 (**a**, **b**): Red and violaceous macules on the lateral canthi, medial canthi and nasal sidewalls, commonly seen in association with the heliotrope sign

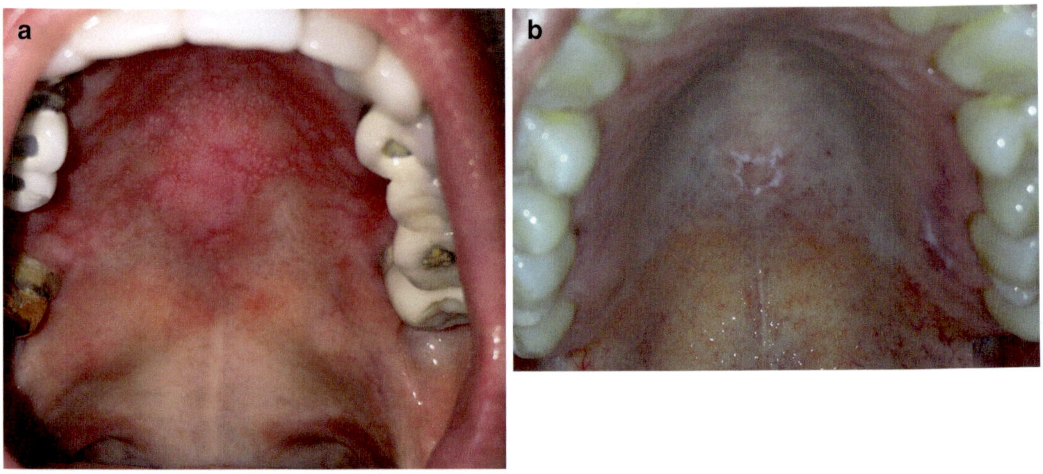

Fig. 4.7 "Red on white" reticulated patch (a) and ovoid palatal patch (b) seen on the posterior hard palate

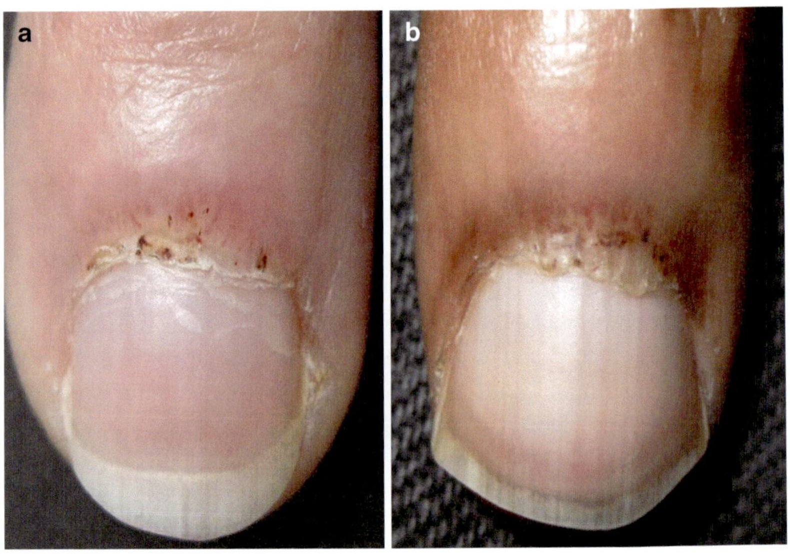

Fig. 4.8 (a, b) Dilated capillary loops, cuticular hemorrhages, and intervening yellow to white avascular areas, with elongated and ragged cuticles

well as cuticular hemorrhages and elongated, ragged cuticles (Fig. 4.8a, b). These changes are a sign of ongoing cutaneous disease activity [22], though persistently ramified capillaries may represent damage in longstanding DM [23].

The vasculopathy that plays an important role in cutaneous DM may sometimes become clinically prominent, causing ulceration, Degos-like lesions, and livedo reticularis. Degos-like lesions are most common on the dorsal fingers and are characterized by a depressed, porcelain-white papule with a rim of bright red erythema. The clinical significance of these lesions in DM is unknown. Ulceration may be present in 30% of patients and typically affects the skin over the extensor joint surfaces, the digital pulp, or the periungal skin [24]. In our U.S. cohort, ulceration was associated with anti-MDA5 antibodies, although it may be noted in other contexts as well. DM patients with anti-MDA5 antibodies display a more severe vasculopathic phenotype.

Calcinosis of the dermis, subcutaneous tissue, fascia, or muscle is a late manifestation of DM, typically involving the trunk, proximal extremities, or areas of previous disease activity. The prevalence of calcinosis is 20% in adult DM [25] and up to 40% in juvenile DM [26]. Calcinosis also occurs more rapidly after disease onset in

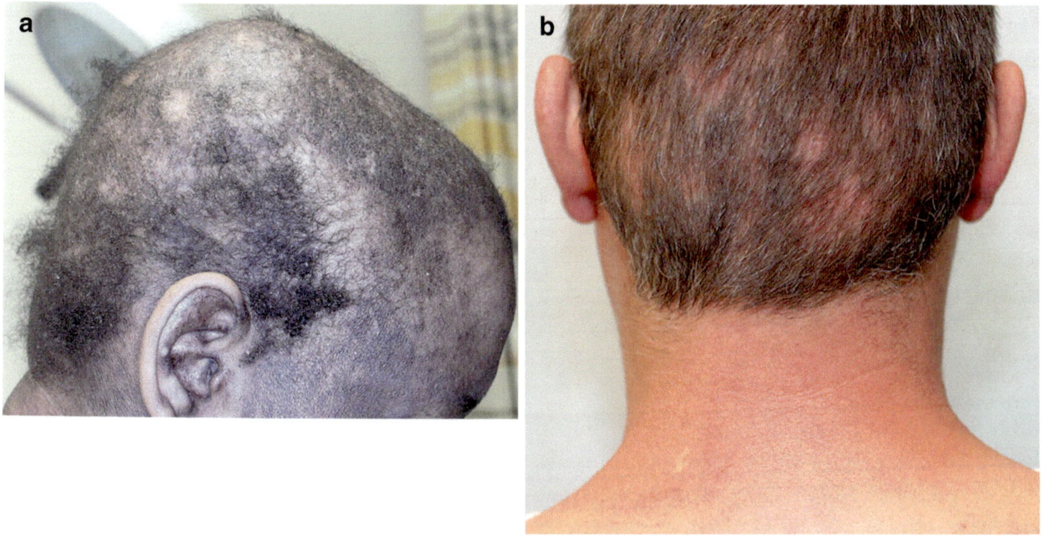

Fig. 4.9 (**a**, **b**) Non-scarring alopecia, seen in DM patients with anti-MDA5 antibodies

juvenile DM compared with adult DM (2.9 years vs. 7.9 years, respectively) [27]. In juvenile DM, risk factors for development of calcinosis include longer disease duration, younger age of disease onset, sustained disease activity, and internal organ involvement [28, 29]. Calcinosis is most frequent on the proximal extremities, buttocks and trunk in DM, an important distinguishing factor from the calcinosis seen in systemic sclerosis, which typically affects the digits and elbows [27]. In both juvenile and adult DM, the presence of anti-nuclear matrix protein 2 (NXP2) antibodies are associated with an increased risk of calcinosis [30, 31]. Calcinosis is also commonly seen in the anti-MDA5 subset (especially those patients with longstanding disease) [31], which is associated with known vasculopathy. In adults with DM, fingertip ulceration has been associated with calcinosis [31], suggesting that vascular insufficiency or damage may be involved in the pathogenesis of calcinosis.

Panniculitis may occur in DM and typically affects the buttocks, trunk, and proximal extremities. It may progress to calcinosis and/or lipoatrophy [32]. Histopathology shows a lobular panniculitis, but lipomembranous change as seen in lupus panniculitis may be present, and septal thickening may be seen, as in deep morphea. Panniculitis appears to be more common among the anti-MDA5 DM group.

Non-scarring alopecia may occur in DM, either secondary to scalp inflammation or due to telogen effluvium. This manifestation is particularly common in the anti-MDA5 group (Fig. 4.9a, b). In this group, alopecia closely mirrors the cutaneous disease activity.

Rare Presentations of Cutaneous DM

There is a subset of DM patients with overlapping features of both psoriasis and DM. Their skin disease may show psoriasiform, well-demarcated, thick plaques over the MCP and PIP joints, elbows and knees, along with dilated nailfold capillaries. Skin biopsies reveal both epidermal hyperplasia and interface dermatitis. Some affected patients have a history of psoriasis, and it is unclear whether these psoriasiform lesions represent concomitant psoriasis or a psoriasiform manifestation of DM. DM and psoriasis share similar interferon gene signatures, which could at least partly explain this presentation[33, 34].

Other rare presentations of DM include subcutaneous edema in the distal extremities and generalized edema, both of which may portend more severe muscle inflammation or aggressive disease [35, 36]. Lastly, DM may rarely present with erythroderma, in which 90% or more of the body surface is involved with confluent erythema.

Cutaneous Signs of Interstitial Lung Disease

Hyperkeratosis and fissuring along the ulnar aspect of the thumb and radial aspect of the index and middle fingers were first described as mechanic's hands by Stahl et al. in 1979, in a series of eight patients with inflammatory myopathies [37]. In 1991, Love et al. found that myositis patients with anti-synthetase antibodies were more likely to have mechanic's hands, ILD, fever, and arthritis [18]. In 2012, Sato et al. noted an increased prevalence of ILD among DM patients with mechanic's hands (7/9 patients, 78%) as compared to those without mechanic's hands (12/30 patients, 40%) [38], suggesting that mechanic's hands may be a cutaneous clue to the presence of ILD. We have observed that additional features of mechanic's hands in anti-synthetase antibody positive DM patients include hyperkeratosis and fissuring of the distal fingertips and palmar fingers.

Japanese case series have suggested that cutaneous ulceration is associated with lung disease in DM [39–41]. In our U.S. cohort, we did not find an association between ulceration and ILD [24]. However, in the presence of anti-MDA5 antibodies, cutaneous ulceration was associated with a markedly increased odds of having ILD (OR 35.19, 95% CI 3.55–3.49, p = 0.0024) [24]. Thus, the significance of ulceration in DM may depend upon the autoantibody status of the patient. Anti-MDA5 antibodies are more commonly seen in Japanese DM patients, and this may explain the data associating ulceration with lung disease in the patients from Japan. In addition, in the anti-MDA5 patients, we have found a correlation between the severity of the ulceration and the severity of ILD (unpublished data). Worsening cutaneous ulceration in a patient with anti-MDA5 DM, therefore, may be a cutaneous sign of worsening ILD.

Because anti-MDA5 antibodies are strongly associated with lung disease, other cutaneous features associated with this serologic group should also raise suspicion for underlying lung inflammation. These include the frankly eroded papules ("inverse Gottron's papules") on the palmar fingers that are virtually pathognomonic for patients with anti-MDA5 antibodies (Fig. 4.10). Patients with these antibodies may also have violaceous reticular erythema over the palmar surfaces and digital pulps. Severe alopecia may also be a sign of anti-MDA5 antibodies.

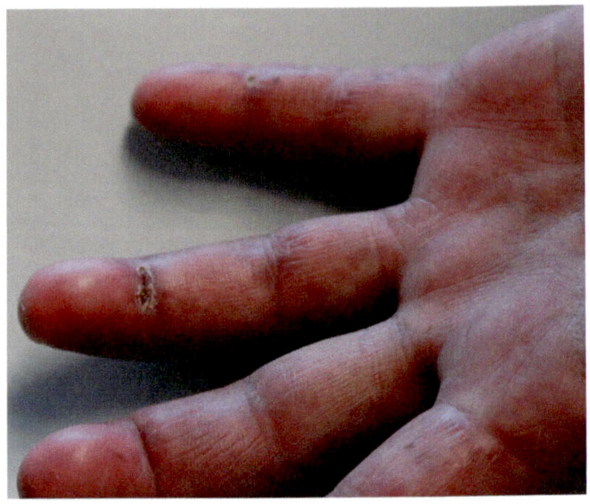

Fig. 4.10 Eroded papules on the palmar fingers overlying the interphalangeal joints in a DM patient with anti-MDA5 antibodies

Cutaneous Signs of Internal Malignancy

Cutaneous necrosis and cutaneous small vessel vasculitis have been reported to be associated with paraneoplastic DM [42, 43]. However, necrosis causing ulceration should raise suspicion for other conditions, such as ILD, as reviewed above. Additionally, vasculitis has been reported in cases not associated with malignancy [44–48]. Acquired ichthyosis, manifesting as a paraneoplastic dermatosis, has been described in association with malignancy and DM [49–51].

Histopathology

Biopsy of involved skin in DM classically shows an interface dermatitis, basement membrane thickening, epidermal atrophy, perivascular lymphocytic infiltrate, increased dermal mucin and vascular ectasia. However, many of these features are often subtle or absent, including the interface dermatitis. Smith et al. reviewed 40 DM skin biopsies and noted that when interface dermatitis was absent (20% of cases), increased dermal mucin was always present [52]. Magro et al. described supervening dermal sclerosis in DM as a sign of more severe endothelial damage and potentially a more severe disease course [53].

Routine histopathology cannot reliably be used to distinguish cutaneous lupus from DM. Likewise, direct immunofluorescence is not always reliable. The presence of immunoreactants along the dermoepidermal junction, a finding often observed in sun-exposed lesional skin in acute cutaneous lupus, has been variably reported in lesional skin in DM. Black et al. found that 65% (19 of 29) of lesional biopsies from DM patients demonstrated positive IgM, IgG or C3 at the basement membrane[54]. Magro et al. suggested a more stringent definition of the DIF findings seen in lupus (sometimes called the lupus band), requiring either a continuous, moderately intense band of IgM and/or presence of IgG (interrupted or continuous) at the dermoepidermal junction [55]; using this definition, DM skin, unlike that from lupus patients, virtually never displayed a positive result. Using these criteria, DIF may be a useful test in distinguishing acute cutaneous lupus from DM. However, it is important to note that DIF may also be negative in lupus patients.

Building on the observations of Mascaró Jr. et al. [56], Magro et al. suggest that the presence of membrane attack complex (C5b-C9) deposits around the dermoepidermal junction and vessels is a characteristic finding in DM. When coupled with the absence of direct immunofluorescence findings seen in lupus, this finding yielded a sensitivity for the diagnosis of DM of 93.5% and a specificity of 78.3% [55]. The absence of lupus direct immunofluorescence findings alone or positive C5b-C9 deposition alone yielded specificities of 64.5% and 78.6%, respectively [55]. The utility of immunofluorescence testing in the diagnosis of DM warrants further evaluation.

Differential Diagnosis

A common differential diagnosis for the cutaneous findings of DM includes cutaneous lupus, psoriasis, acne rosacea, phototoxic or photoallergic drug eruption, atopic dermatitis, and mycosis fungoides.

As compared to cutaneous lupus erythematosus (CLE), the erythema is more violaceous in color in DM than in CLE and has a different distribution, affecting the extensor joint surfaces. Erythema over the dorsal fingers may be seen in acute or subacute cutaneous lupus, but it is typically more prominent over the hair-bearing interphalangeal skin, with relative sparing of the PIP joints, although there are many instances bearing exception to this rule. Periungual erythema and nailfold capillary changes can be seen in both CLE and DM, including dilation, hemorrhage and dropout; however, in our experience, severe capillary changes are more common in DM. Although marked periorbital edema and erythema has been described in discoid lupus and can mimic the heliotrope rash, these findings tend to be unilateral and affect the lower eyelids [57–59].

The extensor surfaces and the scalp may be involved in both psoriasis and DM; however, the heliotrope, V-neck and shawl signs should be absent in psoriasis. Psoriasis also tends to present with more abundant, thick, silvery to whitish scale than is seen in DM. Scalp tightness and dysesthesia are typically absent in psoriasis. As a caveat, as reviewed, DM and psoriasis may present as an overlap syndrome, including clinical and histologic features of both psoriasis and DM.

Facial involvement in erythematotelangiectatic rosacea is most prominent on the midcheeks, chin and glabella, and it tends to spare the upper eyelids, factors that can distinguish it from DM. In neurogenic rosacea, which is a rare variant, there may be intense burning symptoms out of proportion to examination findings. These symptoms may resemble the dysesthesia seen in DM [60, 61]; however, facial disease in DM tends not to be highly symptomatic.

Photoprotected sites are not typically involved phototoxic or photoallergic eruptions, whereas these sites may be involved in DM, e.g., the holster sign on the lateral hips and Gottron's sign on the knees. Nailfold capillary changes are absent in phototoxic or photoallergic eruptions. When a photoeruption becomes chronic, as in chronic actinic dermatitis, the skin becomes lichenified, whereas the chronically involved skin in DM tends to become atrophied.

Periorbital and scalp erythema, edema, and scale may be present in atopic dermatitis, but the eczematous plaques should also involve flexural areas. Additionally, the eruption in atopic dermatitis becomes more lichenified with time, and nailfold capillary changes are absent.

Although DM patients may have puffy fingers and nailfold capillary changes similar to those seen in systemic sclerosis, facial involvement with microstomia is not observed in DM. The dyspigmentation on the face and trunk seen in systemic sclerosis is accompanied by cutaneous sclerosis, which is absent in DM.

Poikilodermatous mycosis fungoides (previously named poikiloderma vasculare atrophicans and parapsoriasis variegata) is a variant of mycosis fungoides presenting with large, violaceous plaques characterized by hyperpigmentation, hypopigmentation, atrophy and telangiectasias, which may be clinically indistinguishable from those of DM. In this variant of MF, however, and in contrast to DM, the majority of the body surface area of the trunk, buttocks and flexural surfaces is involved.

Muscle Disease

Classic Presentation

Myopathy in DM typically presents as symmetrical proximal muscle weakness. Muscle symptoms may occur before, after, or at the same time as cutaneous manifestations [62]. As discussed, approximately 20% of DM patients are classified as clinically amyopathic, such that even with mild muscle enzyme elevations or abnormalities in an electromyogram, magnetic resonance imaging (MRI), or muscle histopathology, there are no signs of objective weakness on physical examination. Those DM patients that do develop weakness often do so within the first year of symptom onset although weakness can present many years after disease onset [63]. The temporal course of myositis is generally acute or subacute, and progressive.

Patients most often experience weakness of the extensor muscles surrounding the shoulder and pelvic girdles and of proximal limbs. Patients with shoulder and upper extremity weakness may experience difficulty washing their hair or reaching for items in overhead cupboards. Quadriceps and gluteal muscle weakness may manifest as difficulty in rising from a seated position, climbing stairs, or stepping onto curbs. Distal muscle weakness in the hands, manifesting as difficulty opening jars or holding onto objects, typically occurs late in the disease, although patients with the anti-NXP2 antibody may develop distal disease early in the course of DM. With neck flexor muscle involvement, patients may have difficulty raising the head off the table while laying supine. Along with neck weakness, patients experiencing difficulty swallowing liquids and/or solids or having dysphonia may portend poor prognosis. Patients with DM may also describe global symptoms of myopathy, such as fatigue or decreased exercise capacity.

Muscle involvement may also result in symptoms other than classic weakness. Involvement of respiratory muscles of the chest wall or diaphragm may lead to respiratory insufficiency and occasionally respiratory failure. Patients may note a hoarse or raspy voice (dysphonia) due to cricoarytenoid muscle involvement, which occurs in up to 40% of DM patients [64]. Dysphagia may occur in 20% to 50% of cases, due to weak pharyngeal musculature and thus an inability to propel food in the pharyngeal phase of swallowing [65]. Dysphagia is often experienced by the patient as having to "think about swallowing" solids, choking on liquids, or a feeling of not being able to clear their throat. The dermatologist must not only ask patients about weakness and myalgias but also about these bulbar symptoms such as dysphagia or dysphonia, as they can be important clues of muscle activity, and, if severe, can portend need for hospitalization or more aggressive care. Significant bulbar symptoms, especially in cases with cranial nerve involvement, should alert the clinician to consider an overlap with myasethenia gravis, which can occur concomitantly with DM. Approximately 30% of patients will complain of muscle pain with or without muscle weakness [66].

Early in the course of myositis, serum muscle enzymes (i.e., creatine kinase [CK], aldolase, lactate dehydrogenase [LDH], aspartate aminotransferase [AST], and alanine aminotransferase [ALT]) are sensitive biomarkers of muscle inflammation. However, in the mid- to late course of myositis, their sensitivities decrease. CK may be elevated as high as over 100 times above the upper limit of normal; alternative benign causes of myositis, by contrast, which include strenuous exercise, viral illness, and muscle trauma, typically result in CK elevations less than 5 times the upper limit of normal. African-Americans and muscular individuals may have baseline CK levels above the reference laboratory range, usually less than three times the upper limit [67].

Histopathology

Classic cutaneous findings along with weakness and muscle enzyme elevation are sufficient for making a clinical diagnosis of DM and for treating. When performed, biopsy of involved muscle in DM typically demonstrates perifascicular atrophy, degenerating and regenerating myofibers, endothelial cell swelling and capillary necrosis, and membrane attack complex deposition in the endomysial capillary walls [68]. The perifascicular pathology has been proposed to result from the destruction of capillaries populating this region, which could result in localized hypoxia and subsequent myofiber injury. An inflammatory infiltrate is present, consisting of CD4+ T cells [69], plasmacytoid dendritic cells secreting interferon alpha [70], B cells, macrophages, and plasma cells.

If muscle biopsy is performed at the time of acute presentation, features of concomitant rhabdomyolysis with overwhelming necrosis may obscure the primary underlying pathologic process. Nonetheless, a muscle biopsy may still be warranted at this time if immunosuppressive therapy is to be initiated. Prednisone and other immunomodulatory therapies will decrease the yield of the muscle biopsy, resulting in a false negative due to the presence of patchy muscle inflammation. If a muscle biopsy is necessary to confirm the diagnosis of DM, we recommend it be performed within 2 weeks of the initiation of immunomodulatory therapy.

Electromyography

In some cases, electromyography (EMG) may be a helpful adjunct in identifying inflammatory myopathy. EMG can suggest the category of disease (i.e., neuropathic vs myopathic) and will identify patterns of abnormalities to allow for further characterization within each category.

On EMG, DM patients demonstrate the classic triad of small amplitude, short duration, polyphasic motor unit potentials; fibrillations and positive sharp waves; and complex repetitive discharges [71]. Similar patterns may be noted in patients with other inflammatory myopathies, such as polymyositis [72].

Early in the course of disease, EMG detects myositis in 70–90% of DM patients. Later in the course, the sensitivity of EMG in detecting myositis decreases. A potential explanation for decreased sensitivity of EMG (as well as muscle enzymes) over time is that longstanding myositis may result in perifascicular muscle atrophy and fibrosis, leading to less dramatic results, even while inflammation persists.

Imaging

MRI may be useful to assess for signs of myositis when muscle enzymes and EMG studies are inconclusive. MRI can also be used to direct the site of a diagnostic biopsy [73] or, in some cases, assess clinical response to treatment [74]. MRI provides a detailed view of the muscle anatomy, allowing for localization and discrimination of pathologic processes, e.g., edema, inflammation, fibrosis, calcifications or atrophy. On short tau inversion recovery (STIR) sequencing, in which normal muscle is dark and inflamed muscle is bright, an increased signal intensity is noted within muscles affected by inflammation, necrosis, and/or degeneration [75]. Yoshida et al. performed MRI studies on 14 newly diagnosed DM patients and noted that on STIR sequences, fasciitis was the predominant finding in the first 2 months after symptom onset. They also analyzed en bloc muscle biopsies from each patient and found histopathologic evidence of fasciitis in 12 of 14 patients, suggesting that the fascial microvasculature may be a primary site of involvement [76]. In T1-weighted MRI images, in which fat is bright and normal muscle is dark, chronic muscle damage may be identified as fatty replacement of skeletal muscle [77].

Differential Diagnosis

The differential diagnosis for weakness is broad. The presence of characteristic cutaneous findings of DM obviously help to point away from other causes. However, in the case of a patient with a photodistributed rash and muscle weakness, the possibility that they are two unrelated conditions must be considered by the clinician before assuming a diagnosis of DM. In cases when the cutaneous eruption is subtle or specific features are in question, other causes of myositis may be considered. It is also essential to distinguish between myopathic and nonmyopathic causes of weakness.

Nonmyopathic etiologies of weakness include other disorders of the motor unit [67] as well as global causes, including chronic pain and chronic fatigue syndromes [78]. Neuromuscular diseases such as myasthenia gravis have been described as co-existing with DM [79]. The presence of ptosis, diplopia, fatiguability, and bulbar symptoms should raise concern for myasthenia gravis. Neuromyelitis optica (Devic's disease), another neuromuscular disease, has been described in a juvenile and adult patient with DM [80, 81].

Myopathic causes may be hereditary and may include channelopathies and muscular dystrophies. Acquired causes of myopathy include autoimmune (DM, polymyositis, inclusion body myositis, immune-mediated necrotizing myopathy, other connective tissue disease associated), toxic (drug-induced) or metabolic myopathies (thyroid and adrenal dysfunction) [67].

Systemic lupus erythematosus (SLE) often presents with a photodistributed eruption, and myositis is present in 4% to 16% of SLE patients [82–86]. Moreover, 50% of SLE patients may complain of myalgias [87]. Symptoms of myositis in these patients, as in DM, frequently include fatigue and proximal muscle weakness [82]. CK levels are elevated in the majority of cases, and electromyographic studies show signs of myositis [88]. Muscle biopsy shows a nonspecific perivascular and perimysial infiltrate of inflammatory cells, without invasion of non-necrotic fibers and type II muscle fiber atrophy [89].

Polymyositis lacks a well-defined clinical phenotype. These patients may present with proximal muscle weakness, elevated muscle enzymes, and myopathic changes on EMG; however, the cutaneous manifestations of DM are, by definition, absent [90]. Muscle biopsy is essential to confirm the diagnosis of polymyositis. Classic histopathologic features include an endomysial inflammatory infiltrate consisting predominantly of CD8+ T cells, as well as muscle fiber necrosis and regeneration [20].

Anti-synthetase antibody syndrome, characterized by fever, arthritis, myositis, ILD, mechanic's hands, Raynaud's phenomenon and the presence of an anti-synthetase autoantibody, may be seen in both DM and polymyositis. Specific histopathologic findings in muscle biopsies of anti-synthetase antibody syndrome have been identified [91], while the ultrastructural findings of myonuclear actin aggregation and intranuclear rod formation have been found to have 81% sensitivity and 100% specificity for anti-synthetase syndrome-myositis [92].

Inclusion body myositis typically affects men older than 40 years and has an insidious onset, preferentially affecting the finger flexors (causing difficulty with fine motor movements) and the quadriceps [93]. Muscle biopsy shows a mixed infiltrate of CD8+ T cells and monocytes surrounding non-necrotic myofibers, rimmed vacuoles and amyloid and p62 inclusions within myofibers [94].

Up to 30% of patients with systemic sclerosis have a myopathy [95–97]. The subset of systemic sclerosis patients with anti-PM-Scl antibodies may have an inflammatory myositis in roughly 50% of cases [98]. Systemic sclerosis patients typically lack classic cutaneous manifestations of DM, however. There are case reports of sclerodermatomyositis [99, 100], however, described in patients with systemic sclerosis and myositis who have anti-PM-Scl antibodies.

Trichinosis is a meat-borne parasitic disease caused by ingestion of roundworm larvae from the Trichinella species, usually found in undercooked pork. Fifteen cases were confirmed in the U.S in 2012 [101]. It manifests with an initial enteral phase with diarrhea and abdominal pain within 1 week of larvae ingestion. In the systemic phase, beginning 1–6 weeks following ingestion, patients develop eosinophilic myositis, characterized by fever, myalgias and periorbital edema [102]. Muscle pain is typically present in the nuchal muscles, masseters, and upper and lower extremities. No cutaneous manifestations are observed. Diagnosis may be made with serum anti-Trichinella antibodies or by a muscle biopsy [103]. The severity of symptoms may range from mild to death from myocarditis or meningoencephalitis, depending on the number of larvae ingested and the host immune response. Treatment for the systemic phase is with albendazole and systemic corticosteroids [101].

Numerous medications have been implicated in drug-induced myopathies, including antidepressants, antipsychotics, anti-retrovirals, anticonvulsants, colchicine and statins [67]. Corticosteroids are the most common cause. Glucocorticoids induce atrophy of type II (predominantly type IIb, fast-twitch) fibers. The clinical presentation may be acute, within 4 weeks of administration of high-dose fluorinated glucocorticoids, such as dexamethasone or triamcinolone. Onset may also be insidious, over weeks to months. Risk factors include older age, malignancy, and poor nutritional status. The pelvic girdle and proximal leg muscles are more commonly affected than the shoulders and arms [104]. Muscle enzymes are normal. EMG testing may be normal early in the course but may show myopathic changes in late stages, such small-amplitude polyphasic action potentials without spontaneous activity upon needle insertion. Muscle biopsy provides the most definitive diagnosis of corticosteroid myopathy, with histology demonstrating nonspecific atrophy of type IIb muscle fibers, absence of inflammatory infiltrates, and variations in fiber size with centrally-placed nuclei [105].

Although myalgias occur in 10% of statin users [106], statin myopathy occurs in 5 in 100,000 persons and is characterized by elevated CK levels greater than 10 times normal [107]. Rhabdomyolysis is a rare, severe form of statin myopathy with an incidence of 0.44 cases per 10,000 person-years, characterized by massive myonecrosis potentially leading to renal failure and death [108]. Risk factors for statin myopathy include higher doses, the particular statins fluvastatin and pravastatin [109], the DRB1*11:01 allele [110], SLCO1B1 gene variants [111], obesity, older age, hypothyroidism, and preexisting liver disease [112]. Statin myopathy is self-limited, with resolution of symptoms seen in an average of 2 months following discontinuation of the drug culprit [113].

Immune-mediated necrotizing myopathy from anti-HMG-CoA reductase antibodies may also present with symmetric proximal muscle weakness in a patient on a statin. However, 25% of patients with this statin-associated immune-mediated necrotizing myopathy will not have a history of statin exposure [114]. The average duration of statin exposure prior to symptom onset is 3 years (range 2 months to 10 years) [115]. Laboratory evaluation reveals highly elevated CK levels (mean 10,000 IU/L) and anti-HMG-CoA reductase antibodies [116]. An irritant myopathy may be evident on EMG; MRI may show muscle edema [116]. Muscle biopsy, which is not diagnostically specific, shows prominent necrosis with minimal inflammatory cell infiltrate. Autoantibody testing is a more direct method of confirming the diagnosis [117]. Myopathic symptoms do not resolve with drug discontinuation.

An important caveat in the differential diagnosis of DM is that hepatic inflammation from a variety of causes, including nonalcoholic steatohepatitis, drug-induced hepatitis, and infectious hepatitis, may cause elevations in any of the muscle enzymes, particularly AST, ALT, and/or aldolase. Therefore, if a DM patient develops such elevations in muscle enzymes without clinical evidence of weakness, it is prudent to exclude hepatic injury. Initial investigation includes obtaining serum gamma glutamyl transferase and alkaline phosphatase as well as a hepatic ultrasound. Further work-up, including anti-smooth muscle antibody, anti-liver/kidney microsomal antibody-1 antibody, and anti-mitochondrial antibody, may be helpful in diagnosing concomitant autoimmune hepatitis, which has been previously described in patients with DM [118, 119].

It is important to consider that continued weakness despite adequate treatment or that is disconnected from improvement in skin activity may be a sign of other myopathy related to ongoing corticosteroid use, hydroxychloroquine-related myopathy, de-conditioning or post-inflmmatoary myopathy.

Systemic Disease

Pulmonary Manifestations

Pulmonary manifestations in DM include ILD, pulmonary hypertension, and aspiration pneumonia. Drug-induced pneumonitis due to agents such as methotrexate is also an important consideration. Prevalence estimates for methotrexate-induced pneumonitis in patients treated for rheumatologic indications range from 0.5% to 1%[120, 121].

Interstitial Lung Disease

Interstitial lung disease (ILD) is a leading cause of morbidity and mortality in DM [122]. ILD affects between 15% and 50% of patients with DM, depending upon the population studied and the autoantibody distribution [123–126]. Large case series have suggested that 75–86% of patients who have an anti-synthetase antibody will develop ILD [127, 128]. Similarly, DM patients with anti-MDA5 antibodies have a marked increase in risk for developing ILD, with 50–100% of these patients developing this manifestation[24, 129]. Rapidly-progressive ILD (RP-ILD) is an aggressive form of ILD that responds poorly to immunosuppressive therapies, having a 6-month survival rate of approximately 40% [130]. RP-ILD affects 40–60% of patients with anti-MDA5 antibodies [129, 131–133]. Serum ferritin is often highly elevated (>500 mg/dl) in anti-MDA5 DM patients [134] and may serve as a useful biomarker in assessing severity and the clinical response of ILD [135, 136].

Symptom onset in ILD is often insidious. Patients present with dry cough, decreased exercise capacity, or dyspnea with relatively minor exertion. Less commonly, acute onset of shortness of breath, hypoxia and respiratory failure may occur. While there are no formal guidelines for ILD screening, it is prudent to obtain baseline pulmonary function tests (PFTs) with diffusion capacity, and then repeat screening annually for at least the first 3–5 years after diagnosis. Screening PFTs may be performed more frequently if new pulmonary symptoms develop.

Diffusion capacity of carbon monoxide (DLCO) and forced vital capacity (FVC) are the two most informative parameters in evaluating for ILD: both are reduced below 80% of the predicted value [137]. In systemic sclerosis patients, who may also develop ILD, DLCO correlates better with disease severity, as assessed by high resolution computed tomography (HRCT) scans, than do lung volumes or other spirometric values [138]. Additionally, in idiopathic pulmonary fibrosis, an absolute change of 10% in FVC or 15% in DLCO signifies disease progression and an increased risk of mortality, and these parameters are reasonably applicable to ILD associated with connective tissue diseases [139]. The significance of isolated reductions in FVC of less than 5% or in DLCO of less than 10% are difficult to interpret in the absence of a clear trend over time. This degree of change may be influenced by patient effort and/or intrinsic variability of the test.

Exertional oxygen desaturation on the 6-minute walk test provides a global assessment of cardiopulmonary function and exercise performance. However, it may not be the most accurate assessment of lung function in patients with CTDs due to confounding factors, such as deconditioning, myopathy, arthritis, respiratory muscle weakness and pulmonary hypertension [140].

When there is a concern for ILD on based on pulmonary function testing or 6-minute walk testing, HRCT scan of the chest should be the next step in evaluation. HCRT of the chest may also be useful in detecting subclinical fibrosis prior to symptom onset, which is noted in up to 65% of patients with polymyositis and DM [141]. The most common pulmonary radiographic and histologic pattern in DM is nonspecific interstitial pneumonia (NSIP), which was reported in 81.8% (18/22 cases) of DM patients in one series [142]. In this study by Douglas et al. there were also two cases of diffuse alveolar damage (9%), one case of usual interstitial pneumonia (UIP, 4.5%) and one case of cryptogenic organizing pneumonia (OP, 4.5%) [142]. Radiographically, basilar and peripheral ground glass opacities and subpleural sparing characterize NSIP. By contrast, UIP is characterized by basilar and peripheral honeycombing and subpleural involvement [139]. More than one pattern may exist in a single patient. Patients with the NSIP and OP patterns experience better responses to systemic corticosteroids than those with UIP [143].

Pulmonary Arterial Hypertension

Pulmonary arterial hypertension (PAH) is a rare manifestation in DM. Symptoms may include increased fatigue, shortness of breath, dyspnea on exertion, palpitations, chest pain, edema, lightheadedness, and, rarely, pre-syncopal or syncopal episodes. A loud pulmonic component of the second heart sound may be audible at the left second intercostal space, corresponding to elevated pressure in the pulmonary arteries and delayed closure of the pulmonic valve [144]. Electrocardiogram may show right axis deviation due to right ventricular (RV) hypertrophy. Pulmonary function testing revealing a disproportionately low DLCO compared to a relatively normal FVC should prompt further screening for PAH. In systemic sclerosis patients, a DLCO of <55% and a normal FVC or an FVC/DLCO ratio of greater than 1.6 were highly associated with PAH [121].

Echocardiographic findings suggestive of pulmonary hypertension include a RV systolic pressure of >40 mmHg, RV enlargement, maximum tricuspid regurgitant velocity > 3.0 m/s, and presence of a pericardial effusion [145]. Tricuspid annular plane systolic excursion (TAPSE, a measure of RV contractility) < 1.7 cm signifies worse RV function and has been associated with higher mortality in systemic sclerosis patients [146]. Transthoracic echocardiogram has a sensitivity of only 82% and specificity of 69% in detecting pulmonary hypertension and cannot be used to differentiate patients with PAH from those with left heart disease or ILD-associated pulmonary hypertension [145]. The gold standard for the diagnosis of PAH is right heart catheterization showing a mean pulmonary artery pressure of ≥25 mmHg at rest and an end-expiratory pulmonary artery wedge pressure (PAWP) ≤15 mm Hg [147].

Cardiac Manifestations

DM-Specific Cardiac Involvement

Cardiac involvement is increasingly recognized as an important clinical feature in DM. It is typically subclinical but can present with electrocardiographic abnormalities, most commonly including ST-T segment changes and conduction abnormalities in 12.5–56.7% and 25–38.5%, respectively, of DM patients [148]. Echocardiographic findings include ventricular hypertrophy and left ventricular diastolic dysfunction in 8–15% and 42%, respectively [149]. Myocarditis may lead to myocardial fibrosis, ventricular dysfunction and thus cardiomyopathy. Rosenbohm et al. screened 11 DM patients with cardiac MRI and found that 54% (6 of 11) displayed evidence of late gadolinium enhancement, consistent with myocardial inflammation [150]. Cardiac troponin I may be a useful biomarker in detecting subclinical cardiac muscle involvement [151], and this topic warrants further inquiry.

DM patients with anti-MDA5 antibodies may be at higher risk for cardiac involvement [152, 153]. We currently follow three anti-MDA5 DM patients with cardiomyopathy; a cardiac muscle biopsy from one of these patients revealed endomyocardial fibrosis. Further studies in this patient subgroup with cardiac MRI and/or biopsies are necessary to determine the true frequency and pathogenesis of cardiac involvement in these patients.

Coronary Artery Disease

DM patients are at increased risk of developing coronary artery disease (CAD) compared with the general population. The etiology for the accelerated atherosclerosis is likely multifactorial. Important factors include the chronic inflammatory state, endothelial dysfunction, hypercoagulability [154], and prolonged exposure to prednisone in the context of traditional cardiovascular disease risk factors [155], such as hypertension, hyperglycemia, and dyslipidemia [156].

A meta-analysis of four large epidemiologic studies of patients with idiopathic inflammatory myopathies showed an increased frequency of cardiovascular events compared to controls with a risk ratio of 2.26 (95% confidence interval 1.02–4.92) [157]. A U.S. retrospective case-control study of 50,322 hospitalization records of DM patients found that 20% of these hospitalizations were associated with a concurrent atherosclerotic cardiovascular diagnosis or procedure. Additionally, DM patients with CAD were twice as likely to die during hospitalization compared to age and sex-matched controls with CAD, and compared to DM patients without CAD [158].

In a prospective case-control study in Taiwan in which 907 DM patients and 4535 age and sex-matched controls were followed over 2 years, 14 patients with DM (1.5%) vs. 18 controls (0.4%) sustained acute myocardial infarctions. After adjustment for cardiovascular risk factors, the hazard ratio for an acute myocardial infarction among patients with DM was 3.37 (95% confidence interval 1.67–6.8, $p = 0.0007$) [159]. In this study, 46 DM patients (5.1%) and 133 controls (2.9%) experienced an ischemic cerebrovascular event, resulting in an adjusted hazard ratio of 1.78 (95% confidence interval 1.29–2.49, $p = 0.0028$) [159].

These studies underscore the importance of recognizing the increased CAD risk in DM patients. Cardiovascular risk factors should be addressed and corticosteroid exposure should be minimized while the underlying inflammation is controlled with corticosteroid-sparing therapies.

Thromboembolic Disease

In a large retrospective study of 355 DM patients and 443 polymyositis patients, an increased risk of deep vein thrombosis (DVT) was found among patients with DM (hazard ratio 9.40 [95% CI 2.88 to 30.68]) and polymyositis (hazard ratio 6.16 [95% CI 2.50 to 13.92])as compared to age- and sex-matched controls [111]. In this study, risk of pulmonary embolism (PE) was significantly increased among polymyositis patients (hazard ratio 9.42 [95% CI 4.59 to 18.70]), but this risk did not reach statistical significance in the DM cohort (hazard ratio 4.70 [95% CI 0.85 to 25.98]) [160].

Similarly, a trend towards increased risk of venous thromboembolism (VTE) was noted in a Spanish cohort of 87 DM patients in whom 6 developed the event (6.8%)[161]. In large epidemiologic studies combing DM and polymyositis patients from Sweden [162] and the United Kingdom [163], the risk of PE was increased (standardized incidence ratio 16.44 [95% CI 11.57–22.69]) compared to the baseline population risk. Thus, while the risk of DVT appears to be elevated in DM, the risk of VTE or PE needs further clarification.

Joint Manifestations

Arthritis is reported in 30–40% of DM patients [164–166]. Although arthritis frequently presents concurrently with the initial presentation of myositis, flares of arthritis affect only 50% of patients during disease relapses [167].

Arthritis and arthralgias are more common among DM patients with anti-MDA5 and anti-synthetase antibodies. Hall et al. found 9 of 11 (81.8%) anti-MDA5 patients exhibited an inflammatory arthritis, as compared to 40 of 149 (26.7%, $p < 0.001$) non-MDA5 DM patients [168]. DM patients with anti-synthetase antibodies, most commonly Jo-1, may also demonstrate non-erosive arthritis in up to 93% of cases [167]. In these patients, the non-erosive arthritis may occur in the setting of "anti-synthetase syndrome" which consists of fever, arthritis, myositis, ILD, mechanic's hands and/or Raynaud's phenomenon, as reviewed above.

Symmetric non-erosive polyarthropathy is the most common arthritis presentation in patients with anti-MDA5 and anti-synthetase antibodies [77, 168]. However, erosive changes have been reported, more commonly in the anti-synthetase antibody subset [169–172]. In these instances, DM patients with arthritis as the presenting symptom may be misdiagnosed with rheumatoid arthritis or a rheumatoid arthritis overlap disease [173].

In general, the arthritis in DM is mild to moderate in severity and typically involves the small joints of the hands (including the wrists and metacarpophalangeal and proximal interphalangeal joints) as well as the shoulders, elbows, and ankles [167]. Signs and symptoms of inflammatory arthritis include joint swelling, morning stiffness for 30 minutes or longer, or joint pain that improves with activity.

On examination, one must first determine if the pain is articular in origin, as opposed to involving the periarticular soft tissue such as tendons, ligaments or bursae. Asking the patient to point and localize the exact area of pain may be helpful. Key points in the rheumatologic exam include inspection for deformity, swelling, and muscle wasting. Examination for synovitis, indicative of active joint inflammation, includes palpation of the small joints of the hands as well as elbows, shoulders, knees and symptomatic joints, evaluating for warmth, range of motion, swelling or palpable fluid, and tenderness. True articular pathology will limit both active and passive range of motion, in contrast to tendonitis, in which pain will be elicited with active range of motion alone. Inflammatory markers (erythrocyte sedimentation rate, C-reactive protein) may or may not be elevated.

The differential diagnosis for joint pain in DM patients includes osteoarthritis, rheumatoid arthritis, polymyalgia rheumatica, infectious arthritis, crystalline arthropathies and chronic pain syndromes.

In osteoarthritis, morning stiffness may last only one to several minutes, and the pain is often worse with activity. Joint swelling is typically absent.

Rheumatoid arthritis is typically associated with elevated acute phase reactants in addition to elevated titers of rheumatoid factor and antibodies to cyclic citrullinated peptide. Rash and myositis are rare.

Polymyalgia rheumatica is characterized by morning stiffness in the shoulder and hip girdles in patients over the age of 50 years. Characteristically, it is associated with an elevated sedimentation rate. Although weakness may be reported, examination will demonstrate normal muscle strength [174].

Infectious arthritis should be considered in any immunosuppressed host presenting with acute onset of monoarticular joint pain and swelling. Fever, tachycardia, malaise, and/or leukocytosis may or may not be present. If the suspicion is high for infectious arthritis, urgent referral for arthrocentesis and evaluation for septic arthritis is necessary.

Crystalline arthropathies include gout and pseudogout or chondrocalcinosis. These entities typically present with acute onset of mono- or polyarticular arthritis with crystals (monosodium urate in gout and calcium pyrophosphate crystals in pseudogout) observed upon arthrocentesis of the involved joints.

Chronic pain syndrome is often seen in combination with rheumatic conditions. Pain is diffuse, and there are multiple tender points, typically over myofascial points instead of over joints.

Patients with joint disease having synovitis / inflammation may benefit from being on hydroxychloroquine and may warrant the choice of methorexate as initial immunosuppressive therapy.

Renal Manifestations

Direct renal involvement in DM is rare and has not been well described. However, renal complications in DM may be more common than previously thought. These complications occur via three broad mechanisms: (1) rhabdomyolysis, (2) presence of an associated glomerulopathy, and (3) drug-induced nephrotoxicity.

In cases of acute fulminant myositis, which typically occurs at disease onset, rhabdomyolysis may result in myoglobin-induced acute tubular necrosis (183,184).

Multiple types of nephropathies have been reported in association with DM, the most common (~50%) of which is immune complex-mediated glomerulonephritis [175]. Other reported glomerulopathies in association with DM include IgA nephropathy [176–178], membranous nephropathy [179–181], diffuse proliferative glomerulonephritis [182], and anti-neutrophil cytoplasmic antibody (ANCA)-associated crescentic glomerulonephritis [183, 184].

A recent French retrospective cohort study by Couvrat-Desvergnes et al. found that among 96 DM patients, 21 (22%) had evidence of chronic kidney disease (CKD) [175]. In 40% of these patients, nephrotoxicity was thought to be medication-induced. Five of the DM patients underwent renal biopsy, which revealed vascular lesions in two patients, minimal change disease in two patients, and focal segmental glomerulosclerosis and vascular lesions in one patient. Risk factors for development of CKD were presence of cardiovascular risk factors such as hypertension and diabetes (HR 16.56, 95% CI 2.56–107.16, $p = 0.0032$), previous episode of acute kidney injury (HR 15.09, 95% CI 6.19–36.79, $p < 0.0001$) and age at myositis onset (HR per year of increased age 1.05, 95% CI 1.02–1.08, $p = 0.0016$). Female sex was protective (HR 0.4, 95% CI 0.18–0.89, $p = 0.0024$).

Further study is needed to validate these associations in DM patients and to characterize the mechanism of renal injury. Nonetheless, it is important to be aware of the potential for renal involvement in DM patients. It is prudent to carefully monitor renal function, particularly early in the disease course, especially in patients with severe myositis, cardiovascular risk factors, previous episodes of acute kidney injury, or exposure to nephrotoxic medications.

Rare Manifestations

Macrophage activation syndrome (MAS), also known as acquired hemophagocytic lymphohistiocytosis (HLH), is a severe and potentially fatal complication or presenting syndrome in DM. MAS is a state of dysregulated immune hyperactivation of macrophages that can lead to multisystem organ failure and death. Clinical features include prolonged high fever, lymphadenopathy, and hepatosplenomegaly, with laboratory findings of hyperferritinemia (>500 mg/dl), cytopenias (hemoglobin <9 g/dl, platelets <100,000/mm^3, neutrophils <1000/mm^3), hypertriglyceridemia (>265 mg/dl), hemophagocytosis in the bone marrow, spleen or lymph nodes, low natural killer cell activity, and elevation of soluble CD25 (> 400 U/l) [185].

Cancer

DM is associated with an internal malignancy in 10–20% of cases [2]. A meta-analysis by Olazagasti et al. analyzed seven population-based and three hospital-based DM cohorts with follow-up of 3.7 to 10.4 years. They found a standardized incidence ratio of 4.79 for cancer development during follow-up (95% confidence interval 3.71–5.87) [1]. Buchbinder et al. retrospectively reviewed 537 patients with biopsy-proven idiopathic inflammatory myopathy. DM was diagnosed in 85 of these cases over an average follow-up period of 5.3 years. A malignancy was observed in 32 (42%) patients, and the risk of cancer diagnosis was greatest within the first 3 years after diagnosis of DM [186].

Although cancer types appear to vary based on population studied, the most common malignancies associated with DM include breast, lung, ovarian, prostate, colorectal, gastric, and pancreatic cancers, as well as non-Hodgkin lymphoma [187–189]. Nasopharyngeal cancer is more common among Southeast Asians [190].

The autoantibodies anti-TIF1-γ and possibly anti-NXP2 are associated with an increased risk of cancer in DM. NXP2 has a role in activating p53 and inducing cellular senescence [191, 192] while TIF1-γ interacts with Smad2/3 in embryonic stem cells to modulate transcriptional elongation and tissue differentiation [192]. In collaboration with researchers at Johns Hopkins, we found that anti-NXP2 and anti-TIF1-γ antibodies were observed in 37 of 213 DM patients (17%) and 82 of 213 (38%), respectively. A cancer was detected in 14% (29/213) of these DM patients. Among the 20 patients with cancer, 24 (83%) had antibodies to either NXP2 or TIF1-γ [193]. In addition, anti-NXP2 antibodies were disproportionately represented among male DM patients having cancer (7 of 9 patients, 78%). Similarly, Ichimura et al. reviewed 457 cases of DM and found that seven patients (1.6%) had anti-NXP2 antibodies [191]. Of those, three (43%) had associated malignancies, all of whom were male. Trallero-Araguas et al. meta-analyzed six studies that included 312 adult DM patients and found a 27-fold higher odds of developing cancer-associated myositis (95% CI 6.59–112.82) among anti-TIF1-γ positive DM patients [194]. Of note, however, at least in the U.S. population, most DM patients with these antibodies still do not harbor a malignancy.

Regardless of autoantibody status, the frequency of cancer-associated DM increases in patients over age 60 years [195]. Other proposed risk factors include male sex, presence of constitutional symptoms [196], highly elevated erythrocyte sedimentation rate, and cutaneous necrosis (208).

There are no existing guidelines for cancer screening in patients with newly diagnosed DM. In a case series of 33 DM patients, 13 of whom had coexisting malignancies, initial routine cancer screening failed to discover 4 malignancies (30%) [196]. In collaboration with the University of Louisville, we have retrospectively examined cancer screening practices at our two institutions in a cohort of 400 DM patients [197]. In this cohort, 16 patients harbored an unknown internal malignancy at the time of DM diagnosis but had no symptoms or signs of cancer based on physical examination and routine blood testing (blood counts, chemistry and urinalysis). Blind testing with CT scan, colonoscopy, mammogram, and prostate-specific antigen evaluation revealed the cancer in these patients. Blind screening may therefore be of benefit in detecting malignancy in at least a proportion of DM patients. Identifying the most appropriate screening tests, the timing and frequency of these screenings, and the population subset most appropriate for these screenings is a high priority.

In addition to a complete history and physical examination, routine age-appropriate cancer screening studies (colonoscopy, mammogram, prostate exam) and relevant screening bloodwork (complete blood count, renal and liver function tests) as well as a urinalysis are indicated at the time of DM diagnosis. The role of other blood tests, including erythrocyte sedimentation rate, C-reactive protein, serum cancer markers, and serum and urine protein immunofixation electrophoresis, is currently not established. Our practice is to perform screening CT scans of the chest, abdomen and pelvis, and to consider screening ultrasound of the thyroid gland and transvaginal ultrasound of the ovaries.

The necessity for annual re-screening for malignancy is even less clear. We recommend that re-screening be considered in clinically high-risk patients whose disease is difficult to control or those who have experienced a substantial disease flare after a sustained quiescent period. Of note, treatment of the associated malignancy may result in disease remission.

Principles of Management

Overview

Appropriate management of DM hinges on ascertaining a comprehensive understanding of the involved organ systems. ILD and underlying malignancies are the leading causes of disease-related death in DM and thus should be prioritized in treatment. Establishing collaborative relationships with co-managing providers (rheumatologist, dermatologist, cardiologist, pulmonologist) is essential to monitor disease activity and optimize therapeutic strategies when multiple organ systems are involved.

Many DM patients ultimately enter a long-term remission, often induced by prolonged immunomodulation and/or immunosuppression [198]. Rarely, DM may spontaneously remit without therapy [199]. In our experience, sustaining immunosuppression or immunomodulation for at least 9–12 months after remission is achieved may decrease the likelihood of relapse.

The evidence for medical therapies in DM is derived largely from single-center, retrospective case series, case reports, and expert opinion. Only 15 randomized clinical trials have been performed on DM treatment, including the Rituximab in Myositis (RIM) trial, which represents the largest clinical trial to date, with 76 adult and 48 juvenile DM patients. Gordon et al. identified 14 additional randomized clinical trials in a Cochrane Review from 2012[200]. Ten of these trials, the largest of which included 62 patients, were analyzed in that review. As such, therapeutic strategies are currently informed mostly by expert opinion [201–204].

Treatment of the skin disease in DM is challenging. In a single patient, multiple systemic immunomodulatory and immunosuppressive agents must often be combined to achieve control. Moreover, skin disease and muscle disease often have discordant response to treatment[205]. In some patients, recalcitrant skin disease may be active for years after remission is achieved for myopathy. Given the chronicity, and in some cases the recalcitrance, of the skin disease, it is worthwhile to weigh the long-term toxicity of the prescribed therapy against the achieved or potential cutaneous benefit. Commonly used systemic agents for cutaneous DM are discussed below, along with other management strategies.

Behavioral Change

Photoprotection is an essential first step in management of the cutaneous disease in DM. However, it is important to note that up to 60% of DM patients are only minimally photosensitive, and as few as 20% report disease exacerbation after UV exposure [205, 206]. Despite this observation, it is prudent to counsel patients on UV protection. Patients should be advised to use broad-spectrum sunscreens that protect against both UVA and UVB radiation, wear sun-protective clothing, avoid exposure during hours of high UV intensity (10 a.m. to 4 p.m.), and seek shade whenever possible.

Physical Medicine and Rehabilitation

Strength training has been shown to improve muscle strength and function in patients with DM[207–209], while aerobic exercise has been shown to improve endurance [210, 211]. In a randomized clinical trial of patients with active disease, a home strength training program was shown to be safe [212] but conferred no benefit in strength or disease control over the control group, who performed range of motion exercises [213]. We advise all patients to enroll in a physical therapy program soon after diagnosis to prevent injury and to maintain mobility and muscle strength.

Topical Agents

Topical Corticosteroids

Topical corticosteroids play a supportive role in suppressing cutaneous inflammation in DM and can provide temporary relief, but they are unlikely to fully control even mild cutaneous disease activity.

For the scalp and body, class I or class II topical corticosteroids, applied twice daily, are typically necessary to ameliorate pruritus, erythema and scale. They can be applied under occlusion with plastic wrap to increase potency, a technique that is particularly helpful for painful nail bed disease or hyperkeratotic plaques on the elbows and knees.

For the face and intertriginous zones, low potency (class VI) topical corticosteroidsare preferred to minimize the risk of atrophy and hypopigmentation. When necessary, class I or class II corticosteroids may be applied to the face or intertriginous area for brief intervals (i.e., 2 weeks) followed by similar periods (i.e., 2 weeks) off therapy.

Topical Calcineurin Inhibitors

Topical calcineurin inhibitors (TCIs), such as tacrolimus 0.1% ointment, have shown modest efficacy in several cases of cutaneous DM [214–217]. One study in 6 patients with cutaneous DM using a split face design with vehicle applied on the contralateral face showed no detectable benefit of tacrolimus ointment 0.1% after 2 months [218]. Pimecrolimus 1% cream used twice daily for 4–6 months was reported to significantly improve cutaneous disease in DM in two patients who were concomitantly treated with hydroxychloroquine, prednisone and methotrexate [219].

There are no studies comparing the efficacy of TCIs to topical corticosteroids in DM. However, unlike potent topical corticosteroids, TCIs may be used safely on the face without concern for atrophy or hypopigmentation. As such, TCIs may represent valuable topical corticosteroid-sparing agents in DM owing to their favorable side effect profile.

Transient application site reactions are the most common adverse effects of TCIs, manifesting as a warm or burning sensation in up to 58% of patients [220]. This burning is likely due to local induction of release of neuropeptides, such as substance P, from sensory nerve endings [221]. The burning sensation typically lasts 10–15 minutes after application and subsides after 3–7 days of regular use [222].

Systemic Medications

Antimalarials

Antimalarials are often used as first-line agents for cutaneous DM. Retrospective studies suggest that improvement is seen in approximately 30–50% of cutaneous DM patients on antimalarials[223]. In our experience, however, this improvement is generally mild. In addition, up to 30% of DM patients may experience a drug eruption (morbilliform or lichenoid) in the days or weeks after initiating hydroxychloroquine [224]. Antimalarials are therefore a reasonable choice for management of cutaneous DM in mild cases where the patient prefers to avoid immunosuppression and is comfortable waiting 4–6 months for a detectable response. The addition of quinacrine to hydroxychloroquine or chloroquine may result in higher efficacy than single-agent therapy [225]. Hydroxychloroquine may also be useful for treating mild symptoms of inflammatory arthritis, and chloroquine was noted to ameliorate arthritis in DM in one case report [226].

Methotrexate

Methotrexate is effective in significantly reducing cutaneous disease severity in 50–100% of DM patients [227–230]. In combination with prednisone, it also represents first-line treatment for myositis; doses of 20–25 mg per week are typically necessary to control muscle inflammation [164, 231]. Methotrexate is also a preferable treatment choice when concomitant arthritis is present [232].

It is important to recognize that elevation of serum transaminases should not preclude the use of methotrexate in a patient with active myositis, as these elevations might be related to the muscle disease. Switching from oral to subcutaneous or intramuscular administration may improve gastrointestinal tolerability [231] and efficacy [228] as compared with oral administration. Splitting the methotrexate dose into two, each 12 hours apart, also improved bioavailability. Patients should be counseled regarding oligospermia, teratogenicity, hepatotoxicity and bone marrow suppression with methotrexate. The cutaneous side effects include mucositis and hair shedding, which are mitigated by increasing folic acid supplementation. When ILD is present, it is prudent to avoid methotrexate due to its potential to induce acute pneumonitis and pulmonary fibrosis [233, 234].

Systemic Corticosteroids

For cutaneous DM, systemic corticosteroids are undesirable agents as monotherapy, as they usually elicit only partial responses, even at moderate to high doses, and require long-term administration. The predictable toxicities associated with prolonged high-dose corticosteroids outweigh the potential cutaneous benefits.

In myositis, by contrast, systemic corticosteroids are considered first-line, though formal, controlled studies regarding dose or tapering regimens have not been performed [235]. Complete clinical responses in muscle inflammation with prednisone monotherapy at doses greater than 0.5 mg/kg/day have been achieved in 27% [236] to 87% [237] of DM patients [238]. Oral or intra-articular corticosteroids are typically highly effective for the arthritis associated with DM [232].

The addition of corticosteroid-sparing agents may improve control of myositis and extramuscular inflammation, but their critical role is to minimize toxicities of oral corticosteroids, including the risk for corticosteroid-induced myopathy [239]. At our institution, a corticosteroid-sparing agent is started simultaneously or soon after oral corticosteroids. Although oral corticosteroids are used as empiric therapy for ILD associated with DM [127], response rates with monotherapy may be as low as 50% [240–243], and thus the addition or substitution of a corticosteroid-sparing agent is usually required.

Mycophenolate Mofetil

Mycophenolate mofetil (MMF) has been shown to be effective in reducing cutaneous disease severity [244, 245] and myositis in DM at doses of 2–3 grams divided daily [246–248]. It is considered the first line oral agent when ILD is present [249–253].

A significant proportion (20%) of patients will experience nausea or diarrhea on MMF at 2 g daily [254]. When gastrointestinal side effects are dose-limiting, switching to enteric-coated mycophenolate sodium is an option for maintaining the current dosing with improved tolerability[255].

Methotrexate and mycophenolate may be combined when either alone is insufficient to achieve disease control. Patients receiving combination therapy may require increased monitoring for bone marrow suppression, infection and neoplasia.

Intravenous Immunoglobulin

Intravenous immunoglobulin (IVIG) appears to be the single most effective agent for cutaneous DM, with up to 70–80% of patients achieving an almost complete or complete response (272,273). IVIG is also effective for myositis [256, 257]. The first randomized placebo-controlled crossover trial of IVIG in DM, including 15 patients in 1993 [258], showed a significant improvement in muscle strength in 9/12 (75%) patients and dramatic improvements in skin disease based on clinical photographs in 8/12 (67%) patients who received IVIG.

The standard dosing regimen is 2 grams/kg divided over 2–3 days, infused monthly. The therapeutic effect may be perceived as early as 2 weeks, but it may not be fully evident until 3–4 months of treatment. Because IVIG works relatively quickly in decreasing muscle inflammation, along with high dose corticosteroids, we often use this agent in hospitalized patients who are rapidly declining or are acutely ill with dysphagia or respiratory muscle involvement. In circumstances in which immunosuppression is relatively contraindicated, such as in patients with a history of malignancy or recurrent infection, IVIG offers a safe and effective means to gain disease control.

There are case reports of IVIG ameliorating ILD in DM [259], polymyositis [260], and systemic sclerosis [261, 262]. Further study is needed to clarify the benefit of IVIG in ILD. There is also interest in transitioning to subcutaneous immunoglobulin due to ease of dosing, particularly to maintain disease control after remission is achieved with IVIG[263–265].

IVIG is generally well-tolerated, though up to 56% of patients may experience headache, which can be severe and debilitating. The rate of infusion, the total dose [266] and the formulation of IVIG [267] may influence the occurrence of headache. Aseptic meningitis is a rare adverse effect of IVIG, manifesting as fever, headache, photophobia, meningismus, and neutrophilic pleocytosis or eosinophilia in the cerebrospinal fluid [268, 269]. It occurs 24–48 hours after infusion and generally resolves spontaneously without sequelae in 2–7 days. Acute kidney injury is another rare complication of IVIG; risk factors include pre-existing renal insufficiency, concomitant administration of nephrotoxic medications or sucrose preparations, and dehydration [269]. Anaphylaxis is also rare but may occur in patients with primary IgA deficiency; checking serum IgA levels prior to infusion is therefore recommended. There is no evidence that having low but detectable immunoglobulin levels confers any increased risk for anaphylaxis [266]. Finally, the risk for thrombotic complications with IVIG must be considered in patients with concomitant hypercoagulable states.

Rituximab

Rituximab has shown mixed results for cutaneous DM [270, 271], and the current evidence does not support its use for cutaneous disease alone. With regard to myositis, the RIM trial randomized 200 patients (76 with polymyositis, 76 DM, 48 juvenile DM) to either rituximab at week 0 (early) or week 8 (late), with the primary endpoint of time to disease improvement. Although there was no significant difference in the time to improvement, 83% of refractory adult and juvenile myositis patients ultimately met criteria for disease improvement [272]. A shorter time to improvement was seen in patients with anti-synthetase antibodies, namely anti-Jo-1 (hazard ratio 3.08, $p < 0.01$) and anti-Mi-2 (hazard ratio 2.5 $p < 0.01$) [273].

Rituximab has been reported to be successful in retrospective studies for the treatment of ILD. Andersson et al. published their experience with 112 patients with anti-synthetase syndrome-related ILD: of the 24 patients with severe ILD who received rituximab, 24% had improvement in FVC and 17% had improvement in diffusion capacity at 1 year [274]. The benefit was most pronounced in the 7 patients with disease duration of less than 12 months and those with acute onset of ILD. Another retrospective cohort study found that 4 of 5 patients with DM or polymyositis-associated ILD exhibited 18% improvement in FVC and 22% in diffusion capacity 9–12 months after receiving rituximab [275].

Rituximab dosing in DM typically follows the rheumatoid arthritis protocol of 1000 mg administered intravenously at day 0 and day 14 [271]. Infectious complications are the most frequent [276] serious adverse effects in DM patients, with rare reports of progressive multifocal leukoencephalopathy [276–278].

Cyclosporine

Cyclosporine, a calcineurin inhibitor, binds cyclophilin, inhibiting interleukin-2 production and T cell activation. The evidence for cyclosporine in cutaneous DM is limited to case reports [279], but it has been found to be a rapidly acting and effective agent for myositis [280]. A randomized clinical trial of 36 patients with DM ($n = 20$) or polymyositis ($n = 16$) comparing cyclosporine (3–3.5 mg/kg/day) with methotrexate (7.5-15 mg weekly) in addition to oral corticosteroids found comparable decreases in CK and improvements in strength between the groups at 6 months [281].

Cyclosporine is utilized in the setting of severe ILD as rescue therapy [241, 282] and has also been shown to improve overall survival in retrospective studies [283]. When used in combination with intravenous cyclophosphamide and pulse dose methylprednisolone, cyclosporine has been found beneficial for rapidly progressive ILD in anti-MDA5 DM patients in Asia [284]. Cyclosporine is dosed based on ideal body weight and has improved bioavailability in its hydrophilic microemulsion [285].

Careful monitoring of renal function and blood pressure is needed for the duration of treatment with cyclosporine; nephrotoxicity risk is highest at doses above 3 mg/kg/day [286, 287]. Cyclosporine may also induce hirsutism, gingival hyperplasia, and increased LDL cholesterol and triglyceride levels.

Tofacitinib

Tofacitinib is an oral Janus kinase (JAK)-1/3 inhibitor approved for use in rheumatoid arthritis, psoriatic arthritis, and ulcerative colitis. It suppresses interferon signaling [288], which is upregulated in DM [289], and it has therefore been investigated as an off-label treatment for this condition.

In a 2016 case series of three patients with refractory cutaneous DM, all subjects demonstrated improvement in the validated Cutaneous Dermatomyositis Disease Area and Severity

Index (CDASI) activity score as well as in pruritus [290]. Similarly, in a 2019 case series, four patients with DM refractory to immunosuppressive and immunomodulatory therapy experienced significant improvement in cutaneous and extracutaneous manifestations when treated with tofacitinib [291].

Adverse effects of tofacitinib include infection, nasopharyngitis, myocardial infarction, stroke, cancer, blood clots, and death. Laboratory monitoring is recommended due to risk of lymphocytopenia, neutropenia, anemia, elevated liver function tests, and increased serum cholesterol.

Tacrolimus

Tacrolimus, another calcineurin inhibitor, binds FK binding protein and is 100 times more potent a T-cell inhibitor than is cyclosporine [292]. There are case reports of improvement in cutaneous DM with tacrolimus [293], most often for patients with juvenile DM [294, 295]. Tacrolimus has been found to be beneficial in treatment of myositis and may allow for accelerated corticosteroid tapering [293]. However, this agent is typically reserved for refractory ILD, with several retrospective reports supporting its efficacy [296–298], particularly in the anti-synthetase antibody group [299]. Tacrolimus has also shown prolonged survival benefit for treatment of ILD compared with prednisone alone [300].

As with cyclosporine, due to a low therapeutic index and high inter-patient variability in pharmacodynamics, close monitoring of renal function is necessary during tacrolimus therapy to avoid nephrotoxicity. In addition, tacrolimus has been associated with GI upset and hypomagnesemia [301].

Nonsteroidal Anti-inflammatory Drugs

Nonsteroidal anti-inflammatory drugs (NSAIDs) have been reported to be useful as initial therapy for arthritis associated with juvenile DM [232]. NSAIDs are typically not effective as monotherapy for moderate or severe arthritis [226] but may be useful adjunctive agents in cases where arthritis becomes more symptomatic as oral corticosteroids are tapered. Cycloxygenase-2 selective NSAIDs such as celecoxib or meloxicam are preferred due to better gastrointestinal tolerability [302, 303], particularly if the patient is on concomitant oral corticosteroids.

Azathioprine

Azathioprine has not been assessed specifically in cutaneous DM. In combined studies of DM and polymyositis, azathioprine has shown efficacy in improving myositis, in up to 75% of cases [304–306], as well as overall survival [307]. The first randomized controlled trial of 28 patients with polymyositis or DM compared prednisolone in combination with azathioprine 2.5 mg/kg/day versus prednisolone in combination with methotrexate 15 mg weekly and found no difference in efficacy for myositis [25]. The second randomized controlled crossover trial of 30 patients with polymyositis or DM showed improved response in the group receiving combination oral methotrexate and azathioprine (8/15, 53%) as compared to the group receiving methotrexate alone (3/15, 20%) [280].

We occasionally combine low dose azathioprine with methotrexate when myositis is persistent with methotrexate alone. Azathioprine is commonly used as maintenance therapy in the treatment of ILD associated with idiopathic inflammatory myopathies [127, 142], typically following induction with cyclophosphamide [308, 309].

Azathioprine has comparable tolerability to methotrexate, with risks of bone marrow suppression and gastrointestinal upset [306]. Initially, thiopurine methyltransferase (TPMT) levels should be checked to avoid severe bone marrow toxicity. Additionally, a rare systemic hypersensitivity reaction, manifesting with fever, myalgia, nausea, vomiting, hypotension and shock, has been reported; it may occur in the first 4 weeks of therapy [310] and resolves with drug discontinuation.

Leflunomide

Leflunomide inhibits pyrimidine synthesis, leukocyte adhesion to vascular endothelium, and nuclear factor kappa-light-chain-enhancer of activated B cells (NF-κB) [311], resulting in immunosuppressive and anti-inflammatory effects. Although leflunomide is used primarily to treat rheumatoid arthritis, there are 4 reported cases of its use to treat DM, with evidence of improvement in both skin and muscle disease at 20 mg daily [312, 313]. We find it useful particularly in the setting of arthritis in DM, or as a corticosteroid-sparing agent for both skin and muscle disease in patients with intolerance or poor response to methotrexate or MMF.

The most commonly reported side effectsof leflunomide are gastrointestinal, with diarrhea, nausea and abdominal pain [314]seen in 10–25% of patients. Less common side effects include alopecia, hypertension and hepatotoxicity [315, 316]. Leflunomide may induce acute interstitial pneumonitis in patients with inflammatory arthritis [317–319] and therefore may not be preferable in patients with ILD.

Dapsone

Dapsone is a sulfone antibiotic that inhibits neutrophil function and complement activation [320]. Its potential for benefit in cutaneous DM has been noted in several case reports [321–323]. In one case report [323], there was concomitant improvement in skin and muscle disease on dapsone 75 mg daily. There is no evidence for the use of dapsone in ILD.

Quantitative glucose-6-phosphate dehydrogenase (G6PD) levels should be checked prior to initiation to prevent methemoglobinemia and severe hemolysis. Common side effects include a dose-dependent hemolysis and gastrointestinal upset [324]. Rarely, hepatotoxicity, agranulocytosis and aplastic anemia have been reported, justifying serial blood monitoring [325].

Thalidomide

Thalidomide is a glutamic acid derivative that inhibits expression of tumor necrosis factor alpha (TNFα) adhesion molecules on neutrophils, TNFα synthesis, neutrophil phagocytosis, and angiogenesis [326]. We noted one case report describing its benefit in cutaneous DM, with 60% improvement [327]. Teratogenicity and increased risk of thrombosis [328] preclude its use in many patients. As many as 25% of patients may develop a dose-dependent sensory peripheral neuropathy [17, 329].

Cyclophosphamide

Skin disease rarely warrants treatment with cytotoxic agents, except perhaps when there is evidence of progressive cutaneous vasculitis [45]. The alkylating agent cyclophosphamide may be used, however, for refractory or rapidly progressive myositis. Most commonly in DM, cyclophosphamide is indicated for the treatment of ILD [45, 309, 330–338].

Although a randomized controlled trial demonstrated efficacy over placebo in the treatment of systemic sclerosis-associated ILD [339], the supportive evidence for the treatment of ILD associated with inflammatory myopathies derives primarily from case reports. In a randomized trial of 10 DM patients with rapidly progressive ILD, Kameda et al. compared a three-drug combination regimen (prednisolone 0.5 mg/kg/day, intravenous cyclophosphamide 10–30 mg/kg every 3–4 weeks, and cyclosporine 2–4 mg/kg/day) with dual agent therapy consisting of corticosteroids plus either agent alone [299]. Yamasaki et al. treated 14 DM patients with refractory ILD with intravenous cyclophosphamide 300–800 mg/m^2 every 4 weeks and observed significant improvements in HRCT, PFTs, and dyspnea [45].

Cyclophosphamide may produce a host of immediate toxicities, including nausea and vomiting, alopecia, myelosuppression, hemorrhagic cystitis and, rarely, interstitial pneumonitis [340]. Long-term toxicities include malignancy (skin, bladder and hematologic) [341], infertility and gonadal failure [342]. Vigilant monitoring with serial blood tests and urinalyses is essential.

Special Cases: Calcinosis Cutis and Ulceration

Calcinosis is the Achilles heel for DM patients and clinicians alike. Surgical excision for localized lesions remains the definitive therapy [312]. Data are lacking to guide medical therapy. Multiple agents have been proposed, including anti-inflammatories and calcium and phosphate modulators, but no single agent is reliably effective [26]. IVIG has been reported to be effective in some cases, especially in juvenile DM, [313, 343, 344] but not others [345]. Bisphosphonates have been cited as effective for calcinosis in juvenile DM, but controlled studies are needed [346, 347]. The editor (AG) of this textbook has observed softening and size reductions of plaques and nodules of calcinosis with both intralesional and intravenous sodium thiosulfate (personal communication). Lastly, a study of risk factors for calcinosis identified that digital ulcers were present in 50% of DM patients with digital ulcers vs. 9% without digital ulcers ($p < .001$), suggesting a common underlying vascular mechanism [31]; given these data, it is plausible that long-term vasodilatory therapy may be effective for the prevention and treatment of calcinosis.

Cutaneous ulceration in anti-MDA5 DM patients can also be challenging to treat. We have found coexisting thrombophilias in several of our patients with this autoantibody. Treatment of any underlying hypercoagulable state may be instrumental in ulcer healing. We speculate that the pathophysiology of ulceration in anti-MDA5 DM is a vasculopathy with endothelial damage and microvascular occlusion. The most common sites of ulceration are the extensor surfaces over the joints or on the digits [24]. We have achieved resolution of chronic ulceration by using potent vasodilators, such as phosphodiesterase inhibitors like sildenafil 20–40 mg three times daily.

Summary

Dermatomyositis (DM) is a systemic autoimmune disease that commonly manifests with inflammation of the skin, muscle and lungs. Patients are at increased risk of malignancy at disease onset and should undergo cancer screening. ILD is another important cause of morbidity and mortality in DM. Collaboration between rheumatology and dermatology, among other disciplines, is essential to ensure appropriate assessment of all possible involved organs and treatment monitoring.

Skin and muscle disease often respond at different rates and require different treatments. Patients may require multiple agents to achieve remission, and the risks and benefits of such treatment must be weighed carefully given the frequent need for long-term treatment.

References

1. Olazagasti JM, et al. Cancer risk in dermatomyositis: a meta-analysis of cohort studies. Am J Clin Dermatol. 2015;16(2):89–98.
2. Madan V, et al. Defining cancer risk in dermatomyositis. Clin Exp Dermatol. 2009;34:451–5.
3. Meyer A, et al. Incidence and prevalence of inflammatory myopathies: a systematic review. Rheumatology (Oxford). 2015;54(1):50–63.
4. Bernatsky S, et al. Estimating the prevalence of polymyositis and dermatomyositis from administrative data: age, sex and regional differences. Ann Rheum Dis. 2009;68:1192–6.
5. Bendewald MJ, et al. Incidence of dermatomyositis and clinically amyopathic dermatomyositis: a population-based study in Olmsted County, Minnesota. Arch Dermatol. 2010;146(1):26–30.
6. See LC, et al. Sex-and age-specific incidence of autoimmune rheumatic diseases in the Chinese population: a Taiwan population-based study. Semin Arthritis Rheum. 2013;43(3):381–6.
7. Hengstman GJ, et al. The relative prevalence of dermatomyositis and polymyositis in Europe exhibits a latitudinal gradient. Ann Rheum Dis. 2000;59:141–2.
8. Okada S, et al. Global surface ultraviolet radiation intensity may modulate the clinical and immunologic expression of autoimmune muscle disease. Arthritis Rheum. 2003;48(8):2285–93.
9. Love LA, et al. Ultraviolet radiation intensity predicts the relative distribution of dermatomyositis and anti-Mi-2 autoantibodies in women. Arthritis Rheum. 2009;60:2499–504.
10. Petri MH, et al. Implications in the difference of anti-Mi-2 and-p155/140 autoantibody prevalence in two dermatomyositis cohorts from Mexico City and Guadalajara. Arthritis Res Ther. 2013;15(2):R48.
11. Shah M, et al. Brief report ultraviolet radiation exposure is associated with clinical and autoantibody phenotypes in juvenile myositis. Arthritis Rheum. 2013;65(7):1934–41.
12. Bohan A, Peter JB. Polymyositis and dermatomyositis (second of two parts). N Engl J Med. 1975;292(8 SRC):403–7.
13. Bohan A, et al. Polymyositis and dermatomyositis (first of two parts). N Engl J Med. 1975;292:344–7.
14. Pearson C. Arthritis and allied conditions: a textbook of rheumatology, Polymyositis and dermatomyositis. 9th ed. Philadelphia: Lea & Febiger; 1972.
15. Euwer RL, Sontheimer RD. Amyopathic dermatomyositis (dermatomyositis sine myositis).

Presentation of six new cases and review of the literature. J Am Acad Dermatol. 1991;24:959–66.
16. Sontheimer RD. Dermatomyositis: an overview of recent progress with emphasis on dermatologic aspects. Dermatol Clin. 2002;20(3):387–408.
17. Bastuji-Garin S, et al. Incidence and risk factors for thalidomide neuropathy: a prospective study of 135 dermatologic patients. J Invest Dermatol. 2002;119:1020–6.
18. Love LA, et al. A new approach to the classification of idiopathic inflammatory myopathy: myositis-specific autoantibodies define useful homogeneous patient groups. Medicine (Baltimore). 1991;70:360–74.
19. Schultz HY, et al. From pathogenesis, epidemiology, and genetics to definitions, diagnosis, and treatments of cutaneous lupus erythematosus and dermatomyositis: a report from the 3rd International Conference on Cutaneous Lupus Erythematosus (ICCLE). J Dermatol. 2015;135(1):7–12.
20. Nousari HC, et al. Centripetal flagellate erythema: a cutaneous manifestation associated with dermatomyositis. J Rheumatol. 1999;26(3):692–5.
21. Bernet L, et al. JAMA Dermatology. 2016;152(9):1049–51. PMID: 27224238.
22. Smith RL, et al. Skin involvement in juvenile dermatomyositis is associated with loss of end row nailfold capillary loops. J Rheumatol. 2004;31(8):1644–9.
23. Manfredi A, et al. Nailfold capillaroscopic changes in dermatomyositis and polymyositis. Clin Rheumatol. 2015;34(2):279–84.
24. Narang NS, et al. Cutaneous ulceration in dermatomyositis: association with anti-melanoma differentiation-associated gene 5 antibodies and interstitial lung disease. Arthritis Care Res (Hoboken). 2015;67(5):667–72.
25. Miller J, et al. Randomised double blind controlled trial of methotrexate and steroids compared with azathioprine and steroids in the treatment of idiopathic inflammatory myopathy. J Neurol Sci. 2002;199:S53.
26. Hoeltzel MF, et al. The presentation, assessment, pathogenesis, and treatment of calcinosis in juvenile dermatomyositis. Curr Rheumatol Rep. 2014;16:467.
27. Balin SJ, et al. Calcinosis cutis occurring in association with autoimmune connective tissue disease: the Mayo Clinic experience with 78 patients. Arch Dermatol. 2012;148:455–62.
28. Sallum AM, et al. Risk factors associated with calcinosis of juvenile dermatomyositis. J Pediatr. 2008;84(1):68–74.
29. Sanner H, et al. Cumulative organ damage and prognostic factors in juvenile dermatomyositis: a cross-sectional study median 16.8 years after symptom onset. Rheumatology (Oxford). 2009;48(12):1541–7.
30. Gunawardena H, et al. Autoantibodies to a 140-kd protein in juvenile dermatomyositis are associated with calcinosis. Arthritis Rheum. 2009;60:1807–14.
31. Valenzuela A, et al. Identification of clinical features and autoantibodies associated with calcinosis in dermatomyositis. JAMA Dermatol. 2014;150(7):724–9.
32. Hansen CB, Callen JP. Connective tissue panniculitis: lupus panniculitis, dermatomyositis, morphea/scleroderma. Dermatol Ther. 2010;23:341–9.
33. Sarin KY, et al. Molecular profiling to diagnose a case of atypical dermatomyositis. J Invest Dermatol. 2013;133(12):2796–9.
34. Wong D, et al. Interferon and biologic signatures in dermatomyositis skin: specificity and heterogeneity across diseases. PLoS One. 2012;7:e29161.
35. Milisenda JC, et al. Dermatomyositis presenting with severe subcutaneous edema: five additional cases and review of the literature. Semin Arthritis Rheum. 2014;44(2):228–33.
36. Tu J, McLean-Tooke A, Junckerstorff R. Increasing recognition of dermatomyositis with subcutaneous edema-is this a poorer prognostic marker? Dermatol Online J. 2014;20(1):21244.
37. Taggart AJ, et al. Anti Jo-1 myositis. 'Mechanic's hands' and interstitial lung disease. Ulster Med. 2002;71(1):68–71.
38. Sato Y, et al. Clinical characterization of dermatomyositis associated with mechanic's hands. J Dermatol. 2012;39(12):1093–5.
39. Ishigaki K, et al. Skin ulcer is a predictive and prognostic factor of acute or subacute interstitial lung disease in dermatomyositis. Rheumatol Int. 2013;33:2381–9.
40. Ideura G, et al. Interstitial lung disease associated with amyopathic dermatomyositis: review of 18 cases. Respir Med. 2007;101:1406–11.
41. Mimori A, et al. Dermatomyositis and cutaneous necrosis: report of five cases. Mod Rheumatol. 2000;10(2):117–20.
42. Di Rollo D, et al. Cancer risk in dermatomyositis: a systematic review of the literature. G Ital Dermatol Venereol. 2014;149(5):525–37.
43. Lu X, et al. Factors predicting malignancy in patients with polymyositis and dermatomyostis: a systematic review and meta-analysis. PLoS One. 2014;9:e94128.
44. Ueda-Hayakawa I, et al. Cutaneous necrotizing vasculitis in a patient with dermatomyositis positive for anti-PL-7 antibody. Eur J Dermatol. 2013;23(6):889–90.
45. Tsujimura S, Saito K, Tanaka Y. Complete resolution of dermatomyositis with refractory cutaneous vasculitis by intravenous cyclophosphamide pulse therapy. Intern Med. 2008;47(21):1935–40.
46. Kawakami T, et al. Histopathological evidence of small-vessel vasculitis within the skin and lungs associated with interstitial pneumonia in an adult patient with dermatomyositis. Clin Exp Dermatol. 2008;33(4):415–7.

47. Kadoya A, et al. Cutaneous vasculitis in a patient with dermatomyositis without muscle involvement. Intern Med. 1994;33:809–12.
48. Martini A, et al. Recurrent juvenile dermatomyositis and cutaneous necrotizing arteritis with molecular mimicry between streptococcal type 5 M protein and human skeletal myosin. J Pediatr. 1992;121(5 Pt 1):739–42.
49. Inuzuka M, et al. Acquired ichthyosis associated with dermatomyositis in a patient with hepatocellular carcinoma. Br J Dermatol. 2001;144:416–7.
50. Roselino AM, et al. Dermatomyositis and acquired ichthyosis as paraneoplastic manifestations of ovarian tumor. Int J Dermatol. 1997;36(8):611–4.
51. Urrutia S, et al. Sanchez acquired ichthyosis associated with dermatomyositis. J Am Acad Dermatol. 1987;16(3 Pt 1):627–9.
52. Smith ES, et al. Dermatomyositis: a clinicopathological study of 40 patients. Am J Dermatopathol. 2009;31(1):61–7.
53. Magro CM, et al. Cutaneous lesions of dermatomyositis with supervening fibrosis. J Cutan Pathol. 2008;35(1):31–9.
54. Jones SA, Black MM. The value of direct immunofluorescence as a diagnostic aid in dermatomyositis-a study of 35 cases. Clin Exp Dermatol. 1997;22(2):77–81.
55. Magro CM, Crowson AN. The immunofluorescent profile of dermatomyositis: a comparative study with lupus erythematosus. J Cutan Pathol. 1997;24(9):543–52.
56. Mascaro JMJ, et al. Membrane attack complex deposits in cutaneous lesions of dermatomyositis. Arch Dermatol. 1995;131(12):1386–92.
57. Serarslan G, Atik E, Sarikaya G. Periorbital edema and erythema: an unusual localization of DLE in a patient with psoriasis. J Dermatol. 2011;38(5):486–8.
58. Braun RP, et al. Periorbital oedema and erythema as a manifestation of discoid lupus erythematosus. Dermatology. 2002;205:194–7.
59. Cyran S, Douglass MC, Silverstein JL. Chronic cutaneous lupus erythematosus presenting as periorbital edema and erythema. J Am Acad Dermatol. 1992;26(2 Pt 2):334–8.
60. Parkins GJ, Maan A, Dawn G. Neurogenic rosacea: an uncommon and poorly recognized entity? Clin Exp Dermatol. 2015;40:930.
61. Scharschmidt TC, et al. Neurogenic rosacea: a distinct clinical subtype requiring a modified approach to treatment. Arch Dermatol. 2011;147(1):123–6.
62. Rockerbie NR, et al. Cutaneous changes of dermatomyositis precede muscle weakness. J Am Acad Dermatol. 1989;20(4):629–32.
63. Cosnes A, et al. Dermatomyositis without muscle weakness. Longterm followup of 12 patients without systemic corticosteroids. Arch Dermatol. 1995;131:1381–5.
64. Pachman LM, et al. Juvenile dermatomyositis at diagnosis: clinical characteristics of 79 children. J Rheumatol. 1998;25(6):1198–204.
65. Parodi A, et al. De La dermatomyositis in 132 patients with different clinical subtypes: cutaneous signs, constitutional symptoms and circulating antibodies. Acta Derm Venereol. 2002;82(1):48–51.
66. Dalakas MC, Hohlfeld R. Polymyositis and dermatomyositis. Lancet. 2003;362:971–82.
67. Barohn RJ, Dimachkie MM, Jackson CE. A pattern recognition approach to patients with a suspected myopathy. Neurol Clin. 2014;32:569–93.
68. Kissel JT, Mendell JR, Rammohan KW. Microvascular deposition of complement membrane attack complex in dermatomyositis. N Engl J Med. 1986;314(6):329–34.
69. Arahata K, Engel AG. Monoclonal antibody analysis of mononuclear cells in myopathies I Quantitation of subsets according to diagnosis and sites of accumulation and demonstration and counts of muscle fibers invaded by T cells. Ann Neurol. 1984;16:193–208.
70. Greenberg SA, et al. Interferon-alpha/beta-mediated innate immune mechanisms in dermatomyositis. Ann Neurol. 2005;57(5):664–78.
71. Bohan A, et al. Computer-assisted analysis of 153 patients with polymyositis and dermatomyositis. Medicine (Baltimore). 1977;56:255–86.
72. Briani C, et al. Update on idiopathic inflammatory myopathies. Autoimmunity. 2006;39:161–70.
73. Del Grande F, et al. Magnetic resonance imaging of inflammatory myopathies. Top Magn Reson Imaging. 2011;22(2):39–43.
74. Curiel RV, Jones R, Brindle K. Magnetic resonance imaging of the idiopathic inflammatory myopathies: structural and clinical aspects. Ann N Y Acad Sci. 2009;1154:101–14.
75. Adams EM, et al. The idiopathic inflammatory myopathies: spectrum of MR imaging findings. Radiographics. 1995;15:563–74.
76. Yoshida K, et al. Fasciitis as a common lesion of dermatomyositis, demonstrated early after disease onset by en bloc biopsy combined with magnetic resonance imaging. Arthritis Rheum. 2010;62(12):3751–9.
77. Mammen AL. Autoimmune myopathies: autoantibodies, phenotypes and pathogenesis. Nat Rev Neurol. 2011;7(6):343–54.
78. Smith BW, McCarthy JC, Dawley CA. Suspect myopathy? Take this approach to the work-up. J Fam Pract. 2014;63(11):631–8.
79. Paik JJ, Corse AM, Mammen AL. The co-existence of myasthenia gravis in patients with myositis: a case series. Semin Arthritis Rheum. 2014;43(6):792–6.
80. Fraga MM, et al. Devic's disease in an adolescent girl with juvenile dermatomyositis. Rev Bras Reumatol. 2015;S0482-5004:00020-0.
81. Delman D, et al. Dermatomyositis as a presentation of neuromyelitis optica spectrum disorder. J Neuroimmunol. 2015;278:108–11.
82. Tsokos GC, Moutsopoulos HM, Steinberg AD. Muscle involvement in systemic lupus erythematosus. JAMA. 1981;246(7):766–8.
83. Jacobsen S, et al. A multicentre study of 513 Danish patients with systemic lupus erythematosus

II. Disease manifestations and analyses of clinical subsets. Clin Rheumatol. 1998;17:468–77.
84. Foote RA, Kimbrough SM, Stevens JC. Lupus myositis. Muscle Nerve. 1982;5(1):65–8.
85. Garton MJ, Isenberg DA. Clinical features of lupus myositis versus idiopathic myositis: a review of 30 cases. Br J Rheumatol. 1997;36(10):1067–74.
86. Font J, et al. Clusters of clinical and immunologic features in systemic lupus erythematosus: analysis of 600 patients from a single center. Semin Arthritis Rheum. 2004;33(4):217–30.
87. Isenber DA, Snaith ML. Muscle disease in systemic lupus erythematosus: a study of its nature, frequency and cause. J Rheumatol. 1981;8(6):917–24.
88. Maazoun F, et al. Systemic lupus erythematosus-myositis overlap syndrome: report of 6 cases. Clin Pract. 2011;1(4):e89.
89. Jakati S, et al. SLE myopathy: a clinicopathological study. Int J Rheum Dis. 2015;18:886.
90. Milisenda JC, Selva-O'Callaghan A, Grau JM. The diagnosis and classification of polymyositis. Autoimmun Rev. 2014;48-49:118–21.
91. Mahler M, Miller FW, Fritzler MJ. Idiopathic inflammatory myopathies and the anti-synthetase syndrome: a comprehensive review. Autoimmun Rev. 2014;13:367–71.
92. Stenzel W, et al. Nuclear actin aggregation is a hallmark of anti-synthetase syndrome-induced dysimmune myopathy. Neurology. 2015;84(13): 1346–54.
93. Griggs RC, et al. Inclusion body myositis and myopathies. Ann Neurol. 1995;38(5):705–13.
94. Brady S, et al. A retrospective cohort study identifying the principal pathological features useful in the diagnosis of inclusion body myositis. BMJ Open. 2014;4:e004552.
95. Hong J, et al. Muscle disease in systemic sclerosis is associated with an increased risk for cardiac involvement. Dent Abstr. 2014;721.
96. Paik JJ, et al. Myopathy in scleroderma, its identification, prevalence, and treatment: lessons learned from cohort studies. Curr Opin Rheumatol. 2014;26(2):124–30.
97. Muangchan C, et al. The 15% rule in scleroderma: the frequency of severe organ complications in systemic sclerosis. A systematic review. J Rheumatol. 2013;40(9):1545–56.
98. Koschik RWN, et al. Anti-PM-Scl antibody in patients with systemic sclerosis. Clin Exp Rheumatol. 2012;30:S12–6.
99. Toll A, et al. Sclerodermatomyositis associated with severe arthritis. Dermatol Online J. 2004; 10(2):18.
100. Garcia-Patos V, et al. Childhood sclerodermatomyositis: report of a case with the anti-PM/Scl antibody and mechanic's hands. Br J Dermatol. 1996;135:613–6.
101. Wilson NO, et al. Trichinellosis surveillance-United States, 2008-2012. MMWR Surveill Summ. 2015;1:2008–12.
102. Kociecka W. Trichinellosis: human disease, diagnosis and treatment. Vet Parasitol. 2000;93(3–4):365–83.
103. Neghina R, Neghina AM, Marincu I. Reviews on trichinellosis (III): cardiovascular involvement. Foodborne Pathog Dis. 2011;8(8):853–60.
104. Gupta A, Gupta Y. Glucocorticoid-induced myopathy: pathophysiology, diagnosis, and treatment. Indian J Endocrinol Metab. 2013;17:913–6.
105. Pereira RM, Freire de Carvalho J. Glucocorticoid-induced myopathy. Joint Bone Spine. 2011;78(1):41–4.
106. Law M, Rudnicka AR. Statin safety: a systematic review. Am J Cardiol. 2006;97:52C–60.
107. Bruckert E, et al. Mild to moderate muscular symptoms with high-dosage statin therapy in hyperlipidemic patients–the PRIMO study. Cardiovasc Drugs Ther. 2005;19(6):403–14.
108. Graham DJ, et al. Incidence of hospitalized rhabdomyolysis in patients treated with lipid-lowering drugs. JAMA. 2004;292:2585–90.
109. Molokhia M, et al. Statin induced myopathy and myalgia: time trend analysis and comparison of risk associated with statin class from. PLoS One. 2008;3(6):1991–2006.
110. Mammen AL, et al. Increased frequency of DRB1*11:01 in anti-hydroxymethylglutaryl-coenzyme a reductase-associated autoimmune myopathy. Arthritis Care Res Hoboken. 2012;64(8):1233–7.
111. Group, S.C, et al. SLCO1B1 variants and statin-induced myopathy–a genomewide study. N Engl J Med. 2008;359(8):789–99.
112. Mammen AL. Toxic myopathies. Continuum (Minneap Min), 2013. 19(6 Muscle Disease): p. 1634–49.
113. Hansen KE, et al. Outcomes in 45 patients with statin-associated myopathy. Arch Intern Med. 2005;165:2671–6.
114. Mammen AL, et al. Autoantibodies against 3-hydroxy-3-methylglutaryl-coenzyme a reductase in patients with statin-associated autoimmune myopathy. Arthritis Rheum. 2011;63(3):713–21.
115. Needham M, et al. Progressive myopathy with up-regulation of MHC-I associated with statin therapy. Neuromuscul Disord. 2007;17(2):194–200.
116. Christopher-Stine L, et al. A novel autoantibody recognizing 200-kd and 100-kd proteins is associated with an immune-mediated necrotizing myopathy. Arthritis Rheum. 2010;62:2757–66.
117. Nance JR, Mammen AL. Diagnostic evaluation of rhabdomyolysis. Muscle Nerve. 2015;51(6):793–810.
118. Pamfil C, et al. Primary biliary cirrhosis-autoimmune hepatitis overlap syndrome associated with dermatomyositis, autoimmune thyroiditis and antiphospholipid syndrome. J Gastrointestin Liver Dis. 2015;24(1):101–4.
119. Noda S, et al. A case of dermatomyositis with "liver disease associated with rheumatoid diseases" posi-

tive for anti-liver-kidney microsome-1 antibody. Clin Rheumatol. 2010;29(8):941–3.
120. Saravanan V, Kelly C. Drug-related pulmonary problems in patients with rheumatoid arthritis. Rheumatology (Oxford). 2006;45(7):787–9.
121. Sathi N, et al. How common is methotrexate pneumonitis? A large prospective study investigates. Clin Rheumatol. 2012;31(1):79–83.
122. Marie I, et al. Short-term and long-term outcomes of interstitial lung disease in polymyositis and dermatomyositis: a series of 107 patients. Arthritis Rheum. 2011;63(11):3439–47.
123. Kang EH, et al. Interstitial lung disease in patients with polymyositis, dermatomyositis and amyopathic dermatomyositis. Rheumatology (Oxford). 2005;44:1282–6.
124. Fiorentino D, et al. The mucocutaneous and systemic phenotype of dermatomyositis patients with antibodies to MDA5 (CADM-140): a retrospective study. Acad Dermatol. 2011;65:25–34.
125. Sun Y, et al. Interstitial lung disease in clinically amyopathic dermatomyositis (CADM) patients: a retrospective study of 41 Chinese Han patients. Rheumatol Int. 2013;33(5):1295–302.
126. Mukae H, et al. Clinical differences between interstitial lung disease associated with clinically amyopathic dermatomyositis and classic dermatomyositis. Chest. 2009;136(5):1341–7.
127. Connors GR, et al. Interstitial lung disease associated with the idiopathic inflammatory myopathies: what progress has been made in the past 35 years? Chest. 2010;138:1464–74.
128. Richards TJ, et al. Characterization and peripheral blood biomarker assessment of anti-Jo-1 antibody-positive interstitial lung disease. Arthritis Rheum. 2009;60(7):2183–92.
129. Cao H, et al. Clinical manifestations of dermatomyositis and clinically amyopathic dermatomyositis patients with positive expression of anti-melanoma differentiation-associated gene 5 antibody. Arthritis Care Res Hoboken. 2012;64:1602–10.
130. Chen Z, et al. Utility of anti-melanoma differentiation-associated gene 5 antibody measurement in identifying patients with dermatomyositis and a high risk for developing rapidly progressive interstitial lung disease: a review of the literature and a meta-analysis. Arthritis Care Res Hoboken. 2013;65:1316–24.
131. Hamaguchi Y, et al. Clinical correlations with dermatomyositis-specific autoantibodies in adult Japanese patients with dermatomyositis: a multicenter cross-sectional study. Arch Dermatol. 2011;147:391–8.
132. Gono T, et al. Clinical manifestation and prognostic factor in anti-melanoma differentiation-associated gene 5 antibody-associated interstitial lung disease as a complication of dermatomyositis. Rheumatology (Oxford). 2010;49:1713 9.
133. Labrador-Horrillo M, et al. Anti-MDA5 antibodies in a large Mediterranean population of adults with dermatomyositis. J Immunol Res. 2014;2014:290797.
134. Horai Y, et al. Serum interferon-alpha is a useful biomarker in patients with anti-melanoma differentiation-associated gene 5 (MDA5) antibody-positive dermatomyositis. Mod Rheumatol. 2015;25:85–9.
135. Gono T, et al. Anti-MDA5 antibody, ferritin and IL-18 are useful for the evaluation of response to treatment in interstitial lung disease with anti-MDA5 antibody-positive dermatomyositis. Rheumatology (Oxford). 2012;51:1563–70.
136. Mimori T, Nakashima R, Hosono Y. Interstitial lung disease in myositis: clinical subsets, biomarkers, and treatment. Curr Rheumatol Rep. 2012;14(3):264–74.
137. Martinez FJ, Flaherty K. Pulmonary function testing in idiopathic interstitial pneumonias. Proc Am Thorac Soc. 2006;3(4):315–21.
138. Wells AU, et al. Fibrosing alveolitis in systemic sclerosis: indices of lung function in relation to extent of disease on computed tomography. Arthritis Rheum. 1997;40(7):1229–36.
139. Raghu G, et al. An official ATS/ERS/JRS/ALAT statement: idiopathic pulmonary fibrosis: evidence-based guidelines for diagnosis and management. Am J Respir Crit Care Med. 2011;183(6):788–824.
140. Silva JA, et al. Da Safety of low dose glucocorticoid treatment in rheumatoid arthritis: published evidence and prospective trial data. Ann Rheum Dis. 2006;65:285–93.
141. Fathi M, et al. Interstitial lung disease, a common manifestation of newly diagnosed polymyositis and dermatomyositis. Ann Rheum Dis. 2004;63(3):297–301.
142. Douglas WW, et al. Polymyositis-dermatomyositis-associated interstitial lung disease. Am J Respir Crit Care Med. 2001;164(7):1182–5.
143. Johkoh T. Nonspecific interstitial pneumonia and usual interstitial pneumonia: is differentiation possible by high-resolution computed tomography? Semin Ultrasound CT MR. 2014;35(1):24–8.
144. Feiner J, et al. Chapter 23, in The second heart sound. In: Clinical methods the history physical and laboratory examinations. 3rd ed. Boston: Butterworths; 1990.
145. Zhang RF, et al. Diagnostic value of transthoracic Doppler echocardiography in pulmonary hypertension: a meta-analysis. Am J Hypertens. 2010;23(12):1261–4.
146. Mathai SC, et al. Tricuspid annular plane systolic excursion is a robust outcome measure in systemic sclerosis-associated pulmonary arterial hypertension. J Rheumatol. 2011;38(11):2410–8.
147. Hoeper MM, et al. Definitions and diagnosis of pulmonary hypertension. J Am Coll Cardiol. 2013;62(25):D42–50.
148. Zhang L, et al. Cardiac involvement in adult polymyositis or dermatomyositis: a systematic review. Clin Cardiol. 2012;35(11):686–91.

149. Gonzalez-Lopez L, et al. Cardiac manifestations in dermato-polymyositis. Clin Exp Rheumatol. 1996;14(4):373–9.
150. Rosenbohm A, et al. Early diagnosis of cardiac involvement in idiopathic inflammatory myopathy by cardiac magnetic resonance tomography. J Neurol. 2015;262(4):949–56.
151. Hughes M, et al. Cardiac troponin testing in idiopathic inflammatory myopathies and systemic sclerosis-spectrum disorders: biomarkers to distinguish between primary cardiac involvement and low-grade skeletal muscle disease activity. Ann Rheum Dis. 2015;74(5):795–8.
152. Pau-Charles I, et al. Anti-MDA5 positive clinically amyopathic dermatomyositis presenting with severe cardiomyopathy. J Eur Acad Dermatol Venereol. 2014;28(8):1097–102.
153. Sakurai N, et al. Anti-CADM-140 antibody-positive juvenile dermatomyositis with rapidly progressive interstitial lung disease and cardiac involvement. J Rheumatol. 2011;38(5):963–4.
154. Esmon CT. The interactions between inflammation and coagulation. Br J Haematol. 2005;131(4):417–30.
155. Limaye VS, et al. Idiopathic inflammatory myositis is associated with a high incidence of hypertension and diabetes mellitus. Int J Rheum Dis. 2010;13(2):132–7.
156. Durante A, Bronzato S. The increased cardiovascular risk in patients affected by autoimmune diseases: review of the various manifestations. J Clin Med Res. 2015;7(6):379–84.
157. Ungprasert P, et al. Risk of coronary artery disease in patients with idiopathic inflammatory myopathies: a systematic review and meta-analysis of observational studies. Semin Arthritis Rheum. 2014;44(1):63–7.
158. Linos E, et al. Atherosclerotic cardiovascular disease and dermatomyositis: an analysis of the Nationwide Inpatient Sample survey. Arthritis Res Ther. 2013;15(1):R7.
159. Lai YT, et al. Dermatomyositis is associated with an increased risk of cardiovascular and cerebrovascular events: a Taiwanese population-based longitudinal follow-up study. Br J Dermatol. 2013;168(5):1054–9.
160. Carruthers EC, et al. Risk of deep venous thrombosis and pulmonary embolism in individuals with polymyositis and dermatomyositis: a general population-based study. Ann Rheum Dis. 2014;75:110.
161. Selva-O'Callaghan A, et al. Venous thromboembolism in patients with dermatomyositis and polymyositis. Clin Exp Rheumatol. 2011;29(5):846–9.
162. Zoller B, et al. Risk of pulmonary embolism in patients with autoimmune disorders: a nationwide follow-up study from Sweden. Lancet. 2012;379(9812):244–9.
163. Ramagopalan SV, et al. Risk of venous thromboembolism in people admitted to hospital with selected immune-mediated diseases: record-linkage study. BMC Med. 2011;9:1–7015.
164. Koh ET, et al. Adult onset polymyositis/dermatomyositis: clinical and laboratory features and treatment response in 75 patients. Ann Rheum Dis. 1993;52(12):857–61.
165. Citera G, et al. Maldonado joint involvement in polymyositis/dermatomyositis. Clin Rheumatol. 1994;13(1):70–4.
166. Porkodi R, et al. Clinical spectrum of inflammatory myositis in South India-a ten year study. J Assoc Physicians India. 2002;50:1255–8.
167. Klein M, et al. Arthritis in idiopathic inflammatory myopathy: clinical features and autoantibody associations. J Rheumatol. 2014;41(6):1133–9.
168. Hall JC, et al. Anti-melanoma differentiation-associated protein 5-associated dermatomyositis: expanding the clinical spectrum. Arthritis Care Res Hoboken. 2013;65(8):1307–15.
169. Wasko MC, et al. Dermatomyositis with erosive arthropathy: association with the anti-PL-7 antibody. J Rheumatol. 1999;26(12):2693–4.
170. Oddis CV, et al. Subluxing arthropathy associated with the anti-Jo-1 antibody in polymyositis/dermatomyositis. Arthritis Rheum. 1990;33(11):1640–5.
171. Schumacher HR, et al. Articular manifestations of polymyositis and dermatomyositis. Am J Med. 1979;67(2):287–92.
172. Levin J, Werth VP. Skin disorders with arthritis. Best Pract Res Clin Rheumatol. 2006;20(4):809–26.
173. Mumm GE, McKown KM, Bell CL. Antisynthetase syndrome presenting as rheumatoid-like polyarthritis. J Rheumatol. 2010;16(7):307–12.
174. Nesher G. Polymyalgia rheumatica-diagnosis and classification. J Autoimmun. 2014;48–49:76.
175. Couvrat-Desvergnes G, et al. The spectrum of renal involvement in patients with inflammatory myopathies. Medicine (Baltimore). 2014;93(1):33–41.
176. Yen TH, et al. Unexpected IgA nephropathy during the treatment of a young woman with idiopathic dermatomyositis: case report and review of the literature. J Nephrol. 2003;16(1):148–53.
177. Barros TB, et al. IgA nephropathy and polymyositis: a rare association. Rev Bras Reumatol. 2014;54(3 SRC):231–3.
178. Civilibal M, et al. Selcuk nephropathy associated with juvenile dermatomyositis. Pediatr Nephrol. 2009;24(10):2073–5.
179. Akashi Y, et al. Dermatomyositis associated with membranous nephropathy in a 43-year-old female. Am J Nephrol. 2002;22(4):385–8.
180. Makino H, et al. Membranous nephropathy developing during the course of dermatomyositis. J Rheumatol. 1994;21(7):1377–8.
181. Rose JD. Membranous glomerulonephritis, dermatomyositis, and bronchial carcinoma. Br Med J. 1979;2(6191):641.
182. Xie Q, et al. Diffuse proliferative glomerulonephritis associated with dermatomyositis with nephrotic syndrome. Rheumatol Int. 2010;30(6):821–5.

183. Kawai H, et al. Myeloperoxidase-antineutrophil cytoplasmic antibody-related crescentic glomerulonephritis after treatment for clinically amyopathic dermatomyositis: a coincidental combination or not? Clin Exp Nephrol. 2011;15(4):577–81.
184. Yuste C, et al. Overlap between dermatomyositis and ANCA vasculitides. Clin Kidney J. 2014;7(1):59–61.
185. Henter JI, et al. HLH-: diagnostic and therapeutic guidelines for hemophagocytic lymphohistiocytosis. Pediatr Blood Cancer. 2007;48(2):124–31.
186. Buchbinder R, et al. Incidence of malignant disease in biopsy-proven inflammatory myopathy. A population based cohort study. Ann Intern Med. 2001;134(12):1087–95.
187. Hill CL, et al. Frequency of specific cancer types in dermatomyositis and polymyositis: a population-based study. Lancet. 2001;357(9250):96–100.
188. Chow WH, et al. Cancer risk following polymyositis and dermatomyositis: a nationwide cohort study in Denmark. Cancer Causes Control. 1995;6(1):9–13.
189. Sigurgeirsson B, et al. Risk of cancer in patients with dermatomyositis or polymyositis. A population based study. N Engl J Med. 1992;326(6):363–7.
190. Huang YL, et al. Malignancies associated with dermatomyositis and polymyositis in Taiwan: a nationwide population-based study. Br J Dermatol. 2009;161(4):854–60.
191. Ichimura Y, et al. Anti-NXP2 autoantibodies in adult patients with idiopathic inflammatory myopathies: possible association with malignancy. Ann Rheum Dis. 2012;71(5):710–3.
192. Cammas F, et al. TRIM involvement in transcriptional regulation. Adv Exp Med Biol. 2012;770:59–76.
193. Fiorentino DF, et al. Most patients with cancer-associated dermatomyositis have antibodies to nuclear matrix protein NXP-2 or transcription intermediary factor 1gamma. Arthritis Rheum. 2013;65(11):2954–62.
194. Trallero-Araguas E, et al. Usefulness of anti-p155 autoantibody for diagnosing cancer-associated dermatomyositis: a systematic review and meta-analysis. Arthritis Rheum. 2012;64(2):523–32.
195. Shah AA, Casciola-Rosen L, Rosen A. Review: cancer-induced autoimmunity in the rheumatic diseases. Arthritis Rheum. 2015;67(2):317–26.
196. Sparsa A, et al. Routine vs extensive malignancy search for adult dermatomyositis and polymyositis: a study of 40 patients. Arch Dermatol. 2002;138(7):885–90.
197. Leatham H, et al. Medicine (Baltimore). 2018;97(2):e9639. PMID: 29480875
198. Kim S, et al. Complete and sustained remission of juvenile dermatomyositis resulting from aggressive treatment. Arthritis Rheum. 2009;60(6):1825–30.
199. Jordan JR, et al. Spontaneously remitting dermatomyositis. Acad Dermatol Venereol. 2004;18(4):495–8.
200. Gordon PA, et al. Immunosuppressant and immunomodulatory treatment for dermatomyositis and polymyositis. Cochrane Database Syst Rev. 2012;(8):CD003643.
201. Femia AN, Vleugels RA, Callen JP. Cutaneous dermatomyositis: an updated review of treatment options and internal associations. Am J Clin Dermatol. 2013;14(4):291–313.
202. Lam C, Vleugels RA. Management of cutaneous dermatomyositis. Dermatol Ther. 2012;25(2):112–34.
203. Strowd LC, Jorizzo JL. Review of dermatomyositis: establishing the diagnosis and treatment algorithm. J Dermatolog Treat. 2013;24(6):418–21.
204. Jorizzo JL, Vleugels RA. Dermatomyositis. In: Bolognia J, Jorizzo JL, Schaefer JV, editors. Dermatology. 3rd ed. Elsevier: Edinburgh; 2012.
205. Dourmishev L, Meffert H, Piazena H. Dermatomyositis: comparative studies of cutaneous photosensitivity in lupus erythematosus and normal subjects. Photodermatol Photoimmunol Photomed. 2004;20(5 SRC):230–4.
206. Cheong WK, et al. Cutaneous photosensitivity in dermatomyositis. Br J Dermatol. 1994;131(2):205–8.
207. Mattar MA, et al. Safety and possible effects of low-intensity resistance training associated with partial blood flow restriction in polymyositis and dermatomyositis. Arthritis Res Ther. 2014;16(5):473–014.
208. Alexanderson H, et al. Benefits of intensive resistance training in patients with chronic polymyositis or dermatomyositis. Arthritis Rheum. 2007;57:768–77.
209. Wiesinger GF, et al. Improvement of physical fitness and muscle strength in polymyositis/dermatomyositis patients by a training programme. Br J Rheumatol. 1998;37(2):196–200.
210. Riisager M, et al. Aerobic training in persons who have recovered from juvenile dermatomyositis. Neuromuscul Disord. 2013;23(12):962–8.
211. Omori CH, et al. Exercise training in juvenile dermatomyositis. Arthritis Care Res (Hoboken). 2012;64(8):1186–94.
212. Alexanderson H, et al. The safety of a resistive home exercise program in patients with recent onset active polymyositis or dermatomyositis. Scandinavica. 2000;29:295–301.
213. Alexanderson H, et al. Resistive home exercise in patients with recent-onset polymyositis and dermatomyositis-a randomized controlled single-blinded study with a 2-year followup. J Rheumatol. 2014;41:1124–32.
214. Peyrot I, et al. Topical tacrolimus and resistant skin lesions of dermatomyositis. Rev Med Interne. 2006;27(10 SRC):730–5.
215. Lampropoulos CE, D'Cruz DP. Topical tacrolimus treatment in a patient with dermatomyositis. Ann Rheum Dis. 2005;64(9):1376–7
216. Hollar CB, Jorizzo JL. Topical tacrolimus 0.1% ointment for refractory skin disease in dermatomyositis a pilot study. J Dermatolog Treat. 2004;15(1):35–9.
217. Yoshimasu T, et al. Topical FK506 (tacrolimus) therapy for facial erythematous lesions of cutaneous lupus erythematosus and dermatomyositis. Eur J Dermatol. 2002;12(1):50–2.

218. Garcia-Doval I, Cruces M. Topical tacrolimus in cutaneous lesions of dermatomyositis: lack of effect in side-by-side comparison in five patients. Dermatology. 2004;209(3):247–8.
219. Kim JE, et al. Successful treatment of cutaneous lesions of dermatomyositis with topical pimecrolimus. Ann Dermatol. 2011;23(3):348–51.
220. Soter NA, et al. Tacrolimus ointment for the treatment of atopic dermatitis in adult patients: part II, safety. J Am Acad Dermatol. 2001;44(1):S39–46.
221. Pereira U, et al. Mechanisms of the sensory effects of tacrolimus on the skin. Br J Dermatol. 2010;163(1):70–7.
222. Rustin MH. The safety of tacrolimus ointment for the treatment of atopic dermatitis: a review. Br J Dermatol. 2007;157(5):861–73.
223. Woo TY, et al. Cutaneous lesions of dermatomyositis are improved by hydroxychloroquine. J Am Acad Dermatol. 1984;10(4):592–600.
224. Pelle MT, Callen JP. Adverse cutaneous reactions to hydroxychloroquine are more common in patients with dermatomyositis than in patients with cutaneous lupus erythematosus. Arch Dermatol. 2002;138(9):1231–3.
225. Ang GC, Werth VP. Combination antimalarials in the treatment of cutaneous dermatomyositis: a retrospective study. Arch Dermatol. 2005;141:855–9.
226. Climent-Albaladejo A, et al. Dermatomyositis sine myositis and antisynthetase syndrome. Joint Bone Spine. 2002;69:72–5.
227. Zieglschmid-Adams ME, et al. Treatment of dermatomyositis with methotrexate. J Am Acad Dermatol. 1995;32(5 Pt 1):754–7.
228. Kasteler JS, Callen JP. Low-dose methotrexate administered weekly is an effective corticosteroid-sparing agent for the treatment of the cutaneous manifestations of dermatomyositis. J Acad Dermatol. 1997;36:67–71.
229. Hornung T, et al. Efficacy of low-dose methotrexate in the treatment of dermatomyositis skin lesions. Clin Exp Dermatol. 2012;37:139–42.
230. Click JW, et al. Methotrexate for the treatment of cutaneous dermatomyositis. Acad Dermatol. 2013;68:1043–5.
231. Metzger AL, et al. Polymyositis and dermatomyositis: combined methotrexate and corticosteroid therapy. Ann Intern Med. 1974;81(2):182–9.
232. Tse S, et al. The arthritis of inflammatory childhood myositis syndromes. J Rheumatol. 2001;28(1):192–7.
233. Camus P, et al. Interstitial lung disease induced by drugs and radiation. Respiration. 2004;71:301–26.
234. Kim YJ, Song M, Ryu JC. Mechanisms underlying methotrexate-induced pulmonary toxicity. Expert Opin Drug Saf. 2009;8:451–8.
235. Iorizzo L Jr, Jorizzo JL. The treatment and prognosis of dermatomyositis: an updated review. J Am Acad Dermatol. 2008;59(1):99–112.
236. Chwalinska-Sadowska H, Maldykowa H. Polymyositis-dermatomyositis: 25 years of follow-up of 50 patients disease course, treatment, prognostic factors. Mater Med Pol. 1990;22(3 SRC):213–8.
237. Troyanov Y, et al. Novel classification of idiopathic inflammatory myopathies based on overlap syndrome features and autoantibodies: analysis of 100 French Canadian patients. Medicine (Baltimore). 2005;84(4):231–49.
238. Marie I, et al. Polymyositis and dermatomyositis: short term and longterm outcome, and predictive factors of prognosis. J Rheumatol. 2001;28(10):2230–7.
239. Dalakas MC. Inflammatory myopathies: management of steroid resistance. Curr Opin Neurol. 2011;24(5):457–62.
240. Schwarz MI, et al. Interstitial lung disease in polymyositis and dermatomyositis: analysis of six cases and review of the literature. Medicine (Baltimore). 1976;55(1):89–104.
241. Nawata Y, et al. Corticosteroid resistant interstitial pneumonitis in dermatomyositis/polymyositis: prediction and treatment with cyclosporine. J Rheumatol. 1999;26(7):1527–33.
242. Schnabel A, et al. Interstitial lung disease in polymyositis and dermatomyositis: clinical course and response to treatment. Semin Arthritis Rheum. 2003;32(5):273–84.
243. Dickey BF, Myers AR. Pulmonary disease in polymyositis/dermatomyositis. Semin Arthritis Rheum. 1984;14:60–76.
244. Edge JC, et al. Mycophenolate mofetil as an effective corticosteroid-sparing therapy for recalcitrant dermatomyositis. Arch Dermatol. 2006;142:65–9.
245. Gelber AC, et al. Mycophenolate mofetil in the treatment of severe skin manifestations of dermatomyositis: a series of 4 cases. J Rheumatol. 2000;27:1542–5.
246. Majithia V, Harisdangkul V. Mycophenolate mofetil (CellCept): an alternative therapy for autoimmune inflammatory myopathy. Rheumatology (Oxford). 2005;44(3):386–9.
247. Pisoni CN, et al. Mycophenolate mofetil treatment in resistant myositis. Rheumatology (Oxford). 2007;46(3):516–8.
248. Rowin J, et al. Mycophenolate mofetil in dermatomyositis: is it safe? Neurology. 2006;66(8):1245–7.
249. Tsuchiya H, et al. Mycophenolate mofetil therapy for rapidly progressive interstitial lung disease in a patient with clinically amyopathic dermatomyositis. Mod Rheumatol. 2014;24(4):694–6.
250. Cozzani E, et al. Amyopathic dermatomyositis with lung involvement responsive to mycophenolate mofetil. Immunopharmacol Immunotoxicol. 2013;35:687–92.
251. Morganroth PA, Kreider ME, Werth VP. Mycophenolate mofetil for interstitial lung disease in dermatomyositis. Arthritis Care Res Hoboken. 2010;62(10):1496–501.
252. Mira-Avendano IC, et al. A retrospective review of clinical features and treatment outcomes in

steroid-resistant interstitial lung disease from polymyositis/dermatomyositis. Respir Med. 2013;107(6):890–6.
253. Saketkoo LA, Espinoza LR. Experience of mycophenolate mofetil in 10 patients with autoimmune-related interstitial lung disease demonstrates promising effects. Am J Med Sci. 2009;337(5):329–35.
254. Kitchin JE, et al. Rediscovering mycophenolic acid: a review of its mechanism, side effects, and potential uses. J Acad Dermatol. 1997;37:445–9.
255. Sterneck M, et al. Improvement in gastrointestinal and health-related quality of life outcomes after conversion from mycophenolate mofetil to enteric-coated mycophenolate sodium in liver transplant recipients. Transplant Proc. 2014;46(1):234–40.
256. Cherin P, et al. Intravenous immunoglobulin for polymyositis and dermatomyositis. Lancet. 1990;116:336.
257. Cherin P, et al. Efficacy of intravenous gammaglobulin therapy in chronic refractory polymyositis and dermatomyositis: an open study with 20 adult patients. Am J Med. 1991;91:162–8.
258. Dalakas MC, et al. A controlled trial of high-dose intravenous immune globulin infusions as treatment for dermatomyositis. N Engl J Med. 1993;329:1993–2000.
259. Suzuki Y, et al. Intravenous immunoglobulin therapy for refractory interstitial lung disease associated with polymyositis/dermatomyositis. Lung. 2009;187(3):201–6.
260. Bakewell CJ, Raghu G. Polymyositis associated with severe interstitial lung disease: remission after three doses of IV immunoglobulin. Chest. 2011;139:441–3.
261. Mauhin W, et al. Improvement in lung fibrosis using intravenous immunoglobulin in systemic sclerosis with myositis. Scand J Rheumatol. 2014;43(2):170–1.
262. Cantarini L, et al. Intravenous immunoglobulins (IVIG) in systemic sclerosis: a challenging yet promising future. Immunol Res. 2015;61:326–37.
263. Danieli MG, et al. Subcutaneous immunoglobulin in polymyositis and dermatomyositis: a novel application. Autoimmun Rev. 2011;10:144–9.
264. Danieli MG, et al. Open-label study on treatment with 20% subcutaneous IgG administration in polymyositis and dermatomyositis. Clin Rheumatol. 2014;33:531–6.
265. Schleinitz N, et al. Subcutaneous immunoglobulin administration: an alternative to intravenous infusion as adjuvant treatment for dermatomyositis? Clin Rheumatol. 2008;27(8):1067–8.
266. Caress JB, Kennedy BL, Eickman KD. Safety of intravenous immunoglobulin treatment. Expert Opin Drug Saf. 2010;9:971–9.
267. Feldmeyer L, et al. Not all intravenous immunoglobulin preparations are equally well tolerated. Acta Derm Venereol. 2010;90:494–7.
268. Sekul EA, Cupler EJ, Dalakas MC. Aseptic meningitis associated with high-dose intravenous immunoglobulin therapy: frequency and risk factors. Ann Intern Med. 1994;121(4):259–62.
269. Obando I, et al. Aseptic meningitis due to administration of intravenous immunoglobulin with an unusually high number of leukocytes in cerebrospinal fluid. Pediatr Emerg Care. 2002;18(6):429–32.
270. Dinh HV, et al. Rituximab for the treatment of the skin manifestations of dermatomyositis: a report of 3 cases. Acad Dermatol. 2007;56:148–53.
271. Chung L, Genovese MC, Fiorentino DF. A pilot trial of rituximab in the treatment of patients with dermatomyositis. Arch Dermatol. 2007;143:763–7.
272. Oddis CV, et al. Rituximab in the treatment of refractory adult and juvenile dermatomyositis and adult polymyositis: a randomized, placebo-phase trial. Arthritis Rheum. 2013;65(2):314–24.
273. Aggarwal R, et al. Predictors of clinical improvement in rituximab-treated refractory adult and juvenile dermatomyositis and adult polymyositis. Arthritis Rheum. 2014;66:740–9.
274. Andersson H, et al. Long-term experience with rituximab in anti-synthetase syndrome-related interstitial lung disease. Rheumatology (Oxford). 2015;54:1420.
275. Keir GJ, et al. Severe interstitial lung disease in connective tissue disease: rituximab as rescue therapy. Eur Respir J. 2012;40:641–8.
276. Marie I, et al. Infectious complications in polymyositis and dermatomyositis: a series of 279 patients. Semin Arthritis Rheum. 2011;41(1):48–60.
277. Belhassen-Garcia M, et al. Atypical progressive multifocal leukoencephalopathy in a patient with antisynthetase syndrome. Intern Med. 2015;54:519–24.
278. Vulliemoz S, et al. Favourable outcome of progressive multifocal leucoencephalopathy in two patients with dermatomyositis. J Neurol Neurosurg Psychiatry. 2006;77(9):1079–82.
279. Mehregan DR, Su WP. Cyclosporine treatment for dermatomyositis/polymyositis. Curtis. 1993;51(1):59–61.
280. Villalba L, et al. Treatment of refractory myositis: a randomized crossover study of two new cytotoxic regimens. Arthritis Rheum. 1998;41(3):392–9.
281. Vencovsky J, et al. Cyclosporine a versus methotrexate in the treatment of polymyositis and dermatomyositis. Scand J Rheumatol. 2000;29(2):95–102.
282. Maeda K, et al. Cyclosporine treatment for polymyositis/dermatomyositis: is it possible to rescue the deteriorating cases with interstitial pneumonitis? Scand J Rheumatol. 1997;26:24–9.
283. Takada K, Nagasaka K, Miyasaka N. Polymyositis/dermatomyositis and interstitial lung disease: a new therapeutic approach with T-cell-specific immunosuppressants. Autoimmunity. 2005;38(5):383–92.
284. Kameda H, et al. Combination therapy with corticosteroids, cyclosporin a, and intravenous pulse cyclophosphamide for acute/subacute interstitial pneumonia in patients with dermatomyositis. J Rheumatol. 2005;32:1719–26.

285. Nagai K, et al. Therapeutic drug monitoring of cyclosporine microemulsion in interstitial pneumonia with dermatomyositis. Mod Rheumatol. 2011;21(1):32–6.
286. Ryan C, Amor KT, Menter A. The use of cyclosporine in dermatology: part II. J Am Acad Dermatol. 2010;63(6):949–72.
287. Amor KT, et al. The use of cyclosporine in dermatology: part I. Acad Dermatol. 2010;63:925–46, quiz 9478
288. Rosengren S, et al. The JAK inhibitor CP-690,550 (tofacitinib) inhibits TNF-induced chemokine expression in fibroblast-like synoviocytes: autocrine role of type I interferon. Ann Rheum Dis. 2012;71(3):440–7.
289. Kao L, Chung L, Fiorentino DF. Pathogenesis of dermatomyositis: role of cytokines and interferon. Curr Rheumatol Rep. 2011;13(3):225–32.
290. Kurtzman DJ, et al. Tofacitinib citrate for refractory cutaneous dermatomyositis: an alternative treatment. JAMA Dermatol. 2016;152(8):944–5.
291. Moghadam-Kia S, et al. Management of refractory cutaneous dermatomyositis: potential role of Janus kinase inhibition with tofacitinib. Rheumatology (Oxford). 2019;58:1011.
292. Dumont FJ. FK506, an immunosuppressant targeting calcineurin function. Curr Med Chem. 2000;7:731–48.
293. Shimojima Y, et al. Coadministration of tacrolimus with corticosteroid accelerates recovery in refractory patients with polymyositis/dermatomyositis: a retrospective study. BMC Musculoskelet Disord. 2012;13:228.
294. Hassan J, van der Net JJ, van Royen-Kerkhof A. Treatment of refractory juvenile dermatomyositis with tacrolimus. Clin Rheumatol. 2008;27:1469–71.
295. Nalda A, et al. Martin Modesto Arnal Boronat Barcelo efficacy of tacrolimus (FK-506) in the treatment of recalcitrant juvenile dermatomyositis: study of 6 cases. Med Clin (Barc). 2006;127(18):697–701.
296. Kurita T, et al. The efficacy of tacrolimus in patients with interstitial lung diseases complicated with polymyositis or dermatomyositis. Rheumatology (Oxford). 2015;54:39–44.
297. Yokoyama Y, et al. Corticosteroid-sparing effect of tacrolimus in the initial treatment of dermatomyositis and polymyositis. Mod Rheumatol. 2015;30:1–5.
298. Rigby AL, Plit M, Glanville AR. Tacrolimus rescue therapy for severe respiratory failure in the anti-synthetase syndrome. Respirol Case Rep. 2014;2(2):70–2.
299. Wilkes MR, et al. Treatment of antisynthetase-associated interstitial lung disease with tacrolimus. Arthritis Rheum. 2005;52(8):2439–46.
300. Gordon P, Gooptu B. Tacrolimus in idiopathic inflammatory myopathy-associated interstitial lung disease: defining roles and responders. Rheumatology (Oxford). 2015;54:3–4.
301. Naesens M, Kuypers DR, Sarwal M. Calcineurin inhibitor nephrotoxicity. Clin J Am Soc Nephrol. 2009;4(2):481–508.
302. McCormack PL. Celecoxib: a review of its use for symptomatic relief in the treatment of osteoarthritis, rheumatoid arthritis and ankylosing spondylitis. Drugs. 2011;71(18):2457–89.
303. Mallen SR, Essex MN, Zhang R. Gastrointestinal tolerability of NSAIDs in elderly patients: a pooled analysis of 21 randomized clinical trials with celecoxib and nonselective NSAIDs. Curr Med Res Opin. 2011;27(7):1359–66.
304. Ramirez G, et al. Adult-onset polymyositis-dermatomyositis: description of 25 patients with emphasis on treatment. Semin Arthritis Rheum. 1990;20(2):114–20.
305. de Vere Hollingworth P, et al. Intensive immunosuppression versus prednisolone in the treatment of connective tissue diseases. Ann Rheum Dis. 1982;41:557–62.
306. Joffe MM, et al. Drug therapy of the idiopathic inflammatory myopathies: predictors of response to prednisone, azathioprine, and methotrexate and a comparison of their efficacy. Am J Med. 1993;94:379–87.
307. Yu KH, et al. Survival analysis of patients with dermatomyositis and polymyositis: analysis of 192 Chinese cases. Clin Rheumatol. 2011;30(12):1595–601.
308. Hoyles RK, et al. A multicenter, prospective, randomized, double-blind, placebo-controlled trial of corticosteroids and intravenous cyclophosphamide followed by oral azathioprine for the treatment of pulmonary fibrosis in scleroderma. Arthritis Rheum. 2006;54:3962–70.
309. Mok CC, C.H. To, Szeto ML. Successful treatment of dermatomyositis-related rapidly progressive interstitial pneumonitis with sequential oral cyclophosphamide and azathioprine. Scand J Rheumatol. 2003;32(3):181–3.
310. Bidinger JJ, et al. The cutaneous and systemic manifestations of azathioprine hypersensitivity syndrome. Acad Dermatol. 2011;65:184–91.
311. Sangle VS, Sangle SR, D'Cruz DP. Leflunomide as a remission-maintaining therapy in difficult-to-treat dermatomyositis. Ann Rheum Dis. 2008;67(5):723.
312. Welborn MC, et al. Juvenile dermatomyositis: of calcinosis cutis of the elbow and review of the literature. J Pediatr Orthop. 2014;35:e43.
313. Schanz S, Ulmer A, Fierlbeck G. Response of dystrophic calcification to intravenous immunoglobulin. Arch Dermatol. 2008;144(5):585–7.
314. Hewitson PJ, et al. Leflunomide and rheumatoid arthritis: a systematic review of effectiveness, safety and cost implications. Pharm Ther. 2000;25:295–302.
315. Alcorn N, Saunders S, Madhok R. Benefit-risk assessment of leflunomide: an appraisal of leflunomide in rheumatoid arthritis 10 years after licensing. Drug Saf. 2009;32(12):1123–34.

316. Osiri M, et al. Leflunomide for treating rheumatoid arthritis. Cochrane Database Syst Rev. 2017;(1):CD002047.
317. Roubille C, Haraoui B. Interstitial lung diseases induced or exacerbated by DMARDS and biologic agents in rheumatoid arthritis: a systematic literature review. Semin Arthritis Rheum. 2014;43(5):613–26.
318. Inokuma S. Leflunomide-induced interstitial pneumonitis might be a representative of disease-modifying antirheumatic drug-induced lung injury. Expert Opin Drug Saf. 2011;10:603–11.
319. Lee MA, Hutchinson DG. HRCT-proven leflunomide pneumonitis in a patient with psoriatic arthritis and normal lung function tests and chest radiography. Rheumatology (Oxford). 2010;49:1206–7.
320. Coleman MD. Dapsone: modes of action, toxicity and possible strategies for increasing patient tolerance. Br J Dermatol. 1993;129:507–13.
321. Kawachi Y, et al. Pruritic poikilodermatous eruption associated with dermatomyositis: successful treatment with dapsone. Eur J Dermatol. 2012;22:289–90.
322. Cohen JB, And J. Cutaneous involvement of dermatomyositis can respond to Dapsone therapy. Int J Dermatol. 2002;41:182–4.
323. Konohana A, Kawashima J. Successful treatment of dermatomyositis with dapsone. Clin Exp Dermatol. 1994;19:367.
324. Mok CC, Lau CS, Wong RW. Toxicities of dapsone in the treatment of cutaneous manifestations of rheumatic diseases. J Rheumatol. 1998;25(6):1246–7.
325. Wolverton SE, Remlinger K. Suggested guidelines for patient monitoring: hepatic and hematologic toxicity attributable to systemic dermatologic drugs. Dermatol Clin. 2007;25(2):195–205.
326. Lenardo TM, Calabrese LH. The role of thalidomide in the treatment of rheumatic disease. J Rheumatol. 2000;6:19–26.
327. Flores-Suarez LF, et al. Drug-induced amyopathic dermatomyositis. Rheumatology. 2002;8:50–4.
328. Piette JC, Sbai A, Frances C. Warning: thalidomide-related thrombotic risk potentially concerns patients with lupus. Lupus. 2002;11(2):67–70.
329. Gaspari A. Thalidomide neurotoxicity in dermatological patients: the next "STEP". J Invest Dermatol. 2002;119(5):987–8.
330. Watanabe R, et al. Successful multi-target therapy using corticosteroid, tacrolimus, cyclophosphamide, and rituximab for rapidly progressive interstitial lung disease in a patient with clinically amyopathic dermatomyositis. Mod Rheumatol. 2015;20:1–6.
331. Hildebrand BAJ, Arroyo R. Evolution of clinically amyopathic dermatomyositis despite aggressive immunosuppression with cyclophosphamide and prednisone. Rheumatology. 2010;16:143–5.
332. Murota H, et al. Successful treatment with regimen of intravenous gamma globulin and cyclophosphamide for dermatomyositis accompanied by interstitial pneumonia, opportunistic infection and steroid psychosis. Allergol Int. 2006;55(2):199–202.
333. Tanaka F, et al. Successful combined therapy of cyclophosphamide and cyclosporine for acute exacerbated interstitial pneumonia associated with dermatomyositis. Intern Med. 2000;39(5):428–30.
334. Takashi S, et al. Amyopathic dermatomyositis with interstitial pneumonia: effective treatment with cyclophosphamide pulse therapy. Nihon Kokyuki Gakkai Zasshi. 1999;37(8):647–51.
335. Yoshida T, et al. Pulse intravenous cyclophosphamide treatment for steroid-resistant interstitial pneumonitis associated with polymyositis. Intern Med. 1999;38(9):733–8.
336. Shinohara T, et al. Rapidly progressive interstitial lung disease associated with dermatomyositis responding to intravenous cyclophosphamide pulse therapy. Intern Med. 1997;36(7):519–23.
337. Takizawa H, Ito K. Cyclophosphamide pulse therapy for rapidly progressive interstitial pneumonia in dermatomyositis. A new possibility for rescue? Intern Med. 1997;36(7):448–9.
338. Yamasaki Y, et al. Intravenous cyclophosphamide therapy for progressive interstitial pneumonia in patients with polymyositis/dermatomyositis. Rheumatology (Oxford). 2007;46(1):124–30.
339. Tashkin DP, et al. Cyclophosphamide versus placebo in scleroderma lung disease. N Engl J Med. 2006;354(25):2655–66.
340. Fraiser LH, Kanekal S, Kehrer JP. Cyclophosphamide toxicity. Characterising and avoiding the problem. Drugs. 1991;42:781–95.
341. Radis CD, et al. Effects of cyclophosphamide on the development of malignancy and on long-term survival of patients with rheumatoid arthritis. A 20year followup study. Arthritis Rheum. 1995;38(8):1120–7.
342. Kenney LB, et al. High risk of infertility and long term gonadal damage in males treated with high dose cyclophosphamide for sarcoma during childhood. Cancer. 2001;91:613–21.
343. Shahani L. Refractory calcinosis in a patient with dermatomyositis: response to intravenous immune globulin. BMJ Case Rep. 2012;2012:bcr2012006629.
344. Penate Y, et al. Calcinosis cutis associated with amyopathic dermatomyositis: response to intravenous immunoglobulin. J Am Acad Dermatol. 2009;60(6):1076–7.
345. Kalajian AH, Perryman JH, Callen JP. Intravenous immunoglobulin therapy for dystrophic calcinosis cutis: unreliable in our hands. Arch Dermatol. 2009;145(3):334.
346. Palaniappan P, Lionel AP, Kumar S. Successful treatment of calcinosis cutis in juvenile dermatomyositis with pamidronate. J Clin Rheumatol. 2014;20(8):454–5.
347. Tayfur AC, et al. Bisphosphonates in juvenile dermatomyositis with dystrophic calcinosis. Mod Rheumatol. 2015;24:1–6.

348. Casciola-Rosen L, Mammen AL. Myositis autoantibodies. Curr Opin Rheumatol. 2012;24:602–8.
349. Tansley SL, McHugh NJ. Myositis specific and associated autoantibodies in the diagnosis and management of juvenile and adult idiopathic inflammatory myopathies. Curr Rheumatol Rep. 2014;16(12):464.
350. Yamasaki Y, et al. Unusually high frequency of autoantibodies to PL-7 associated with milder muscle disease in Japanese patients with polymyositis/dermatomyositis. Arthritis Rheum. 2006;54(6):2004–9.
351. Targoff IN, Arnett FC. Clinical manifestations in patients with antibody to PL-12 antigen (alanyl-tRNA synthetase). Am J Med. 1990;88(3):241–51.
352. Hirakata M, et al. Clinical and immunogenetic features of patients with autoantibodies to asparaginyl-transfer RNA synthetase. Arthritis Rheum. 2007;56:1295–303.
353. Sato S, Kuwana M, Hirakata M. Clinical characteristics of Japanese patients with anti-OJ (anti-isoleucyl-tRNA synthetase) autoantibodies. Rheumatology (Oxford). 2007;46(5):842–5.
354. Gunawardena H, Betteridge ZE, McHugh NJ. Myositis-specific autoantibodies: their clinical and pathogenic significance in disease expression. Rheumatology (Oxford). 2009;48:607–12.
355. Komura K, et al. Prevalence and clinical characteristics of anti-Mi-2 antibodies in Japanese patients with dermatomyositis. J Dermatolog Sci. 2005;40(3):215–7.
356. Targoff IN, Reichlin M. The association between Mi-2 antibodies and dermatomyositis. Arthritis Rheum. 1985;28:796–803.
357. Sato S, et al. RNA helicase encoded by melanoma differentiation-associated gene 5 is a major autoantigen in patients with clinically amyopathic dermatomyositis: association with rapidly progressive interstitial lung disease. Arthritis Rheum. 2009;60:2193–200.
358. Koga T, et al. The diagnostic utility of anti-melanoma differentiation-associated gene 5 antibody testing for predicting the prognosis of Japanese patients with DM. Rheumatology (Oxford). 2012;51:1278–84.
359. Ceribelli A, et al. Anti-MJ/NXP-2 autoantibody specificity in a cohort of adult Italian patients with polymyositis/dermatomyositis. Arthritis Res Ther. 2012;R97:14.
360. Tarricone E, et al. Anti-SAE antibodies in autoimmune myositis: identification by unlabelled protein immunoprecipitation in an Italian patient cohort. J Immunol Methods. 2012;384:128–34.
361. Fujimoto M, et al. Autoantibodies to small ubiquitin-like modifier activating enzymes in Japanese patients with dermatomyositis: comparison with a cohort. Ann Rheum Dis. 2013;72:151–3.
362. Bodoki L, et al. Four dermatomyositis-specific autoantibodies-anti-TIF1gamma, anti-NXP2, anti-SAE and anti-MDA5-in adult and juvenile patients with idiopathic inflammatory myopathies in a Hungarian cohort. Autoimmun Rev. 2014;13:1211–9.
363. Muro Y, Sugiura K, Akiyama M. Low prevalence of anti-small ubiquitin-like modifier activating enzyme antibodies in dermatomyositis patients. Autoimmunity. 2013;46:279–84.
364. Betteridge Z, et al. Identification of a novel autoantibody directed against small ubiquitin-like modifier activating enzyme in dermatomyositis. Arthritis Rheum. 2007;56:3132–7.

5 Morphea

Ada Man, M. Kari Connolly, and Robert W. Simms

Key Points

- Distribution and spread of sclerosis can help distinguish generalized morphea from systemic sclerosis (SSc).
- Approximately half of patients with plaque morphea will experience spontaneous regression after 3 years.
- Linear morphea may involve deeper tissues and may result in contractures and other extremity abnormalities that impart worse long-term outcomes than other subtypes.
- Methotrexate, sometimes in combination with glucocorticoids, is the preferred systemic option to treat progressive subtypes of morphea.

Interdisciplinary Introduction

Morphea is an inflammatory disorder characterized by sclerosis of the dermis and subcutaneous fat. While it shares histopathological characteristics with systemic sclerosis (SSc), it is a distinct entity with a generally better prognosis. (See Chap. 6 for a full discussion of SSc.) It is important to distinguish the two entities to provide accurate prognosis and to avoid causing unnecessary anxiety for patients.

A. Man
University of Manitoba, Winnipeg, MB, Canada

M. K. Connolly (✉)
University of California San Francisco, Dermatology and Medicine, San Francisco, CA, USA
e-mail: Connolly@ucsf.edu

R. W. Simms
Boston University School of Medicine, Boston, MA, USA

Nomenclature

Inconsistent nomenclature has contributed to confusion about the relationship between morphea and SSc. Outside the dermatologic literature, morphea has been referred to as localized scleroderma and circumscribed scleroderma, among other misleading names. To minimize confusion, we will use the term morphea exclusively wherever possible.

Epidemiology

There are no large population-based epidemiology studies evaluating the burden of disease in morphea, and the existing small retrospective studies may underestimate true incidence and prevalence of the disease. According to the best available data, morphea is rare, with an incidence of 0.4–2.7 per 100,000 people and a prevalence of up to 200 per 100,000 by age 80 [1, 2].

Adults and children have the same overall prevalence [1, 3], but prevalence of morphea subsets differs by age. Linear morphea, for example,

A. Garg et al. (eds.), *Interdisciplinary Approaches to Overlap Disorders in Dermatology & Rheumatology*,
https://doi.org/10.1007/978-3-319-18446-3_5

is the most common subset in children and comprises 65% of cases in this demographic [4]. Both the en coup de sabre (ECDS) and progressive hemifacial atrophy (PHA) variants of linear morphea have median onset at age of 10 and 13.6 years, respectively [5].

There is a female to male predominance in morphea of approximately 3 to 1 [1]. Morphea is somewhat more common among whites than other races [1, 3].

Pathogenesis

The etiology of morphea appears to involve complex interactions between the vascular, immune and inflammatory systems, as well as the extracellular matrix, which lead to excessive collagen deposition with end organ damage and dysfunction [6–8]. Specifying this fibrotic pathway and its upstream drivers is essential to developing effective therapies in morphea. Current hypotheses suggest that morphea is an autoimmune disease that may be initiated by an environmental trigger in genetically susceptible individuals.

Evidence for Autoimmunity

Several associations suggest that morphea is an autoimmune disease. Morphea is associated with personal and family history of autoimmune disease, including systemic lupus erythematosus, vitiligo, primary biliary cirrhosis, autoimmune hepatitis, Hashimoto thyroiditis and myasthenia gravis [3, 4]. Moreover, autoimmune serologies are often positive in morphea. A positive ANA has been reported in 20–80% of morphea patients [1, 9, 10]. Dharamsi et al. observed a prevalence of 12% for anti-histone antibodies and 8% for anti-single-stranded DNA antibodies in their cohort [10]. Additional autoantibodies reported in morphea patients include anti-fibrillin-1, rheumatoid factor, anti-cardiolipin and anti-topoisomerase II alpha [1, 11]. Of note, morphea patients are negative for autoantibodies specific for SSc, i.e., anti-centromere, anti-Scl-70, and anti-RNA polymerase III [3].

Genetic Susceptibility

The genetics of morphea have not been fully elucidated, although there is evidence to suggest genetic susceptibility in some patients. Approximately 20 familial cases of morphea have been reported. Most kindreds include a parent and a child, but morphea has also been reported to occur in monozygotic twins [12, 13]. Additionally, in a study of Major Histocompatibility Complex class I and II alleles, Jacobe et al. observed specific risk alleles for morphea. The strongest associations were with *DRB1*04:04* (in HLA class II) and *HLA-B*37* (in HLA class I) [14].

Environmental Triggers

As in many autoimmune diseases, environmental triggers may play a role in a subset of morphea cases. Suggested triggers include trauma, infection, drugs, vaccinations and radiation therapy [1, 11]. In a cohort of 750 children, 13% of children reported some kind of environmental trigger [4]. These included mechanical factors (67%, most commonly trauma, as well as insect bites or vaccinations), infections (25%), drugs (5%), and psychological distress (3%) [4]. Similar findings have been observed in adults: 16% of patients in one cohort noted triggers including surgery, penetrating trauma, injections, herpes zoster, radiation therapy, diagnostic x-ray, and extreme exercise [15].

One controversial environmental trigger implicated in morphea that deserves particular attention is infection, particularly with *Borrelia burgdorferi* [1, 11]. In a review of 19 studies from 1993 to 2007, six studies involving 40 patients showed an association between Borrelia and morphea, while 13 studies involving 240 patients failed to show the association [16]. Borrelia as a trigger for morphea in some patients is plausible but it remains unproven. Moreover, the association has not been observed in the U.S. In addition to Borrelia, a variety of viral infections have been noted as possible triggers, including CMV and hepatitis B and C [1, 11].

Drugs have rarely been implicated as a trigger in morphea [1, 17]. Implicated drugs and drug regimens include the following: balicatib, bisoprolol, bleomycin, peplomycin, D-penicillamine, bromocriptine, L-5 hydroxytryptophane plus carbidopa, L-5 hydroxytryptophane plus carbidopa and flunitrazepam, bromocriptine and clobazam, pentazocine and vitamin B12, vitamin K, and TNF alpha inhibitors [10, 17, 18]. Drugs that may cause local injection site reactions, including vaccines, represent a special case since they induce local trauma.

Morphea has also been reported to occur in association with radiation therapy [1, 11]. A recent review summarized 66 cases of morphea, which represented approximately 0.2% of breast cancer patients undergoing radiation therapy [18]. Morphea may occur within months of initiating radiation therapy, or as long as 20 years later [11]. When occurring in the setting of radiation, morphea may be mistaken for recurrent breast cancer or radiation dermatitis. It also tends to be painful and it does not respond well to usual therapies for morphea [19].

Further characterizing potential triggers in morphea may lead to insight into the underlying disease mechanism and therapeutic options.

Histopathology

Skin biopsy is an important tool in the diagnosis of morphea. Histological examination can help characterize the degree of inflammation and depth of sclerosis, and it can help rule out other entities in the differential diagnosis (Table 5.1).

Table 5.1 Differential diagnosis of morphea

Chronic graft versus host disease (GVHD)
Lipodermatosclerosis
Injection site reactions
Porphyria cutanea tarda
POEMS syndrome (Polyneuropathy, Organomegaly, Endocrinopathy, Monoclonal protein, Skin changes)
Radiation dermatitis
Stiff skin syndrome
Cutaneous malignancies
Vitiligo
Port wine stains
Hypertrophic scar

The key histopathologic findings in morphea include altered collagen in the dermis and subcutis as well as microvascular changes and inflammatory infiltrates in early lesions [1, 20]. Broad, sclerotic collagen bundles extend from the reticular dermis to the subcutis, replacing the subcutaneous fat (Fig. 5.1a, b). These changes give the gross specimen from a punch biopsy the characteristic so-called "squared off" or "cookie cutter" shape [11]. Additional findings include atrophy of adnexal structures including pilosebaceous units and eccrine glands, along with occasional endothelial cell swelling with thickening of small blood vessel walls. There is a perivascular lymphocytic infiltrate composed of both CD4+ and CD8+ cells, with some plasma cells and macrophages admixed.

Classification

Patients with morphea often are not diagnosed with the disease until 2 years into their course, which has implications for controlling the disease [21]. In part, this delay may result from a lack of published diagnostic criteria or widely accepted method of classifying the disease.

Existing classification schemes are typically based on morphology [1, 22]. We review two frequently cited classification schemes herein. Our proposed modified classification, with aspects drawn from both, is delineated in Table 5.2.

Peterson Criteria (1995)

The Peterson criteria delineate five subtypes of morphea: (1) plaque, (2) generalized (involving >2 body areas), (3) bullous, (4) linear, and (5) deep [4]. In this scheme, guttate morphea, keloidal morphea, atrophoderma of Pasini and Pierni, and lichen sclerosus et atrophicus (LS) are classified as variants of plaque morphea. We have separated out these four conditions in our classification scheme to create a rare variants group.

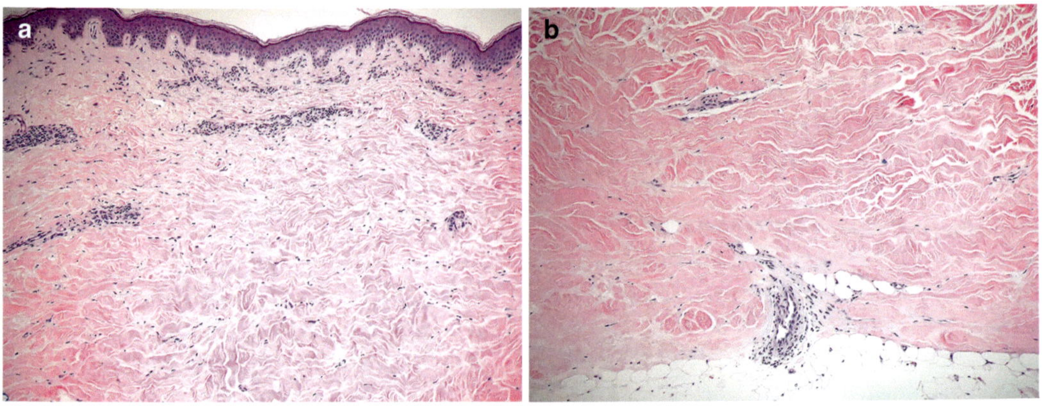

Fig. 5.1 (**a**, **b**) Histopathology of morphea. (**a**) Low power: There is marked sclerosis with diminished space between collagen bundles throughout the reticular dermis. A concurrent perivascular and interstitial infiltrate is present (H&E, × 100). (**b**) High power: Strikingly sclerotic collagen bundles are present at the juncture between the dermis and subcutis. Perivascular lymphocytes and rare plasma cells are present (H&E, ×200). (Courtesy of Silvija P. Gottesman, MD)

Table 5.2 Morphea subsets. Proposed modified criteria, based on the classifications by Peterson (1995) and Laxer and Zulian (2006)

Variant	Frequency	Characteristics
1. Plaque morphea	40–50% (adults)	Asymmetric, round-oval, sclerotic plaques, 2–16 cm Lilac borders Hyperpigmented
2. Generalized morphea	10%	>4 individual indurated plaques >3 cm, involving $\geq$2 of 7 anatomic sites (head-neck, left upper extremity, right upper extremity, left lower extremity, right lower extremity, anterior trunk, posterior trunk)
3. Linear morphea (Includes en coup de sabre, Parry-Romberg, progressive facial hemiatrophy)	20% in adults (65% in children)	Sclerotic plaque in linear configuration
4. Deep morphea (Includes morphea profunda, disabling pansclerotic morphea, eosinophilic fasciitis	<5%	Involves underlying fascia and muscle and may spare the overlying skin
5. Mixed morphea	15%	2 or more subtypes
Rare/controversial variants: Bullous morphea Guttate morphea Atrophoderma of Pasini and Pierini Keloidal (nodular) morphea Lichen sclerosis	<5%	

Of note, although bullous morphea is included as a separate category in the Peterson classification criteria [22], there were no cases of bullous morphea in their population study [4]; we have therefore included bullous morphea in our rare variants category.

Laxer and Zulian (2006)

The Laxer and Zulian criteria describe subtypes of juvenile localized scleroderma (JLS), a term synonymous with morphea that is often used in the rheumatology literature [23]. (As discussed above, instead of using the term JLS we will refer to this entity as morphea.) The Laxer and Zulian scheme includes five categories of morphea: (1) circumscribed, (2) linear, (3) generalized, (4) pansclerotic, and (5) mixed.

Within these five categories, circumscribed morphea, which is the same as plaque morphea, is divided into superficial and deep subtypes. Generalized morphea is defined as four or more individual indurated plaques >3 cm each, involving >2 of 7 anatomic sites (head-neck, each extremity, anterior trunk and posterior trunk); we believe this definition is an improvement over Peterson's and have incorporated it into our classification. Mixed morphea refers to the simultaneous presence of two or more morphea subtypes in a single patient. Of note the Laxer and Zulian classification does not include bullous morphea as a separate category.

Clinical Features

We review the clinical features of morphea subtypes according to our modified classification. In addition to the cutaneous manifestations reviewed below, morphea patients commonly experience a variety of extracutaneous symptoms such as arthralgias, myalgias and fatigue [1, 3, 4, 10]

Plaque Morphea

We define plaque morphea as three or fewer plaques on the trunk or extremities. The plaques are typically painless, round or oval, edematous, firm and indurated; they can range in size from a few centimeters to up to 30 centimeters [1, 9, 11]. Early, active lesions have a characteristic lilac to dusky violaceous erythematous color surrounding the plaque (Fig. 5.2a). As the lesions expand, they may develop yellow-white sclerotic shiny centers. As plaques of morphea age, they become sclerotic, with hyperpigmentation or hypopigmentation; there may be loss of hair and sweat glands within the plaques (Fig. 5.2b).

Generalized Morphea

Generalized morphea accounts for approximately 10% of the adult morphea patients [2]. We define generalized morphea as four or more individual plaques, each >3 cm, involving ≥2 anatomic sites, and sparing the face and hands [1, 22]. When the chest wall is involved, the nipples are characteristically spared [1]. Patients with generalized morphea often have extracutaneous symptoms, including mylagias, arthralgias and fatigue [3].

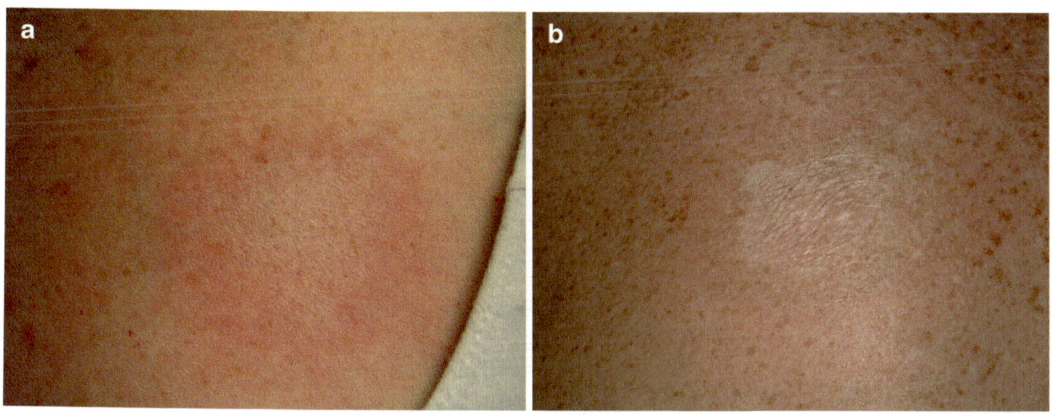

Fig. 5.2 (**a**, **b**) Plaque morphea. (**a**) Acute plaque of morphea with an indurated sclerotic center and lilac colored erythema at the periphery. Chronic sclerotic plaque of morphea with a characteristic whitish color and a wrinkled appearance on the surface, which represents epidermal atrophy. (Courtesy of Amit Garg, MD)

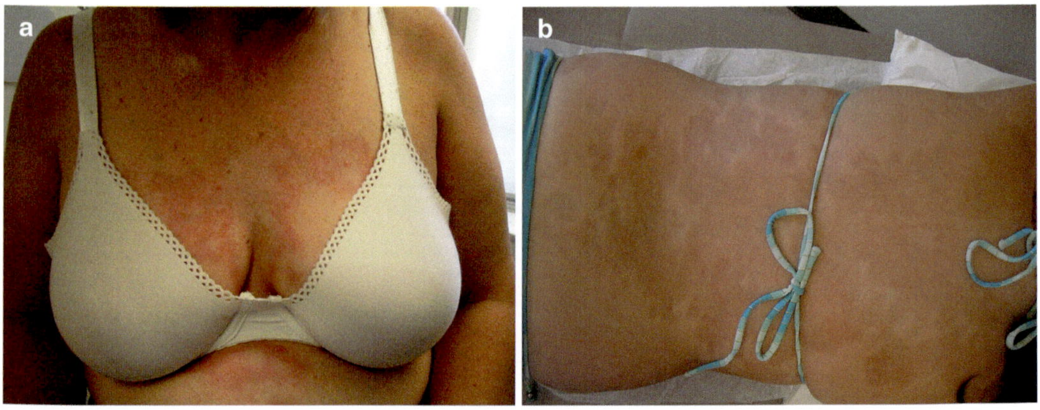

Fig. 5.3 (**a**) Generalized morphea. Rounded indurated plaques with central sclerosis and peripheral lilac colored erythema on the trunk. Face and hands are spared. (Courtesy of Amit Garg, MD). (**b**) Generalized morphea. Multiple brownish colored indurated plaques coalescing to form larger plaques over the trunk. Face and hands are spared. (Courtesy of Amit Garg, MD)

The presentation of generalized morphea may initially appear concerning for SSc, but the two entities can readily be distinguished based on their clinical features. Generalized morphea typically begins on the trunk area (Fig. 5.3a, b) and spreads outward, sparing the face, hands and feet. In contrast, diffuse SSc typically begins on the hands and spreads proximally. In addition, patients with generalized morphea do not have Raynaud's phenomenon, nailfold capillary abnormalities, or sclerodactyly. (See Chap. 6 for a full discussion of SSc.)

Linear Morphea

Linear morphea presents with a linear, indurated plaque that may follow the lines of Blaschko. It can involve a single limb (Fig. 5.4), multiple limbs, the trunk or the head. In addition to the skin, linear morphea may involve deeper tissues, including subcutaneous fat, muscle and bone. Plaques of linear morphea may result in contractures, atrophic limbs and limb length discrepancies. Partly for this reason, linear morphea is associated with worse long-term outcomes than other subtypes, both functionally and from a quality-of-life standpoint [24].

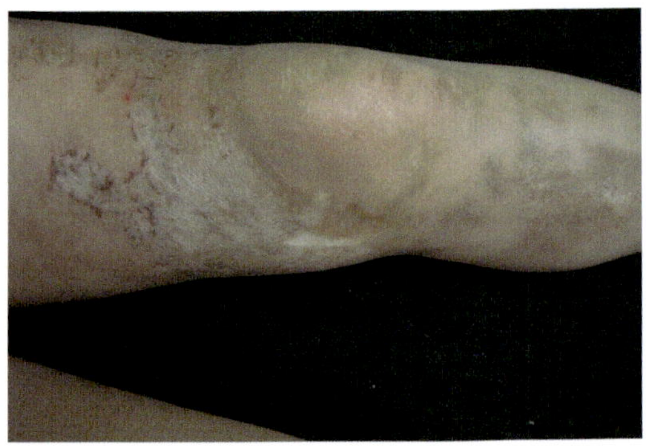

Fig. 5.4 Linear morphea. Sclerotic plaques arranged linearly involving the leg and knee joint of an adolescent. (Courtesy of Amit Garg, MD)

Two important types of linear morphea deserve special mention. En coup de sabre (ECDS; "the cut of the sabre") presents with an erythematous, sclerotic, atrophic linear plaque of morphea on the face, most commonly the paramedian forehead (Fig. 5.5). Progressive hemifacial atrophy (PHA, Parry-Romberg syndrome) affects the face and head and may also affect the eye and brain [4, 5]. In PHA, the overlying skin is normal but the deep facial structures on one side of the face, including bone, muscle and fat, fail to develop. The normal overlying skin allows PHA to be readily distinguished from ECDS.

It is important to note that both ECDS and PHA may be associated with ocular or neurological abnormalities, and thus it is of particular importance to identify patients having these sub-

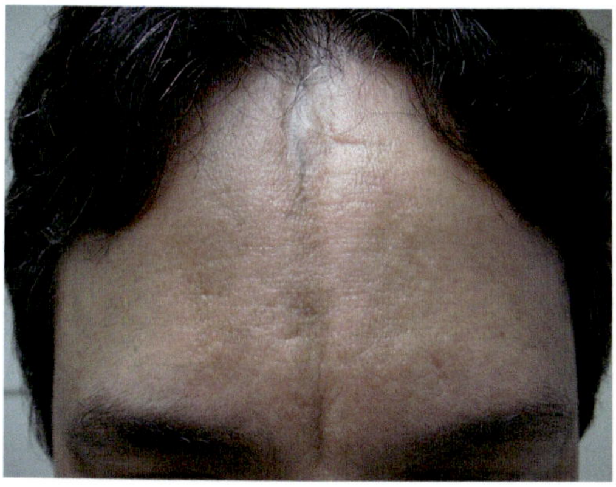

Fig. 5.5 Linear morphea (en coup de sabre). A linear atrophic sclerotic plaque of morphea on the paramedian forehead. (Courtesy of Amit Garg, MD)

types to facilitate monitoring. In a cohort of 750 pediatric morphea patients, 23% had head-face localization (99 ECDS, 8 PHA, 6 a combination); of those, 21 patients (19%) had neurologic manifestations, including seizures, headaches, vascular malformations and behavioral changes [4]. Headaches, including migraine headaches, were the presenting sign in four ECDS patients in one study [25]. There were also neuroimaging abnormalities noted in ECDS patients, including white matter abnormalities, calcifications, and EEG abnormalities. Ocular findings in these variants have been found to include anterior uveitis, episcleritis, glaucoma and keratitis [4].

Deep Morphea

Deep morphea (also called morphea profunda or subcutaneous morphea) involves underlying fascia and muscle and may spare the overlying skin [2]. Two variants of deep morphea, disabling pansclerotic morphea (DPM) and eosinophilic fasciitis (EF), deserve particular attention.

Disabling Pansclerotic Morphea

DPM of children is a variant of deep morphea described in 1980 by Winkelmann and colleagues in a series of 14 patients (10 girls and 4 boys) [26]. The clinical features were varied: 12 of 14 patients had generalized morphea, and some had esophageal or pulmonary involvement. On biopsy, however, all patients shared the common finding of pansclerosis extending from the dermis down to the panniculus, fascia, muscle and in some cases also to bone. Nine patients had a progressive course unresponsive to therapy, and two patients died from complications of the disease. The Winklemann series highlighted the important point that while morphea typically takes a benign course, more fulminant presentations with worse outcomes are possible.

Subsequent classification schemes have offered different definitions for DPM. In the Laxer and Zulian classification criteria, pansclerotic morphea (no longer referred to as "disabling") is defined as: "circumferential involvement of the limbs involving epidermis, dermis, subcutaneous tissue, muscle and bone; may affect other areas of the body with full depth sclerosis [23]." In their study of 750 children with morphea, two patients (0.3%) had DPM [4]; of these, one child developed severe atrophy of the right leg, ultimately resulting in auto-amputation. The second child developed a squamous cell carcinoma in a chronic leg ulcer and subsequently died. Other studies have found an association between DPM and recalcitrant skin ulcers as well as an increased incidence of squamous cell carcinomas [27, 28].

More recently, it has been recognized that DPM may occur in adults [29, 30]. Kim et al. reported 13 cases of adult DPM, representing a 3.6% prevalence in their adults and children cohort; mean age of onset was 54 years [30]. Seven were female and 6 were male; all patients had a generalized distribution with a more rapid onset and severe progression than in other subtypes [30].

Eosinophilic Fasciitis

A second important variant of deep morphea is eosinophilic fasciitis (EF, also called Shulman syndrome). EF is characterized by rapid-onset, symmetric, subcutaneous sclerosis, typically involving the distal extremities but sparing the hands and feet [31]. There is limb edema, associated with discomfort and pain. After the edema subsides, the surface of the skin takes on a characteristic "peau d'orange" appearance. Some patients may manifest a so-called "groove sign," in which a depression appears in the skin along the course of a vein. In about one third of patients, there is a history of antecedent intense physical exercise or trauma. The hands are not typically involved, and patients do not develop Raynaud's phenomenon.

A deep incisional biopsy to fascia is the gold standard for diagnosis of EF. MRI to assess for fascial inflammation may be helpful in supporting a clinical diagnosis of EF, guiding biopsy site selection, judging the extent of disease and monitoring response to therapy [32]. Associated laboratory findings include peripheral eosinophilia, elevated inflammatory markers and hypergammaglobulinemia [31]. Hematologic malignancies have been reported in EF patients. Different from forms of SSc, this condition tends to be responsive to oral glucocorticoids,

Mixed Morphea

Mixed morphea is characterized by the simultaneous presence of two or more subtypes of morphea. The clinical features of each type are consistent with those reviewed above.

Rare Variants

Our rare variants group includes five entities: bullous morphea, guttate morphea, atrophoderma of Pasini and Pierini, keloidal morphea, and lichen sclerosus et atrophicus. Bullous morphea is characterized by one or more tense blisters overlying a morphea plaque [22]. Guttate (or "drop-like") morphea appears as multiple, small (less than a centimeter) sclerotic papules that tend to be more superficial and lighter in color than those in other variants [9, 22]. Atrophoderma of Pasini and Pierini is characterized by multiple, depressed, atrophic, well-demarcated, hyperpigmented patches with a predilection for the posterior trunk [22]. A lack of sclerosis and dermal atrophy results in characteristic "cliff-drop borders" [22]. Some authors view this variant as burned-out morphea, while others characterize it as a distinct entity [33]. Keloidal (nodular) morphea is characterized by nodules indistinguishable from classic keloids, arising within a morphea lesion [1]. Lastly, lichen sclerosis (LS) is an idiopathic, inflammatory condition affecting the skin and mucosa, which manifests on the anogenital (85% of cases) as well as extragenital skin [9]. The eruption appears as sclerotic, white, flat-topped papules with atrophic overlying skin, fine wrinkling and follicular plugging. Studies have pointed to an association between all types of morphea and genital LS, though the frequency reported varies [34–36]. Lutz et al. found genital LS was present in 38% of morphea patients, as compared to 3% of controls [34]. Kreuter et al. noted a frequency 5.7% of LS in a retrospective study of their German morphea cohort of 472 [36]. These studies highlight the importance of genital exams in all morphea patients, particularly as genital LS may be asymptomatic and therefore patients may not be aware of it or bring it to the physician's attention. Untreated genital LS may cause unnecessary scarring, and vulvar LS carries a 5% increased lifelong risk of squamous cell carcinoma [35].

Natural History

The natural history of morphea is variable and depends, to some extent, on subtype. In approximately 50% of patients with plaque morphea, plaques will spontaneously regress and soften 3 years into the course [2]. Similarly, deep morphea may soften in 5–6 years [2]. Those lesions that do spontaneously remit may also recur, sometimes years later: in one study, children had a recurrence rate of 27%, while recurrence in adults occurred in 17% [37]. In a small group of patients, lesions of morphea stay active and persist throughout life; this is the especially true of the linear and deep subsets.

Prognosis for patients with morphea is generally good. In one study, although 11% of morphea patients had some form of long-term disability related to joint involvement, overall survival rates were the same as the general population and they had a normal life expectancy [2]. As discussed above, DPM is an important potential exception which warrants further study.

Disease Assessment

A variety of non-conventional tools have been used to assess extent and activity of skin involvement in morphea, including computerized skin scores, durometers, cutometers, infrared thermography, ultrasound and MRIs [38–40]. There is an ongoing need for better quantitative disease measurements, especially those that may be used to measure improvement from treatment over time.

Many of the existing ancillary studies of morphea disease activity require specialized tools, training, time and expense to carry out and are neither widely available nor used routinely in the clinical setting. Skin scoring systems represent one of the best available disease assessment tools for morphea, because they require no specialized equipment and rely instead on physical examination and forms that can readily be completed and scored.

One of these is the Localized Scleroderma Cutaneous Assessment Tool (LoSCAT), developed and validated by Arkachaisri et al., who integrated the modified Localized Scleroderma Skin Activity Index (mLoSSI) and the Localized Scleroderma Skin Damage Index (LoSDI) with the physician global assessment of disease damage; this tool has been demonstrated to have good inter- and intra-rater reliability [41, 42].

Comorbidities

As reviewed above, morphea patients, especially those with generalized morphea, have been found to have higher rates of autoimmune and rheumatic disease than the general population [3]. The most prevalent of these comorbidities were psoriasis, systemic lupus erythematosus, multiple sclerosis and vitiligo [3].

Morphea patients of both sexes have a high incidence of genital LS. Additionally, in a large Swedish cancer registry that looked at incidence of female cancers (breast, ovarian, uterine, and other genital cancer) in patients with 33 different autoimmune diseases, morphea patients had the highest risk of "other genital cancers" with a standard incidence ratio of 35.88 [43]. Lastly, adults and children with morphea have higher rates of depression and anxiety than age matched controls [44].

Approach to Screening and Monitoring

All morphea patients, including children, should have annual genital exams to evaluate for genital LS [34–36] (Table 5.3).

Children with linear morphea of the head (ECDS or PHA) require monitoring for ocular and central nervous system (CNS) involvement [1, 4]. Based on their finding that 14.2% of children with ECDS had ocular involvement, which was often asymptomatic even when requiring aggressive therapy to prevent irreversible damage,

Table 5.3 Workup for morphea

Morphea subset	Test/exam
All morphea patients (men and women, adults and children)	Annual genital exam to rule out LS
Patients with linear morphea of the face, head and neck (ECDS; Parry-Romberg; Progressive hemifacial atrophy)	Ophthalmologic screening every 3–4 months in the first 3 years to detect asymptomatic inflammatory eye disease Consider MRI of the head to identify and track underlying brain involvement
Generalized morphea	Although these patients can experience some external chest constriction with breathing, they do not need a full systemic sclerosis (SSc) pulmonary workup, including pulmonary function tests and high-resolution computed tomography to rule out SSc-associated interstitial lung disease (See Chap. 6 for discussion of SSc management)

Zannin et al. recommended ophthalmologic screening every 3–4 months for the first 3 years after diagnosis in patients with ECDS [45].

Monitoring for CNS involvement in patients with linear morphea of the head is less straightforward. In one series of 21 cases, 4 patients (19%) had abnormalities on head MRI, although abnormal imaging did not correlate with neurologic symptoms. The authors noted that abnormal imaging changed management in two asymptomatic patients [46]. Obtaining an MRI often requires sedation in children and may not always have management implications. As such, head MRIs in children with ECDS remain controversial.

Principals of Management

Treatment of morphea has been attempted with a wide variety of topical and systemic modalities (Table 5.4), although evidence for efficacy is limited by the quality of available studies. In particular, treatment studies suffer from a lack of validated outcome measures, small sample sizes, and a lack of controlled trials. Those randomized, controlled trials that do exist are often underpowered [47]. We review our overall approach to treating morphea as well as evidence for use of available treatment modalities.

Our approach to treating morphea is guided by the following principles [38, 40, 47]. First, it is important to establish which category of disease the patient belongs to—i.e., plaque, linear, generalized, deep or mixed—because therapy may be tailored to subtype. It is particularly important to establish depth of the lesions, since superficial lesions may respond to topicals and phototherapy, while deeper lesions usually do not and often require systemic medications. Second, it is important to note number and location of lesions: greater number of lesions overall and the presence of lesions located over joints are indications for more aggressive therapy. Third, it is critical to distinguish lesions that are active (less than 6 months old), inflammatory, and growing, from those that are burned-out, scarred and fixed, since this may guide therapeutic approach. Finally, photography is helpful to document changes in lesions during therapy.

Regardless of subtype, residual damage may result in significant morbidity and sometimes disfigurement. Physical therapy is essential to maintaining mobility and strength, especially if patients develop contractures over joints. Cosmetic treatments including fillers, fat transfers, and reconstructions may be considered when it is clear the disease has remitted [48]. Further research is needed on the outcomes of these treatments.

Table 5.4 Treatment of morphea

Modality		Subtype
Topical therapy	Class I topical corticosteroids bid for 8 to 12 weeks Tacrolimus 0.1% ointment (Protopic) Imiquimod 5% cream (Aldara) Calcipotriene (Dovonex) Calcipotriene/betamethasone dipropionate (Taclonex)	Plaque
UV phototherapy	NBUVB UVA1 (low, medium, high doses) Broadband UVA PUVA	Linear Generalized
Systemic therapy	Methotrexate in combination with systemic steroids Methotrexate Mycophenolate mofetil	Linear (ECDS; over a joint) Generalized
Experimental	Pirfenidone gel Fractional Carbon Dioxide Laser Rituximab and methotrexate HSCT	

Topical Therapy

Topical or intralesional corticosteroids are frequently used to treat morphea initially, but there is minimal evidence to support their use [9]. The highest quality studies are for genital lichen sclerosus, in which prospective and retrospective studies have shown that class I corticosteroids are effective in treating the condition [49, 50].

For lesions not responding to topical corticosteroids, topical tacrolimus 0.1% ointment (Protopic) may be used twice daily [51]. Other treatments that have been found to be effective in some studies include topical imiquimod 5% cream three times weekly, calcipotriene ointment, and a combination ointment of calcipotriol and betamethasone [52–54].

Pirfenidone 8% gel is a novel anti-fibrotic topical treatment which demonstrated improvement in the mLoSSI in a phase II trial conducted in 12 patients over 6 months [55]. Further studies are needed to clarify the optimal topical management in morphea.

Phototherapy

With anti-inflammatory and anti-fibrotic properties, phototherapy may be an efficacious and safe treatment for morphea, especially in children and pregnant women [56]. Kerscher et al. introduced UVA1 therapy for morphea [57]. Subsequently, Kreuter et al. demonstrated that narrow-band UVB (NBUVB) was comparable to low- and medium-dose UVA1 [58].

There is no consensus in the literature on the optimal phototherapy modality for treatment of morphea, i.e., NBUVB, UVA1, broadband UVA or PUVA; rather, this choice is largely a function of body location, regional preference, and access to devices. We do not have UVA1 at our institution but have good success with NBUVB for superficial lesions and PUVA for deeper ones. In our experience it takes longer than 8 weeks to achieve an initial response, and we do not evaluate treatment success or failure until 3–6 months into therapy.

Systemic Therapy

Methotrexate, sometimes in combination with glucocorticoids, is the preferred systemic option to treat progressive subtypes of morphea. Linear morphea in children and adults has been shown to respond to this combination in several trials, including a randomized controlled trial [38, 47, 59, 60]. The dose of methotrexate is 0.3–0.4 mg/kg per week in children or 15–25 mg/week in adults. The prednisone dose is 1 mg/kg daily. Pulse dosing of intravenous corticosteroids followed by a taper may also be used [38, 61]. If there is inadequate response to methotrexate and prednisone after 8–12 weeks, then mycophenolate mofetil may be considered [38]. Evidence for remaining systemic treatment options is anecdotal.

Summary

Morphea is a rare sclerosing skin disease that is not associated with visceral organ involvement, although generalized, linear and pansclerotic subtypes may be associated with significant morbidity. Approximately half of patients will experience spontaneous regression, and prognosis for patients with morphea is generally good. Management involves establishing subtype, depth and extent of lesions, and activity of lesions. Methotrexate, sometimes in combination with glucocorticoids, is the preferred systemic option to treat severe or progressive disease. Physical therapy is an essential component of the management of patients with deep lesions and those with lesions overlying joints.

References

1. Fett N, Werth VP. Update on morphea: part I. Epidemiology, clinical presentation, and pathogenesis. J Am Acad Dermatol. 2011;64(2):217–28; quiz 229–30.
2. Peterson LS, et al. The epidemiology of morphea (localized scleroderma) in Olmsted County 1960–1993. J Rheumatol. 1997;24(1):73–80.

3. Leitenberger JJ, et al. Distinct autoimmune syndromes in morphea: a review of 245 adult and pediatric cases. Arch Dermatol. 2009;145(5):545–50.
4. Zulian F, et al. Juvenile localized scleroderma: clinical and epidemiological features in 750 children. An international study. Rheumatology (Oxford). 2006;45(5):614–20.
5. Tolkachjov SN, Patel NG, Tollefson MM. Progressive hemifacial atrophy: a review. Orphanet J Rare Dis. 2015;10:39.
6. Gabrielli A, Avvedimento EV, Krieg T. Scleroderma. N Engl J Med. 2009;360(19):1989–2003.
7. Katsumoto TR, Whitfield ML, Connolly MK. The pathogenesis of systemic sclerosis. Annu Rev Pathol. 2011;6:509–37.
8. Varga J. Overview: pathogenesis integrated. In: Varga J, Denton CP, Wigley FM, editors. Scleroderma: from pathogenesis to comprehensive management. New York: Springer Science+Business Media LLC; 2012. p. 163.
9. Rocken M, Ghoreschi K, Morphea and lichen sclerosus In: Bolognia J, Jorizzo J, Schaffer J, editors. Dermatology. Elsevier Saunders, Amsterdam, The Netherlands; 2012. p. 657–70.
10. Dharamsi JW, et al. Morphea in adults and children cohort III: nested case-control study--the clinical significance of autoantibodies in morphea. JAMA Dermatol. 2013;149(10):1159–65.
11. Gilliam AE, Gilliam AC. Localized scleroderma. In: Varga J, Denton CP, Wigley FM, editors. Scleroderma. Springer, New York City, NY, USA; 2012. p. 113–35.
12. Pham CM, Browning JC. Morphea affecting a father and son. Pediatr Dermatol. 2010;27(5):536–7.
13. Dubois EL, et al. Progressive systemic sclerosis (PSS) and localized scleroderma (morphea) with positive LE cell test and unusual systemic manifesstations compatible with systemic lupus erythematous (SLE): presentation of 14 cases including one set of identical twins, one with scleroderma dn the other with SLE. Review of the literature. Medicine (Baltimore). 1971;50(3):199–222.
14. Jacobe H, et al. Major histocompatibility complex class I and class II alleles may confer susceptibility to or protection against morphea: findings from the Morphea in Adults and Children cohort. Arthritis Rheumatol. 2014;66(11):3170–7.
15. Grabell D, et al. The role of skin trauma in the distribution of morphea lesions: a cross-sectional survey of the Morphea in Adults and Children cohort IV. J Am Acad Dermatol. 2014;71(3):493–8.
16. Zollinger T, et al. Borrelia in granuloma annulare, morphea and lichen sclerosus: a PCR-based study and review of the literature. J Cutan Pathol. 2010;37(5):571–7.
17. Peroni A, et al. Drug-induced morphea: report of a case induced by balicatib and review of the literature. J Am Acad Dermatol. 2008;59(1):125–9.
18. Ramírez J, et al. Morphea associated with the use of adalimumab: a case report and review of the literature. Mod Rheumatol. 2012;22(4):602–4.
19. Spalek M, Jonska-Gmyrek J, Gałecki J. Radiation-induced morphea - a literature review. J Eur Acad Dermatol Venereol. 2015;29(2):197–202.
20. Weedon D. Disorders of collagen. In: Weedon's skin pathology. Churchill, Livingstone, Elsevier, London, United Kingdom; 2010. p. 304–29.
21. Johnson W, Jacobe H. Morphea in adults and children cohort II: patients with morphea experience delay in diagnosis and large variation in treatment. J Am Acad Dermatol. 2012;67(5):881–9.
22. Peterson LS, Nelson AM, Su WP. Classification of morphea (localized scleroderma). Mayo Clin Proc. 1995;70(11):1068–76.
23. Laxer RM, Zulian F. Localized scleroderma. Curr Opin Rheumatol. 2006;18(6):606–13.
24. Saxton-Daniels S, Jacobe HT. An evaluation of long-term outcomes in adults with pediatric-onset morphea. Arch Dermatol. 2010;146(9):1044–5.
25. Polcari I, et al. Headaches as a presenting symptom of linear morphea en coup de sabre. Pediatrics. 2014;134(6):e1715–9.
26. Diaz-Perez JL, Connolly SM, Winkelmann RK. Disabling pansclerotic morphea of children. Arch Dermatol. 1980;116(2):169–73.
27. Wollina U, et al. Disabling pansclerotic morphea of childhood poses a high risk of chronic ulceration of the skin and squamous cell carcinoma. Int J Low Extrem Wounds. 2007;6(4):291–8.
28. Grewal I, Khan O, Davis W. Squamous cell carcinoma and eosinophilia in a long-term course of pansclerotic morphea. BMJ Case Rep. 2014;2014:bcr2014205737.
29. Maragh SH, et al. Disabling pansclerotic morphea: clinical presentation in two adults. J Am Acad Dermatol. 2005;53(2 Suppl 1):S115–9.
30. Kim A, et al. Clinical features of patients with morphea and the pansclerotic subtype: a cross-sectional study from the morphea in adults and children cohort. J Rheumatol. 2014;41(1):106–12.
31. Pinal-Fernandez I, Selva-O'Callaghan A, Grau JM. Diagnosis and classification of eosinophilic fasciitis. Autoimmun Rev. 2014;13(4–5):379–82.
32. Kirchgesner T, et al. Eosinophilic fasciitis: typical abnormalities, variants and differential diagnosis of fasciae abnormalities using MR imaging. Diagn Interv Imaging. 2015;96(4):341–8.
33. Provost, T., A. Greenberg, and V. Falanga, Localized cutaneous sclerosis. In: Sontheimer R, Provost T, editors. Cutaneous manifestations of rheumatic diseases. Philadelphia: Lippincott, Williams & Wilkins: Philadelphia; 2004. p. 125–34.
34. Lutz V, et al. High frequency of genital lichen sclerosus in a prospective series of 76 patients with morphea: toward a better understanding of the spectrum of morphea. Arch Dermatol. 2012;148(1):24–8.
35. Schlosser BJ. Practice gaps. Missing genital lichen sclerosus in patients with morphea: don't ask? Don't tell?: comment on "High frequency of genital lichen sclerosus in a prospective series of 76 patients with morphea". Arch Dermatol. 2012;148(1):28–9.

36. Kreuter A, et al. Coexistence of lichen sclerosus and morphea: a retrospective analysis of 472 patients with localized scleroderma from a German tertiary referral center. J Am Acad Dermatol. 2012;67(6):1157–62.
37. Mertens JS, et al. Disease recurrence in localized scleroderma: a retrospective analysis of 344 patients with paediatric- or adult-onset disease. Br J Dermatol. 2015;172(3):722–8.
38. Fett N, Werth VP. Update on morphea: part II. Outcome measures and treatment. J Am Acad Dermatol. 2011;64(2):231–42; quiz 243–4.
39. Zulian F. Juvenile localized scleroderma. In: Varga J, Denton CP, Wigley FM, editors. Scleroderma. Springer, New York City, NY, USA; 2012. p. 85–92.
40. Nouri S, Jacobe H. Recent developments in diagnosis and assessment of morphea. Curr Rheumatol Rep. 2013;15(2):308.
41. Arkachaisri T, et al. The localized scleroderma skin severity index and physician global assessment of disease activity: a work in progress toward development of localized scleroderma outcome measures. J Rheumatol. 2009;36(12):2819–29.
42. Arkachaisri T, et al. Development and initial validation of the localized scleroderma skin damage index and physician global assessment of disease damage: a proof-of-concept study. Rheumatology (Oxford). 2010;49(2):373–81.
43. Hemminki K, et al. Effect of autoimmune diseases on risk and survival in female cancers. Gynecol Oncol. 2012;127(1):180–5.
44. Kroft EB, de Jong EM, Evers AW. Psychological distress in patients with morphea and eosinophilic fasciitis. Arch Dermatol. 2009;145(9):1017–22.
45. Zannin ME, et al. Ocular involvement in children with localised scleroderma: a multi-centre study. Br J Ophthalmol. 2007;91(10):1311–4.
46. Chiu YE, et al. A significant proportion of children with morphea en coup de sabre and Parry-Romberg syndrome have neuroimaging findings. Pediatr Dermatol. 2012;29(6):738–48.
47. Zwischenberger BA, Jacobe HT. A systematic review of morphea treatments and therapeutic algorithm. J Am Acad Dermatol. 2011;65(5):925–41.
48. Cavusoglu T, et al. Reconstruction of coup de sabre deformity (linear localized scleroderma) by using galeal frontalis muscle flap and demineralized bone matrix combination. J Craniofac Surg. 2011;22(1):257–8.
49. Funaro D, et al. A double-blind, randomized prospective study evaluating topical clobetasol propionate 0.05% versus topical tacrolimus 0.1% in patients with vulvar lichen sclerosus. J Am Acad Dermatol. 2014;71(1):84–91.
50. Goldstein AT, et al. A double-blind, randomized controlled trial of clobetasol versus pimecrolimus in patients with vulvar lichen sclerosus. J Am Acad Dermatol. 2011;64(6):e99–104.
51. Kroft EB, et al. Efficacy of topical tacrolimus 0.1% in active plaque morphea: randomized, double-blind, emollient-controlled pilot study. Am J Clin Dermatol. 2009;10(3):181–7.
52. Dytoc M, et al. Evaluation of the efficacy and safety of topical imiquimod 5% for plaque-type morphea: a multicenter, prospective, vehicle-controlled trial. J Cutan Med Surg. 2015;19(2):132–9.
53. Cunningham BB, et al. Topical calcipotriene for morphea/linear scleroderma. J Am Acad Dermatol. 1998;39(2 Pt 1):211–5.
54. Dytoc MT, Kossintseva I, Ting PT. First case series on the use of calcipotriol-betamethasone dipropionate for morphoea. Br J Dermatol. 2007;157(3):615–8.
55. Rodríguez-Castellanos M, et al. Pirfenidone gel in patients with localized scleroderma: a phase II study. Arthritis Res Ther. 2015;16(6):510.
56. Walker D, Jacobe H. Phototherapy in the age of biologics. Semin Cutan Med Surg. 2011;30(4):190–8.
57. Kerscher M, Dirschka T, Volkenandt M. Treatment of localised scleroderma by UVA1 phototherapy. Lancet. 1995;346(8983):1166.
58. Kreuter A, et al. A randomized controlled study of low-dose UVA1, medium-dose UVA1, and narrowband UVB phototherapy in the treatment of localized scleroderma. J Am Acad Dermatol. 2006;54(3):440–7.
59. Zulian F, et al. Methotrexate treatment in juvenile localized scleroderma: a randomized, double-blind, placebo-controlled trial. Arthritis Rheum. 2011;63(7):1998–2006.
60. Zulian F, et al. A long-term follow-up study of methotrexate in juvenile localized scleroderma (morphea). J Am Acad Dermatol. 2012;67(6):1151–6.
61. Martini G, et al. Successful treatment of severe or methotrexate-resistant juvenile localized scleroderma with mycophenolate mofetil. Rheumatology (Oxford). 2009;48(11):1410–3.

Systemic Sclerosis

6

Ada Man, M. Kari Connolly, and Robert W. Simms

Key Points

- Systemic sclerosis (SSc) is an autoimmune connective tissue disease with internal organ involvement that carries significant morbidity and mortality
- SSc is a disorder distinct from morphea, with a different presentation and graver prognosis; the two entities should not be conflated
- SSc patients must be monitored and treated for pulmonary, renal, gastrointestinal (GI), and cardiac involvement
- Highly specific autoantibodies may be present in SSc patients, with diagnostic and prognostic implications
- Recent therapeutic advances indicate that immunosuppressive therapy can prevent progression of severe systemic disease in SSc

Interdisciplinary Introduction

Systemic sclerosis (SSc, also called scleroderma) is an autoimmune connective tissue disease characterized by cutaneous sclerosis. It commonly progresses to involve fibrosis of one or more internal organs, with pulmonary involvement as the leading cause of death. In many ways, SSc is the prototype disease for which optimal management requires streamlined collaboration between multiple subspecialists, including dermatologists, rheumatologists, pulmonologists, nephrologists, gastroenterologists, nursing and support staff. Patients may be best served at academic centers with a focus on SSc patients, such as the Scleroderma Centers of Excellence, which may also offer participation in clinical trials. Rheumatologists often function as the coordinating physicians for these patients, while dermatologists have a role in managing cutaneous sclerosis, pruritus and digital ulcers.

To reflect the optimal interdisciplinary approach to SSc, this chapter reviews the classification, clinical features, pathogenesis, treatment and monitoring of SSc, with equal attention paid to all organ systems. The goal is to provide a text that may serve as a resource for physicians of all disciplines.

A. Man
University of Manitoba, Winnipeg, MB, Canada

M. K. Connolly (✉)
University of California San Francisco, Dermatology and Medicine, San Francisco, CA, USA
e-mail: Connolly@ucsf.edu

R. W. Simms
Boston University School of Medicine, Boston, MA, USA

A. Garg et al. (eds.), *Interdisciplinary Approaches to Overlap Disorders in Dermatology & Rheumatology*,
https://doi.org/10.1007/978-3-319-18446-3_6

Nomenclature

We draw a clear distinction between morphea and SSc, which are increasingly understood as separate entities rather than findings on a spectrum. Morphea is a disorder characterized by increased collagen deposition leading to localized cutaneous sclerosis that, unlike SSc, does not typically progress to involve internal organs, even when there is diffuse cutaneous disease. Misdiagnosis of morphea as SSc may expose patients to undue anxiety and unnecessary testing.

Clarity in the nomenclature surrounding these distinct entities is essential to facilitating diagnostic specificity. Unfortunately, the nomenclature is often confusing, as illustrated by the use of the terms "localized scleroderma" and "limited scleroderma." Localized scleroderma is synonymous with morphea; to avoid any confusion we will use the term "morphea" exclusively to describe this entity, as many dermatologists do. Limited scleroderma, by contrast, is a type of SSc that can progress to involve internal organs. It is also known as limited cutaneous (lcSSc) and was previously called CREST syndrome, an acronym standing for calcinosis, Raynaud's phenomenon, esophageal dysmotility, sclerodactyly and telangiectasia. To avoid confusion, we will use the term limited SSc to describe this entity. (See Chap. 5 for a complete discussion on morphea.)

Epidemiology

Reliable epidemiological studies of SSc have been difficult to execute due to the rarity of the condition and heterogeneity in clinical presentation. Incidence is estimated at 3.7 to 23 cases per million people, while prevalence is estimated at 31 to 443 per million people. The wide range relates to variations in diagnostic criteria used, time period surveyed, and geographic location [1]. Moreover, prevalence estimates drawn from populations with milder and earlier disease, and in times with improved survival rates, may yield higher rates. Incidence and prevalence estimates from United States, Australia, and Southern Europe have been higher than those from Japan, Taiwan, and Northern Europe. Of note, there have been no new epidemiological surveys since the establishment of the 2013 American College of Rheumatology (ACR)/European League Against Rheumatism (EULAR) classification criteria for SSc [2]. These new criteria are expected to lead to higher estimates given their increased sensitivity and inclusion of earlier disease manifestations.

SSc affects people of all ages, though the peak age of onset is between 30 and 50 years [3]. As with many other autoimmune diseases, SSc disproportionately affects women, particularly women of reproductive age, with the female to male ratio ranging from 5:1 to 12:1 [4]. The reasons for this sex disparity are incompletely understood, but sex hormones, epigenetics, occupational exposures, and lifestyle differences may all play a role [4, 5]. Males who do develop SSc have been consistently shown to have a worse prognosis when compared to their female counterparts [6–8]. Males tend to have more diffuse disease and higher frequencies of digital ulcers, pulmonary arterial hypertension (PAH), heart failure, and all-cause mortality [9].

There are also variations in the epidemiology of SSc by race and ethnicity. Incidence and prevalence of SSc are greater among African-Americans than whites [6, 10, 11], with a younger age of onset (peak in the third decade of life) [12]. African-Americans are also almost twice as likely to have diffuse SSc, which is often associated with more severe disease [10, 11]. African-Americans with SSc have a higher frequency of autoantibodies to topoisomerase and U3 RNP, a higher risk of interstitial lung (ILD), and 1.8 times the risk of mortality as compared with Caucasians with SSc [6, 13, 14].

Hispanics with SSc have also been noted to have more diffuse skin involvement and digital ulcers than Caucasians [15]. There is a paucity of information on Asians with SSc, though estimates from China and Japan have placed prevalence rates between 21 and 100 cases per million [16, 17].

SSc Classification Criteria

The American Rheumatism Association (now the ACR) established criteria for the classification criteria of SSc in 1980 [18]. One major or two minor criteria were required for a diagnosis of SSc. The major criterion was skin thickening proximal to the metacarpal phalangeal joints, and the minor criteria included sclerodactyly, digital pitting scars, and bibasilar pulmonary fibrosis.

The 1980 ACR criteria were not sensitive enough to detect early disease and also excluded a large portion of limited SSc patients. To correct these deficits, the ACR collaborated with the EULAR to create new criteria, which were published in 2013 (Table 6.1) [2]. These criteria have higher sensitivity (91% as compared to 75% for the 1980 criteria) because they include more disease manifestations, including those that present early in the disease course. They also have improved specificity (92% as compared to 72%), likely due to the weighting of each item. The 2013 criteria are applicable to any patient considered for inclusion in a study on SSc. They do not apply to patients with skin thickening that spares the fingers or to patients who have a SSc-like disorder that better explains their manifestations (Table 6.2).

SSc Subsets

SSc is traditionally divided into two subsets: limited cutaneous SSc (lcScc) and diffuse cutaneous SSc (dcSSc) [19]. Classification is based on the

Table 6.2 Differential diagnosis of systemic sclerosis (SSc)

Generalized morphea
Scleredema
Scleromyxedema
Nephrogenic systemic fibrosis
Eosinophilic fasciitis
Lipodermatosclerosis
Malignancy-related palmar fasciitis
Chronic graft versus host disease
Diabetic cheiroarthropathy
Frostbite
Erythromelalgia
Lichen sclerosus et atrophicus

Table 6.1 The 2013 ACR/EULAR criteria for the classification of SSc [2]

Item	Sub-item(s)	Weight/score*
Skin thickening of the fingers of both hands extending proximal to the metacarpophalangeal joints *(single criterion sufficient for diagnosis)*	–	9
Skin thickening of the fingers *(only count the higher score)*	Puffy fingers	2
	Sclerodactyly of the fingers (distal to the metacarpophalangeal joints but proximal to the proximal interphalangeal joints)	4
Fingertip lesions *(only count the higher score)*	Digital tip ulcers	2
	Fingertip pitting scars	3
Telangiectasia	–	2
Abnormal nailfold capillaries	–	2
Pulmonary arterial hypertension and/or interstitial lung disease *(maximum score is 2)*	Pulmonary arterial hypertension	2
	Interstitial lung disease	2
Raynaud's phenomenon	–	3
SSc-related autoantibodies *(maximum score is 3)*	Anticentromere Anti-topoisomerase I Anti-RNA polymerase III	3
Total score	The total score is determined by adding the maximum weight (score) in each category.	Patients with a total score of ≥9 are classified as having definite SSc.

ACR American College of Rheumatology, *EULAR* European League Against Rheumatism, *SSc* systemic sclerosis extent of skin involvement, with lcSSc being restricted to the face and distal extremities (distal to elbows and knees), and dcSSc also involving the skin proximal to the elbows and knees and/or the trunk. Hand involvement is characteristic of both subsets; without it, the diagnosis of SSc should be reconsidered.

The two SSc subsets tend to take distinct courses. Patients with lcSSc typically have a more prolonged and slower progression of disease: they may first develop Raynaud's phenomenon, and then years later progress to sclerodactyly with possible digital ulcers and pits, accompanied by facial skin thickening, telangectasias and/or calcinosis. Gastroesophageal reflux disease is common, and esophageal dysmotility may be seen. Pulmonary hypertension (PH) can occur in the lcSSc group even many years after stable disease. Many lcSSc patients also have ILD, although it may be milder than that seen in dcSSc and exacerbated by prolonged esophageal reflux, possibly related to recurrent silent aspiration of gastric acids. The lcSSc group is also characterized by positive anti-centromere antibodies, which are associated with improved survival.

Patients with dcSSc tend to have a much more acute and rapidly progressive course than those with lcSSc, including short duration of Raynaud's before the onset of other symptoms. They often develop edema and pruritus of the hands and legs as skin begins to thicken, which progresses from the distal extremities to the trunk within months. Arthralgias, arthritis, carpal tunnel syndrome, tendon friction rubs and constitutional symptoms are characteristic. Renal, cardiac, and intestinal involvement is more common for dcSSc than lcScc.

Beyond the limited and diffuse subsets, there is also a rarer subset called SSc sine scleroderma, which is defined by characteristic SSc-like internal organ involvement plus or minus SSc antibodies, but without cutaneous manifestations.

Individuals with SSc often also have features of other connective tissue diseases, such as myositis or SLE, in which case they would be considered to have an overlap syndrome or mixed connective tissue disease.

New classifications based on clinical features in combination with serological markers are an area of active research.

Clinical Features

SSc is a disease characterized by the triad of vasculopathy, fibrosis, and autoimmunity. These pathogenic categories provide a useful framework for considering the clinical features of the disease. In particular, vasculopathy and fibrosis are apparent in the majority of the organ manifestations, leading to irreversible organ dysfunction.

The natural history of SSc is for most organ involvement to occur within 2–5 years of onset. For dcSSc, peak skin thickness also occurs within 2–5 years, whereas it progresses less rapidly in lcSSc and never reaches as high a peak. After skin thickness peaks, the skin begins to soften. It is rare for new organs to become involved after this time, with the exception that PAH and gastrointestinal (GI) malabsorption may be late manifestations in lcSSc (Fig. 6.1). It is important to recognize that spontaneous skin softening is part of the natural history of SSc, a phenomenon sometimes misattributed to treatment effect.

Here we review clinical manifestations of SSc by organ system.

Cutaneous

In early SSc, an inflammatory, edematous phase often occurs before fibrosis is apparent. In this stage, the hands and fingers may appear puffy, characterized by widened digits with loss of skin creases. Edema may also involve the legs and feet. Pruritus is common during this phase secondary to the production of histamine and bradykinins and possibly irritation of nerve fibers.

After the inflammatory phase, patients typically develop progressive fibrosis over 2–5 years. Some patients may initially appear to have limited-type skin involvement but will progress

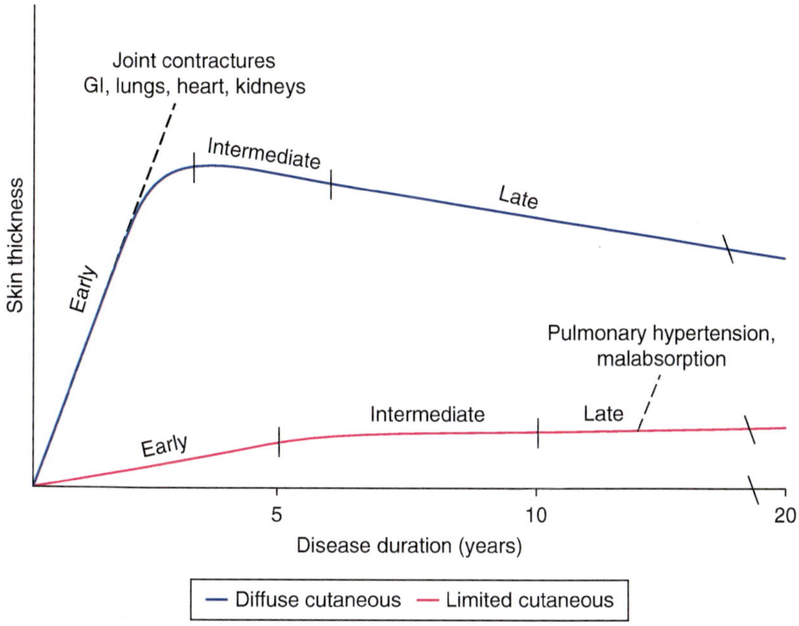

Fig. 6.1 Stages of systemic sclerosis (SSc) [20]. Schematic representation of the stages of diffuse and limited cutaneous SSc over time, including the usual relation between skin thickening and various organ system involvements. (GI, gastrointestinal)

during this period to have clinically apparent dcSSc. Progression of fibrosis usually occurs from distal to proximal, although patches of skin thickening can also occur outside this distribution. As the skin fibrosis progresses, sebaceous and eccrine glands may atrophy, resulting in xerosis and cracking of the skin. Hair loss in involved areas is also common. Rapid progression of skin thickening is associated with poor survival [21].

Skin thickening and tightening can develop in all parts of the body. Sclerodactyly, or thickening and tightening of the skin of the fingers, which are tapered distally, is the hallmark of SSc (Fig. 6.2). When the involved skin extends from the fingers to skin proximal to the metacarpophalangeal (MCP) joints, as reviewed above, this finding alone is enough for diagnosis of SSc (Fig. 6.3). Many SSc patients also have digital skin thickening only distal to the MCP joints, generally accompanied by other features that define the disease. Skin thickening proximal to the MCP joints without involvement of the fingers, by contrast, should prompt the consideration of an alternative diagnosis, including SSc mimics such as morphea or eosinophilic fasciitis. (See Table 6.2 for the differential diagnosis of SSc.) In long-standing SSc, skin on the fingers may become atrophic and appear thinner, sometimes becoming tethered to the underlying soft tissue (Fig. 6.4).

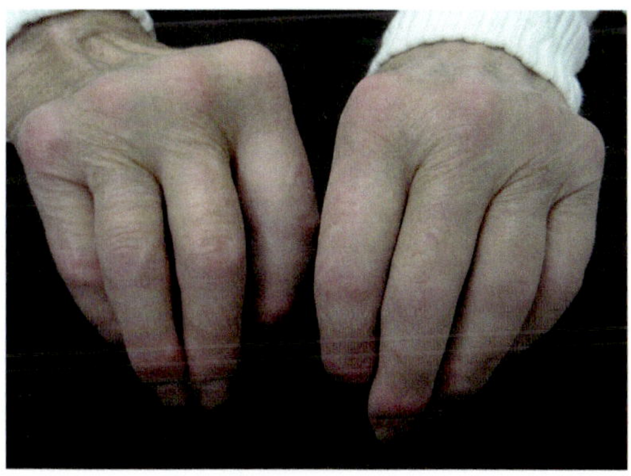

Fig. 6.2 Systemic sclerosis. Sclerodactyly. Thickening and tightening of the skin of fingers, which are tapered distally. (Courtesy of Amit Garg, MD)

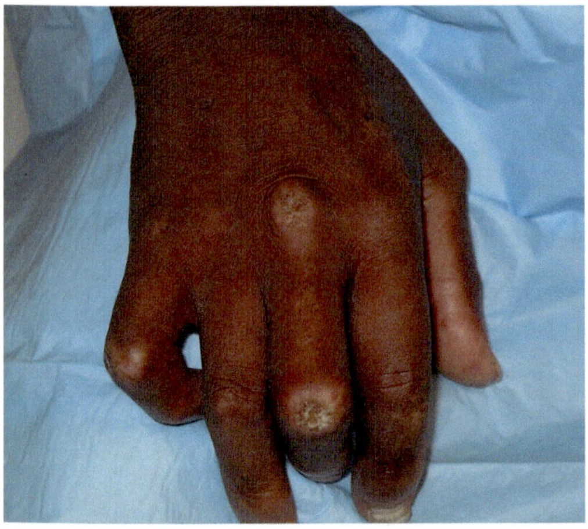

Fig. 6.3 Systemic sclerosis. Ulcerated cutaneous calcinosis involving the fingers over the metacarpophalangeal and proximal interphalangeal joints. (Courtesy of Amit Garg, MD)

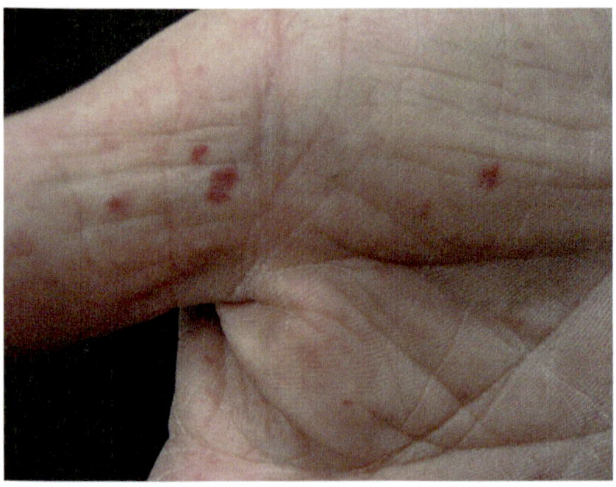

Fig. 6.4 Limited cutaneous systemic sclerosis. Matted telangiectasias on the palm of a patient with limited cutaneous systemic sclerosis. (Courtesy of Amit Garg, MD)

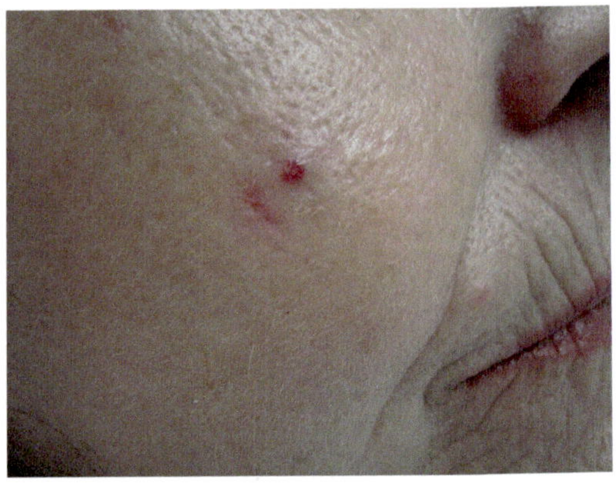

Fig. 6.5 Limited cutaneous systemic sclerosis. Telangiectasia, thinning of the lips and tethering of the skin in the perioral area to create a wrinkled appearance in a patient with limited cutaneous systemic sclerosis. (Courtesy of Amit Garg, MD)

In lcSSc, skin thickening on the extremities occurs distal to the elbows and knees, while in dcSSc, it involves skin proximal to these joints, and may involve the trunk and back. Both subsets may have facial and neck involvement.

On the face, characteristic skin changes in SSc include tethering of the skin in the perioral area to create a wrinkled appearance, along with thinning of the lips and a reduced oral aperture (Fig. 6.5). Gum retraction may occur as well, leading to prominent front teeth. In the neck, Barnett's sign is characterized by a visible and palpable tight band over the platysma when the neck is extended [22]. On the chest and abdomen, the skin may be thickened in a band-like distribution along pressure areas, such as at the bra line and the waist.

Approximately 2–5 years into the course of SSc, the final stage of cutaneous disease is skin softening. This phenomenon occurs to some extent in most patients, though the skin may not always return to its baseline quality. Cutaneous improvement tends to begin in areas that have been affected last. Sweat and oil glands as well as hair follicles may return as well. Patients may note a decrease in fatigue, arthralgias, tendon friction rubs, and pruritus at this stage [23]. There is evidence that those who have significant improvement in skin thickening have improved survival [24]. Late exacerbations of skin thickening can rarely occur [23].

Beyond fibrosis and skin thickening, other cutaneous findings in SSc include hyperpigmentation, hypopigmentation, telangectasias, and calcinosis. Hyperpigmentation commonly occurs in skin creases, but pigmentary alterations may occur anywhere on the body and often have a "salt and pepper" appearance, due to perifollicular sparing of pigment loss (Fig. 6.6). Telangectasias are more common in lcSSc and are usually seen on the face, although they can also be found in other areas, such as the oral mucosa and the tongue. The presence of telan-

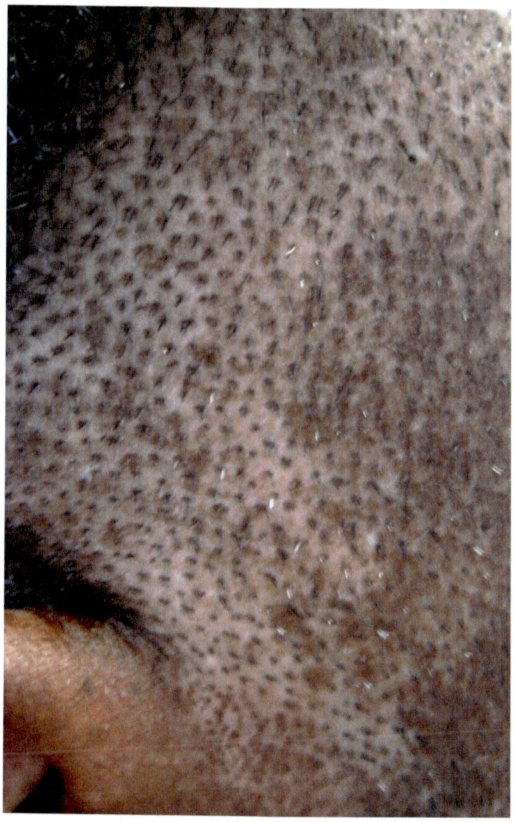

Fig. 6.6 Systemic sclerosis. Pigmentary alterations related to sclerosis often have a "salt and pepper" appearance due to perifollicular sparing of pigment loss. (Courtesy of Joseph Merola, MD)

gectasias in SSc may be associated with presence of PH [25]. Calcinosis, or the subcutaneous deposition of calcium hydroxyapatite, occurs both in lcScc and dcSSc and commonly involves the fingers and extensor surfaces of the limbs, possibly related to mechanical pressure and microtrauma. Involved areas may ulcerate and drain, and they may become infected.

Vascular

Raynaud's Phenomenon

Raynaud's phenomenon is present in greater than 95% of SSc patients. This finding is classically described as triphasic, where pallor of the fingers or toes is followed by ischemia, characterized by bluish duskiness, followed by reactive hyperemia with red erythema. However, many SSc patients do not report all three phases. The color changes typically end at a sharp cutoff at the proximal part of the fingers.

The mechanism behind Raynaud's phenomenon in SSc is thought to be vasospasm occurring in fixed, narrowed blood vessels. This is distinct from the vasospasm that occurs in normal caliber vessels among patients with primary Raynaud's disease. The typical trigger for Raynaud's is cold temperature, though stress or strong emotion may less commonly be implicated.

Digital Ischemia

The digital vasculopathy that precipitates Raynaud's phenomenon in SSc may also lead to persistent digital ischemia and poorly healing digital ulcers, acro-osteolysis (bony resorption of the terminal digital tufts seen on X-rays and shortened fingers seen clinically, loss of bulk from the finger pads, and occasionally gangrene and digital amputation (Fig. 6.7). Digital pits are common in SSc and represent ischemic insults presenting as tiny atrophic depressions at the fingertips. Digital ulcers also occur at the distal fingertips and may be seen in association with necrotic debris underneath the fingernail or overlying the knuckles. This debris is secondary to minor repeated trauma in the setting of poorly healing skin due to flexion contractures and tautness. Digital ulcers are very painful and can take a long time to heal, or they may not heal at all. They often become infected, requiring oral antibiotics. Experts differ in their opinions on whether or not debridement helps with healing. Uncommonly, severe ischemic disease may result in digital amputation [26].

The digital vasculopathy in SSc is mostly microvascular, although overlying macrovascular disease, such as within the ulnar arteries, may exacerbate the ischemic insult and should be ruled out, especially in cases of refractory ischemic complications.

Microvascular disease may be evident in characteristic nailfold capillary abnormalities observed with a widefield microscope or videocapillaroscopy, or a dermatoscope. Characteristic nailfold changes include dilated capillaries, loss of capillary loops ("drop-out"), architectural

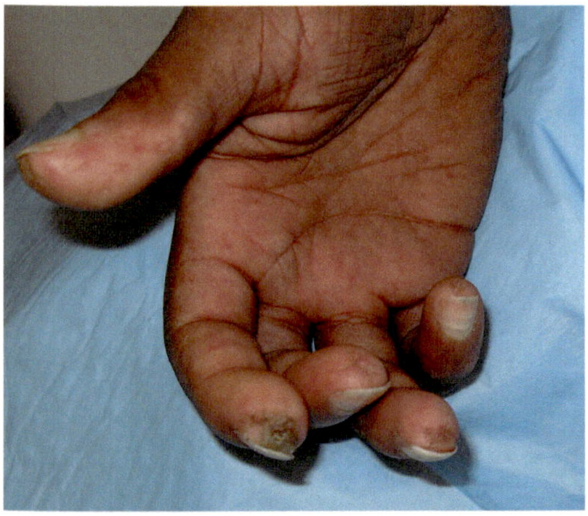

Fig. 6.7 Systemic sclerosis. Finger pad ulcers, pits and loss of bulk secondary to vasculopathy and persistent digital ischemia. (Courtesy of Amit Garg, MD)

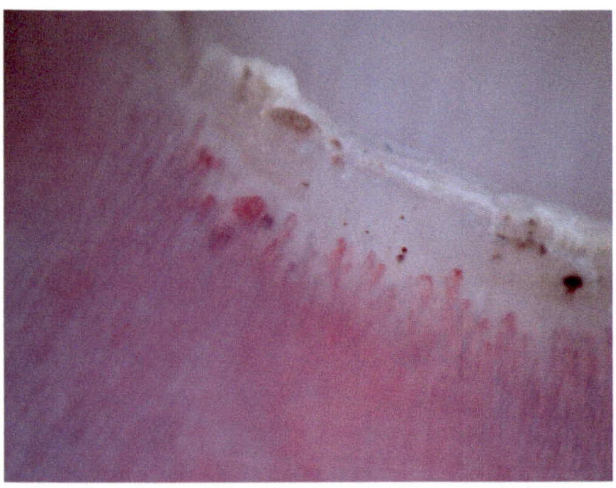

Fig. 6.8 Systemic sclerosis. Proximal nailfold changes including dilated capillaries, loss of capillary loops ("drop-out"), architectural derangement of capillaries, and microhemorrhages. (Courtesy of Joseph Merola, MD)

derangement of capillaries, and microhemorrhages (Fig. 6.8). Several studies have shown that detection of capillary abnormalities may allow for early SSc diagnosis when other SSc features are present. The presence of capillary abnormalities may also allow early differentiation of primary versus secondary Raynaud's. One study including 152 patients with sclerodactyly and Raynaud's phenomenon showed that the addition of visualized dilated capillaries improved the sensitivity of the 1980 ACR criteria for the diagnosis of SSc from 33.6% to 74.3% [27]. While capillaroscopy can clearly be useful, widefield microscopes and videocapillaroscopes are not readily available to most clinicians and require specific training for use. The ophthalmoscope has been used in their place with some success but still requires oil or immersion gel, which may hinder its use in clinical practice. Fortunately, a handheld dermatoscope may be used effectively to detect nailfold capillary changes, and dermatoscope-based studies have shown good concordance with standard methods [28, 29]. The dermatoscope is relatively inexpensive and mean examination time is only 4 minutes [30].

Gastrointestinal

The entire GI tract, anywhere from the mouth to the anus, may be involved in SSc. GI involvement is the most frequent internal complication of SSc, with a prevalence of up to 90% [31]. The pathogenesis of GI abnormalities relates to microvascular derangement, which is thought to lead to neurological dysfunction, causing smooth muscle malfunction with subsequent atrophy and fibrosis of the smooth muscles [32]. GI manifestations vary widely in severity, ranging from mild gastroesophageal reflux to severe malabsorption leading to death. Severe GI involvement affects about 8% of SSc patients and is associated with high mortality (9-year survival rate of 15%) [33].

Oropharynx

Oropharyngeal involvement in SSc begins with complications from a reduced oral aperture and rigidity of the facial skin and tongue, which may lead to difficulty with eating and maintaining dental hygiene. Reduced salivary flow, which can occur with SSc alone or from secondary Sjogren's syndrome, may exacerbate problems with dental health. Oropharyngeal dysphagia occurs in up to 26% of patients win SSc [34].

Esophagus

Esophageal involvement is common in SSc but can be clinically silent in up to 50% of affected patients [35]. Involvement of the smooth muscle of the lower two-thirds of the esophagus results in loss of peristaltic action and symptoms of acid reflux symptoms and dysphagia. The upper third of the esophagus may also be affected in patients with myositis, which may be seen in SSc or overlap syndromes. A weakened lower esophageal sphincter compounds the problem, with acidic gastric contents refluxing into an esophagus that already has poor antegrade motility. Esophageal damage may ensue, manifesting as esophagitis and sometimes ulcers and GI bleeding. Long-term complications may include strictures and Barrett's esophagus, with a possible increase in the risk of esophageal malignancy [36]. In addition to reflux and dysphagia, patients may experience regurgitation, hoarseness, and weight loss.

Gastric

Gastric manifestations in SSc include delayed emptying and vascular abnormalities leading to bleeding. Delayed gastric emptying results in early satiety, nausea, bloating, and weight loss, and it may exacerbate existing reflux disease. Gastric vascular abnormalities include mucosal telangectasias in the stomach or gastric antral vascular ectasia (GAVE), both of which can lead to bleeding varying from occult to large amounts. GAVE is also known as "watermelon stomach" due to its unique endoscopic appearance, with erythematous blood vessels occurring in stripes from the pylorus to the antrum. Histologically, GAVE is characterized by mucosal capillary dilatations containing fibrin thrombi and fibromuscular hyperplasia [37].

Small Intestine

Impaired small intestine mobility can lead to distended bowel loops, manifesting as early satiety, bloating, cramping, nausea, and vomiting. A characteristic sign of small bowel SSc seen on barium studies is a "hide-bound" or "wire-spring" appearance caused by closely packed valvulae in dilated bowel. The intestinal stasis and pooling that occurs may also lead to small intestine bacterial overgrowth (SIBO), which can cause malabsorption, a serious complication in SSc patients. Patients with SIBO and malabsorption often suffer from diarrhea, steatorrhea, weight loss, and malnutrition. Small intestinal hypomotility may also provoke luminal dilatation and lead to pseudo-obstruction caused by functional ileus, which can present as abdominal pain, bloating, and vomiting. Patients may also develop pneumatosis cystoides intestinalis, or gas in the bowel wall, a finding often identified incidentally on abdominal CT performed for other reasons. In SSc, this is usually a benign process, but pneumoperitoneum is a potential complication.

Large Intestine and Anorectum

Involvement of the large intestine in SSc leads to reduced contractile activity and resultant constipation. Patients who have these findings comorbid with SIBO may present with diarrhea alternating with constipation. Refractory constipation can rarely lead to colonic perforation. Muscular atrophy of the intestinal mucosa can lead to characteristic wide-mouth diverticulae on the antimesenteric border, which can be detected on barium enema. Anorectal involvement leads to decreased compliance and reduced anal sphincter tone. These changes mirror the changes seen in the lower esophageal sphincter. Fecal incontinence, and less frequently, rectal prolapse can occur as a result.

Liver

The liver is rarely involved in SSc, although there is an association with primary biliary cirrhosis (PBC), especially among patients with lcSSc. SSc patients with PBC are often anti-centromere antibody positive; compared non-SSc patients with PBC, their hepatic disease tends to progress more slowly [38, 39].

Pulmonary

Pulmonary disease is the leading cause of morbidity and mortality in patients with SSc. The clinical presentation of pulmonary SSc may be completely silent or can include chronic cough and dyspnea on exertion. Severity ranges widely, from limited, non-progressive lung involvement to major pulmonary inflammation and fibrosis ultimately leading to respiratory failure and death.

The two most common pulmonary manifestations of SSc are ILD and PH. These complications may occur simultaneously, or PH can be a consequence of ILD. Less common pulmonary manifestations of SSc include pleuritis, malignancy, bronchiolitis obliterans, and bronchiectasis. SSc patients may also be at a higher risk of aspiration pneumonia due to oropharyngeal and esophageal dysfunction. In addition, patients with myositis due to SSc or overlap syndromes may develop respiratory muscle weakness.

Interstitial Lung Disease

In a recent report from the EULAR SSc Trials and Research database, the overall prevalence of ILD as identified on high resolution CT among patients with SSc was 51.9% [40]. ILD was present in 43.5% of patients with lcSSc and 64.1% of patients with dcSSc. On autopsy, however, the prevalence of ILD is as high as 80% [41].

ILD in SSc (or SSc-ILD) is characterized by basilar-predominant fibrosis, which is detectable on X-ray or high-resolution CT, the latter being a more sensitive imaging modality. The pattern seen on CT is usually consistent with non-specific interstitial pneumonia (NSIP), or less commonly, usual interstitial pneumonia (UIP). UIP has findings consistent with end-stage fibrosis, including honeycombing and traction bronchiectasis, whereas NSIP presents with ground glass opacities and has a better prognosis [42]. Pulmonary function assessment in ILD demonstrates restrictive physiology with approximately equivalent decline in forced vital capacity (FVC) and forced expiratory volume in one second (FEV1) [43, 44].

Risk factors for ILD include diffuse subset, presence of anti-topoisomerase I antibodies, and African-American ethnicity. Male sex, cardiac involvement and African-American ethnicity are additional poor prognostic factors for pulmonary disease [14]. Approximately 10–15% of patients with SSc will experience more severe ILD and progressive decline in lung function [14, 45]. SSc-ILD accounts for 33% of all SSc-related deaths [46].

Pulmonary Hypertension

In one report on patients with SSc, PH occurred in 21.1% of patients, with almost the same frequency in the limited and diffuse subsets [40]. PH in SSc can be of several different forms: (1) PAH due to SSc involvement of the small pulmonary arterioles (most common); (2) PH due to hypoxemia from advanced ILD; and (3) PH caused by myocardial dysfunction. Patients with PH may be asymptomatic in early stages. Later, there is increasing dyspnea on exertion, reduced exercise tolerance, and fatigue. Late-stage signs and symptoms include syncope, chest pain, jugular vein distention, and edema, indicating the development of right heart failure.

Isolated PAH can present even after years of mild, stable disease, highlighting the importance of long-term monitoring in these patients. Risk factors for PAH include greater than 10 cutaneous telangectasias, reduced capillary nailfold density, and the presence of anti-centromere antibodies [25, 47].

PAH associated with SSc is more aggressive than non-SSc PAH, with a median survival time of 1 year following diagnosis if left untreated. PAH accounts for 30% of deaths among SSc patients [48, 49]. SSc-ILD with PH has a much worse prognosis than SSc-ILD alone [50].

Cardiac

Cardiac involvement occurs frequently in both lcSSC and dcSSc but is more common in the latter. Risk factors include rapidly progressive skin disease, presence of anti-U3RNP antibodies, and presence of myositis. In the EULAR SSc Trails and Research (EUSTAR) database, 26% of SSc-related deaths were due to cardiac involvement, making it the third leading cause of death in SSc [51]. SSc may affect any part of the heart; however, pericardial disease, myocardial disease, and arrhythmias are the major SSc-related cardiac manifestations.

Pericardial disease results in symptomatic pericarditis and small or large pericardial effusions. The prevalence of clinically symptomatic cardiac involvement has been estimated at 30–35% [52]. However, pericardial abnormalities may be observed in up to 78% of SSc patients at autopsy [53]. The presence of pericardial effusion can be a clue to impending SSc renal crisis, and when observed with PAH, it may be associated with poor prognosis.

With regard to myocardial disease, microvascular dysfunction leading to recurrent ischemic injury and myocardial fibrosis is thought to be the cause of systolic and diastolic dysfunction observed in SSc patients. In one study in 570 SSc patients, left ventricular systolic and diastolic dysfunction were present in 1% and 18%, respectively [54]. Recent studies have also indicated an increased risk of atherosclerosis and myocardial infarctions in SSc patients, for which the pathophysiology remains unclear [55, 56].

Ventricular and supraventricular arrhythmias are common in SSc and result in a range of symptoms, from transient palpitations to syncope and sudden death. Conduction abnormalities are thought to result from myocardial fibrosis and injury to the conduction system [53].

Renal

Scleroderma renal crisis (SRC) is the most important renal complication in SSc. Rarely, other abnormalities can occur, including interstitial nephritis, glomerulonephritis, chronic proteinuria and chronic renal vasculopathy [57].

SRC has a prevalence of 10% in the entire SSc population and occurs in approximately 20% of patients with dcSSc. It is defined as the new onset of rapidly progressive oliguric renal failure and/or accelerated hypertension. Patients may present with signs and symptoms of malignant hypertension, such as headache, dyspnea, visual disturbance, seizure, and lower extremity edema. However, because patients developing SRC may be normotensive, the diagnosis requires a high index of suspicion.

Additional features of SRC include microangiopathic hemolytic anemia on blood smear, retinopathy typical of acute hypertensive crisis, new onset hematuria, flash pulmonary edema, and renal biopsy with typical features (i.e., onion skin proliferation within the walls of intra-renal arteries and arterioles, fibrinoid necrosis, and glomerular shrinkage). SRC may sometimes be the presenting feature of SSc.

SRC results from renal vasculopathy rather than inflammation and is accompanied by a high renin state. Risk factors for SRC include diffuse subset, rapidly progressive skin thickening, anti-RNA polymerase III antibodies, and pericardial effusion. Poor prognostic factors include older age, male sex, and lower blood pressure at presentation. Prior to the introduction of angiotensin converting enzyme inhibitors (ACEi) for the treatment of this disease, SRC was the leading cause of mortality in patients with SSc. Outcomes have improved significantly with earlier diagnosis and prompt treatment, but SRC still carries a high mortality and morbidity rate: 1-year survival is estimated at 78%, and 40% of affected patients require chronic hemodialysis [58].

Musculoskeletal

The muscles, tendons, joints, and bones can all be involved in SSc. A large proportion of patients with SSc have arthropathy (46–97%) or myositis complicating their skin disease, which may contribute substantially to extremity dysfunction and disability [59–61]. The most common musculoskeletal manifestations are pain and joint contractures resulting from fibrosis around tendons and other periarticular structures. It is important to distinguish joint pain due to contractures from joint pain caused by true synovitis. Joint contractures most frequently involve the fingers, although larger joints including elbows, and knees may also be affected in dcSSc.

An erosive arthropathy involving the proximal and distal interphalangeal joints, resembling psoriatic arthritis, occurs in 15–20% of SSc patients [61]. In some cases, articular involvement may the presenting feature and result in diagnostic confusion, often with rheumatoid arthritis [60]. Further clouding the picture is the fact that up to 30% of SSc patients have a positive serum rheumatoid factor (though its presence does not distinguish those with articular manifestations from those without), and between 1% and 15% have serum anti-citrullinated peptide antibodies [61].

With regard to bones, approximately 20% of SSc patients develop acro-osteolysis, with resorption of bony tuft at the distal phalaynx [62]. As is the case for patients with other chronic inflammatory diseases, SSc patients are at higher risk of osteoporosis; this risk is compounded by immobility from the SSc itself.

Muscle weakness is a prominent symptom in SSc, although not all those with weakness have an identifiable myopathy. One type of SSc-associated myopathy is "bland" myopathy in which there is no significant necrosis or inflammation and creatine kinase levels are normal or only mildly elevated. The second type of SSc myopathy presents similarly to inflammatory myositis, in which patients have significant CK elevations and electrodiagnostic and biopsy findings suggestive of inflammatory myopathy.

Certain musculoskeletal findings can be early signs of SSc. Tendon friction rubs occur in up to 20% of patients with early dcSSc and appear to be associated with more rapid disease progression [63–66]. These can be felt and/or heard using a stethoscope over tendons of the fingers and wrists, elbows, knees, and ankles. Carpal tunnel syndrome is another common presenting manifestation of SSc; patients with bilateral carpal tunnel syndrome together with Raynaud's phenomenon should be evaluated for SSc.

Pathophysiology of Systemic Sclerosis

SSc is thought to result from the complex interplay of three principle pathophysiologic processes in a genetically susceptible individual: (1) vascular phenomena and vasculopathy; (2) autoimmunity or immune dysregulation; and (3) fibrosis [67]. We will review each of these proposed pathophysiologic mechanisms in detail.

Vascular Injury and the Initiation of SSc

The endothelial cell (EC) appears to play a key role in the initial cascade of molecular events that ultimately leads to both vascular damage or vasculopathy and tissue fibrosis in SSc [67, 68]. The prevailing pathophysiologic paradigm proposes that microvascular injury and subsequent EC activation incite increased expression of vascular cell adhesion protein (VCAM), intercellular adhesion molecule (ICAM) and E-selectin, which in turn promote inflammatory cell recruitment from blood into surrounding tissue [69–71]. The accumulation of these inflammatory cells in tissue leads to increased expression of profibrotic mediators, such as transforming growth factor beta (TGfβ), platelet-derived growth factor (PDGF), IL-1, and IL-6, which in turn stimulate increased extracellular matrix protein by tissue-residing myofibroblasts [69].

Progressive vascular injury results in activation and apoptosis of ECs with associated intimal thickening, smooth muscle proliferation, and vessel narrowing to varying degrees depending on the vascular bed [67, 72]. Endothelial cells release a variety of factors including the potent vasoconstrictor, endothelin 1 (ET-1), but also other cytokines, such as TGfβ, which work in concert to promote smooth muscle cell proliferation and luminal narrowing [68]. The role of inflammation in the early vascular events that characterize SSc is controversial but may be important in specific vascular complications such as PAH [73–76].

Modification of angiogenesis also appears to play an important role in the pathogenesis of vascular disease in SSc. Early in SSc, videocapillaroscopy has shown a proinflammatory state, leading to increased production of pro-angiogenic factors that stimulate angiogenesis, leading to new abnormal and tortuous capillaries [28, 77].

Later in disease, the early pro-angiogenic response is followed by loss of angiogenesis, resulting in a reduction in capillary density and development of extensive avascular areas that have been demonstrated by videocapillaroscopy. This latter pathogenic pattern appears to correlate with increased levels both of E-selectin and junctional adhesion molecules (JAMs). JAMs function in the regulation of leukocyte recruitment to sites of inflammation, ischemia reperfusion injury, vascular permeability and angiogenesis.

They appear to be critical in EC motility, EC directional movement and focal content formation during angiogenesis. In early SSc skin disease, JAMs appear to be upregulated in MVECs but have reduced expression in later stage disease, suggesting that JAMs play an important role in the modulation of angiogenesis in the different stages of SSc [78, 79].

Accumulating evidence suggests that deficiency of the transcription factor Friend leukemia integration factor-1 (Fli-1) plays a key role in the process of both skin fibrosis and microvascular injury in SSc. Fli-1 pathway interruption in SSc may connect both this early impairment of angiogenesis and the development of skin fibrosis, since Fli-1 is a transcription factor which appears to regulate many genes in both fibroblasts and ECs [80]. Fli-1 deficiency in dermal fibroblasts, for example, upregulates the expression of type 1 collagen, connective tissue derived growth factor (CTGF or CCN2) and alpha smooth muscle actin, facilitating the transition to predominance of myofibroblasts and uncontrolled deposition of ECM.

In microvascular ECs, Fli-1 deficiency leads to altered expression of a number of molecules involved in vascular homeostasis and angiogenesis, such as vascular endothelial (VE) cadherin, platelet-endothelial cell adhesion molecule (PECAM)-1, CXCL5, cathepsin V, CCN1 and cathepsin B, leading to loss of vascular integrity that manifests clinically as nailfold capillary abnormalities [81]. Asano and colleagues have shown that CCN1 expression in dermal microvessels in patients with SSc was markedly reduced and that Fli-1 deficiency plays a key role in the down-regulation of CCN1 [82]. Furthermore, lower circulating levels of CCN1 could be correlated with the presence of digital ulcers [82].

Autoimmunity

Several lines of evidence point to both innate and adaptive immune dysregulation or autoimmunity in SSc [71]. First, early in the disease, infiltrating immune effector cells (including CD4+ T cells, macrophages, activated B cells and plasmacytoid dendritic cells) consistently display a Type 1 interferon gene signature, a prominent marker of innate immune activation. Effector T cells, particularly Th17 and regulatory T cells (Treg), appear to be critical regulators of this initial inflammation; the presence of Th17 cells in particular has been shown to correlate with clinical parameters, such as disease duration and ILD score. An increase in activated T cells and a reduction in Treg is thought to cause excess production of cytokines that drive the synthesis of extracellular matrix proteins by fibroblasts, resulting in fibrosis [83]. While Th17 cells have been mostly found to be increased in SSc, Treg cells have been reported to be reduced in number or functionally defective in SSc [83, 84]. Additionally, Zhou and colleagues found elevated expression of Th17-related cytokines and receptors to be associated with skin lesion severity in early SSc. This included IL-17A, IL-21, IL-22, IL-26, IL-17RA, IL-21R and IL-22R, which correlated with modified Rodnan skin score (mRss) [85]. Thus recent evidence has revealed a crucial role for immune cells in the establishment and maintenance of fibrosis, with Th1 and Th2 cells contributing to the induction of pro-inflammatory and pro-fibrotic responses. These findings provide a rationale for therapy to decrease T cell activation.

Additional evidence pointing to the role of immune dysregulation in SSc includes evidence from genome wide association studies (GWAS), which have shown polymorphisms in *IRF5* (interferon regulatory factor 5) and *STAT 4* (signal transducer and activator of transcription 4), which are dysregulated in other autoimmune diseases [86–88]. Additionally, as reviewed in detail later in this chapter, SSc is associated with distinctive autoantibodies, such as anti-centromere, anti-Scl 70, and anti-RNA polymerase III, among others [89]. With the possible exception of antibodies to PDGF, the role of autoantibodies in the pathogenesis of SSc remains uncertain. Autoantibodies associated with SSc, however, do appear to have diagnostic importance [90–93].

Other evidence of immune activation in SSc includes elevation of Th2 cytokines such as IL-4, IL-13 and IL-6 [69, 94]. IL-6 in particular plays an important role in Th2-dominant immunity, inflammation and fibrosis [95]. IL-6 is a pleiotropic, pro-inflammatory, multi-functional cytokine produced by a variety of cell types, including lymphocytes, monocytes and fibroblasts [95]. IL-6 levels are elevated in the serum of patients with SSc, and isolated lymphocytes spontaneously produce elevated levels of IL-6 [96]. IL-6 induction of collagen gene expression appears to involve mechanisms dependent on STAT3, TGfβ and Smad 3, mediated through Gremlin-1 protein [95]. IL-6 could thus be considered a molecular target with biologic rationale in SSc; clinical trials of tocilizumab, a humanized monoclonal anti-IL-6 receptor antibody, are underway [97].

Fibrosis

Fibrosis as distinct from wound healing is a complex pathologic process characterized by the extracellular accumulation of a matrix made up of collagen, elastin, glycosaminoglycan and fibronectin [98]. In wound healing following injury, collagen and matrix deposition result in scar formation, which is then downregulated before excess accumulation of scar causes disruption of normal tissue [99–101]. The accumulation of this matrix, which permanently alters the tissue architecture, is the result of increased synthesis by activated fibroblasts or myofibroblasts as well as defective degradation [102–106]. Myofibroblasts may originate from several different locations, including from pericytes from the circulation and from transdifferention of telocytes and ECs. A recent study suggested that myofibroblasts populating fibrotic dermis also derive from adipocytic progenitors [107]. Increasing evidence suggests that matrix stiffness resulting from pathologic deposition of collagen in fibrosis induces a feedback loop via a process termed mechanotransduction, which further enhances fibroblast recruitment and activation at sites of fibrosis [108].

The molecular signaling events that characterize the fibrotic process in SSc have long been linked to TGfβ, considered the master cytokine of fibrosis and wound healing [109, 110]. Recent evidence suggests that, along with genes regulated by type I interferon, gene expression regulated by TGfβ drives the fibrotic process in SSc lung disease [109]. TGfβ is secreted as an inactive precursor bound to TGfβ binding protein by macrophages and other cells and converted to its biologically active form by integrins [111, 112]. Canonical signaling via phosphorylation of the type I TGfβ receptor (also known as ALK5) via the SMAD pathway eventually leads to increased profibrotic gene expression. TGfβ can also activate profibrotic gene expression via non-SMAD pathways via early growth response 1 (ERG1), ABL1 (previously known as c-ABL) and FAK, as well as by inactivation of transcriptional repressors such as peroxisome proliferator-activated receptor δ (PPAR δ), Fli-1 and kruppel-like factor family members. As indicated above, the transcription factor Fli-1 appears to play a particularly important function in SSc pathogenesis because of its dual role in preventing both fibroblast and EC gene transcription. Fli-1 deficiency has multiple downstream effects in fibroblasts and ECs that favor the development of fibrosis and vasculopathy in animal models and human disease [81].

In addition to TGfβ signaling, canonical Wnt signaling also appears to play a central role in fibrosis and has been implicated in pulmonary, renal and liver fibrosis in additional to keloid formation [113]. Wnt proteins stimulate the differentiation of resting fibroblasts into myofibroblasts and increase the release of ECM in vitro. In vivo, overexpression of Wnt 10b, stabilization of β-catenin, or inhibition of GSK3 β produce rapid and progressive skin fibrosis [113]. Wnt signaling is also closely linked to TGFβ-driven myofibroblast activation and upregulation of collagen gene expression: TGfβ induction of canonical Wnt signaling with β-catenin accumulation leads to matrix gene expression in murine skin and cultured fibroblasts, resulting in a negative feedback loop that inhibits TGfβ, in turn reducing Wnt signaling.

PDGF is the term for a family of mesenchymal mitogens with important functions during the embryonal development and in the control of tissue homeostasis in the adult [114]. The PDGF isoforms exert their effects by binding to α–and β-tyrosine kinase receptors. Overactivity of PDGF signaling has been linked to the development of certain malignant and non-malignant diseases, including atherosclerosis and various fibrotic diseases, including SSc [114]. A causative role of PDGF receptor activity in SSc is suggested by the finding that tyrosine kinase inhibitors, e.g., imatinib, dasatinib and nilotinib, ameliorate symptoms in mouse models of SSc [114]. Activating autoantibodies against the PDGFα receptor have been demonstrated in the serum of patients with SSc [115], though this observation has been questioned in other studies [116, 117]. Another report noted PDGFα receptor autoantibodies in 29% of patients with SSc but found that these autoantibodies did not have any agonistic activity [118].

Connective tissue growth factor (CTGF, CCN2) is overexpressed in lung fibroblasts isolated from patients with SSc and ILD and is considered to be a molecular marker of fibrosis [119, 120]. Recent studies suggest that CTGF is important in lung tissue repair and fibrosis and indicate that CTGF-induced migration of lung fibroblasts to the damaged tissue is mediated via the IQGAP1 and MAPK signaling pathways, which are upregulated in SSc lung tissue [119]. IQGAP1 is a scaffold protein that plays a pivotal role in regulating migration of endothelial and epithelial cells. LPA-1, via CTGF, also appears to play a significant role in CTGF-mediated events governing tissue fibrosis [121].

Risk Factors for Systemic Sclerosis

Like many autoimmune diseases, SSc may in some cases be precipitated by an environmental trigger in a genetically susceptible individual. Here we review environmental and genetic risk factors identified to date.

Genetic Risk Factors

The genetic basis for SSc has not yet been fully elucidated. The twin concordance rate in SSc is only 4.7%, with no difference in concordance rates between monozygotic and dizygotic twins [122]. The disease occurs in only 0.4% of siblings [123], compared to 8% and 7% of siblings in RA and ankylosing spondylitis, respectively [124]. However, certain genetic susceptibility loci have been identified. The highest reported prevalence of SSc is in a Choctaw Native American group in Oklahoma, with a prevalence estimated at 4690 cases per million (based on 12 cases) [125]. Within the population who developed SSc, there was strong homogeneity of features, including diffuse disease, anti-topoisomerase I antibodies and pulmonary fibrosis. Several genetic loci were identified within this population that showed highly significant associations with SSc [126]. Further investigation in this vein may help shed light on the overall genetic basis for SSc [127].

Occupational and Environmental Risk Factors

Environmental factors have drawn particular attention in SSc, in part due to reports of geographic clustering. In a rural area in the province of Rome, for example, there were five patients with SSc in a village of 572 persons, while an additional 10 would have met criteria for SSc by today's definition [128]. Counting all 15, this would have represented a prevalence of 15/572, or 26,223 cases per million people, far greater than the expected prevalence based on population-level data. No disease-associated HLA antigen was observed, although there was a higher frequency of HLA B51 and DR2 haplotypes in the entire village population. Similar geographic clustering has been reported in the United Kingdom, Canada, and Australia [129–131]. In the Australian cluster, SSc cases were noted mostly in male farm workers, raising the possibility of dust storm-related silica exposure as being a potential contributor.

Indeed, silica as a potential environmental factor has been a major focus of SSc epidemiological studies. Several countries, including Germany, South Africa, and Canada, consider silica-induced SSc an occupational disease covered under worker's compensation policies [132]. The first report of a possible association between silica exposure and SSc was in a 1914 series of nine Scottish patients, five of whom were stonemasons [133]. Subsequently, disease clustering was identified in miners from South Africa and coal miners from North America [134, 135]. Many other silica-associated cases have been reported, including one recent report of limited SSc in a French winegrower who frequently filtered wine using diatomaceous earth, which is >80% silica [136]. A meta-analysis including 16 studies (9 case-control, 3 cohort, 4 other) examining the relationship between silica and SSc found the combined estimator of relative risk (CERR) in silica exposed versus non-exposed individuals to be 3.2 [137]. The risk was higher in males than females.

Organic solvents have also been implicated in precipitating SSc. A 2007 meta-analysis of 11 studies found that occupational exposure to solvents conferred an adjusted relative risk for developing SSc of 1.8, with male sex conferring excess risk [138]. These findings echo those of a prior study of 2227 patients, in which self-reported solvent exposure was associated with twice the risk of developing SSc [139]. Exposures to epoxy resins or pesticides have also been implicated as possible environmental triggers, but the evidence for these links is limited to case reports. For the majority of SSc cases, no occupational or environmental risk factors can be identified.

Autoantibodies

Several antibodies specific to SSc have been identified and are associated with particular clinical features. The presence of these antibodies provides further prognostic and clinical information beyond the limited and diffuse subsets. Prevalence of individual antibodies has varied by testing method used and differences in cohort characteristics, including ethnicity and country of origin.

In general, anti-nuclear antibodies, which are not specific for SSc, are present in up to 90% of SSc patients. The two most commonly observed SSc-specific antibodies are anti-centromere and anti-topoisomerase I antibodies, each occurring in approximately 30% of patients with SSc of all types [140]. Anti-centromere antibodies are more common among in lcSSc, whereas anti-topoisomerase I antibodies are more common among patients with dcSS. Both antibodies are widely available as commercial tests. Anti-RNA polymerase III antibodies are present in approximately 10% of SSc patients, and their presence correlates with renal crisis and malignancy risk [141, 142]. Anti-centromere, anti-topoisomerase I, and anti-RNA polymerase III are all included as part of the 2013 SSc classification criteria, as previously reviewed in detail.

Other antibodies related to SSc include those targeting Th/To, PmScl, U1 RNP, U3 RNP, Ku, U11/U12 RNP, and RuvBL1/2. Estimated prevalence for each of these antibodies in the SSc population as well as associated clinical features are described in Table 6.3.

Diagnostic Considerations

SSc is a clinical diagnosis based on the history, physical features, and laboratory findings. Skin biopsy is generally not needed for diagnosis. Diagnostic considerations of SSc should mirror the classification criteria (Table 6.1), however, these criteria were developed for research purposes and thus the classification criteria need not be met to make the diagnosis of SSc. For example, a patient with tendon friction rubs and calcinosis, items which are not part of the 2013 SSc classification criteria, may still be diagnosed as SSc if they have other features consistent with the diagnosis, such as Raynaud's and sclerodactyly. In the

Table 6.3 Autoantibody prevalence, clinical associations, and prognosis [3, 140, 143–145]

	Prevalence	Disease subset	Clinical associations	Prognosis
Anti-centromere	16–41%	Limited	Pulmonary hypertension, digital ulcers	Better
Anti-topoisomerase I	9–39%	Diffuse	Interstitial lung disease, cardiac involvement, digital ulcers	Worse
Anti-RNA polymerase III	2–25%	Diffuse	Renal crisis, tendon friction rubs, malignancy, GAVE	Worse
Anti-PM/Scl	0–9%	Limited/overlap	Myositis, calcinosis, digital ulcers	Better
Anti-U1 RNP	5–35%	Limited/overlap	Mixed connective tissue disease, myositis, arthritis, interstitial lung disease, pulmonary hypertension	Better
Anti-U3 RNP (fibrillarin)	1–10%	Diffuse	African-American patients, younger age of onset, pulmonary hypertension, gastrointestinal involvement, cardiac involvement, renal crisis	Worse
Anti-Th/To	1–7%	Limited	Interstitial lung disease, pulmonary hypertension	Worse
Anti-Ku	1–10%	Limited/overlap	Myositis, dysphagia, SLE overlap	–
Anti-U11/U12 RNP [146]	1–5%	Limited and diffuse	Severe interstitial lung disease, gastrointestinal involvement	Worse
Anti-RuvBL1/2 [143]	1–2%	Diffuse/overlap	Male patients, older age of onset, myositis	–

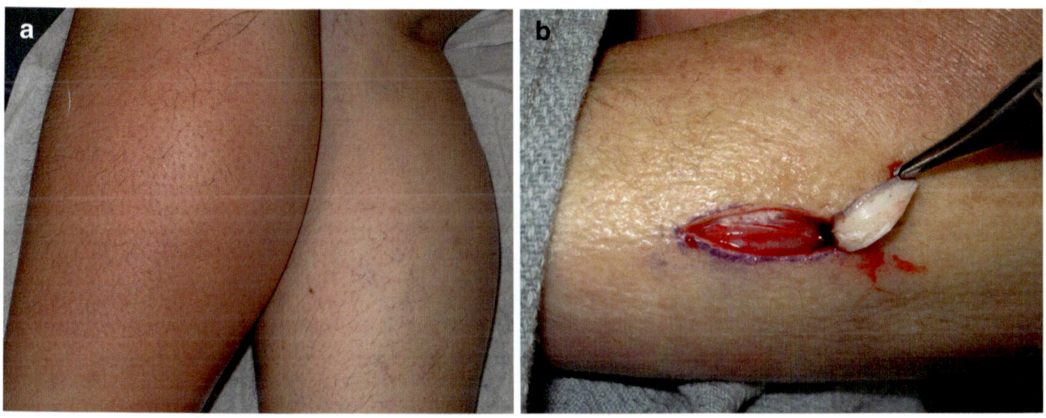

Fig. 6.9 (**a**, **b**) Eosinophilic fasciitis. (**a**) Erythema, swelling and induration of the lower extremity with the characteristic peau d'orange (orange-peel) appearance over the surfaces of the skin. (**b**) Gross specimen demonstrating significant thickening of the fascial layer due to inflammatory involvement with replacement of the subcutis. (Courtesy of Amit Garg, MD)

same way, patients may be diagnosed with SSc based on visceral manifestations and autoantibody profile, even when there is no skin thickening (SSc sine scleroderma). SSc should be suspected in patients with severe Raynaud's phenomenon, especially when there are digital ulcers and/or pits. Bilateral carpal tunnel syndrome may also be a presenting feature. Certainly, any patient with skin thickening and tightness, puffiness or swelling of the fingers should be suspected of having SSc.

Differential diagnosis of SSc includes diffuse morphea, scleredema, scleromyxedema, nephrogenic systemic fibrosis, eosinophilic fasciitis, lipodermatosclerosis, malignancy related palmar fasciitis and chronic graft versus host disease (Table 6.2) (Figs. 6.9, 6.10, and 6.11). A more common mimic of SSc is diabetic cheiroarthropathy, characterized by thickened waxy skin of the hands and fingers and sclerosis of the tendon sheaths with inability to fully flex or extend the

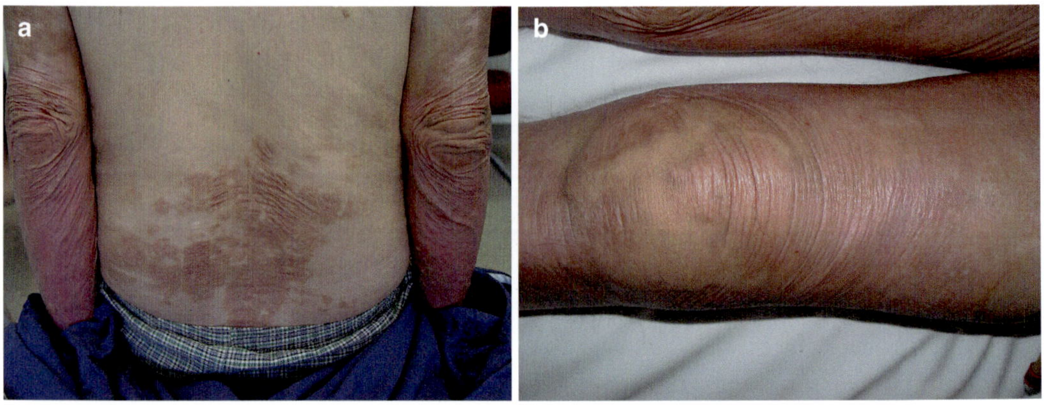

Fig. 6.10 (**a**, **b**) Nephrogenic systemic fibrosis. Symmetric, sharply demarcated, brawny plaques which are indurated and may have a cobblestone or texture. Thickened plaques typically involve trunk and extremities and usually spare the face. This patient has chronic kidney disease and has had imaging with Gadolinium containing contrast. (Courtesy of Amit Garg, MD)

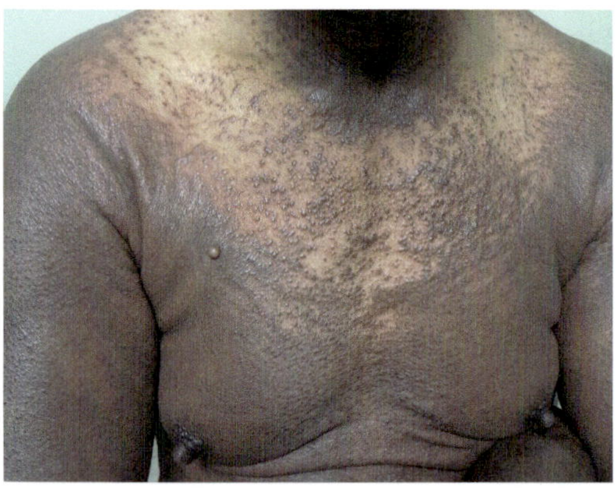

Fig. 6.11 Scleromyxedema. Numerous waxy appearing and firm discrete papules which are also coalescing to plaques on the trunk and extremities. (Courtesy of Amit Garg, MD)

fingers. Frostbite may cause SSc-like changes in a few, rather than all, fingers.

Physical Examination

On physical examination, the clinician should look for features unique to SSc, including puffy fingers (characterized by non-pitting edema), skin thickening and tightening (especially of the fingers, hands, neck, face, and perioral skin), digital pits, loss of digital pulp tissue (with skin often distally tethered to the nail), digital ulcers, telangectasias, and calcinosis. Examination of nailfold capillaries, especially of the fourth fingers, using a dermatoscope, widefield microscope, or videocapillaroscope is likely to aid in the diagnosis.

In addition to a cutaneous examination, careful evaluation of the cardiovascular and respiratory systems is essential to assess for cardiac, pulmonary and renal involvement. A thorough musculoskeletal examination is also needed to assess for joint contractures and synovitis as well as general mobility and joint range of motion.

Laboratory Testing

Routine laboratory testing, including complete blood count and differential, serum creatinine, urinalysis, and serum creatine kinase, may provide information about possible organ involvement. Serological tests including antinuclear, anti-topoisomerase I, anti-centromere, and anti-RNA polymerase III antibodies can support the diagnosis and provide prognostic information (Table 6.3). When there is suspicion of an alternative rheumatological diagnosis or overlap syndrome, other tests may be considered based on the specific presenting clinical features. Some of these may include rheumatoid factor, anti-citrullinated peptides, other extranuclear antigens, anti-double stranded DNA, and complement levels.

Table 6.4 Investigations for complications of SSc

Problem	Investigation
Dysphagia/reflux	Manometry, cine esophagogram, barium swallow, esophagogastroduodenoscopy, 24-hour pH monitoring
Gastric dysmotility	Gastric emptying study, esophagogastroduodenoscopy
Bacterial overgrowth	Glucose hydrogen breath test, D-xylose test, small bowel aspiration
Malabsorption/ Malnutrition	Malnutrition questionnaire, e.g. "Malnutrition universal screening tool," [148] hemoglobin, folic acid, serum carotene, vitamin B12, iron, zinc, vitamin D, INR, serum methylmalonic acid
Renal insufficiency	Blood pressure, blood smear, electrolytes and creatinine, urinalysis, hemolysis workup, consider renal biopsy

Cardiopulmonary Studies

Because ILD and PH are common in SSc and represent leading causes of morbidity and mortality in this population, the authors routinely perform high resolution computed tomography of the chest to evaluate for these conditions. A chest radiograph may be a reasonable first study to limit radiation exposure, but sensitivity is lower. SSc patients with respiratory symptoms and a negative chest radiograph should undergo additional testing. Pulmonary function tests should also be performed as a non-invasive screen for restrictive ventilatory defect and/or decrease in diffuse capacity for carbon monoxide (DLCO), the latter of which may be a sign of either ILD or PH. Echocardiography is also useful to evaluate for PH (in addition to cardiac involvement of SSc).

When echocardiography is suggestive of PH, right heart catheterization (RHC) may be performed to confirm the diagnosis. The most appropriate approach to selecting patients for RHC using other supportive information such as echocardiographic features, electrocardiography and NT-proBNP levels is being investigated [147]. In general, a pulmonary artery systolic pressure (PASP, estimated from echocardiogram) greater than 40 mmHg should trigger suspicion for PH. Other clinical features such as dyspnea, fatigue, reduced DLCO (especially if isolated or out of proportion to FVC reduction in cases of ILD, i.e., FVC%/DLCO% >1.6), and elevated NT-proBNP may warrant further investigation for PH, even when PASP is lower than 40 mmHg. Lastly, a baseline electrocardiogram should also be performed to screen for conduction abnormalities and arrhythmias.

Other Studies

Investigations for other organ involvement may be guided by patient symptoms. Table 6.4 lists some common tests performed for the unique symptoms and complications of SSc.

Disease and Comorbidity Assessment

Measurement of Disease Activity and Severity

The traditional disease activity measurement tool used in virtually all SSc clinical trials is the mRSS [149]. It measures the extent of skin involvement and has been shown to correlate well with internal organ involvement as well as survival. The mRSS assesses 17 body parts, including the face, anterior chest, abdomen, fingers, dorsum of the hands, forearms, upper arms, thighs, lower legs, and dorsum of the feet. In each area, skin with normal thickness is assigned a value of 0, while values of 1, 2 and 3 correspond to mild, moderate, and severe skin thickness, respectively. The total maximum score that can be assigned is 51. mRSS may be measured over time to track the skin thickness progression rate (STPR). A rapid STPR has been associated with reduced short-term survival and renal crisis within 2 years of first evaluation [150]. The durometer has also been tested as a valid and responsive method to measure skin hardness [151]. It may have higher intraobserver reproducibility than mRSS [152], but its use may be limited by cost.

Multiple other SSc outcome measures have been used in clinical trials. These include both patient-reported and investigator-reported outcomes. Most are instruments that are also used for other diseases, such as Short Form-36 Health Survey, while some were specifically developed for SSc, such as the SSc health assessment questionnaire (SHAQ) [153], the UCLA SSc clinical trial consortium gastrointestinal instrument 2.0 [154], and the Raynaud's condition score [155]. Assessments of disease activity in individual organs utilize traditional organ-specific measures, such as FVC for pulmonary function assessment and tender joint count for musculoskeletal evaluation.

In the clinical setting, there are no widely and routinely used disease activity scales for SSc. The European SSc Study Group proposed a 10-point index based on organ system involvement and relevant laboratory findings [156]. However, the index has not yet been studied for early SSc and sensitivity for change in disease activity has not been established.

To assess disease severity, international SSc experts developed a revised Medsger severity index assessing 9 organ systems [157]. While individual item severity scores have been shown to predict survival [158], the entire severity index is not weighed and therefore it is not designed to render a total severity score.

Monitoring

In addition to regular cutaneous examinations, all patients with SSc require screening at routine intervals for the development of systemic manifestations, including pulmonary, cardiac, and renal disease. We recommend following patients with SSc at 3–6 month intervals. Review of systems at each visit should include assessment for difficulty swallowing, reflux, bloating, constipation, diarrhea, Raynaud's phenomenon, digital ulcers, dyspnea, fatigue, syncope, palpitations, chest pain, and blood pressure abnormalities.

For the first 5 years after the initial onset of symptoms, we obtain pulmonary function tests every 6–12 months and annual echocardiograms to assess for ILD and PH. Patients with mild respiratory impairment (FVC > 70%) or mild HRCT fibrosis (<20%) should have PFTs more frequently (every 3–6 months), until stabilization is documented on FVC and DLCO, especially during the first 3–5 years after disease onset. After 5 years, if there are no abnormal features (e.g. low DLCO, dyspnea, decreasing FVC), we decrease the frequency of pulmonary function testing. There are no clear guidelines with regards to frequency of echocardiography, as PH can occur many years after the onset of disease. Some experts choose to repeat echocardiography only in those who are symptomatic or at high risk for PH or with a decrease in DLCO, while others perform this exam on an annual basis indefinitely.

A yearly electrocardiogram is also advised to screen for cardiac involvement. For patients at high risk of renal crisis (male, African-American, anti-RNA polymerase III positive, with early disease, on prednisone), regular home blood pressure monitoring may be indicated.

Comorbidities

Comorbidities of SSc include increased cumulative risk of cardiovascular disease, including myocardial infarction and stroke [56, 159], deep vein thrombosis and pulmonary thromboembolisms [160], and malignancies (especially lung) [161]. A study using two large U.S. datasets to retrospectively assess comorbidities in SSc patients showed that they have a higher chronic disease burden, as defined by higher risks of overall cardiovascular, renal, hepatic, and neuropsychiatric disease [162]. The large epidemiological studies that have produced the above findings are limited by uncertainty with regard to their case and outcome definitions, as all of them are based on administrative codes. Detection bias may also be an issue, as SSc patients have more medical care contact and undergo more testing than do healthy patients. In spite of these limitations, such findings are noteworthy, and more research is taking place to delineate the causes as well as mechanisms to prevent and/or improve outcomes for these comorbidities.

Management of SSc

No single approach to treatment has proven uniformly effective in SSc, and therapeutic studies are limited by the lack of adequate outcome measures and the variable natural history of the disease, including the tendency towards skin softening over time [163]. Future studies promise to utilize potentially more sensitive and specific biomarkers in the assessment of optimal therapeutic approaches [164–166].

Current therapeutic approaches largely focus on interventions tailored to specific organ involvement [86]. Therefore the essential first step in optimal management of SSc is to determine the disease phenotype and stage [167], because as reviewed above, limited and diffuse SSc differ in their natural history and complications. Later stage fibrotic disease of either phenotype may remain stable and therefore not require intervention [167].

Organ-Specific Therapy

Skin Disease

A large multicenter trial of methotrexate compared to placebo in patients with dcSSc showed a trend toward significance in skin score improvement in the methotrexate arm at the end of 24 months [168]. As a secondary outcome in the landmark Scleroderma Lung Study I (SLS I), the mRSS showed statistically significant improvement in patients with dcSSc treated with cyclophosphamide (CYC) as compared to controls, though the clinical significance of this finding was unclear [169]. Currently, there are several ongoing or recently completed studies of biologic therapies in SSc, both open label and randomized, in which changes in either mRSS or a gene expression biomarker in skin is a primary outcome (Table 6.5). Biologic therapies for skin disease alone should be considered experimental, and administration of these therapies is thus best conducted in the context of a clinical trial.

Vascular: Raynaud's Phenomenon and Digital Ischemic Ulcers

First line therapy for symptomatic Raynaud's phenomenon includes calcium channel blockers. Resistant or severe Raynaud's is best treated with PDE-5 inhibitors such as tadalafil or sildenafil, which have also shown to be of benefit in randomized trials of digital ischemic ulcers [170, 171]. ET-1 antagonists appear helpful in prevention of digital ischemic ulcers but not in healing established ulcers [172, 173].

Gastrointestinal

Treatment of GI complications of SSc focuses on symptom management. The mainstays of therapy are pro-motility agents (such as metachlopramide, octreatide, and erythromycin), antibiotics for bacterial overgrowth, and argon laser ablation for GAVE [174].

Table 6.5 Ongoing or recently completed trials of biologic therapy with mRSS or skin biomarkers as the primary outcome

Agent	Target	Design	NIH#
Fresolimumab	TGfβ	Phase I, open label	NCT01284322
Rilonacept	IL-1	Phase II, randomized, placebo controlled	NCT01538719
Abatacept	CTLA-4	Phase II, double blind, randomized, placebo controlled	NCT02161406
Tocilizumab	IL-6	Phase II/III randomized, double blind placebo controlled	NCT01532869
Anti-type I interferon	Type 1 interferon	Phase I, open label	NCT00930683

Pulmonary

Interstitial Lung Disease

ILD of all types has historically been difficult to treat. Recent efforts to treat SSc-associated ILD have focused on immune ablation with CYC. The SLS I was a pivotal trial comparing oral CYC to placebo over the course of 12 months in patients with SSc-associated ILD [169]. The trial showed a statistically significant benefit in FVC in patients treated with CYC, although a follow-up study showed that its benefit waned after 2 years [175].

Another randomized, placebo-controlled trial evaluated a regimen consisting of low-dose prednisolone with intravenous CYC monthly for 6 months followed by oral azathioprine for 6 months. It showed a trend toward statistical improvement in the treatment group, with change in FVC and single breath diffusion capacity for carbon dioxide (DLCO) as the primary outcomes [176].

SLS-II, a randomized, placebo-controlled trial of mycophenylate mofetil (MMF) versus oral CYC for 12 months, showed that MMF was equivalent to CYC in preventing FVC decline over the course of the trial, with lower toxicity. These results suggest that MMF should be considered standard of care in treating progressive ILD associated with SSc [177].

Other therapies currently under evaluation include pirfenidone (anti-fibrotic), palmolidomide (anti-fibrotic), nilotinib (anti-fibrotic) and rituximab (anti-CD20). The standard of care for SSc-associated ILD should involve assessment of stage and chronology of disease—i.e., stability or progression by imaging of the lung with high resolution CT scanning, and assessment of pulmonary function with spirometry and DLCO. Immunosuppressive therapy should then be considered for patients with disease progression or early stage disease. For end-stage progressive disease, lung transplantation may be required [178].

Pulmonary Arterial Hypertension

Virtually all trials of therapy of PAH include patients with SSc; however, to date there is only one randomized trial exclusively in patients with SSc-associated PAH [179]. Perhaps as a result, vasodilatory agents are the mainstay of therapy, in contrast to other manifestations of SSc, which are managed largely with immunomodulators. Still, therapy of PAH has undergone dramatic advances over the past several years.

There are two primary pharmacologic approaches to achieving vasodilation in PAH. The first approach is blocking the vasoconstrictive effects of ET-1. ET-1 antagonists include bosentan, ambrisentan and macitentan. The second approach is enhancing the vasodilatory effects of nitric oxide. Agents that accomplish this include phosphodiesterase (PDE) inhibitors (sildenafil and tadalafil), inhaled nitric oxide, and prostaglandin analogs (epoprostenol and treprostinil).

Both endothelin antagonists and PDE inhibitors have been shown to lead to statistically significant hemodynamic and symptomatic improvement in PAH. Only the most recent ET-1 inhibitor, macitentan, however, has shown a significant event-free survival (with event defined as death or hospitalization from PAH) as compared to placebo [180]. Recent studies suggest that combination therapies may offer improvements in efficacy when compared to monotherapies [181, 182].

The current standard of care for PAH patients falling into symptomatic New York Heart Association (NYHA) functional class II (mild to moderate impairment) is to begin an ET-1 inhibitor or PDE-5 inhibitor. For patients with advanced disease or in NYHA functional class III-IV, continuous intravenous infusion with prostacyclin derivatives such as epoprostenol is considered standard of care [183]. Lung transplantation may also be required for end stage disease [178].

Renal

Prior to the advent of angiotensin converting enzyme (ACE) inhibitors, SRC was associated with high risk of progression to end stage renal disease and high mortality secondary to complications of severe hypertension. ACE inhibitors have significantly improved outcomes in SRC, although the risk of progression to ESRD remains high even with early use of ACE inhibitors [184,

185]. Approximately 30% of patients with SRC who require renal replacement may be able to discontinue hemodialysis within a year if ACE inhibitors are continued during hemodialysis [186].

Musculoskeletal

Despite the frequent occurrence of musculoskeletal complications in SSc, there are no randomized controlled trials of SSc-associated arthropathy. Weekly methotrexate is considered standard of care, the first line disease-modifying therapy for musculoskeletal disease. Open label studies of anti-TNF agents as well as abatacept and tocilizumab suggest that these agents may also be of benefit [59, 167].

Low-dose prednisone may provide some symptomatic and functional benefit for both inflammatory arthritis and myositis. Prednisone at doses higher than 20 mg daily in patients with dcSSc, however, should generally be avoided due to concern about potentially precipitating SRC [187]. Physical and occupational therapy to maintain finger mobility are important adjunctive therapies.

Immune Modulation and Targeted Therapies

Beyond treating organ-specific manifestations, studies have shown benefit from immunomodulatory therapy in treating SSc overall. The 2014 Autologous Stem cell Transplantation International Scleroderma (ASTIS) trial showed that high-dose immunosuppressive therapy and autologous hematopoietic stem cell transplantation (HSCT) in patients with early diffuse SSc and poor prognosis (most of whom had either ILD or a history of renal crisis) conferred a significant survival benefit over lower level conventional immune suppression with monthly intravenous CYC [188]. This approach is not without substantial risk, however, given the 10% mortality associated with the stem cell transplantation [188]. HSCT should be viewed as a potential therapeutic option for patients with aggressive disease, but until treatment-associated mortality can be significantly reduced, it should not be considered a standard of care.

More targeted therapy is urgently needed in SSc, as conventional immunosuppression appears to confer modest benefit that wanes with time, and immune ablative approaches are risky. No such therapy yet exists, but there are number of promising therapies in development targeting potential drivers of disease pathogenesis, including fresolimumab (anti-TGfβ), rilonacept (IL1 inhibitor), tocilizumab (anti-IL6) and abatacept (T cell activation inhibitor).

Survival

Survival in SSc greatly depends on the clinical subtype and antibody profile, type of organ involvement, and patient demographics. Old age, male sex, African-American race, and poor socioeconomic status are associated with worse outcome. Other factors generally accepted as poor prognostic indicators include the diffuse cutaneous subset, anti-topoisomerase I antibody and presence of severe organ involvement (skin, lung, heart, GI tract, kidney) [33, 189]. In a recent analysis of 234 deaths in the EUSTAR database, the independent risk factors for mortality in SSc were proteinuria, PAH, restrictive pulmonary disease, dyspnea greater than NYHA Class II, decreased diffusion capacity, greater age of Raynaud's onset, and greater (mRSS) [51].

Encouragingly, survival in SSc has improved in the last few decades. In a large longitudinal study of a U.S. SSc cohort from Pittsburgh, PA, the 10-year survival rate improved from 54% in the 1970s to 66% in the 1990s [46]. More recent survival estimates in 1999–2010 report in a Brazilian cohort showed overall survival rate to be 90% over 5 years and 84% over 10 years [8]. The 10-year survival rate was lower for those with dcSSc (77%) vs. lcSSc (87%).

The improvement in SSc survival over time is largely attributable to the implementation of effective therapy for SRC, which historically had been the primary cause of death in SSc. Pulmonary fibrosis and PAH have since supplanted SRC as the leading causes of mortality

[46]. Additionally, more SSc patients are dying from non-SSc causes than in previous decades. In the EUSTAR database report, 55% of SSc deaths were directly related to SSc and 41% were secondary to non-SSc causes [51]. Top causes of non-SSc related deaths included infections, malignancies, and cardiovascular disease.

Summary

SSc is a debilitating connective tissue disease that disproportionately afflicts women and African-Americans and carries significant morbidity and mortality. However, recent therapeutic advances indicate that immunosuppressive therapy can prevent progression of severe cutaneous and visceral fibrosis. Patients must be evaluated for cutaenous, pulmonary, renal, GI, and cardiac involvement. Coordinated interdisciplinary care is essential in the evaluation and management of patients with systemic sclerosis.

References

1. Barnes J, Mayes MD. Epidemiology of systemic sclerosis: incidence, prevalence, survival, risk factors, malignancy, and environmental triggers. Curr Opin Rheumatol. 2012;24(2):165–70.
2. van den Hoogen F, et al. 2013 classification criteria for systemic sclerosis: an American College of Rheumatology/European League against Rheumatism collaborative initiative. Arthritis Rheum. 2013;65(11):2737–47.
3. Steen V. Epidemiology and classification of scleroderma. In: Rheumatology. London: Elsevier Ltd; 2008.
4. D'Amico F, Skarmoutsou E, Mazzarino MC. The sex bias in systemic sclerosis: on the possible mechanisms underlying the female disease preponderance. Clin Rev Allergy Immunol. 2014;47(3):334–43.
5. Tiniakou E, Costenbader KH, Kriegel MA. Sex-specific environmental influences on the development of autoimmune diseases. Clin Immunol. 2013;149(2):182–91.
6. Mayes MD, et al. Prevalence, incidence, survival, and disease characteristics of systemic sclerosis in a large US population. Arthritis Rheum. 2003;48(8):2246–55.
7. Hoffmann-Vold AM, et al. Survival and causes of death in an unselected and complete cohort of Norwegian patients with systemic sclerosis. J Rheumatol. 2013;40(7):1127–33.
8. Sampaio-Barros PD, et al. Survival, causes of death, and prognostic factors in systemic sclerosis: analysis of 947 Brazilian patients. J Rheumatol. 2012;39(10):1971–8.
9. Elhai M, et al. A gender gap in primary and secondary heart dysfunctions in systemic sclerosis: a EUSTAR prospective study. Ann Rheum Dis. 2016;75(1):163–9.
10. Reveille JD. Ethnicity and race and systemic sclerosis: how it affects susceptibility, severity, antibody genetics, and clinical manifestations. Curr Rheumatol Rep. 2003;5(2):160–7.
11. Laing TJ, et al. Racial differences in scleroderma among women in Michigan. Arthritis Rheum. 1997;40(4):734–42.
12. Steen VD, et al. Incidence of systemic sclerosis in Allegheny County, Pennsylvania. A twenty-year study of hospital-diagnosed cases, 1963-1982. Arthritis Rheum. 1997;40(3):441–5.
13. Gelber AC, et al. Race and association with disease manifestations and mortality in scleroderma: a 20-year experience at the Johns Hopkins Scleroderma Center and review of the literature. Medicine (Baltimore). 2013;92(4):191–205.
14. Steen VD, et al. Severe restrictive lung disease in systemic sclerosis. Arthritis Rheum. 1994;37(9):1283–9.
15. Reveille JD, et al. Systemic sclerosis in 3 US ethnic groups: a comparison of clinical, sociodemographic, serologic, and immunogenetic determinants. Semin Arthritis Rheum. 2001;30(5):332–46.
16. Li R, et al. Epidemiology of eight common rheumatic diseases in China: a large-scale cross-sectional survey in Beijing. Rheumatology (Oxford). 2012;51(4):721–9.
17. Tamaki T, Mori S, Takehara K. Epidemiological study of patients with systemic sclerosis in Tokyo. Arch Dermatol Res. 1991;283(6):366–71.
18. Preliminary criteria for the classification of systemic sclerosis (scleroderma). Subcommittee for scleroderma criteria of the American Rheumatism Association Diagnostic and Therapeutic Criteria Committee. Arthritis Rheum. 1980;23(5):581–90.
19. LeRoy EC, et al. Scleroderma (systemic sclerosis): classification, subsets and pathogenesis. J Rheumatol. 1988;15(2):202–5.
20. Medsger T Jr. Classification, prognosis. In: Systemic sclerosis. Philadelphia: Lippincott Williams & Wilkins; 2004.
21. Perera A, et al. Clinical subsets, skin thickness progression rate, and serum antibody levels in systemic sclerosis patients with anti-topoisomerase I antibody. Arthritis Rheum. 2007;56(8):2740–6.
22. Barnett AJ. The "neck sign" in scleroderma. Arthritis Rheum. 1989;32(2):209–11.
23. Medsger TA. Natural history of systemic sclerosis and the assessment of disease activity, severity, functional status, and psychologic well-being. Rheum Dis Clin N Am. 2003;29(2):255–73, vi.

24. Steen VD, Medsger TA. Improvement in skin thickening in systemic sclerosis associated with improved survival. Arthritis Rheum. 2001;44(12):2828–35.
25. Shah AA, Wigley FM, Hummers LK. Telangiectases in scleroderma: a potential clinical marker of pulmonary arterial hypertension. J Rheumatol. 2010;37(1):98–104.
26. Caramaschi P, et al. Digital amputation in systemic sclerosis: prevalence and clinical associations. A retrospective longitudinal study. J Rheumatol. 2012;39(8):1648–53.
27. Lonzetti LS, et al. Updating the American College of Rheumatology preliminary classification criteria for systemic sclerosis: addition of severe nailfold capillaroscopy abnormalities markedly increases the sensitivity for limited scleroderma. Arthritis Rheum. 2001;44(3):735–6.
28. Hughes M, et al. A study comparing videocapillaroscopy and dermoscopy in the assessment of nailfold capillaries in patients with systemic sclerosis-spectrum disorders. Rheumatology (Oxford). 2015;54(8):1435–42.
29. Mazzotti NG, et al. Assessment of nailfold capillaroscopy in systemic sclerosis by different optical magnification methods. Clin Exp Dermatol. 2014;39(2):135–41.
30. Bauersachs RM, Lössner F. The poor man's capillary microscope. A novel technique for the assessment of capillary morphology. Ann Rheum Dis. 1997;56(7):435–7.
31. Forbes A, Marie I. Gastrointestinal complications: the most frequent internal complications of systemic sclerosis. Rheumatology (Oxford). 2009;48 Suppl 3:iii36–9.
32. Sjogren RW. Gastrointestinal features of scleroderma. Curr Opin Rheumatol. 1996;8(6):569–75.
33. Steen VD, Medsger TA. Severe organ involvement in systemic sclerosis with diffuse scleroderma. Arthritis Rheum. 2000;43(11):2437–44.
34. Montesi A, et al. Oropharyngeal and esophageal function in scleroderma. Dysphagia. 1991;6(4):219–23.
35. Savarino E, et al. Gastroesophageal reflux and pulmonary fibrosis in scleroderma: a study using pH-impedance monitoring. Am J Respir Crit Care Med. 2009;179(5):408–13.
36. Wipff J, et al. Outcomes of Barrett's oesophagus related to systemic sclerosis: a 3-year EULAR Scleroderma Trials and Research prospective follow-up study. Rheumatology (Oxford). 2011;50(8):1440–4.
37. Watson M, et al. Gastric antral vascular ectasia (watermelon stomach) in patients with systemic sclerosis. Arthritis Rheum. 1996;39(2):341–6.
38. Assassi S, et al. Primary biliary cirrhosis (PBC), PBC autoantibodies, and hepatic parameter abnormalities in a large population of systemic sclerosis patients. J Rheumatol. 2009;36(10):2250–6.
39. Rigamonti C, et al. Clinical features and prognosis of primary biliary cirrhosis associated with systemic sclerosis. Gut. 2006;55(3):388–94.
40. Meier FM, et al. Update on the profile of the EUSTAR cohort: an analysis of the EULAR Scleroderma Trials and Research group database. Ann Rheum Dis. 2012;71(8):1355–60.
41. D'Angelo WA, et al. Pathologic observations in systemic sclerosis (scleroderma). A study of fifty-eight autopsy cases and fifty-eight matched controls. Am J Med. 1969;46(3):428–40.
42. Gyger G, Baron M. Gastrointestinal manifestations of scleroderma: recent progress in evaluation, pathogenesis, and management. Curr Rheumatol Rep. 2012;14(1):22–9.
43. Wells AU. Interstitial lung disease in systemic sclerosis. Presse Med. 2014;43(10 Pt 2):e329–43.
44. Wells AU, et al. Fibrosing alveolitis in systemic sclerosis: indices of lung function in relation to extent of disease on computed tomography. Arthritis Rheum. 1997;40(7):1229–36.
45. Man A, et al. Changes in forced vital capacity over time in systemic sclerosis: application of group-based trajectory modelling. Rheumatology (Oxford). 2015;54(8):1464–71.
46. Steen VD, Medsger TA. Changes in causes of death in systemic sclerosis, 1972-2002. Ann Rheum Dis. 2007;66(7):940–4.
47. Ong YY, et al. Decreased nailfold capillary density in limited scleroderma with pulmonary hypertension. Asian Pac J Allergy Immunol. 1998;16(2–3):81–6.
48. Kawut SM, et al. Hemodynamics and survival in patients with pulmonary arterial hypertension related to systemic sclerosis. Chest. 2003;123(2):344–50.
49. Steen V, Medsger TA. Predictors of isolated pulmonary hypertension in patients with systemic sclerosis and limited cutaneous involvement. Arthritis Rheum. 2003;48(2):516–22.
50. Koh ET, et al. Pulmonary hypertension in systemic sclerosis: an analysis of 17 patients. Br J Rheumatol. 1996;35(10):989–93.
51. Tyndall AJ, et al. Causes and risk factors for death in systemic sclerosis: a study from the EULAR Scleroderma Trials and Research (EUSTAR) database. Ann Rheum Dis. 2010;69(10):1809–15.
52. Ferri C, et al. Systemic sclerosis: demographic, clinical, and serologic features and survival in 1,012 Italian patients. Medicine (Baltimore). 2002;81(2):139–53.
53. Champion HC. The heart in scleroderma. Rheum Dis Clin N Am. 2008;34(1):181–90; viii.
54. de Groote P, et al. Evaluation of cardiac abnormalities by Doppler echocardiography in a large nationwide multicentric cohort of patients with systemic sclerosis. Ann Rheum Dis. 2008;67(1):31–6.
55. Au K, et al. Atherosclerosis in systemic sclerosis: a systematic review and meta-analysis. Arthritis Rheum. 2011;63(7):2078–90.
56. Man A, et al. The risk of cardiovascular disease in systemic sclerosis: a population-based cohort study. Ann Rheum Dis. 2013;72(7):1188–93.

57. Steen VD, et al. Kidney disease other than renal crisis in patients with diffuse scleroderma. J Rheumatol. 2005;32(4):649–55.
58. Teixeira L, et al. Mortality and risk factors of scleroderma renal crisis: a French retrospective study of 50 patients. Ann Rheum Dis. 2008;67(1):110–6.
59. Elhai M, et al. Outcomes of patients with systemic sclerosis-associated polyarthritis and myopathy treated with tocilizumab or abatacept: a EUSTAR observational study. Ann Rheum Dis. 2013;72(7):1217–20.
60. Avouac J, et al. Characteristics of joint involvement and relationships with systemic inflammation in systemic sclerosis: results from the EULAR Scleroderma Trial and Research Group (EUSTAR) database. J Rheumatol. 2010;37(7):1488–501.
61. Avouac J, et al. Articular involvement in systemic sclerosis. Rheumatology (Oxford). 2012;51(8):1347–56.
62. Avouac J, et al. Radiological hand involvement in systemic sclerosis. Ann Rheum Dis. 2006;65(8):1088–92.
63. Steen VD, Medsger TA. The palpable tendon friction rub: an important physical examination finding in patients with systemic sclerosis. Arthritis Rheum. 1997;40(6):1146–51.
64. Shulman LE, Kurban AK, Harvey AM. Tendon friction rubs in progressive system sclerosis (scleroderma). Trans Assoc Am Phys. 1961;74:378–88.
65. Khanna PP, et al. Tendon friction rubs in early diffuse systemic sclerosis: prevalence, characteristics and longitudinal changes in a randomized controlled trial. Rheumatology (Oxford). 2010;49(5):955–9.
66. Avouac J, et al. Joint and tendon involvement predict disease progression in systemic sclerosis: a EUSTAR prospective study. Ann Rheum Dis. 2016;75(1):103–9.
67. Abraham DJ, et al. Overview of pathogenesis of systemic sclerosis. Rheumatology (Oxford). 2009;48 Suppl 3:iii3–7.
68. Abraham D, Distler O. How does endothelial cell injury start? The role of endothelin in systemic sclerosis. Arthritis Res Ther. 2007;9 Suppl 2:S2.
69. Pattanaik D, et al. Pathogenesis of systemic sclerosis. Front Immunol. 2015;6:272.
70. Altorok N, Wang Y, Kahaleh B. Endothelial dysfunction in systemic sclerosis. Curr Opin Rheumatol. 2014;26(6):615–20.
71. Dumoitier N, Lofek S, Mouthon L. Pathophysiology of systemic sclerosis: state of the art in 2014. Presse Med. 2014;43(10 Pt 2):e267–78.
72. Silver RM. Endothelin and scleroderma lung disease. Rheumatology (Oxford). 2008;47 Suppl 5:v25–6.
73. Tuder RM, et al. Relevant issues in the pathology and pathobiology of pulmonary hypertension. J Am Coll Cardiol. 2013;62(25 Suppl):D4–12.
74. Morrell NW, et al. Cellular and molecular basis of pulmonary arterial hypertension. J Am Coll Cardiol. 2009;54(1 Suppl):S20–31.
75. Hassoun PM, et al. Inflammation, growth factors, and pulmonary vascular remodeling. J Am Coll Cardiol. 2009;54(1 Suppl):S10–9.
76. Stenmark KR, Tuder RM, El Kasmi KC. Metabolic reprogramming and inflammation act in concert to control vascular remodeling in hypoxic pulmonary hypertension. J Appl Physiol (1985). 2015;119(10):1164–72.
77. Rossi D, et al. The role of nail-videocapillaroscopy in early diagnosis of scleroderma. Autoimmun Rev. 2013;12(8):821–5.
78. Manetti M, et al. Differential expression of junctional adhesion molecules in different stages of systemic sclerosis. Arthritis Rheum. 2013;65(1):247–57.
79. Jiang N, Li M, Zeng X. Correlation of Th17 cells and CD4+CD25+ regulatory T cells with clinical parameters in patients with systemic sclerosis. Chin Med J. 2014;127(20):3557–61.
80. Asano Y, Bujor AM, Trojanowska M. The impact of Fli1 deficiency on the pathogenesis of systemic sclerosis. J Dermatol Sci. 2010;59(3):153–62.
81. Manetti M. Fli1 deficiency and beyond: a unique pathway linking peripheral vasculopathy and dermal fibrosis in systemic sclerosis. Exp Dermatol. 2015;24(4):256–7.
82. Saigusa R, et al. A possible contribution of endothelial CCN1 downregulation due to Fli1 deficiency to the development of digital ulcers in systemic sclerosis. Exp Dermatol. 2015;24(2):127–32.
83. Brembilla NC, Chizzolini C. T cell abnormalities in systemic sclerosis with a focus on Th17 cells. Eur Cytokine Netw. 2012;23(4):128–39.
84. MacDonald KG, et al. Regulatory T cells produce profibrotic cytokines in the skin of patients with systemic sclerosis. J Allergy Clin Immunol. 2015;135(4):946–e9.
85. Zhou Y, et al. The elevated expression of Th17-related cytokines and receptors is associated with skin lesion severity in early systemic sclerosis. Hum Immunol. 2015;76(1):22–9.
86. Elhai M, et al. Systemic sclerosis: recent insights. Joint Bone Spine. 2015;82(3):148–53.
87. Assassi S, et al. Genetics of scleroderma: implications for personalized medicine? BMC Med. 2013;11:9.
88. López-Isac E, et al. A genome-wide association study follow-up suggests a possible role for PPARG in systemic sclerosis susceptibility. Arthritis Res Ther. 2014;16(1):R6.
89. Hamaguchi Y. Autoantibody profiles in systemic sclerosis: predictive value for clinical evaluation and prognosis. J Dermatol. 2010;37(1):42–53.
90. Grassegger A, et al. Autoantibodies in systemic sclerosis (scleroderma): clues for clinical evaluation, prognosis and pathogenesis. Wien Med Wochenschr. 2008;158(1–2):19–28.
91. Mehra S, et al. Autoantibodies in systemic sclerosis. Autoimmun Rev. 2013;12(3):340–54.
92. Steen VD. Autoantibodies in systemic sclerosis. Semin Arthritis Rheum. 2005;35(1):35–42.

93. Steen VD, Powell DL, Medsger TA. Clinical correlations and prognosis based on serum autoantibodies in patients with systemic sclerosis. Arthritis Rheum. 1988;31(2):196–203.
94. Greenblatt MB, Aliprantis AO. The immune pathogenesis of scleroderma: context is everything. Curr Rheumatol Rep. 2013;15(1):297.
95. O'Reilly S, et al. Interleukin-6 (IL-6) trans signaling drives a STAT3-dependent pathway that leads to hyperactive transforming growth factor-β (TGF-β) signaling promoting SMAD3 activation and fibrosis via Gremlin protein. J Biol Chem. 2014;289(14):9952–60.
96. Needleman BW, Wigley FM, Stair RW. Interleukin-1, interleukin-2, interleukin-4, interleukin-6, tumor necrosis factor alpha, and interferon-gamma levels in sera from patients with scleroderma. Arthritis Rheum. 1992;35(1):67–72.
97. Fernandes das Neves M, et al. Treatment of systemic sclerosis with tocilizumab. Rheumatology (Oxford). 2015;54(2):371–2.
98. Rockey DC, Bell PD, Hill JA. Fibrosis – a common pathway to organ injury and failure. N Engl J Med. 2015;373(1):96.
99. Eaglstein WH. Wound healing and aging. Clin Geriatr Med. 1989;5(1):183–8.
100. Brown GL, et al. Enhancement of wound healing by topical treatment with epidermal growth factor. N Engl J Med. 1989;321(2):76–9.
101. Babu M, Diegelmann R, Oliver N. Fibronectin is overproduced by keloid fibroblasts during abnormal wound healing. Mol Cell Biol. 1989;9(4): 1642–50.
102. Zhang K, et al. Myofibroblasts and their role in lung collagen gene expression during pulmonary fibrosis. A combined immunohistochemical and in situ hybridization study. Am J Pathol. 1994;145:114–25.
103. Masur SK, et al. Myofibroblasts differentiate from fibroblasts when plated at low density. Proc Natl Acad Sci U S A. 1996;93:4219–23.
104. Kissin EY, Merkel PA, Lafyatis R. Myofibroblasts and hyalinized collagen as markers of skin disease in systemic sclerosis. Arthritis Rheum. 2006;54(11):3655–60.
105. Kirk TZ, et al. Myofibroblasts from scleroderma skin synthesize elevated levels of collagen and tissue inhibitor of metalloproteinase (TIMP-1) with two forms of TIMP-1. J Biol Chem. 1995;270(7):3423–8.
106. Desmouliere A, et al. Transforming growth factor-beta 1 induces alpha-smooth muscle actin expression in granulation tissue myofibroblasts and in quiescent and growing cultured fibroblasts. J Cell Biol. 1993;122(1):103–11.
107. Marangoni RG, et al. Myofibroblasts in murine cutaneous fibrosis originate from adiponectin-positive intradermal progenitors. Arthritis Rheumatol. 2015;67(4):1062–73.
108. Liu F, et al. Mechanosignaling through YAP and TAZ drives fibroblast activation and fibrosis. Am J Physiol Lung Cell Mol Physiol. 2015;308(4):L344–57.
109. Christmann RB, et al. Association of Interferon- and transforming growth factor β-regulated genes and macrophage activation with systemic sclerosis-related progressive lung fibrosis. Arthritis Rheumatol. 2014;66(3):714–25.
110. Leask A. Scar wars: is TGFbeta the phantom menace in scleroderma? Arthritis Res Ther. 2006;8(4):213.
111. Robertson IB, et al. Latent TGF-β-binding proteins. Matrix Biol. 2015;47:44–53.
112. Brand OJ, et al. Transforming growth factor-β and interleukin-1β signaling pathways converge on the chemokine CCL20 promoter. J Biol Chem. 2015;290(23):14717–28.
113. Dees C, Distler JH. Canonical Wnt signalling as a key regulator of fibrogenesis - implications for targeted therapies? Exp Dermatol. 2013;22(11):710–3.
114. Iwayama T, Olson LE. Involvement of PDGF in fibrosis and scleroderma: recent insights from animal models and potential therapeutic opportunities. Curr Rheumatol Rep. 2013;15(2):304.
115. Baroni SS, et al. Stimulatory autoantibodies to the PDGF receptor in systemic sclerosis. N Engl J Med. 2006;354(25):2667–76.
116. Loizos N, et al. Lack of detection of agonist activity by antibodies to platelet-derived growth factor receptor alpha in a subset of normal and systemic sclerosis patient sera. Arthritis Rheum. 2009;60(4):1145–51.
117. Balada E, et al. Anti-PDGFR-alpha antibodies measured by non-bioactivity assays are not specific for systemic sclerosis. Ann Rheum Dis. 2008;67(7):1027–9.
118. Kurasawa K, et al. Autoantibodies against platelet-derived growth factor receptor alpha in patients with systemic lupus erythematosus. Mod Rheumatol. 2010;20(5):458–65.
119. Bogatkevich GS, et al. Proteomic analysis of CTGF-activated lung fibroblasts: identification of IQGAP1 as a key player in lung fibroblast migration. Am J Physiol Lung Cell Mol Physiol. 2008;295(4):L603–11.
120. Abraham D. Connective tissue growth factor: growth factor, matricellular organizer, fibrotic biomarker or molecular target for anti-fibrotic therapy in SSc? Rheumatology (Oxford). 2008;47 Suppl 5:v8–9.
121. Sakai N, et al. LPA1-induced cytoskeleton reorganization drives fibrosis through CTGF-dependent fibroblast proliferation. FASEB J. 2013;27(5):1830–46.
122. Feghali-Bostwick C, Medsger TA, Wright TM. Analysis of systemic sclerosis in twins reveals low concordance for disease and high concordance for the presence of antinuclear antibodies. Arthritis Rheum. 2003;48(7):1956–63.
123. Arnett FC, et al. Familial occurrence frequencies and relative risks for systemic sclerosis (scleroderma) in three United States cohorts. Arthritis Rheum. 2001;44(6):1359–62.
124. Roberts-Thomson PJ, Walker JG. Stochastic processes in the aetiopathogenesis of scleroderma. Intern Med J. 2012;42(3):235–42.

125. Arnett FC, et al. Increased prevalence of systemic sclerosis in a Native American tribe in Oklahoma. Association with an Amerindian HLA haplotype. Arthritis Rheum. 1996;39(8):1362–70.
126. Zhou X, et al. Genome-wide association study for regions of systemic sclerosis susceptibility in a Choctaw Indian population with high disease prevalence. Arthritis Rheum. 2003;48(9):2585–92.
127. Tan FK, et al. Association of microsatellite markers near the fibrillin 1 gene on human chromosome 15q with scleroderma in a Native American population. Arthritis Rheum. 1998;41(10):1729–37.
128. Valesini G, et al. Geographical clustering of scleroderma in a rural area in the province of Rome. Clin Exp Rheumatol. 1993;11(1):41–7.
129. Silman AJ, et al. Geographical clustering of scleroderma in south and west London. Br J Rheumatol. 1990;29(2):93–6.
130. Thompson AE, Pope JE. Increased prevalence of scleroderma in southwestern Ontario: a cluster analysis. J Rheumatol. 2002;29(9):1867–73.
131. Englert H, et al. Systemic scleroderma: a spatiotemporal clustering. Intern Med J. 2005;35(4):228–33.
132. Archer C, Gordon DA. Silica and progressive systemic sclerosis (scleroderma): evidence for workers' compensation policy. Am J Ind Med. 1996;29(5):533–8.
133. Bramwell B. Diffuse scleroderma: its frequency; its occurrence in stonemasons, its treatment by fibrinolysis: elevations of temperature due to fibrinolysis injections. Edinb Med J. 1914;12:387–401.
134. Erasmus LD. Scleroderma in goldminers on the Witwatersrand with particular reference to pulmonary manifestations. S Afr J Lab Clin Med. 1957;3(3):209–31.
135. Rodnan GP, et al. The association of progressive systemic sclerosis (scleroderma) with coal miners' pneumoconiosis and other forms of silicosis. Ann Intern Med. 1967;66(2):323–34.
136. Moisan S, et al. Silica-associated limited systemic sclerosis after occupational exposure to calcined diatomaceous earth. Joint Bone Spine. 2010;77(5):472–3.
137. McCormic ZD, et al. Occupational silica exposure as a risk factor for scleroderma: a meta-analysis. Int Arch Occup Environ Health. 2010;83(7):763–9.
138. Kettaneh A, et al. Occupational exposure to solvents and gender-related risk of systemic sclerosis: a metaanalysis of case-control studies. J Rheumatol. 2007;34(1):97–103.
139. Garabrant DH, et al. Scleroderma and solvent exposure among women. Am J Epidemiol. 2003;157(6):493–500.
140. Domsic RT. Scleroderma: the role of serum autoantibodies in defining specific clinical phenotypes and organ system involvement. Curr Opin Rheumatol. 2014;26(6):646–52.
141. Joseph CG, et al. Association of the autoimmune disease scleroderma with an immunologic response to cancer. Science. 2014;343(6167):152–7.
142. Nikpour M, et al. Prevalence, correlates and clinical usefulness of antibodies to RNA polymerase III in systemic sclerosis: a cross-sectional analysis of data from an Australian cohort. Arthritis Res Ther. 2011;13(6):R211.
143. Kaji K, et al. Autoantibodies to RuvBL1 and RuvBL2: a novel systemic sclerosis-related antibody associated with diffuse cutaneous and skeletal muscle involvement. Arthritis Care Res (Hoboken). 2014;66(4):575–84.
144. Kayser C, Fritzler MJ. Autoantibodies in systemic sclerosis: unanswered questions. Front Immunol. 2015;6:167.
145. Nihtyanova SI, Denton CP. Autoantibodies as predictive tools in systemic sclerosis. Nat Rev Rheumatol. 2010;6(2):112–6.
146. Fertig N, et al. Anti-U11/U12 RNP antibodies in systemic sclerosis: a new serologic marker associated with pulmonary fibrosis. Arthritis Rheum. 2009;61(7):958–65.
147. Coghlan JG, et al. Evidence-based detection of pulmonary arterial hypertension in systemic sclerosis: the DETECT study. Ann Rheum Dis. 2014;73(7):1340–9.
148. Baron M, et al. Malnutrition is common in systemic sclerosis: results from the Canadian scleroderma research group database. J Rheumatol. 2009;36(12):2737–43.
149. Clements P, et al. Inter and intraobserver variability of total skin thickness score (modified Rodnan TSS) in systemic sclerosis. J Rheumatol. 1995;22(7):1281–5.
150. Domsic RT, et al. Skin thickness progression rate: a predictor of mortality and early internal organ involvement in diffuse scleroderma. Ann Rheum Dis. 2011;70(1):104–9.
151. Merkel PA, et al. Validity, reliability, and feasibility of durometer measurements of scleroderma skin disease in a multicenter treatment trial. Arthritis Rheum. 2008;59(5):699–705.
152. Kissin EY, et al. Durometry for the assessment of skin disease in systemic sclerosis. Arthritis Rheum. 2006;55(4):603–9.
153. Steen VD, Medsger TA. The value of the Health Assessment Questionnaire and special patient-generated scales to demonstrate change in systemic sclerosis patients over time. Arthritis Rheum. 1997;40(11):1984–91.
154. Khanna D, et al. Reliability and validity of the University of California, Los Angeles scleroderma clinical trial consortium gastrointestinal tract instrument. Arthritis Rheum. 2009;61(9):1257–63.
155. Merkel PA, et al. Measuring disease activity and functional status in patients with scleroderma and Raynaud's phenomenon. Arthritis Rheum. 2002;46(9):2410–20.
156. Valentini G, et al. European multicentre study to define disease activity criteria for systemic sclerosis. II. Identification of disease activity variables and development of preliminary activity indexes. Ann Rheum Dis. 2001;60(6):592–8.

157. Medsger TA, et al. A disease severity scale for systemic sclerosis: development and testing. J Rheumatol. 1999;26(10):2159–67.
158. Geirsson AJ, Wollheim FA, Akesson A. Disease severity of 100 patients with systemic sclerosis over a period of 14 years: using a modified Medsger scale. Ann Rheum Dis. 2001;60(12):1117–22.
159. Chu SY, et al. Increased risk of acute myocardial infarction in systemic sclerosis: a nationwide population-based study. Am J Med. 2013;126(11):982–8.
160. Chung WS, et al. Systemic sclerosis increases the risks of deep vein thrombosis and pulmonary thromboembolism: a nationwide cohort study. Rheumatology (Oxford). 2014;53(9):1639–45.
161. Bonifazi M, et al. Systemic sclerosis (scleroderma) and cancer risk: systematic review and meta-analysis of observational studies. Rheumatology (Oxford). 2013;52(1):143–54.
162. Robinson D, et al. Systemic sclerosis prevalence and comorbidities in the US, 2001-2002. Curr Med Res Opin. 2008;24(4):1157–66.
163. Amjadi S, et al. Course of the modified Rodnan skin thickness score in systemic sclerosis clinical trials: analysis of three large multicenter, double-blind, randomized controlled trials. Arthritis Rheum. 2009;60(8):2490–8.
164. Chora I, et al. Vascular biomarkers and correlation with peripheral vasculopathy in systemic sclerosis. Autoimmun Rev. 2015;14(4):314–22.
165. Castelino FV, Varga J. Current status of systemic sclerosis biomarkers: applications for diagnosis, management and drug development. Expert Rev Clin Immunol. 2013;9(11):1077–90.
166. Avouac J, et al. Cardiac biomarkers in systemic sclerosis: contribution of high-sensitivity cardiac troponin in addition to N-terminal pro-brain natriuretic peptide. Arthritis Care Res (Hoboken). 2015;67(7):1022–30.
167. Shah AA, Wigley FM. My approach to the treatment of scleroderma. Mayo Clin Proc. 2013;88(4):377–93.
168. Pope JE, et al. A randomized, controlled trial of methotrexate versus placebo in early diffuse scleroderma. Arthritis Rheum. 2001;44(6):1351–8.
169. Tashkin DP, et al. Cyclophosphamide versus placebo in scleroderma lung disease. N Engl J Med. 2006;354(25):2655–66.
170. Tingey T, et al. Meta-analysis of healing and prevention of digital ulcers in systemic sclerosis. Arthritis Care Res (Hoboken). 2013;65(9):1460–71.
171. Chung L. Therapeutic options for digital ulcers in patients with systemic sclerosis. J Dtsch Dermatol Ges. 2007;5(6):460–5.
172. Matucci-Cerinic M, et al. Bosentan treatment of digital ulcers related to systemic sclerosis: results from the RAPIDS-2 randomised, double-blind, placebo-controlled trial. Ann Rheum Dis. 2011;70(1):32–8.
173. Korn JH, et al. Digital ulcers in systemic sclerosis: prevention by treatment with bosentan, an oral endothelin receptor antagonist. Arthritis Rheum. 2004;50(12):3985–93.
174. Domsic R, Fasanella K, Bielefeldt K. Gastrointestinal manifestations of systemic sclerosis. Dig Dis Sci. 2008;53(5):1163–74.
175. Tashkin DP, et al. Effects of 1-year treatment with cyclophosphamide on outcomes at 2 years in scleroderma lung disease. Am J Respir Crit Care Med. 2007;176(10):1026–34.
176. Hoyles RK, et al. A multicenter, prospective, randomized, double-blind, placebo-controlled trial of corticosteroids and intravenous cyclophosphamide followed by oral azathioprine for the treatment of pulmonary fibrosis in scleroderma. Arthritis Rheum. 2006;54(12):3962–70.
177. Tashkin DP, et al. Mycophenolate mofetil versus oral cyclophosphamide in scleroderma-related interstitial lung disease (SLS II): a randomised controlled, double-blind, parallel group trial. Lancet Respir Med. 2016;4(9):708–19.
178. Schachna L, et al. Lung transplantation in scleroderma compared with idiopathic pulmonary fibrosis and idiopathic pulmonary arterial hypertension. Arthritis Rheum. 2006;54(12):3954–61.
179. Badesch DB, et al. Continuous intravenous epoprostenol for pulmonary hypertension due to the scleroderma spectrum of disease. A randomized, controlled trial. Ann Intern Med. 2000;132(6):425–34.
180. Pulido T, et al. Macitentan and morbidity and mortality in pulmonary arterial hypertension. N Engl J Med. 2013;369(9):809–18.
181. Pugh ME, Hemnes AR, Robbins IM. Combination therapy in pulmonary arterial hypertension. Clin Chest Med. 2013;34(4):841–55.
182. Buckley MS, Staib RL, Wicks LM. Combination therapy in the management of pulmonary arterial hypertension. Int J Clin Pract Suppl. 2013;179:13–23.
183. Badesch DB, et al. Longterm survival among patients with scleroderma-associated pulmonary arterial hypertension treated with intravenous epoprostenol. J Rheumatol. 2009;36(10):2244–9.
184. Penn H, Denton CP. Diagnosis, management and prevention of scleroderma renal disease. Curr Opin Rheumatol. 2008;20(6):692–6.
185. Mouthon L, et al. Scleroderma renal crisis. J Rheumatol. 2014;41(6):1040–8.
186. Steen VD. Scleroderma renal crisis. Rheum Dis Clin N Am. 2003;29(2):315–33.
187. Steen VD, Medsger TA. Case-control study of corticosteroids and other drugs that either precipitate or protect from the development of scleroderma renal crisis. Arthritis Rheum. 1998;41(9):1613–9.
188. van Laar JM, et al. Autologous hematopoietic stem cell transplantation vs intravenous pulse cyclophosphamide in diffuse cutaneous systemic sclerosis: a randomized clinical trial. JAMA. 2014;311(24):2490–8.
189. Elhai M, et al. Trends in mortality in patients with systemic sclerosis over 40 years: a systematic review and meta-analysis of cohort studies. Rheumatology (Oxford). 2012;51(6):1017–26.

Psoriasis and Psoriatic Arthritis

7

Laura Ferris and Soumya Reddy

Key Points

- While plaque psoriasis is most common, there are a number of psoriasis phenotypes that warrant recognition.
- Psoriatic arthritis (PsA) is defined as an inflammatory articular disease, associated with psoriasis, involving the peripheral joints, entheses, or spine.
- Up to one third of psoriasis patients may develop PsA, and most patients have psoriasis 7–10 years prior to the onset of arthritis.
- Patterns of articular involvement in PsA include asymmetric oligoarthritis, symmetric polyarthritis, distal interphalangeal (DIP) predominant, axial disease or spondyloarthritis, and arthritis mutilans.
- Enthesitis, a characteristic feature of PsA, is present in 30–50% of patients.
- Dactylitis, also known as "sausage digit," is a classic finding in PsA that occurs in approximately 30% of patients.
- A sensitive and specific biomarker does not exist in PsA.
- Rates of erosive disease in PsA are similar to rates in rheumatoid arthritis (RA), and approximately 50% of PsA patients will have at least one erosion after 2 years of diagnosis.
- PsA has unique radiographic findings that distinguish it from RA, including new bone formation (periostitis).
- Targeted biologic therapies have significantly improved outcomes in both psoriasis and PsA.

Interdisciplinary Introduction

The partnership between dermatologist and rheumatologist in the evaluation and management of psoriatic disease may represent a prototype in the interdisciplinary approach to care. This partnership allows the specification of optimal treatment of phenotypes in psoriasis while also supporting the early detection and streamlined management of inflammatory musculoskeletal disease.

Epidemiology & Classification

The prevalence of psoriasis among adults in the United States is estimated to be 2.2–3.15%. In general the prevalence of psoriasis increases with

L. Ferris
University of Pittsburgh, Pittsburgh, PA, USA
e-mail: ferrlk@UPMC.EDU

S. Reddy (✉)
NYU Langone School of Medicine,
New York, NY, USA
e-mail: Soumya.Reddy@nyulangone.org

A. Garg et al. (eds.), *Interdisciplinary Approaches to Overlap Disorders in Dermatology & Rheumatology*,
https://doi.org/10.1007/978-3-319-18446-3_7

distance from the equator. Psoriasis has very low prevalence (less than 0.5% of the population) in Taiwan, India, and Africa, and higher prevalence in Australia (2.3–6.6%) and in Northern Europe (3.73% in Denmark and 8.5% in Norway). Psoriasis affects males and females similarly. While psoriasis can occur at any age, there appears to be an increasing incidence up until about age 39 years, followed by a reduction in incidence starting at around age 40 years, and then another peak in incidence in the sixth and seventh decades [1].

Psoriasis may be classified as type I (early onset, before age 40) vs. type II (later onset, after age 40), although this is generally not a distinction used in clinical practice. More commonly, psoriasis is classified by disease severity with percentage of body surface area (BSA) involvement used to aid in classification. Disease severity can be mild (<5% BSA), moderate (5–10% BSA), or severe (>10% BSA). It is important to note, however, that BSA involvement is not the only component that contributes to assessment of disease severity and that a low BSA involvement on sensitive areas such as the face, scalp, palms, or genitalia can contribute significantly to the qualitative disease burden and may prompt more aggressive therapy. Psoriasis can also be classified by phenotype, as discussed in the clinical features section.

The association of psoriasis and arthritis was recognized as early as the 1800s but it was not until 1964 that psoriatic arthritis (PsA) was recognized as a distinct entity by the American Rheumatism Association [2]. This association is supported by epidemiologic evidence that the incidence of inflammatory arthritis is increased in patients with psoriasis compared with the general population and that psoriasis is noted to occur more commonly in patients with early inflammatory arthritis than expected in the general population [3, 4].

The exact prevalence of PsA is not known, but the estimated prevalence in the US is between 0.1% and 0.25% [5, 6]. Prevalence of PsA worldwide varies from 0.02% to 0.42% and, similar to psoriasis, appears to be higher in northern European populations and lower in Asia, particularly Japan (0.00001%) [7, 8]. The incidence rate of PsA also varies from 3/100,000 in Greece to as high as 7/100,000 per year in the US [5]. Both prevalence and incidence of PsA have been rising over time. It remains unclear if this represents greater recognition of PsA, the availability of more clear diagnostic criteria, or a true change in disease burden [9].

While PsA may occur at any age, mean age at diagnosis is in the early to mid-40s with peak incidence occurring between ages 30–55 years. Average duration from onset of psoriasis to PsA is longer for Type I psoriasis than Type II psoriasis patients, which may be a function of when PsA risk occurs [10]. The vast majority of patients develop PsA after psoriasis onset. The average duration of psoriasis prior to PsA is approximately 7–10 years. In 15–20% of patients, PsA may precede or occur concurrently with the onset of psoriasis. As is the case with psoriasis, both sexes are equally affected by PsA.

PsA is estimated to occur in 7–42% of psoriasis patients. The wide range of estimates may be due to differences among different studied populations and lack of clearly accepted definition prior to 2006. Recent studies have suggested the true estimate to be between 20–30% [11–13].

PsA can be classified according to the original Moll and Wright Criteria into five subtypes or patterns: symmetric polyarticular, asymmetric oligoarticular, distal interphalangeal (DIP) predominant, spine, and arthritis mutilans [14]. The presence of enthesitis and dactylitis are also important features not captured in the original Moll and Wright Criteria. PsA is often considered as part of the broader category of seronegative spondyloarthropathies (SpA) due to several shared characteristics. This group includes conditions such as reactive arthritis, inflammatory bowel disease (IBD) associated arthritis, and ankylosing spondylitis (AS). PsA may also be classified based on disease severity. Currently there is no accepted definition of mild, moderate, or severe disease in PsA.

Pathogenesis

The clear role of genetics in the pathophysiology of psoriasis is demonstrated in twin studies, which show a concordance rate of 35–72% in monozygotic twins and 12–30% in dizygotic twins [15]. While genetics play a strong role in psoriasis susceptibility, this is not a monogenic disease and several loci have been identified, although the particular gene or genes of interest within these loci are not all well-defined. One gene strongly associated with psoriasis susceptibility is the class I molecule *HLA-Cw*0602*, which associated with early-onset, severe disease. However, most patients with psoriasis lack this allele and have other genetic polymorphisms that contribute to their psoriasis susceptibility. While polymorphisms in genes involved in skin barrier function, specifically late cornified envelope proteins, can increase psoriasis susceptibility, most polymorphisms identified to date are in proteins involved in the immune response, including nuclear-factor kappa B and interferon signaling and the IL-23 and IL-17 signaling pathways (*NFKBIA, CARD14, REL, TYK2, IFIH1, IL28RA, TNIP1, TRAF3IP2, IL23A, IL23, IL12B*and *TNFAIP3*) [15].

Beyond genetics, there are environmental factors that play a role in the pathogenesis of psoriasis and PsA. One area of intense research in inflammatory disease has focused on the microbiome, the flora that populate the skin and gut. While this field is still evolving, there seem to be significant differences in the concentration of some types of bacteria, including those of the phylum*firmicutes*, in the skin of psoriatic patients in comparison to healthy controls. Studies of the gut microbiome in PsA also reveal diminished intestinal diversity compared to healthy controls and similar to psoriasis patients. In addition, the PsA gut mircobiota was characterized by a reduction of several species, namely *Akkermansia, Ruminococcus, and Pseudobutyrivibrio,* compared to both healthy control and psoriasis patients [16, 17]. Interestingly similar imbalances in the gut microbiota were detected in patients with obestity and Crohn's disease (CD), both of which are found in higher prevalence in individuals with psoriasis and PsA [18].

Several epidemiologic and genetic studies suggest a strong genetic contribution to PsA, one of the strongest among the rheumatic diseases. The genetic contribution is thought to be complex and multigenic, and as in psoriasis, does not fully explain the risk for development of PsA. The development of PsA is estimated to be 27–49 times more likely in patients with a family history of PsA compared to controls [19, 20]. Approximately 15% of patients with PsA also have a relative with PsA and 30–45% have a family member with psoriasis [21]. The majority of genes implicated in PsA susceptibility are shared with psoriasis and consistent with the proposed pathogenic link between these two conditions. Studies in PsA confirm the frequency of *HLA-Cw*0602* is lower in PsA; it is associated with a long interval between onset of psoriasis and arthritis (>10 years). *HLA B*27* is associated with increased frequency of arthritis and a short interval between the onset of skin and joint disease [22]. In addition, the *B*0v8, B*38,* and *B*39* alleles are more highly associated with the development of PsA as compared to psoriasis [22, 23]. Some genes are associated with specific phenotypes, such as *HLA B*27* with axial involvement; *HLA B*38* and *HLA B*39* with peripheral polyarticular involvement. Polymorphisms in genes involved in the inflammatory cascade have also been found that confer susceptibility to PsA and response to treatments, including a TNF-α gene [24], the IL-23 receptor gene and IL-12-beta [25].

Infections have long been hypothesized to have a role in the development of autoimmune diseases. In PsA there has been no definitive evidence of a viral or other infectious precipitant, with the exception of HIV, which is known to exacerbate Ps and PsA. Interestingly, the microbiome has received much attention recently for a possible pathogenic role in autoimmune diseases [16, 17].

The Koebner phenomenon, described as the ability of trauma to unaffected skin to induce the development of a plaque in a psoriasis patient, is well established and there is evidence to suggest a similar, deeper Koebner phenomenon occurring in PsA. Case series suggest that recent trauma precedes the onset of PsA in approximately 9% of patients [26, 27]. In addition, biomechanical forces at the entheses are thought to play a role in the development of initial inflammation in PsA at these sites.

Clinically, psoriatic plaques are characterized by erythema, induration, and scale. Histologically, psoriasis is characterized by increased vascularity (resulting in erythema), an acanthotic epidermis due to rapid proliferation of keratinocytes (resulting in induration or thickening in plaques), and hyperkeratosis, loss of the granular layer, and parakeratosis (resulting in scaling) due to the impaired maturation of keratinocytes resulting from this rapid proliferation. While historically these findings led to the presumption that psoriasis was primarily a disorder of keratinocytes, it has become clear that these changes are primarily driven by dysregulation of the immune system. Specifically, psoriasis is driven by increased activity of the Th17, Th22, and to a lesser extent, the Th1 pathways.

The cytokine IL-17 plays a pivotal role in the pathogenesis of psoriasis. IL-17 is produced by Th17 T cells and also by γδT cells, a subset of T cells with limited diversity of the T cell receptor that is found in the skin, primarily in the dermis. The IL-17 family consists of 6 soluble cytokines (IL-17A-F), which can form homo- and heterodimers, and the receptors that bind them (IL-17RA-IL-17RE). IL-17A is strongly expressed by T cells within psoriatic plaques and binds directly to keratinocytes and induces proliferation, particularly in the presence of TNF-α [28]. Dermal γδ T cells can also produce TNF-α and IL-22, both of which play roles in psoriasis pathogenesis [29].

Another key cytokine in the Th17 pathway is IL-23, which drives the differentiation and proliferation of Th17 T cells, which amplify the production of IL-17. In addition, IL-23 drives the activation of γδ T cells [30]. TNF-α also plays a clear role in driving disease activity in several inflammatory diseases, including psoriasis and PsA. In the skin, TNF-α is produced by both T cells and antigen presenting cells. TNF-α works in synergy with IL-17 to promote keratinocyte proliferation by stabilizing IL-17 mRNA and by increasing expression of IL-17R on keratinocytes [31].

The cellular and cytokine patterns in psoriatic skin and psoriatic joints share many similarities. In PsA, joints are characterized histologically by synovial tissue hypertrophy and a prominent lymphocytic infiltrate of activated CD4+ and CD8+ cells. CD4+ cells predominate in the sub-lining layer of the joints, while CD8+ cells are more prominent in the enthesis. Neutrophils are also increased in the synovial tissue of joints. PsA synovium is characterized by overexpression of many cytokines similar to those seen in psoriasis skin, including TNF-α, IL-6, and IL-1 and others which stimulate production of metalloproteinases and other enzymes, resulting in cartilage degradation. TNF-α also increases the expression of vascular endothelial growth factor (VEGF) in skin and synovium and may contribute to the increased vascularity characteristic of PsA synovium [32]. Not surprisingly, a polymorphism in the TNF-α gene that confers both susceptibility to PsA and response to TNF-α antagonists has also been identified [24]. TNF-α, via RANK pathways, also stimulates osteoclast precursor differentiation and infiltration into synovium, ultimately resulting in bone erosions and osteolysis. Chronic inflammation in PsA results in a paradoxical increase in new bone formation, manifesting as osteophytes, syndesmophytes, periosititis, and ankylosis. The wingless (Wnt), transforming growth factor (TGF)-beta, bone morphogenic protein (BMP), and prostaglandin (PG) E2 pathways have all been implicated in the development of new bone formation. IL-22 may promote bone formation in animal models of PsA [33].

Experimental evidence for the role of IL-17A in PsA is less robust than in psoriasis. The number of Th17 (IL-17 producing) cells is increased in the synovium of PsA patients and they demonstrate high levels of IL-17RA expression. Synovial fibroblasts from patients with PsA can be stimulated to produce pro-inflammatory cytokines and proteinases in the presence of IL-17A and this can be blocked with an anti-IL17RA monoclonal antibody [34]. Studies have also demonstrated increased levels of circulating Th17 cells in PsA patients [35, 36]. IL-17 also acts on osteoblasts and osteoclast precursors to promote bone resorption. These findings, in conjunction with data from psoriasis studies, highlight the important role of IL-17 in PsA. IL-23 is also found to be increased in PsA synovial tissue.

The enthesis has increasingly been recognized as having a central role in the pathogenensis of PsA. Interestingly, animal models of enthesitis have demonstrated a unique IL-23 receptor positive T cell subset that is resident at the entheseal insertion; IL-23 may stimulate these resident T cells to promote a change to a Th 17 phenotype, resulting in the increased production of IL-17A. This idea supports the functional link of drugs targeting the IL-23 and IL-17 pathway for psoriasis and PsA [37].

Clinical Features

Clinically, psoriasis is characterized by the presence of pink to red scaling plaques on the skin. Disease severity can vary greatly, with some patients having mild disease and others experience severe debilitating disease activity. There are several subtypes of psoriasis and in some cases more than one subtype can be present in one patient [38].

The most common subtype of psoriasis is plaque-type psoriasis, which constitutes about 90% of all cases [38]. This subtype of psoriasis is characterized by the presence of red, indurated, scaling plaques that can occur anywhere but have a predilection for the elbows, knees, and other extensor surfaces in particular (Fig. 7.1). BSA involved with plaque type psoriasis can be highly variable, with some patients presenting with only a few small plaques and others with the majority of the body surface being involved. Scalp psoriasis (Fig. 7.2) can be considered a variant of plaque-type psoriasis and can be present exclusively in the scalp or along with plaques on the trunk and/or extremities. Psoriasis that primarily involves the face and scalp may be referred to as

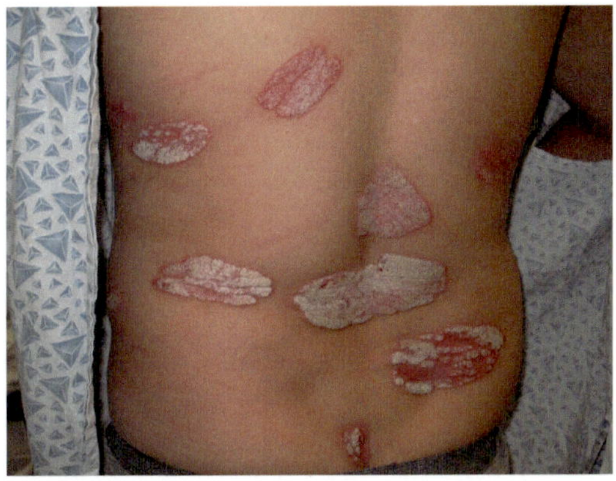

Fig. 7.1 Plaque psoriasis. Well demarcated, red, erythematous, indurated plaques with whitish scale on the trunk. (Courtesy of Amit Garg, MD)

'sebopsoriasis' because of its seborrheic distribution tendency.

Guttate psoriasis is associated with the acute onset of small, usually <1 cm in diameter, plaques that are small, thin, scaly and widely distributed, particularly over the trunk (Fig. 7.3). Often, the onset of guttate psoriasis follows closely after a streptococcal infection, most commonly pharyngitis. Onset of guttate psoriasis occurs most frequently among adolescents [39]. The course of this form of psoriasis is variable, with many cases self-limited, lasting for less than a year. However, some cases of guttate psoriasis will progress to chronic plaque-type psoriasis and even in those individuals who recover from an initial episode of guttate psoriasis, the risk of subsequently developing plaque-type psoriasis is increased.

Generalized pustular psoriasis is characterized by many small pustules on an erythematous base (Fig. 7.4). Pustules can vary in morphology and may be small and diffuse or larger and distributed primarily along the lesion periphery. Patients with plaque-type psoriasis may develop a flare of pustular psoriasis, and this has been reported to occur in the context of withdrawal of from a course of systemic steroids. Following an initial improvement in lesions, and once systemic steroids are discontinued, patients may have a rapid exacerbation of disease with a transition to a pustular morphology. This is uncommon however. In

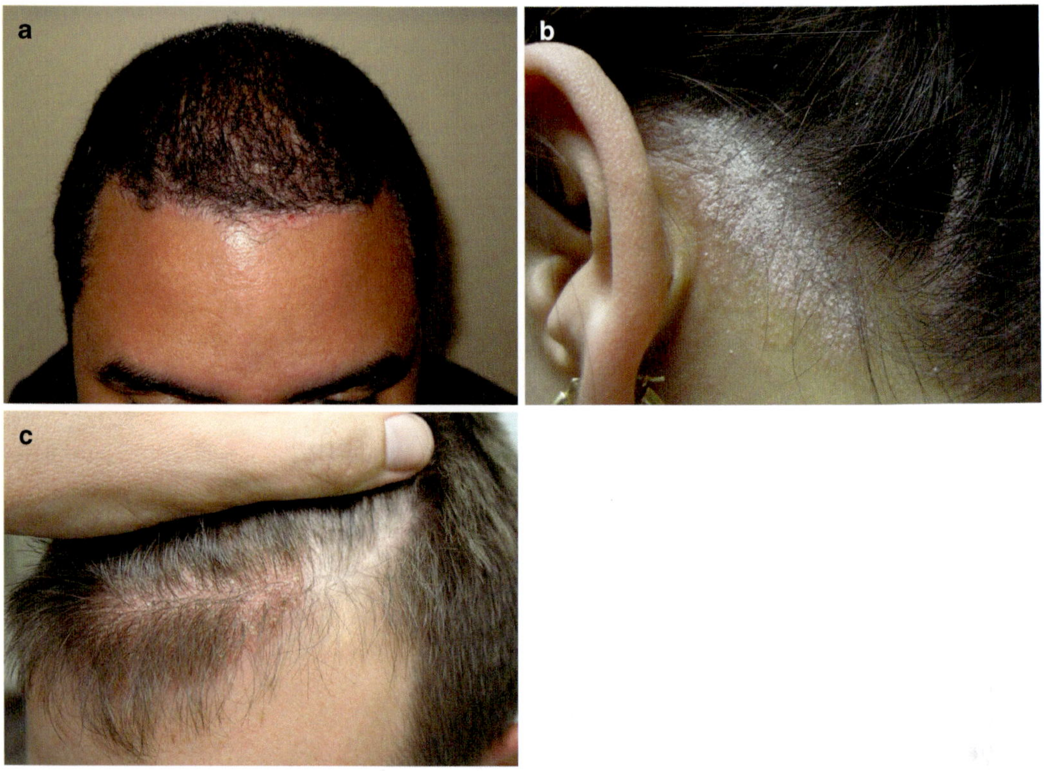

Fig. 7.2 (**a–c**) Scalp psoriasis. Well demarcated, red, erythematous, indurated plaques with whitish scale characteristically involving the hair line. (Courtesy of Amit Garg, MD)

addition to skin findings, pustular psoriasis can be associated with systemic findings such as fever, leukocytosis, hypovolemia, and hypocalcemia. Often patients will require inpatient hospitalizations for severe flares of pustular psoriasis. *Impetigo herpetiformis* is sudden onset of pustular psoriasis in the first 6 months of pregnancy [38]. The more common presentation of pustular psoriasis is the localized form involving the palms and soles. Pustules may be apparent, however patients may only present with tiny collarettes of scale in the involved areas. (Fig. 7.5). Both forms of pustular psoriasis tend to be more recalcitrant and often require systemic treatment to manage. Psoriasis involving the palms and soles most commonly presents as the hyperkeratotic type (Fig. 7.6). Plaques on the palms and soles may not always be well-circumscribed, making the distinction from hand eczema more difficult. Pustules and scale on the palms and soles may be more yellowish in color than white.

Erythrodermic psoriasis is used to describe psoriasis that involves all, or nearly all, of the body (Fig. 7.7). Most commonly erythrodermic psoriasis develops as part of a severe flare in a patient with plaque psoriasis. In addition to gradual worsening of severe psoriasis, potential triggers of erythrodermic psoriasis include drugs, such as lithium or systemic steroids, and systemic infection. Patients with erythrodermic psoriasis need to be carefully monitored for temperature dysregulation and often need replacement of fluids and dietary protein due to the high levels of transepidermal water loss and rapid keratinocyte turnover that occur in erythrodermic psoriasis [38].

Inverse psoriasis is seen in intertriginous and flexural areas of skin including the axillae, groin, inframammary area, and perianal area (Fig. 7.8). Plaques in these areas are red and may be slightly indurated but generally lack significant scale.

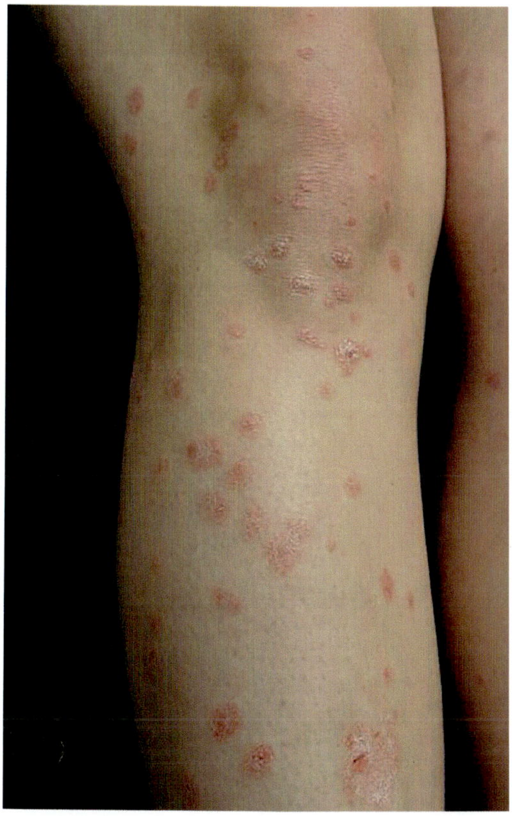

Fig. 7.3 Guttate psoriasis. Small, well-demarcated, red erythematous plaques with scale on the leg. (Courtesy of Amit Garg, MD)

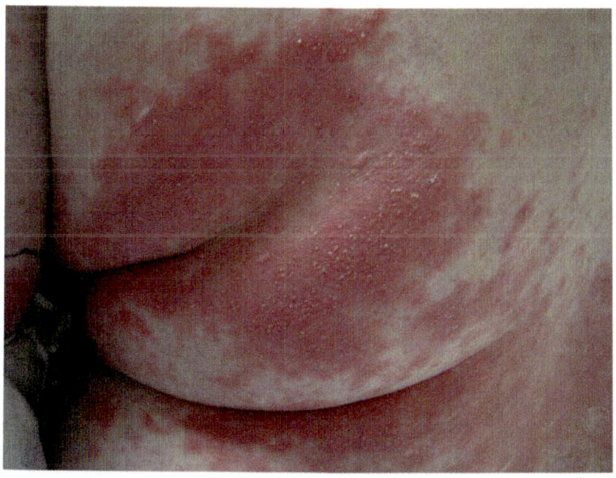

Fig. 7.4 Generalized pustular psoriasis. Less well-circumscribed, deep red erythematous plaques with numerous pustules. In some instances, pustules may coalesce to form "lakes" of pus. (Courtesy of Amit Garg, MD)

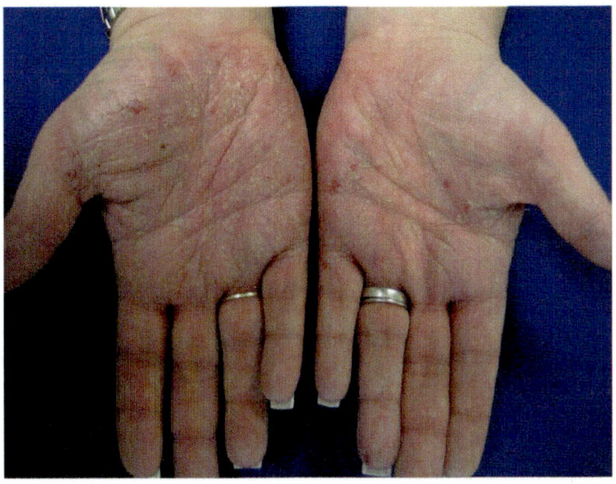

Fig. 7.5 Pustular palmoplantar psoriasis. Poorly circumscribed red erythematous patches with numerous yellowish pustules and collaretes of scale on the palms. (Courtesy of Amit Garg, MD)

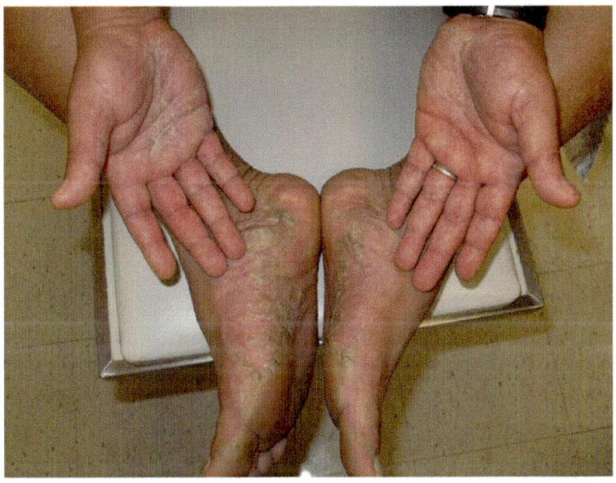

Fig. 7.6 Hyperkeratotic palmoplantar psoriasis. Erythematous plaques with yellowish hyperkeratosis on the palms and soles. Some plaques retain demarcation. (Courtesy of Amit Garg, MD)

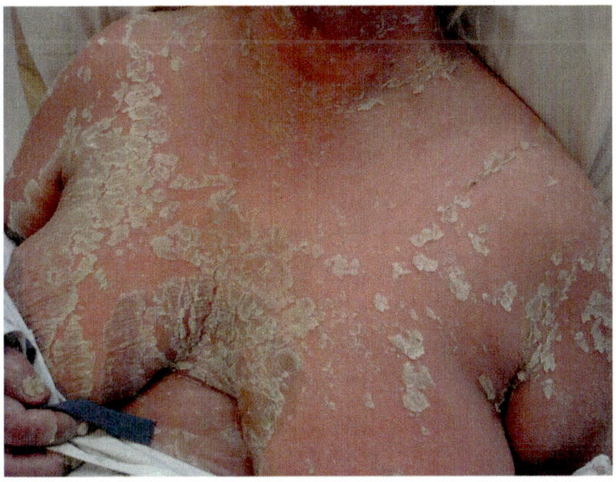

Fig. 7.7 Erythrodermic psoriasis. Pink to red erythema diffusely involving nearly the entire skin surface. The barrier of the skin is perturbed and loses some of its functionality. (Courtesy of Amit Garg, MD)

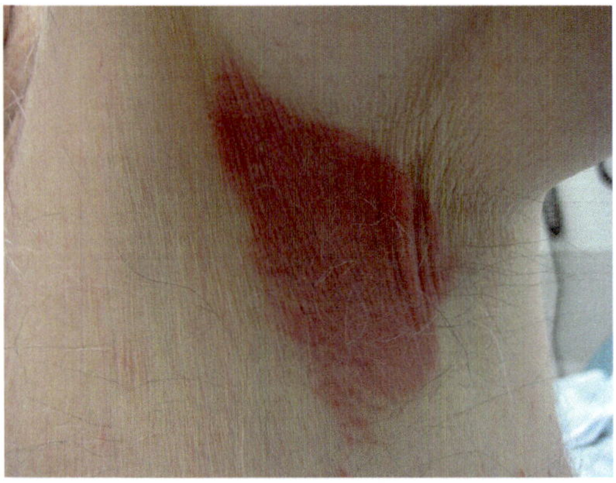

Fig. 7.8 Inverse psoriasis. Well-demarcated, red, erythematous patch in the axilla. There is usually minimal induration and little to no scale. (Courtesy of Amit Garg, MD)

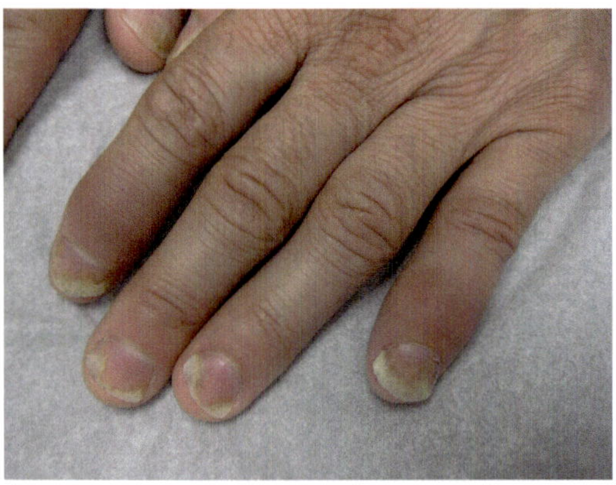

Fig. 7.9 Nail psoriasis, onycholysis. Yellowish discoloration of the distal nail plates due to separation of the nail plate from the nail bed. (Courtesy of Amit Garg, MD)

This form of psoriasis can occur in isolation or as part of another morphology of psoriasis [40].

Nail psoriasis is seen in a significant proportion of psoriasis patients, although the exact prevalence is not known, with reports of 10% to over 80% in the published literature [41]. The most common nail findings in psoriasis are onycholysis (distal separation of the nail plate from the nail bed), the resulting oil spots (a brown-yellow discoloration of the nail plate), and pitting (small indentations in the nail caused by parakeratosis in the nail matrix) (Fig. 7.9). Other findings include nail bed hyperkeratosis, leukonychia, and red spots in the lunula. Nail psoriasis is seen more commonly in those patients who also have PsA. Nail psoriasis can cause significant functional impairment and pain [42].

Clinically, PsA is a heterogeneous condition defined as an inflammatory articular disease, associated with psoriasis, involving the peripheral joints, entheses, or spine. Typically the arthritis develops after the onset of psoriasis in the majority of patients, but it may precede skin disease in approximately 15% [43]. The activity of skin and joint involvement does not always correlate in most patients, but studies do suggest that PsA occurs more frequently in patients with more severe skin psoriasis [43, 44]. Although PsA was previously considered a mild disease, recent evidence suggests that half of patients develop erosive or deforming arthritis in the first years of disease [45, 46]. Patients suffer from a decreased quality of life and an increase in mortality related to PsA [47].

PsA may be described by the pattern of articular involvement as originally described by Moll and Wright: asymmetric oligoarthritis (asymmetric involvement of five or fewer joints), symmetric polyarthritis (similar to rheumatoid arthritis [RA], with more than five joints involved in a symmetric fashion), DIP predominant (predominantly involves the DIP joints of the hands and feet), axial disease or spondyloarthritis (involvement of sacroiliac [SI] joint or the spine), and arthritis mutilans (deforming and destructive arthritis) [14] (Table 7.1). More than one pattern may occur concurrently and patterns may change over time. Most patients present with an oligoarthritis or polyarthritis pattern, but over time polyarthritis becomes more common. Additional important clinical features include enthesitis and dactylitis.

Table 7.1 Moll and Wright criteria

Moll and Wright criteria for psoriatic arthritis (PsA)
Polyarticular "rheumatoid arthritis-like"
Oligoarticular
Distal interphalangeal (DIP) predominant
Spondylitis predominant
Arthritis mutilans

Peripheral joint involvement may present with characteristic joint pain, tenderness, swelling, erythema, and warmth. Stiffness in the joints that is worse in the morning, lasting more than 30 minutes, and improving with activity is a feature of inflammatory arthritis that may be seen in half of PsA patients. Virtually any joint may be involved in PsA, including the DIPs (Fig. 7.10), which are rarely involved in RA. It is important to note that DIP involvement often occurs with psoriasis involvement of the adjacent nail. Patients with PsA may present with an asymmetric oligoarthritis, often in a "ray pattern" involving all joints in an affected digit (Fig. 7.11). In some patients, the arthritis may gradually involve more joints over time, transforming into a polyarticular pattern, while others may present with a symmetric polyarthritis that may resemble RA. Generally it has been observed that patients with PsA have less joint tenderness than RA patients [48].

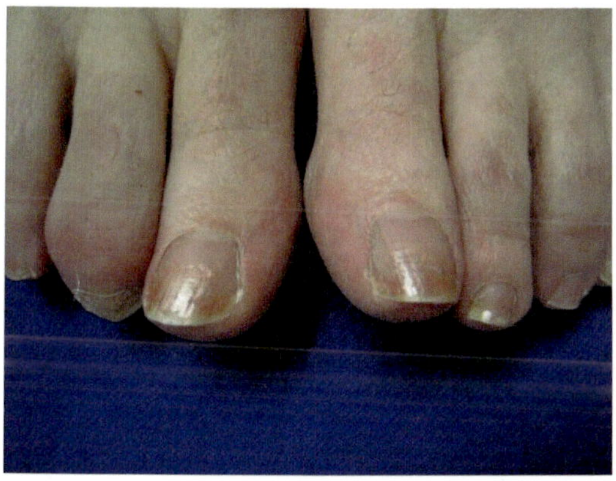

Fig. 7.10 Psoriatic arthritis (PsA). Erythema and swelling of the right second distal interphalangeal (DIP) joint in a patient with psoriasis. (Courtesy of Amit Garg, MD)

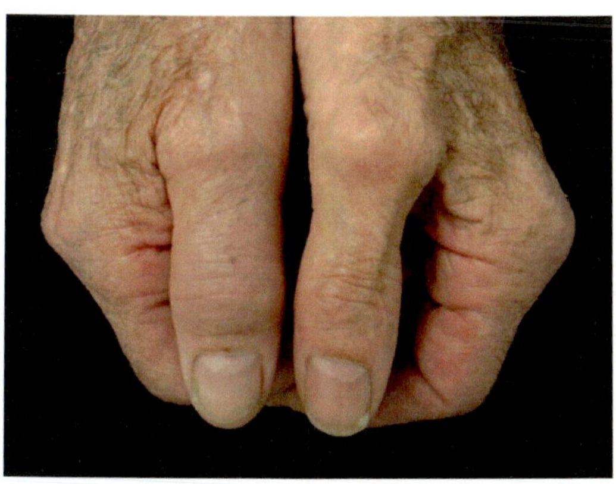

Fig. 7.11 Swelling of the metacarpophalangeal and interphalangeal joints in a ray pattern of the right thumb and sparing of the same joints of the left thumb. (Courtesy of Amit Garg, MD)

Evaluations of peripheral joint disease activity that were developed for RA have largely been adopted for use in PsA. The major method of evaluation is the American College of Rheumatology (ACR) joint count, which records 66/68 clinically involved joints as painful or tender with pressure or passive movement, and swollen other than bony proliferation [49]. It has been modified for PsA to include 76/78 joints with the addition of DIP joints. The modified 28 joint count has also been used in PsA but it should be noted that the 28 joint count excludes the lower extremity joints as well as the DIP joints, which are commonly involved in PsA.

Enthesitis is a characteristic feature of (PsA) and other SpA, and is present in 30–50% of patients. Enthesopathy is defined as inflammation at the sites of tendon, ligament, or joint capsule fiber insertion into bone. It is increasingly recognized that the "enthesis organ" plays a central role in the pathogenesis of PsA and may be the site of initial inflammation [50]. Enthesitis can occur anywhere in the body but lower extremity enthesopathy is especially common in PsA. The most frequently involved sites in PsA include the Achilles tendon, plantar fascia, and ligamentous attachments in the spine, pelvis, and ribs (involvement of which presents as costochondritis). Some patients may present with predominant enthesitis without arthritis. Enthesitis is clinically difficult to detect and imaging studies suggest that it is more prevalent than previously recognized in PsA. Studies have shown that ultrasound is more sensitive for the detection of enthesitis than clinical examination for tenderness and swelling [51]. The significance of asymptomatic enthesitis is not known. Currently, there are several measures available for the clinical assessment of enthesitis in SpA that have been borrowed for use in PsA, including the modified Mander Enthesis Index (MEI), the modified Maastricht Ankylosing

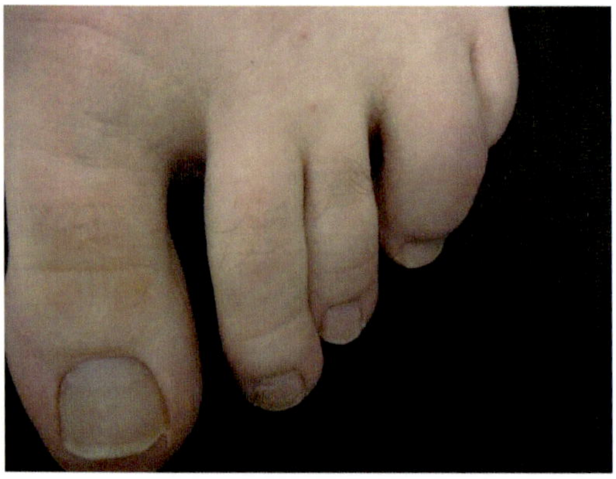

Fig. 7.12 Uniform swelling of the fourth digit on left foot, which is a reflection of inflammation involving both the joints and corresponding attachments. (Courtesy of Amit Garg, MD)

Spondylitis Enthesis Score (MASES), and the Infliximab Multinational Psoriatic Arthritis Controlled Trial index. The Leeds Enthesitis Index (LEI) has been developed and validated for PsA specifically [52].

Dactylitis, also known as "sausage digit," (Fig. 7.12) is a classic finding in PsA and may occur in approximately 30% of patients. Dactylitis results from a combination of tenosynovitis and interphalangeal synovitis of an entire digit, resulting in a uniform diffuse swelling of an entire digital ray. Synovitis occurs in about half of dactylitis joints on imaging but it is not possible to distinguish on clinical exam. The presence of dactylitis in PsA has been associated with increased radiographic damage compared to that seen in unaffected digits in some studies [53, 54]. Ultrasound and Magnetic Resonance Imaging (MRI) both may be helpful to detect tendon structures that are not visualized on plain radiographs. There are many proposed methods of measuring dactylitis but no measures have been accepted for standard use in PsA. Dactylitis is often recorded as present or notated by absent or notated by the number of digits involved. It is not clear if swelling of an entire digit in the absence of tenderness or erythema should be classified separately as chronic dactylitis.

Axial involvement in PsA occurs in up to 40–50% of patients and is an under-recognized manifestation. Axial involvement may include the SI joints and facet joints of the spine. This is another distinguishing feature from RA, which does not typically involve the SI joints and only involves the synovial portion of the C1-C2 axis of the cervical spine. The axial manifestations of PsA support its classification as part of the larger group of SpA. Although the axial disease in PsA shares similarities with AS and SpA, it is typically milder, more heterogeneous, and results in less limitation of range of motion as compared to AS spine disease. Currently there are no outcome measures specific for PsA axial disease and measures for AS are borrowed for assessment.

Arthritis mutilans is a rare, severely destructive form of PsA originally described by Moll and Wright [14]. It is characterized by digital "telescoping" or "shortening" (bones of the hands and feet are destroyed and result in folds of skin that can be pulled out to their original length). Severe osteolysis of the distal digits and pencil and cup deformities can be seen on radiographs. Severe bony ankylosis can also occur in arthritis mutilans.

Fatigue is a prominent manifestation in patients with active PsA. Fatigue contributes to significant morbidity for many patients with psoriasis and PsA.

Diagnostic Considerations

The diagnosis of psoriasis is generally made clinically, and if the presentation is classic, this is sufficient. Clinical findings include classic plaque morphology, distribution on elbows and knees, nail findings of psoriasis, and joint tenderness or changes consistent with PsA. Other entities in the differential diagnosis of psoriasis may include mycosis fungoides (cutaneous T cell lymphoma), tinea corporis, or atopic dermatitis. Physical examination findings can help in making the diagnosis, particularly plaque location (elbow/knee for psoriasis, buttocks for mycosis fungoides, flexural surfaces for atopic dermatitis). Skin biopsy may be helpful in making the diagnosis, though it is rarely necessary. Biopsy of the palms and soles in particular is not likely to yield classic findings that may specify diagnosis.

The diagnosis of PsA is made based primarily on the characteristic clinical features of inflammatory arthritis and psoriasis. Specific patterns of arthritis, taken together with the absence of rheumatoid factor (RF), and the presence of skin or nail lesions of psoriasis or a family history of psoriasis, aid in the diagnosis of PsA. Laboratory data and radiographic findings may be useful in some cases. Currently a sensitive and specific biomarker does not exist for PsA as is available for RA. The CASPAR (ClASsification of Psoriatic Arthritis) criteria were established in 2006 based on a study of 588 patients with PsA and 536 patients with other forms of inflammatory arthritis. The CASPAR criteria are the most widely accepted classification criteria for PsA [55]. The CASPAR criteria can only be applied in patients who have been determined to have an inflammatory articular disease (joints, entheses, or spine) and meant for use by rheumatologists. The CASPAR criteria have a sensitivity of 91.4% and a specificity of 98.7% for the classification of PsA [Table 7.2]. Given its high performance, the instrument may prove useful as a diagnostic tool in the clinics.

Laboratory findings are not specific in PsA. Acute phase reactants, such as erythrocyte sedimentation rate (ESR) and C-reactive protein (CRP) may be elevated in up to 40% of patients with PsA [43, 56, 57]. Elevated inflammatory markers are seen more often with polyarticular disease and may be markers of more severe disease [56, 58]. ESR and CRP levels have been shown to be responsive to treatment and markers of good response in clinical trials of TNF inhibitors.

Table 7.2 CASPAR criteria

Established presence of inflammatory arthritis, enthesitis, or spondylitis with at least 3 points from below:	
Feature	Points
Psoriasis	
Current psoriasis OR	2
Personal history of psoriasis OR	1
Family history of psoriasis	1
Current or history of dactylitis documented by a rheumatologist	1
Nail dystrophy (onycholysis, pitting)	1
Negative rheumatoid factor (RF)	1
Evidence of juxta-articular new bone formation on radiographs	1

RF and anti-cyclic citrullinated peptides (anti-CCP) antibodies have high specificity and moderate sensitivity for the diagnosis of RA. Positive RF can be seen in approximately 2–10% of patients with PsA. Anti-CCP antibodies can be seen in approximately 3–17% of patients with PsA [43, 59–62], although typically they are not high titer when they are detected. Positive antinuclear antibodies (ANA) in low titer are also seen in almost half of patients with PsA; only 14% have a titer >1:80. Generally the incidence of lupus-specific antibodies is very low [59].

Patients with PsA were previously thought to have milder disease and less radiographic damage compared to those with RA. Recent studies have suggested that this is not the case. PsA and RA patients have similar rates of erosive disease [63]. Approximately 50% of patients with PsA will have at least one erosion after 2 years of diagnosis. PsA has unique radiographic findings that distinguish it from RA. One distinguishing feature of PsA is the concurrent presence of erosive changes and new bone formation (periostitis), sometimes even affecting the same joint. PsA radiographic changes (Fig. 7.13) include erosions, terminal osteolysis of the distal phalanges, frank destruction, "pencil-in-cup" changes and new bone formation manifesting as periostitis, enthesophytes, and bony anklyosis [43, 64]. MRI may be more sensitive than plain radiographs for detection of inflammatory changes in the joints, peri-articular structures, entheses, bone marrow edema, and soft tissue. As in SpA, PsA can also result in SI joint findings of sacroiliitis, erosions, and fusion although typically the findings are more asymmetric and milder in nature (even when bilateral involvement occurs) compared to AS (Fig. 7.14). MRI, although more sensitive for detection of sacroiliitis, does not correlate well with clinical symptoms [65]. In the spine, syndesmophytes (Fig. 7.15) can be seen in PsA but are typically more asymmetric and not continuous, in contrast to AS. Also, the syndes-

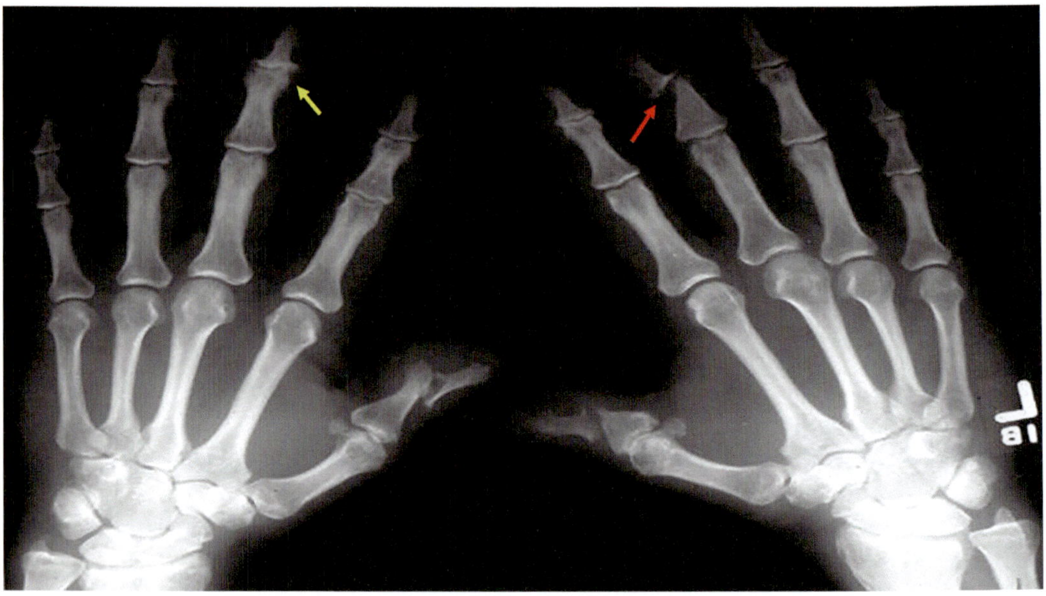

Fig. 7.13 Plain film demonstrating marginal erosions progressing centrally into a pencil in cup deformity (red arrow) as well as new bone formation (periostitis, yellow arrow), changes, which are both specific to PsA. (Courtesy of Amit Garg, MD)

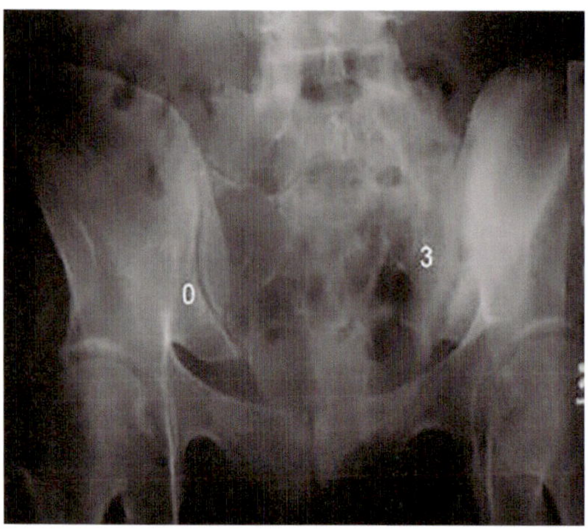

Fig. 7.14 Asymmetric sacroiliitis with grade 3 inflammation with erosions and sclerosis of the left sacroiliac (SI) joint. In contrast, inflammation of the right SI joint is not evident. (Courtesy of Amit Garg, MD)

mophytes seen in PsA are paramarginal, compared to marginal in AS. Although the joint destruction in PsA has some similarities to RA, including erosions and joint space narrowing, the unique features of PsA, notably DIP involvement, periostitis, new bone formation, and anky-

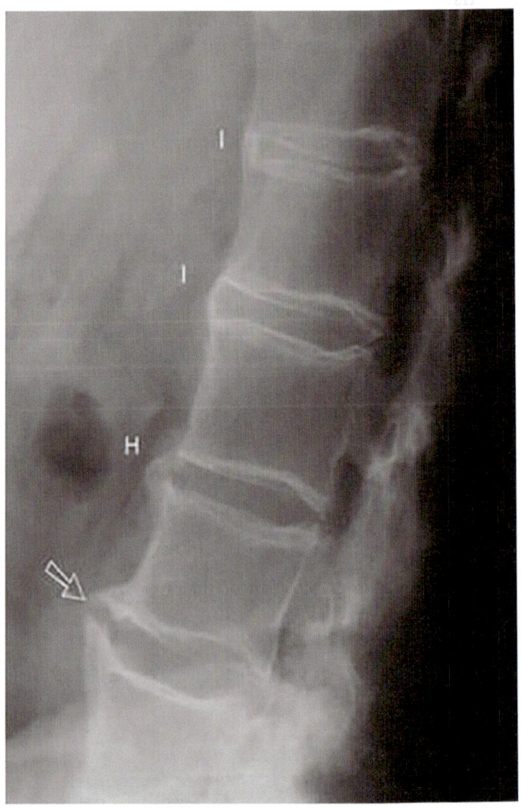

Fig. 7.15 Asymmetric paramarginal syndesmophytes resulting from ossification of fibers attaching intervertebral discs. (Courtesy of Amit Garg, MD)

losis, are not captured using standard assessment tools for RA.

PsA can be difficult to diagnose and can present with findings similar to other arthritides. Major considerations in the differential diagnosis of PsA include RA, AS, IBD associated arthritis, reactive arthritis, gout, fibromyalgia, and osteoarthritis (OA). Patients with RA often present with a symmetric polyarthritis involving the small joints of the hands and feet that may appear identical to the symmetric polyarthritis pattern of PsA. One distinguishing feature is that RA does not typically affect the DIP joints, SI, or thoracic and lumbar spine. In addition, RA patients commonly have an elevated RF or CCP antibody not usually seen in PsA. OA may be difficult to distinguish from PsA in a patient with psoriasis. OA may also involve the DIP joints but manifests with bony hypertrophy of the joints and Heberden's and Bouchard's nodes as opposed to inflammatory arthritis changes. Gout is another condition to be considered in the differential diagnosis of PsA and can coexist with psoriasis, as psoriasis is associated with elevated uric acid levels. Gout often affects the toes first, a presentation known as podagra, and can be confused with PsA dactylitis. The detection of uric acid crystals in the synovial fluid may help confirm the diagnosis of gout.

Screening Tools

The recognition that damage may occur early in the disease course in PsA, and the awareness that delays in diagnosis and treatment have a negative impact on patients' quality of life and disability, combined with the difficulty in diagnosing PsA, have led to increased efforts to identify PsA patients early. Several screening questionnaires have been developed to identify PsA patients, namely the Psoraisis and Arthritis Screening Questionnaire (PASQ), Psoriasis Epidemiology Screening Tool (PEST), and Psoriatic Arthritis Screening Evaluation (PASE) [3, 66–68]. One tool, the Toronto Psoriatic Arthritis Screen (ToPAS), was developed to identify patients with psoriasis or PsA in a general practice [69]. These measures all have similar sensitivity and specificity and help to identify patients that warrant further evaluation by a rheumatologist [70].

Disease and Comorbidity Assessment

In addition to arthritis, psoriasis is associated with several diseases and medical comorbidities. These comorbidities may be due to the presence of chronic inflammation or due to a common immunologic etiology. Managing comorbid conditions, often as part of a multidisciplinary team, is an important aspect of caring for the patient with psoriasis and PsA.

Gastrointestinal Disease

Studies show that among patients with CD, the likelihood of having a family member with psoriasis is about three-to four-fold higher than it is for individuals without CD. Similarly, families with psoriasis have a higher incidence of CD than families without psoriasis. The psoriasis susceptibility locus, *PSORS-1*, and the CD susceptibility locus, *IBD-3*, are both located in the portion of chromosome 6 encoding the gene for TNF-α, supporting the important role of this cytokine in both diseases [71].

Similarly, the incidence of IBD, including CD and ulcerative colitis, is estimated to be up to six-fold higher in patients with PsA, although these data are based on limited, small studies [72]. Interestingly, asymptomatic PsA patients have also been reported to have high rates of subclinical bowel inflammation on colonoscopy, again suggesting a pathogenic link [73].

Several studies have shown an increased prevalence of Celiac disease among patients with psoriasis. Interestingly, adherence to a gluten-free diet seems to improve skin disease severity in some patients as well [74, 75].

Autoimmune Ophthalmic Disease

Autoimmune ophthalmic disease is associated with PsA as well as with other SpA. Although there is some evidence that patients with psoriasis are also at increased risk of ocular involvement, this is not well-characterized [76]. In PsA, the prevalence of uveitis may be as high as 7–25% [77, 78]. Other autoimmune ophthalmic diseases that may occur in association with PsA include episcleritis, scleritis, conjunctivitis, and keratitis. As these conditions are associated with significant morbidity, early recognition and treatment are important.

Psychiatric Disease

Several psychiatric comorbidities are associated with psoriasis. Alcoholism is nearly nine times more common among patients with psoriasis than among those with other skin conditions and generally precedes disease onset [79]. Depression, anxiety, and suicidal ideation are more common among patients with psoriasis than in the general population [80].

Metabolic Syndrome and Cardiovascular Disease

The presence of metabolic syndrome (type II diabetes, obesity, central adiposity, and dyslipidemia) is more common in patients with psoriasis and PsA than the general population. Psoriasis is an independent risk factor for diabetes (OR of diabetes, 1.59 [95% CI, 1.38–1.83]), with the risk increasing with psoriasis severity [81]. Type II diabetes is also more prevalent in women with PsA compared to the general population and estimated to occur in approximately 15% of patients with PsA [82]. Similarly, the risk of cardiovascular disease is also increased among patients with psoriasis and PsA, with risk of a major adverse cardiovascular event (myocardial infarction, cerebrovascular accident, or cardiovascular death) being greatest among those patients with PsA without a DMARD (HR 1.25, 95% CI 1.03–1.49) and those with psoriasis also taking a DMARD (i.e. more severe psoriasis) (HR 1.42, 95% CI 1.1–.173) [83]. Despite the greater prevalence of metabolic syndrome among psoriasis patients, psoriasis is an independent risk factor for coronary artery, cerebrovascular, and peripheral vascular disease and for cardiovascular mortality. Interestingly, as in CD and psoriatic plaques, atherosclerotic plaques contain elevated levels of VEGF, TNF-α, IL-6, IL-8, and IL-17, suggesting a common etiology of these diseases and the crucial role of inflammation.

Obesity is also linked to psoriasis and PsA at the molecular level. Adipose tissue is endocrinologically active and secretes mediators that regulate inflammation, including adiponectin and leptin. Adiponectin, which is decreased in obese patients, downregulates the production and activity of TNF-α. By contrast, leptin, which is elevated in obese individuals, increases pro-inflammatory mediators [84]. Psoriasis and PsA patients have a greater risk of obesity compared to patients with RA and the general population, and individuals with PsA in particular have the highest risk [85]. Obesity has been found to be an incident risk factor for the development of psoriasis and PsA in recent studies highlighting the potential pathogenic link [86, 87]. Interestingly, obesity may also have a negative impact on treatment response and the likelihood of achieving minimal disease activity (MDA) [88].

Fatty liver disease or nonalcoholic steatohepatitis (NASH) is more prevalent in patients with psoriasis and PsA and may be related to the associated metabolic syndrome and to medication use. There is limited data in PsA, but studies in psoriasis suggest that the development of NASH in methotrexate (MTX) users was increased in the presence of obesity, diabetes, and with an increasing cumulative dose of MTX [89].

Principles in Management

Disease Outcome Measures

Skin disease severity in patients with psoriasis can be measured in several ways. BSA measures the percentage of the patient's body involved with psoriasis, with the general guideline that the area covered by one of the patient's handprints is roughly 1% of the total BSA. While this metric can generally be quickly assessed, it does not take into account plaque severity nor the distribution of disease; plaques on the face, scalp, palms, soles, and genitalia can often cause significant impairment that is proportionally more burdensome than similar BSA involvement on the trunk or extremities.

The psoriasis area and severity index (PASI) score is frequently used in clinical trials to measure response to an intervention. The PASI score is a scale from 0 to 72 that incorporates the extent of BSA involved with psoriasis as well as the erythema, induration, and scaling of plaques [90]. Response to an intervention can be expressed as the percentage of subjects who achieve at least a given level of improvement in their PASI score; for example, if 60% of subjects have an improvement of 75% or greater reduction in PASI score between baseline and week 12, this would be referred to as 60% of subjects achieving a PASI 75 response at week 12. The physician's global assessment (PGA, sometimes called the static PGA, or sPGA) can also be used to measure disease severity. This is a score, on either a 5 or 6 point scale, in which a 0 indicates the patient's skin is clear and a 1 indicates the patient's skin is almost clear; a higher PGA score indicates increasing severity of skin disease. Notably, the PGA score takes into account plaque erythema, induration, and scale but not BSA. While this method is more understandable to those outside the research setting, the fact that it does not quantify BSA may be problematic as it can result in over- or under-estimation of disease severity [90].

Nail psoriasis can be measured by several different scales. The most commonly reported in clinical trials is the Nail Psoriasis Severity Index (NAPSI). This tool, which scores on a scale of 0–80 for fingernails, measures both nail matrix and bed disease, taking into account features such as nail pitting, onycholysis, splinter hemorrhages, oil spots, nail crumbling, and subungual hyperkeratosis. The mean percent improvement in the NAPSI score from baseline to endpoint is usually given as a measure of improvement in psoriatic fingernail disease in response to therapy [91].

Scalp psoriasis can be graded using the Psoriasis Scalp Severity Index (PSSI), which is similar to the PASI but adapted for the scalp. To calculate the PSSI, a score ranging from 0 (absent) to 4 (very severe) for each of the three categories of erythema, desquamation and thickness, is given. These individual scores are then added together and multiplied by a score based on the area of the scalp that is covered by psoriasis, giving a final PSSI score that ranges from 0 to 72.

Composite measures provide a way to assess all relevant clinical outcomes with a single instrument. One of the most commonly used outcome measures in clinical trials to assess response in PsA is the American College of Rheumatology (ACR) Response Criteria, initially created for RA [92]. An ACR response is defined as a 20%, 50%, or 70% improvement in the tender <u>and</u> swollen joint count <u>plus</u> improvement in 3 out of 5 additional ACR core set measures (Visual Analog Scales [VAS] scores of patient pain, patient and physician global assessments, patient assessed disability measure [HAQ], and an acute phase reactant [ESR or CRP]). The ACR response criteria may be modified for PsA by including DIP joints of the feet and carpometacarpal joints of the hand (total of 78 tender and 76 swollen joints counted). This ACR Response Criteria have been validated in PsA clinical trials [93, 94]. It is important to note, however, that most clinical trials require patients to have an elevated joint count and/or ESR or CRP for entry. Whether the ACR criteria perform equally well in PsA patients with less severe disease or without elevation of inflammatory markers is not known.

The Disease Activity Score (DAS) is another outcome measure borrowed from RA clinical trials and was developed using a calculated weighting system of key clinical variables. The DAS allows assessment of aggregate disease activity at any point in time because it is a continuous variable. In addition, the DAS can be used to evaluate changes in disease activity over time, so that a response to a therapeutic intervention can be classified as good, moderate, or none by European League Against Rheumatism (EULAR) criteria [95]. The DAS and DAS 28, a modification with 28 joints counted, have also been used in PsA clinical trials. It is important to note that the DAS 28 excludes the joints of the lower extremity and DIP joints that are commonly involved in PsA and although performs well in clinical trials, may not be suitable for PsA assessment in other settings. The DAS has been reported in trials of infliximab in PsA and discriminated between placebo and treatment [96].

Composite measures have been developed specifically for PsA. The Psoriatic Arthritis Response Criteria (PsARC) were developed for the evaluation of clinical response to therapy in PsA and although shown to perform well in a few PsA clinical trials, they have not gained widespread use [97]. The Disease Activity Index for Psoriatic Arthritis (DAPSA) is another PsA measure adapted from a tool created for reactive arthritis. Unlike other composite measures utilized in PsA that largely focus on peripheral arthritis manifestations, newer measures that include other domains have been developed [98]. The Psoriatic Arthritis Disease Activity Score (PASDAS), includes measures for peripheral arthritis, enthesitis, and dactylitis; the Arithmetic Mean of Desirability Function (AMDF) includes measures of peripheral arthritis and skin. The Composite Psoriatic Disease Activity Index (CPDAI) measures disease involvement in the five key domains of PsA: peripheral arthritis, skin, enthesitis, dactylitis, and spinal manifestations. The performance of these measures in clinical trials and practice is under investigation [98].

Minimal Disease Activity State and Treat to Target

MDA refers to a state of disease activity deemed a useful and meaningful target by both patients and physicians. MDA criteria for PsA were developed in 2009 and are defined in Table 7.3 [99]. The MDA criteria have been validated using clinical trial data and support the concept that achieving MDA is associated with a reduction in radiographic progression [100].

The concept of treat to target refers to a management strategy to achieve a specified disease target. The PsA MDA criteria were used in a randomized trial to evaluate a treat to target strategy on PsA outcomes, the Tight Control of PsA study (TICOPA). Patients were randomized to a tight control arm with escalation of therapies according to a protocol until MDA was achieved, versus standard of care. Greater improvements in peripheral arthritis activity, skin disease activity, and quality of life measures was noted in the tight control group [101, 102].

Table 7.3 Minimal disease activity (MDA) criteria in PsA

MDA in PsA requires 5 out of the following 7 criteria being met:
Tender joint count ≤1
Swollen joint count ≤1
Psoriasis area and severity index (PASI) ≤ 1 or body surface area (BSA) ≤ 3%
Patient pain by visual analog scale (VAS) ≤ 15
Patient global activity by VAS ≤ 20
Health assessment questionnaire (HAQ) ≤ 0.5
Tender entheseal points ≤ 1

Therapeutic Interventions

Lifestyle Modifications

Obesity is known to be associated with an increased risk of developing psoriasis and PsA as well as with greater severity of psoriasis. Several studies have examined the impact of weight loss on psoriasis severity. Weight loss through strict adherence to a low energy diet has been shown to result in improvement in psoriasis symptoms and also to improve responsiveness to several medications for the treatment of psoriasis. Many patients who have undergone weight loss surgery have also seen an improvement in psoriasis [103]. In another study, individuals with an inadequate response to 4 weeks of systemic therapy were randomized to receive either a 20-week dietary and physical exercise plan for weight loss or simple informative counseling about the utility of weight loss for control of psoriatic disease. Those who received the dietary and exercise plan were more likely to lose 5% or more of their baseline weight and showed a greater mean reduction in PASI score than those randomized to counseling alone [104].

Few studies have evaluated the effect of weight loss in PsA. In one study, obese patients with PsA starting treatment with a TNF-α inhibitor were randomized to a hypocaloric diet or a free managed diet. Regardless of the type of diet, weight loss of 5% or more was significantly associated with a higher chance of achieving MDA for PsA [88]. Studies also suggest that PsA patients with higher BMI were less likely to achieve MDA compared to those with lower BMI even after adjusting for possible confounding variables [105].

Given the increased prevalence of celiac disease and the presence of anti-gliadin antibodies (AGA) among individuals with psoriasis, there has been some interest in what role a gluten-free diet may play in altering psoriasis severity. In one small open-label study, a decrease in PASI score was observed among 73% of patients who were AGA positive, but none who were AGA negative, after following a gluten-free diet for 3 months [74].

Patients with psoriasis are more likely to smoke than control patients without psoriasis. In one small, non-randomized study of patients with palmoplantar pustulosis, smoking cessation was associated with a reduction in disease severity [106].

Topical Therapy for Psoriasis

Topical therapy is often used alone for the treatment of mild to moderate psoriasis or may be used in conjunction with systemic or phototherapy for the treatment of moderate to severe psoriasis. Topical therapy has the advantage of having minimal impact on comorbid conditions such as diabetes and renal or hepatic disease and requires no laboratory monitoring. However, application of topical medicines can be messy and time-consuming. Topical therapies most commonly used to treat psoriasis include topical steroids and topical vitamin D3 analogs. Higher potency topical steroids, such as clobetasol 0.05% preparations, are generally used to treat psoriasis of the scalp, trunk, and extremities. Lower potency preparations, such as hydrocortisone or desonide, are used to treat psoriasis of the face, flexural areas and groin. Topical vitamin D3 preparations can be used on any area of the body safely, but they can cause irritation, particularly when used on the face or flexural areas [107]. Combination therapies that include both a high potency topical steroid and a vitamin D3 analog are generally more effective than either component alone. The primary risks of treatment with topical steroids are the development of skin thinning and striae.

Other topical therapies used to treat psoriasis include topical tar and salicylic acid preparations, particularly incorporated into shampoos for the treatment of scalp psoriasis. These can cause irritation and are modestly effective in the treatment of psoriasis. The topical retinoid tazarotene can also result in some improvement in psoriasis, but its use is limited by the irritation it causes; for this reason topical tazarotene is best used in combination with topical steroids [108].

Phototherapy

Ultraviolet light exposure has long been noted to improve psoriasis severity, and patients often find that their disease severity is reduced in the summer months due to exposure to sunlight. Phototherapy can be a relatively safe and effective treatment option for some psoriasis patients. Phototherapy likely works by downregulating the activity of Langerhans cells in the skin and by shifting the local cutaneous cytokine profile from that which is predominated by Th1 or Th17 cytokines to one that is Th2 polarized. Initial phototherapy protocols in psoriasis primarily focused on the combination of ultraviolet A (UVA) light (320–400 nm) with an oral photosensitizing agent, primarily 8-methoxypsoralen in the United States and 5-methoxypsoralen in Europe, a treatment known as psoralen plus UVA (PUVA). Patients are generally treated 2–3 times weekly initially and clearance rates of 89–100% have been reported with various PUVA regimens. Disadvantages of PUVA include prolonged photosensitization requiring eye protection, inconvenience to the patient due to the need to visit a physician's office multiple times per week, and an increased risk of skin cancers, including squamous cell carcinomas and possibly melanoma. For these reasons, PUVA is infrequently used in the United States and has been largely replaced by treatment with UVB. Studies have shown that 313 nm light is the most effective wavelength for treating psoriasis; this is referred to as narrow band UVB (NB-UVB). Studies comparing NB-UVB to PUVA in treatment of plaque psoriasis show somewhat conflicting results, but NB-UVB is likely equivalent in efficacy and side effects while more convenient [109]. The excimer laser, which delivers 308 nm monochromatic light, is also used as a targeted therapy to treat plaques of psoriasis. Because unaffected skin is not treated, more intense therapy can be delivered directly to psoriatic plaques. Studies measuring the efficacy of the excimer laser vary in design but generally show high efficacy, with 85% achieving a PASI 90 response in one study. Remission generally lasts 3–4 months.

Phototherapy can be used in patients with medical comorbidities who are not good candidates for systemic therapies. Phototherapy, without psoralen, can also be used safely in women who are pregnant or lactating. It is important to review the patient's medication list prior to starting phototherapy, as concurrent use of photosensitizing medication can result in severe burning. Phototherapy should not be used in patients who have medical conditions in which exposure to UV light may be deleterious, such as lupus or xeroderma pigmentosum. Caution should be used in using phototherapy in patients with a history of melanoma or multiple non-melanoma skin cancers, and these patients should be followed regularly with full body skin examinations [110].

Oral Therapy

Non-steroidal Anti-inflammatory Drugs and Corticosteroids

Non-steroidal anti-inflammatory drugs (NSAIDs) are often utilized in the treatment of arthritis, including PsA, despite concern that NSAIDs may worsen psoriasis, which has not been demonstrated in prospective studies. There are only two randomized clinical trials of COX 2 inhibitors in PsA, only one of which showed improvement in the number of tender and swollen joints and patient and physician global assessments compared to placebo [111]. It is important to recognize that although NSAIDs may be effective in treating the symptoms of PsA, they do not have a disease-modifying effect and therefore do not prevent structural damage to joints.

Systemic steroids are commonly used in the treatment of inflammatory arthritis, often as a bridge to more definitive treatment or to control a flare of disease activity, including PsA. Steroid use in PsA is undertaken with caution, given the concern for possible rebound flare of generalized pustular psoriasis after steroid withdrawal, although there are only a few reports to support this [112]. There are few data regarding the efficacy of steroids in PsA. Intra-articular steroids may be a useful option in PsA patients with monoarthritis or limited joint involvement, a treatment supported largely by clinical experience rather than standardized studies [113].

Methotrexate

MTX inhibits the enzymes dihydrofolate reductase and thymidylate synthetase. MTX is often used as a first-line systemic agent to treat psoriasis and PsA because of its low cost and relatively high efficacy and safety. Although little is known about its exact mechanism of action, small studies have demonstrated reductions in the serum levels of IL-6 and IL-22 in psoriasis patients treated with MTX. Additional studies suggest MTX may also exert its effects though an increase in extracellular adenosine, which has anti-inflammatory properties [114]. MTX may be effective in the treatment of psoriasis and PsA, although it was FDA approved for psoriasis prior to the widespread use of large randomized, double blind, placebo-controlled studies. MTX is usually given at doses of 10–25 mg weekly, either orally, subcutaneously, or intramuscularly with folic acid supplementation. In one study comparing MTX to cyclosporine A (CsA) in which MTX was dosed at 15–22.5 mg weekly, 60% of 43 subjects treated with MTX had a PASI 75 response and 40% had a PASI 90 response. Notably, in this study, 12 patients had to be discontinued from MTX due to transaminitis. This is a higher rate than what would be expected in clinical practice; one advantage of MTX is that it can be used at a wide range of doses to balance efficacy and toxicity [115].

MTX is one of the most commonly used drugs in PsA by rheumatologists worldwide and is central to the treatment recommendations of several organizations [116, 117]. In RA there is abundant evidence regarding the efficacy of MTX. In contrast, in PsA there are limited studies and only a handful of randomized clinical trials with conflicting results but generally suggesting that weekly doses of at least 15 mg or higher may have efficacy [118, 119]. The most widely quoted randomized double-blind placebo controlled trial, the MIPA (Methotrexate in Psoriatic Arthritis) trial, followed 221 patients with PsA treated with up to 15 mg of MTX weekly versus placebo. The study only showed statistically significant responses for skin scores (PASI) and physician global assessment (PGA). The study did not show significant differences in response for the peripheral arthritis outcome measures (PsARC, ACR, DAS28). The study had several limitations that may account for the lack of efficacy seen, including the low dose of MTX used and high drop-out rates [120]. An open label study of 115 PsA patients treated with MTX versus MTX plus infliximab showed ACR 20/50/70 responses of 67%, 40%, and 19% in the MTX group, which were lower than the combination group but still suggested efficacy for MTX [121]. As a result of lack of convincing randomized placebo controlled data, the most recent treatment guidelines for PsA published by the American College of Rheumatology and the National Psoriasis Foundation did not include MTX as first-line therapy [122].

More recently, the Study of Etanercept and Methotrexate in Combination or as Monotherapy in Subjects with Psoriatic Arthritis (SEAM-PsA) evaluated the efficacy of etanercept monotherapy, MTX monotherapy, and the combination of both agents in patients with MTX and biologic-naive active PsA in a large randomized placebo-controlled study [123]. Within the etanercept monotherapy arm, an ACR20 response rate of 61% and MDA response of 36% were seen. These responses were significantly higher than those achieved in the MTX monotherapy arm (ACR20 response 50.7% and MDA 22.9%). Although it is not possible to definitively evaluate the effectiveness of MTX in this trial given the lack of a placebo arm, the ACR 20 response rates noted in the MTX monotherapy arm suggest that MTX is an effective therapy in PsA. Additional measures evaluated in the SEAM-PsA study included achievement of clear or almost clear skin (66.3% for MTX monotherapy versus 72.3% in the etanercept monotherapy arm) and resolution of enthesitis (43.1% versus 52.6% respectively). There was no significant benefit in response rates noted in the combination of MTX and etanercept arm versus the etanercept monotherapy arm, in contrast to the synergistic effects noted in RA with such combination therapy. The study showed less radiographic progression in the etanercept-containing arms versus MTX but there was little progression overall in all groups at 24 months. The SEAM-PsA study provides additional important data suggesting efficacy of MTX in several domains in PsA, but given the lack of placebo arm in this study, it is not possible to determine the true effects of MTX. There are currently no data to suggest MTX efficacy for axial disease in PsA.

The most common serious laboratory abnormalities seen with MTX use are elevated transaminases and decreased white blood cell counts. Prior to starting MTX, it is recommended to check a complete blood count (CBC), a hepatic function panel, hepatitis B and C serologies, and a pregnancy test in women of child-bearing potential. Blood counts and liver enzymes are generally monitored monthly for the first 3 months and, if stable, then every 3 months. Risk factors for methotrexate-induced hepatotoxicity include type II diabetes, obesity, viral hepatitis, and alcohol consumption. Because MTX can cause liver fibrosis that does not cause significant changes in liver enzyme serum values, some experts advocate for liver biopsies once a patient has reached a cumulative dose of 3–4 g. Other non-invasive tests for liver damage from MTX have been proposed, including procollagen-3 N-terminal peptide levels, liver ultrasound, and a liver elastrography test known as Fibroscan [124]. However, none of these had sufficiently high enough sensitivity and specificity relative to liver biopsy in one meta-analysis to recommend routine use in clinical practice, although others suggest that these tests may be ideal for monitoring liver toxicity. Additionally, MTX is an abortifactant and teratogen and thus must be used with caution in women who may become pregnant, although it is safe for women to become pregnant once they have discontinued MTX for 1 month. Because MTX may be associated with a higher rate of teratogenicity in babies born to fathers taking MTX, it is conservatively recommended that men taking MTX not father a child until they have discontinued the drug for at least 3 months [125].

Leflunomide

Leflunomide inhibits pyrimidine synthesis via dihydroorotate dehydrogenase and is approved for use in RA. The Treatment of Psoriatic Arthritis Study (TOPAS) was a randomized, double-blind, placebo-controlled study evaluating patients with PsA treated with leflunomide or placebo. At 24 weeks, the leflunomide group showed a statistically significant improvement compared to the placebo group as defined by the PsARC (59% vs 30% respectively) measuring peripheral arthritis [93]. However it should be noted that leflunomide it is not officially approved for use in PsA. Leflunomide's side effects include diarrhea and transaminitis, which may occur in up to 10% of patients. Leflunomide has teratogenic effects, and females of childbearing potential need to be counseled prior to initiation. Due to the long half-life of leflunomide's active metabolites, the drug must be discontinued 2 years prior to becoming pregnant. Leflunomide may be modestly effective in treating psoriasis [126], but it is generally not used to treat cutaneous disease.

Sulfasalazine

Sulfasalazine (SSA) has shown only modest efficacy in PsA, with one placebo-controlled study of 221 patients showing peripheral arthritis improvement in 59% compared to 47% of control patients [97]. SSA is not considered to be effective in skin psoriasis and there are no studies demonstrating inhibition or slowing of radiographic progression in PsA treated with SSA.

Acitretin

Acitretin is an oral retinoid that modulates keratinocyte proliferation and differentiation but also seems to alter the immune response through downregulation of Th1 and Th17, but not Th2, responses in the skin of psoriasis patients [127]. Acitretin is modestly effective in the treatment of psoriasis, although large randomized studies are not available for this drug. In one study, among patients with plaque-type psoriasis treated with 50 mg/d of acitretin for 8 weeks, 23% achieved a PASI 75 response [128]. While modestly effective as monotherapy, acitretin can be quite effective as when used together with phototherapy. In one retrospective study, 72.5% of patients who were treated with acitretin and NB-UVB had a PASI 75 response [129]. Acitretin can also be particularly effective in treating patients with pustular psoriasis [130].

Acitretin cannot be used in women of childbearing potential due to its teratogenicity and its prolonged retention in adipose tissue (up to 3 years) if the patient consumes alcohol. Other side effects of acitretin include inflammatory hepatitis, elevation of triglycerides, dry skin and lips, and hair loss [131].

Cyclosporine

CsA is a systemic immunosuppressive drug that was developed to prevent rejection in organ transplant patients but was incidentally found to greatly improve the coexisting psoriasis in a few transplant patients afflicted with the disease. This observation helped to fuel the paradigm shift in thinking of psoriasis as an immunologic disease rather than a keratinocyte disease [132].

CsA binds to cyclophilin, forming a complex that inhibits the calcineurin-mediated dephosphorylation of NFAT, blocking the differentiation and activation of T cells and the production of multiple cytokines including IL-4, IFN-gamma, IL-17, and IL-2 [31]. CsA is usually dosed at 3–5 mg/kg/day. While highly effective in treating psoriasis, with PASI 75 responses at a dose of 5 mg/kg in 50–97% of patients noted in one systematic review, the use of CsA is limited by its side effects, including impaired renal function, hyperlipidemia, and hypertension. Duration of treatment over 2 years can result in a 30% or greater impairment in creatinine clearance in more than half of patients. For this reason, and because of its rapid onset of action, it is usually recommend that CsA be used in the initial treatment of more severe psoriasis but that patients are eventually transitioned to another therapy for long-term maintenance [133]. Although there are data suggesting modest efficacy of CsA in PsA, it is not a commonly used drug for PsA.

Apremilast

Apremilast is an oral small molecule inhibitor of phosphodiesterasetype 4 that reduces production of several cytokines, including TNF-α, IL-2, IL-12, and IL-23. It is dosed at 30 mg orally twice a day, which is reached gradually to increase tolerability. Data from a phase 2b study showed that 41% of patients given 30 mg twice daily, versus 11% of patients given placebo, achieved a PASI 75 response after 16 weeks of treatment [134].

Apremilast was approved for the treatment of PsA based on several clinical trials, named PALACE 1, 2, 3, and 4. In PALACE 1, a Phase III study of apremilast 30 mg twice daily, ACR 20 response was achieved in 40% of patients in the apremilast group compared to only 19% in the placebo group at 16 weeks [135]. There was no significant differences in improvement in PsA patients who continued on background stable MTX compared to those treated with apremilast alone noted. Long term follow up studies of apremilast to 52 weeks showed 54.6% of patients maintained an ACR 20 response [136].

Reported adverse events associated with apremilast were mild to moderate, limited, and included headache, nasopharyngitis, nausea, and diarrhea. Rare adverse events of weight loss, increased depression, and suicidal ideation have also been reported [134].

Biologic Therapy

TNF-α Antagonists

TNF-α antagonists are among the first biologics approved in the treatment of psoriasis and PsA and thus as a class have the greatest amount of long-term safety and efficacy data. TNF-α is secreted by and acts upon several cells in the immune response, as well as keratinocytes, and thus blocking this cytokine improves psoriasis severity in most patients. It is well established that TNF-α antagonists have substantial efficacy in treating various aspects of PsA, including peripheral joint disease, axial involvement, enthesitis, and dactylitis. The efficacy of the TNF-α antagonists exceeds that of traditional DMARDs and these are the first therapeutic agents to demonstrate significant inhibition of radiographic progression. Long-term follow-up studies that are available thus far for the TNF-α antagonists suggest that clinical and radiographic efficacy are maintained. Currently there are four TNF-α antagonists approved by the FDA for the treatment of psoriasis and five for the treatment of PsA. Although there are limited data for head-to-head comparisons of the TNF-α antagonists in PsA, a meta-analysis of four TNF-α antagonists in psoriasis and PsA suggested there were no significant differences in outcomes for skin and peripheral joint involvement [137].

Etanercept

Etanercept is a soluble dimeric fusion protein that links the p75 TNF-α receptor protein to the Fc portion of IgG1 and binds to soluble TNF-α, decreasing its free concentration in serum. Because etanercept contains the binding region of the p75 TNF-α receptor, it also binds to the other natural ligand of the p75 receptor, lymphotoxin B. Etanercept is dosed subcutaneously at 50 mg twice a week for 12 weeks, followed by a maintenance dose of 50 mg weekly for the treatment of psoriasis. At this dosing, a PASI 75 response was reached by 49% of subjects at week 12 and by 54% of subjects at week 24 in a randomized, double-blind, placebo-controlled study (vs. 3% at week 12 in the placebo arm) [138]. Additionally, at this dosing, in patients with scalp psoriasis, mean severity of scalp disease decreased by over 90% at week 24 [139], and in patients with nail psoriasis, an improvement of greater than 70% in severity of disease was noted after 24 weeks of treatment [140]. Although no biologics are currently FDA-approved for the treatment of pediatric psoriasis, in a randomized double-blind, placebo-controlled study of 211 patients age 4–17 years with psoriasis, at week 12 of treatment 57% of patients treated with etanercept 0.8 mg/kg/week and 11% of those treated with placebo achieved a PASI 75 response [141].

Etanercept for PsA is dosed subcutaneously either at 25 mg biweekly or 50 mg weekly. Significant improvement measured by ACR 20 response was noted in 59% of PsA subjects at 12 weeks treated with etanercept (vs 15% in the placebo group). Improvements were also noted in Health Assessment Questionnaire (HAQ) scores. Radiographic disease progression was also significantly diminished in the etanercept group as measured by modified Sharp scores (−0.03 unit) compared to a slight increase in the control group (+1.00 unit) [94].

Adalimumab

Adalimumab is a fully human monoclonal antibody that binds to both cell-bound and soluble TNF-α. In a 52 week randomized, double-blind, placebo-controlled study, after 16 weeks of treatment with adalimumab 40 mg subcutaneously every other week, with an initial loading dose of 80 mg subcutaneously, 71% of adalimumab-treated patients reached a PASI 75 response (vs. 7% of subjects who received placebo). After 52 weeks of continuous treatment, 5% of patients who had initially responded lost their response to adalimumab [142]. In a head-to-head study with MTX, after16 weeks of treatment, 79.6% of adalimumab-treated patients achieved a PASI 75 response, compared with 35.5% for MTX. This study had a notably high placebo response rate (18.9% with PASI 75 response). More adalimumab-treated patients than MTX or placebo-treated patients achieved complete clearance of disease [143]. Additionally, adalimumab has been shown to be effective in the treatment of scalp and nail psoriasis, with median reductions of 100% from the baseline PSSI and 39.5% from the baseline NAPSI, respectively, after 16 weeks of treatment [144].

In PsA, the Adalimumab Effectiveness in Psoriatic Arthritis Trial (ADEPT) demonstrated significant improvement in ACR 20 responses at 12 weeks in active PsA subjects who were DMARD naïve, treated with adalimumab 40 mg subcutaneously every other week compared to placebo treated subjects (ACR 20 58% vs 14%) [145, 146]. The study also demonstrated a significant decrease in radiographic progression in the adalimumab-treated group at 24 weeks. Additional studies have demonstrated efficacy of adalimumab in PsA subjects who had a prior inadequate response to a DMARD [147].

Infliximab

Infliximab is a chimeric antibody that is 75% human and 25% murine in composition. Although infliximab was originally developed and indicated for the treatment of IBD, it was noted that a patient with CD and psoriasis had dramatic clearance of her psoriasis after initiating therapy with infliximab [148]. In fact, this observation sparked interest in TNF-α antagonists as a therapy for psoriasis. A subsequent double-blind, placebo-controlled study demonstrated a PASI 75 response at week 10 in 88% of patients treated with the currently used dosing of 5 mg/kg IV at weeks 0, 2, and 6, with responses noted as early as 2 weeks [149]. The recommended maintenance dosing for infliximab is 5 mg/kg IV every 8 weeks following this initial loading dose. In a meta-analysis of studies of infliximab treatment of patients with nail psoriasis for 6–12 months, a significant improvement in nail psoriasis (57.2% improvement in disease severity) was noted [150].

Infliximab is also approved for use in PsA at the same dose as in psoriasis. In practice, doses of up to 10 mg/kg of infliximab may be used in some patients, similar to its dosing in RA. The IMPACT evaluated subjects with PsA treated with infliximab versus placebo. The infliximab group achieved ACR 20 responses in 65% compared to only 10% of placebo subjects at week 16 of the study [96]. A subsequent study, IMPACT

2, demonstrated similar significant improvements of ACR scores in PsA subjects who had inadequate response to prior treatments compared to placebo patients [151]. Radiographic progression was inhibited in the infliximab group compared to controls at 24 weeks (PsA modified Sharp score, −0.70 vs +0.82, respectively) [152].

Golimumab

Golimumab is a human monoclonal antibody that binds to human TNF-α and is currently approved for PsA. Golimumab is dosed subcutaneously at 50 mg once monthly. Studies in PsA demonstrate improvement of ACR 20 responses in subjects treated with golimumab 50 mg subcutaneously monthly as compared to placebo (51% vs 9%) at 14 weeks [153]. Statistically significant inhibition of radiographic progression was also demonstrated with golimumab versus placebo at 24 weeks [153, 154]. Golimumab intravenous formulation, dosed at 2 mg/kg at week 0 and 4, followed by every 8 weeks, is also FDA-approved for the treatment of PsA. Intravenous Golimumab has demonstrated significant efficacy in active PsA in the GO-VIBRANT trial, with achievement of ACR 20/50/70 responses of 75/44/25% in the golimumab arm versus 22/6/2% in the placebo arm at 14 weeks [155]. Although golimumab is not approved currently for the treatment of psoriasis, as a secondary endpoint in one study, PASI 75 response was assessed in subjects with PsA who also had ≥3% BSA involvement with psoriasis. After 14 weeks of treatment, PASI 75 response was reached by 40% of subjects who received the 50 mg dose of golimumab. However, it is important to note that PASI scores are less accurate in patients with low BSA involvement. Furthermore, some patients in this study were concomitantly taking MTX. Also, after 24 weeks of treatment with 50 mg of golimumab monthly, patients with nail psoriasis at baseline had a median improvement of 33% in NAPSI scores [156]. In the GO-VIBRANT trial of intravenous golimumab in active PsA, PASI 75 response was seen in 59% of golimumab treated patients compared to 14% of placebo group patients [155].

Certolizumab

Certolizumab is a pegylated human anti-TNF-α monoclonal antibody Fab' fragment that neutralizes both membrane-bound and soluble TNF. It is approved for the treatment of PsA. Certolizumab is injected subcutaneously with an initial loading dose of 400 mg every 2 weeks for three doses followed by a maintenance dose of 200 mg every 2 weeks or 400 mg every month. Certolizumab was shown to be effective in PsA patients who had failed at least one DMARD compared to placebo at 12 weeks (ACR 20 of 58% for 200 mg every 2 weeks and 51% for 400 mg once a month vs 24% placebo), and sustained improvement in enthesitis and dactylitis were also seen [157]. Certolizumab also demonstrated efficacy in PsA patients who had prior treatment with another TNF-α inhibitor. Additionally, certolizumab has been approved for use in psoriasis at a higher dose of 400 mg subcutaneously every 2 weeks based on efficacy in a Phase III study, with significantly higher PASI 75 responses at 16 weeks of 82% in the 400 mg group and, 76.7% in the 200 mg group compared to 9.9% in subjects receiving placebo every 2 weeks [158, 159].

It should be noted that all five of the currently FDA-approved TNF-α antagonists for use in PsA are also approved for use in AS and by extension presumed to be effective for clinical axial disease in PsA as well, although specific data are not available. In addition, unlike in RA no clear synergistic effect of combining MTX with TNF-α antagonists has been noted. Data from small studies suggest that the addition of MTX may prolong drug survival in the case of adalimumab and infliximab [160].

Risks and Benefits of Using TNF-α Antagonists

One of the risks of treatment with TNF-α antagonists is an increased incidence of both serious and non-serious infection [161]. Of particular concern is reactivation of latent tuberculosis, and it is standard to screen for latent tuberculosis in all patients prior to initiating therapy with any of the biologic agents [162]. There is also an increased risk of herpes zoster among patients taking TNF-α antagonists [163]. Other uncommon risks include worsening of congestive heart failure, central demyelinating disease, new onset of psoriasis (either among patients taking these drugs for another indication or as a new type of psoriasis in those with pre-existing psoriasis), and drug-induced lupus [164].

There are also potential additional benefits to the use of TNF-α antagonists, particularly in the psoriasis population, including a reduction in the risk of cardiovascular disease and diabetes. In one study, among patients with RA or psoriasis, the adjusted risk of developing type II diabetes was lower for individuals starting a TNF inhibitor compared with those starting other non-biologic treatments [165]. Also, the risk of cardiovascular disease, particularly myocardial infarction, appears to be reduced by approximately half in patients with psoriasis who are treated with a TNF inhibitor compared to those treated with topical medicines [166].

IL-12 / IL-23 Antagonists

Ustekinumab

Ustekinumab is a fully human monoclonal antibody to the common p40 subunit shared by the cytokines IL-12 and IL-23 that is FDA-approved for the treatment of moderate to severe plaque type psoriasis as well as PsA. Like infliximab, dosing of ustekinumab is based upon the patient's weight, with patients who weigh less than 100 kg receiving 45 mg per dose and those who are 100 kg or greater receiving 90 mg per dose. Ustekinumab is dosed subcutaneously at week 0, week 4, and then every 12 weeks. Ustekinumab was found to be effective in two nearly identical phase III, double-blind, placebo-controlled studies. In these two studies, PASI 75 responses were reached at week 12 by 66.7% and 67.1% of subjects who received the 45 mg dose, by 75.7% and 66.4% of those who received the 90 mg dose, and by 3.7% and 3.1% of those who received placebo [167, 168]. In one phase III study, among those patients with nail psoriasis who received ustekinumab, at week 24, the percentage improvement from baseline NAPSI score was 46.5% (ustekinumab 45 mg) and 48.7% (ustekinumab 90 mg) [169]. In a head to head study, the efficacy of ustekinumab was statistically superior to that of etanercept (at standard initial dosing regimens) over a 12-week period in patients with psoriasis, with PASI 75 responses at week 12 being reached in 67.5% of patients who received 45 mg of ustekinumab, 73.8% of patients who received 90 mg ustekinumab, and 56.8% of those who received etanercept. Also, 65.1% of patients who received 45 mg of ustekinumab, 70.6% of patients who received 90 mg of ustekinumab, and 49.0% of those who received etanercept were determined to be clear or had minimal disease according to the PGA [170].

In a randomized, placebo-controlled trial of PsA subjects, PSUMMIT 1, ustekinumab 45 mg and 90 mg demonstrated efficacy at 24 weeks with ACR 20 responses of 42.4% and 49.5%, respectively, versus 22.8% for the placebo group [171]. Improvement is enthesitis and dactylitis were also demonstrated [171]. PSUMMIT 2 evaluated PsA patients previously treated with a TNF inhibitor and demonstrated similar responses to PSUMMIT 1 (ACR 20 43% for ustekinumab vs 20% for placebo) [172]. Long-term studies pooled from both PSUMMIT 1 and PSUMMIT 2 show inhibition of radiographic progression with ustekinumab versus placebo in PsA patients [173]. Ustekinumab was not shown to be effective in a study of active AS and as result it is inferred that it would not likely be effective for PsA axial disease [174]. Currently there are no specific studies on ustekinumab in axial PsA.

Guselkumab

Guselkumab is the first drug that specifically targets IL-23 by binding to the p19 subunit present in IL-23 (but not IL-12) to receive FDA approval for the treatment of plaque psoriasis. Guselkumab is dosed at 100 mg administered subcutaneously at weeks 0, 4, and every 8 weeks thereafter. In an active comparator study, more subjects achieved a PGA of 0 or 1 at week 16 with guselkumab than with adalimumab (85.1% vs 65.9%, $p < 0.001$), both using their respective FDA-approved doses [175]. Guselkumab has also been shown to be effective in patients with psoriasis who did not achieve an adequate response (defined as an IGA 0 or 1 response at week 16) to ustekinumab [176]. Guselkumab appears to be effective and approved for use in PsA. In a phase and III trials, patients who received gesulkumab at the same approved psoriasis dosing at week 24 achieved significantly better ACR responses compared to the placebo group [177].

Risankizumab and Tildrakizumab

Risankizumab is a monoclonal antibody against IL-23, which targets the p19 subunit of IL-23. Risankizumab showed superior efficacy to ustekinumab (at FDA-approved dosing) for the treatment of moderate to severe plaque psoriasis in phase II and phase III trials [178, 179]. In the Phase III studies, an impressive PASI 90 response was seen in 75% of risankizumab patients compared to 2% and 5% in placebo treated patients. Risankizumab was recently approved for use in psoriasis at a dose of 150 mg injected subcutaneously at week 0 and 4, followed by 150 mg every 12 weeks. Another antibody to IL-23, tildrakizumab, is FDA-approved for psoriasis and was found to result in a higher PASI 75 response than both placebo and etanercept (at FDA-approved dosing) in patients with moderate to severe plaque psoriasis [180]. These agents are currently undergoing investigation for use in PsA.

Safety Concerns with IL-12/23 Antagonists

Inhibition of IL-12/23 may confer an increased risk of cardiovascular events. Despite impressive efficacy, the IL-12/23 p40 antagonist briakinumab was ultimately withdrawn from further investigation due to an observed increase in major adverse cardiovascular events (MACE) in treated subjects in early clinical trials [181]. [182], A meta-analysis pooling the data from published studies of briakinumab and ustekinumab showed that 10 of 3179 patients receiving anti-IL-12/23 therapies experienced MACE; no events were seen in 1474 patients receiving placebo. However, this difference did not reach statistical significance [181]. Analysis of a large registry of over 12,095 psoriasis patients, of whom 3,308 had ever received ustekinimab, did not show an increased risk of MACE relative to patients who received other psoriasis therapy. However, this was not a randomized study, reported results were not age-adjusted, and patients on ustekinumab were younger than those on non-biologic therapy [183].

Additional theoretical risks in patients treated with IL-12/23 antagonists are based on the fact that individuals who lack p40 entirely due to mutations in the *IL12B* gene have increased susceptibility to infection with Salmonella species, bacteria Calmette–Guérin (BCG), and other non-tuberculous mycobacteria [184]. Although no cases of these infections were observed in clinical studies, they remain theoretical risks and patients taking ustekinumab are advised to avoid vaccination with BCG.

IL-17 Antagonists

Secukinumab

Secukinumab is a monoclonal antibody to IL-17A that is dosed subcutaneously at 300 mg given as a loading dose at weeks 0, 1, 2, 3, and 4, followed by dosing every 4 weeks for maintenance. Two phase III, double-blind, placebo-controlled studies of secukinumab showed efficacy of this drug for the treatment of psoriasis, one of which included an active comparator, etanercept. In these studies, subjects received secukinumab or placebo subcutaneously at weeks 0, 1, 2, 3, and 4 and then every 4 weeks thereafter. Etanercept was dosed at the FDA-approved regimen of 50 mg subcutaneously twice weekly for 12 weeks then once weekly thereafter. PASI 75 responses at week 12 were achieved by 81.6% and 77.1% of subjects who received the 300 mg dose of secukinumab and in 4.5% and 4.9% of those received placebo. In the study that included an etanercept treatment arm, 44.0% of subjects treated with etanercept achieved a PASI 75 response. Secukinumab was found to be superior in efficacy to both placebo and etanercept. In addition, maintenance of a PASI 75 response was seen in the majority of patients in both studies, with a higher rate of maintained response seen among those treated with the 300 mg dose of secukinumab than those treated with etanercept [185]. A head-to-head study of secukimab vs. ustekinumab, both at FDA-approved doses, showed that secukinumab demonstrated IGA 0/1, PASI 90, and PASI 100 responses that were superior to those of ustekinumab [186].

Secukinumab is also approved for use in PsA in the US, with dosing of 150 mg subcutaneously given as a loading dose at weeks 0, 1, 2, 3, and 4, followed by dosing every 4 weeks for maintenance. Patients with concurrent psoriasis may use the higher psoriasis dosing regimen. A phase III randomized controlled trial of PsA patients treated with secukinumab demonstrated significantly higher ACR 20 responses of 54% compared to 15% in placebo-treated patients at 24 weeks and results were maintained to week 52. The study also demonstrated improvement in enthesitis, dactylitis and inhibition of radiographic joint damage [187].

Ixekizumab

Ixekizumab is a humanized monoclonal antibody to IL-17A that is FDA-approved for the treatment of psoriasis and PsA. The FDA-approved dosing for psoriasis is 160 mg subcutaneously at week 0, then 80 mg subcutaneously at weeks 2, 4, 6, 8, 10, 12, then 80 mg subcutaneously every 4 weeks. In two phase III studies in which ixekizumab at this dosing was compared to placebo and etanercept (at FDA-approved dosing), ixekizumab was superior to both placebo and etanercept as measured by IGA 0/1, PASI 75, PASI 90, and PASI 100 responses [188]. Among those who initially responded to ixekizumab with a PGA 0/1 response, this response was maintained in 73.8% at 60 weeks of treatment [189].

The FDA-approved dose of ixekizumab for PsA is 160 mg subcutaneously at week 0 followed by 80 mg subcutaneously every 4 weeks. Patients with both PsA and moderate-to-severe psoriasis should be dosed with the psoriasis regimen. In a phase 3 study with both a placebo and active comparator (adalimumab, at FDA-approved dosing for PsA), SPIRIT P1, ACR 20 response was achieved at week 24 by 30.2% of subjects who received placebo, 57.9% of subjects who receive ixekizumab 80 mg every 4 weeks (after an initial 160 mg dose), 62.1% of subjects who receive ixekizumab 80 mg every 2 weeks (after an initial 160 mg dose), and 57.4% of subjects who receive adalimumab. Ixekizumab has also demonstrated efficacy for reduction of enthesitis and dactylitis in PsA. Progression of structural damage at week 24, measured by changes from baseline in mTSS, was significantly less in the ixekizumab every 4 weeks (0.17), ixekizumab every 2 weeks (0.08) and adalimumab (0.10) groups than in the placebo group (0.49) ($p \leq 0.01$) [190].

Brodalumab

Brodalumab is a human monoclonal antibody to the IL-17 receptor. It is FDA-approved for the treatment of moderate to severe plaque type psoriasis at a dose of 210 mg subcutaneously at weeks 0, 1, and 2, and every 2 weeks thereafter. In a phase III, double-blind, placebo-controlled study, at week 12, 83% of subjects receiving this dose of brodalumab vs. 3% of subjects receiving placebo achieved PASI 75, and 76% who received brodalumab vs. 1% who received placebo achieved an sPGA of 0 or 1 [191]. In two phase III head-to-head studies with ustekinumab, PASI 75, PASI 100, and IGA 0/1 responses at week 12 were greater in subjects assigned to take brodalumab than in those assigned to ustekinumab at the FDA-approved dose [192].

Brodalumab also demonstrated efficacy in PsA in a double-blind, randomized, placebo-controlled trial. ACR 20 responses at week 12 in the Brodalumab 140 mg and 280 mg groups were seen in 37 and 39%, respectively, versus 18% in the placebo group. Similar response rates were seen in PsA patients previously treated with biologics as well [193]. However, further studies with brodalumab in PsA were put on hold due to safety concerns.

Similar to the situation with TNF inhibitors, the evidence for effectiveness of secukinumab and ixekizumab in AS enables us to feel comfortable with extrapolating its presumed efficacy for axial PsA. Again, specific data regarding the efficacy of these agents in axial disease in PsA is not available.

Safety Concerns with IL-17 Antagonists

Cases of mucocutaenous candidiasis and neutropenia have been reported in patients taking IL-17 pathway antagonists, although none were serious or required systemic therapy [185, 194, 195]. Deficiency of IL-17RA and IL-17F is associated with the development of chronic mucocutaneous candidiasis, warranting concern about the risk of candidal infection when the IL-17 pathway is blocked in the treatment of psoriasis [196]. Although brodalumab has been approved for the treatment of moderate to severe plaque type psoriasis, due to concerns about suicidality associated with this drug, it carries a black box warning about the risk of suicidal ideation and behavior and is only available from providers who participate in a risk evaluation and mitigation program. Despite initial hopes that IL-17 may be a useful target in the treatment of IBD based on preclinical data, a clinical trial of secukinumab in moderate-to-severe CD was ineffective and ended early due to an increased number of flares noted in patients in the treatment arm compared to placebo arm, raising concerns about IL-17 inhibition and exacerbation of IBD. Clinical trial and post-marketing safety data suggest that the incidence rates of IBD in psoriasis, PsA, and AS patients treated with secukinumab are low and in the ranges expected in these conditions due to the known associations. Regardless, further long-term safety data is needed to investigate this issue and it preferable to avoid IL-17 inhibitors in patients with IBD [197, 198].

Janus Kinase Inhibitors

The janus kinase (JAK) family of tyrosine kinases, including JAK1, JAK2, JAK3, and TYK2, are key signaling proteins important in intracellular signal transduction. Tofacitinib is an oral small molecule that specifically targets JAK3 and JAK1. Tofacitinib is the first JAK inhibitor approved for the treatment of active PsA in patients with an inadequate response to MTX or other DMARDs. The recommended dose for PsA is 5 mg orally twice daily [199]. The efficacy of tofacitinib in PsA has been demonstrated in two Phase III trials. The first study, the Oral Psoriatic Arthritis trial (OPAL)- Broaden, evaluated TNFi-naïve patients who had an inadequate response to DMARD therapy, randomizing subjects to treatment with tofacitininb at 5 mg orally twice daily, tofacitinib 10 mg orally twice daily, adalimumab 40 mg subcutaneously every 2 weeks, or placebo. ACR 20/50/70 responses were significantly higher for the tofacitinib 5 mg (50/28/17%) and tofacitinib 10 mg (61/40/14%) groups compared to placebo (33/10/5%). The adalimumab group had an ACR 20 response rate of 52% [199]. The OPAL-Beyond study evaluated PsA patients with inadequate response to at least one TNFi. Patients were randomized to three groups: tofacitinib 5 mg twice daily, 10 mg twice daily, or placebo. ACR 20 response rates at 3 months were significantly higher for the tofacitinib 5 mg and 10 mg groups (50% and 48%, respectively) compared to placebo (24%). The tofacitinib 5 mg and 10 mg twice daily group also demonstrated significantly higher PASI 75 responses (21% and 43%, respectively) compared to placebo (14%) in the OPAL-Beyond study. A greater reduction in LEI score with tofacitinib as compared to placebo was also noted [200]. Tofacitinib is not currently approved for psoriasis due to safety concerns at the higher dose.

Other promising selective JAK inhibitors currently under investigation for both psoriasis and PsA include barcitinib, upadacitinib and filgotinib.

Safety Concerns with JAK Inhibitors

As with the biologic agents, JAK inhibitors carry an increased risk of infections, including opportunistic infection, viral reactivation, and herpes zoster. Additional concerns with inhibition of the JAK-STAT pathway include cytopenias and increased risk of malignancy. In the OPAL-Broaden study there were four malignancies seen in the tofacitinib groups and none in the placebo group; however, so far, long-term studies of tofacitinib have not shown an increased risk of cancer [199, 201]. Further long-term studies are needed to clarify this risk. Recently a black box warning was added to the label for tofacitinib for increased risk of pulmonary embolism and death at the higher dose of 10 mg orally twice daily, which is currently approved for ulcerative colitis but not PsA [202].

T Cell Costimulation Blockade

Abatacept is a soluble fusion protein of the extracellular domain of cytotoxic T lymphocyte-associated antigen 4 (CTLA-4) linked to the Fc portion of an immunoglobulin. Abatacept exerts its effects by blocking T cell activation and the downstream inflammatory cascade by competing with CD28 for binding to CD80/CD86 which is required for T cell activation and subsequent production of inflammatory cytokines. Abatacept was been shown to be effective for the treatment of PsA in two clinical trial studies. A randomized, placebo-controlled, phase III study of subcutaneous abatacept in active PsA demonstrated significantly higher ACR 20 responses of 39.4% vs 22.3% for placebo at 24 weeks [203]. Similar results were noted for a Phase II study of intravenous abatacept in active PsA patients at 24 weeks (ACR 20 responses of 47.5% in the highest-dose, abatacept 10mg/kg arm, versus 19% in placebo) [204]. It should be noted that the ACR responses for abatacept are generally lower than those seen with other biologic agents currently approved for PsA. Enthesitis and dactylitis also demonstrated modest improvements in the abatacept treatment group compared to placebo. Effects on axial disease were not evaluated in these studies and generally abatacept is not thought to be effective for axial disease in PsA based on disappointing results in an open-label pilot study in AS [205]. Abatacept is currently approved for use in active PsA for both subcutaneous dosing (125 mg every week) and intravenous dosing based on weight (500 mg–1000 mg at weeks 0, 2, and 4 followed by every 28 days). Psoriasis outcomes did not demonstrate significant improvement in the treatment arm compared to placebo in both of these studies and currently abatacept is not approved for use in psoriasis.

Safety Concerns with T Cell Co-stimulation Blockade

Generally, abatacept is considered to be well-tolerated with a favorable safety profile including low rates of infection and malignancy. Similar to other biologics, however, monitoring is needed for increased risk of infection, particularly respiratory infections.

Monitoring in Biologics

While biologics are generally safe, the risk of infection, particularly reactivation of latent TB, is well-documented. In addition, patients with chronic hepatitis B are at risk of developing fulminant infection when treated with TNF-antagonists. Lab abnormalities are rare but can occur: the use of biologics has been associated with isolated cytopenias and pancytopenia as well as elevated transaminases. Prior to starting any biologic, patients should be screened for latent TB, generally with a tuberculin skin test (TST) or interferon gamma release assay (IGRA). It is recommended that this testing is repeated annually while a patient is taking a biologic. In addition, prior to starting a biologic, appropriate baseline testing includes hepatitis B serology (for hepatitis B surface antigen, surface antibody, and core antibody) [206], a CBC, and liver transaminases. Most guidelines recommend that the CBC and liver transaminases be repeated every 6 months [207]. For patients who have evidence of past, acute, or chronic hepatitis B, a biologic should only be started in collaboration with the patient's hepatologist [206].

It is recommended that, if possible, patients receive updated vaccinations prior to starting a biologic or other immunosuppressive therapy for psoriasis or PsA. Live vaccines are not recommended while taking biologics or other immunosuppressive therapies such as cyclosporine or high dose MTX (particularly at doses >0.4 mg/kg/wk). The two live vaccines most likely to be offered to psoriatic patients in the past were the intranasal influenza vaccine and the herpes zoster vaccine (for patients 60 years and older), but the intranasal influenza vaccine is no longer in use and a new inactivated zoster vaccine has been approved. Given the increased risk of developing zoster associated with use of TNF-α antagonists and JAK inhibitors, vaccination in patients 60 or older is recommended. Also, because vaccine responses may be slightly diminished in patients taking biologics and other immunosuppressive agents, administration prior to starting therapy may be beneficial [207].

Combining Psoriasis Therapies

Often, patients will require a combination of two or more psoriasis treatments. Topical therapies can generally be combined with any systemic therapy and are a good option for the treatment of recalcitrant plaques. While patients undergoing phototherapy can also use topical therapies, they should make sure to apply them after their light treatments. MTX is frequently used in combination with biologics, particularly TNF-α antagonists. In one study, the combination of MTX and etanercept was found to be superior to treatment with etanercept alone [208]. MTX may decrease the production of anti-drug antibodies in patients taking biologics [209]. Either acitretin or MTX can be used in combination with cyclosporine, although transaminase levels and, in the case of acitretin, lipid profiles, must be closely monitored. Concurrent use of MTX and acitretin should be avoided due to hepatotoxicity.

Few studies have examined the efficacy of adding NB-UVB to biologics. In two randomized studies of etanercept as monotherapy vs. with concomitant NB-UVB, there was not a significant benefit, in terms of patients reaching PASI 75 responses, to adding phototherapy [210]. In a split-body study in which patients were given ustekinumab and only one half of the body was treated with NB-UVB, for the body half treated with NB-UVB, there was an 82% mean PASI reduction compared with a 54% mean PASI reduction in the other body half at week 6 [211]. It should be noted, however, that the ustekinumab prescribing information recommends against the concurrent use of phototherapy due to a theoretical increase in risk of skin cancer.

Combining therapies for PsA is a common practice, although few data exist to support these combinations, and regimens are largely borrowed from experience in RA. Oral DMARDs may be used in combination (SSA with MTX; MTX with leflunomide). In apremilast clinical studies, patients were allowed to continue MTX but no additional benefit was noted with the combination versus apremilast alone [212]. Although the combination of MTX and TNF inhibitors has shown a synergistic effect in RA and psoriasis, studies in PsA do not suggest improved outcomes for this combination versus TNF-α inhibitor alone [213, 214]. There is evidence, though, that this combination improves retention rates, likely due its effect on decreasing anti-drug antibodies in patients on certain biologics [213]. In general, it is not recommended to combine biologic agents due to potential safety concerns in regards to infections and the lack of overall data on this approach. Several case reports have been published, however, as dual biologic therapy is being increasingly tried as an option in refractory psoriatic disease or in patients with differential responses for skin and joint disease [215].

Cost of Psoriasis and Psoriatic Arthritis Therapies

Biologic therapies generally offer good efficacy and safety and have revolutionized the treatment of psoriasis and PsA. However, this comes at a significant financial cost, with the average wholesale price of most biologic therapies reaching tens of thousands of dollars per year. By contrast, MTX is relatively inexpensive, costing only a few dollars per week. To help adjust cost for efficacy, a recent study examined the cost of several drugs in terms of the cost per month per patient who reaches a PASI 75 response. Even when cost-adjusted for recommended lab monitoring,

Table 7.4 Efficacy of DMARDS and biologics for the treatment of psoriasis and PsA

Drug	Molecular Target	Psoriasis dosing	Evidence for efficacy in psoriasis	FDA approved for psoriasis	PsA dosing	Evidence for efficacy in PsA	FDA-approved for PsA
Methotrexate	Dihyrofolate reductase and thymidylate synthetase	10-25 mg PO/IM/SC qwk	Yes	Yes	10-25 mg PO/IM/SC qwk	Yes	No
Acitretin	Retinoic acid receptors	10–50 mg PO daily	Yes	Yes	N/A	No	No
Leflunomide	Dihydroorotate dehydrogenase	N/A	Minimal	No	20 mg daily	Yes	No
Cyclosporine	Cyclophilin	2–5 mg/kg PO daily	Yes	Yes	N/A	No	No
Apremilast	PDE4	30 mg PO BID	Yes	Yes	30 mg PO BID	Yes	Yes
Etanercept	TNF-α	50 mg SC BIW × 12wks, then qwk	Yes	Yes	50 mg SC qwk	Yes	Yes
Adalimumab	TNF-α	80 mg SC ×1 then in 7 days 40 mg SC q2wks	Yes	Yes	40 mg SC q2wks	Yes	Yes
Infliximab	TNF-α	5 mg/kg IV at weeks 0, 2, 6 then q8wks	Yes	Yes	5 mg/kg IV at weeks 0, 2, 6 then q8wks	Yes	Yes
Golimumab	TNF-α	50 mg SC q4wks or 2 mg/kg IV at week 0, 4 and then q8wks	Yes	No	50 mg SC q4wks or 2 mg/kg IV at week 0, 4 and then q8wks	Yes	Yes
Certolizumab	TNF-α	400 mg SC q2wks	Yes	Yes	400 mg SC q2wks × 3 doses then 200 mg q2wks OR 400 mg q4wks	Yes	Yes

Table 7.4 (continued)

Drug	Molecular Target	Psoriasis dosing	Evidence for efficacy in psoriasis	FDA approved for psoriasis	PsA dosing	Evidence for efficacy in PsA	FDA-approved for PsA
Ustekinumab	IL-12/23 p40	45 mg SC at week 0, 4 then q12wks (if >100 kg, use 90 mg)	Yes	Yes	45 mg SC at wk 0, 4 then q12wks (if >100 kg, use 90 mg)	Yes	Yes
Secukinumab	IL-17A	300 mg SC qwk ×5 wks then q4wks	Yes	Yes	150–300 mg SC qwk ×5 wks then q4wks	Yes	Yes
Ixekizumab	IL-17A	160 mg SC at week 0, then 80 mg SC at weeks 2, 4, 6, 8, 10, 12, then q4wks	Yes	Yes	160 mg SC at wk 0, then 80 mg SC q4wks	Yes	Yes
Brodalumab	IL-17 receptor	210 mg SC at wks 0, 1, 2 then q2wks	Yes	Yes	140 mg or 280 mg SC at wks 0, 1, 2, then q2wks	Yes	No
Abatacept	CD80/CD86	N/A	No	No	125 mg SC q1wk OR 500–1000 mg IV q4wks	Yes	Yes
Guselkumab	IL-23 p19	100 mg SC at wk 0 and 4, then q8wks	Yes	Yes	100 mg SC at wk 0 and 4, then q8wks	Yes	Yes
Risankizumab	IL-23 p19	150 mg SC at wk 0 and 4, then q12wks	Yes	Yes	N/A	N/A	No
Tofacitinib	JAK1/JAK3	N/A	No	No	5 mg PO BID OR 11 mg daily	Yes	Yes

MTX was the most cost-effective option at $794.05-1,502.51 per month. The most expensive therapies were infliximab and ustekinumab 90 mg, costing $8,704.68-15,235.52 and $12,505.26-14,256.75 monthly, respectively (Table 7.4) [216].

References

1. Parisi R, Symmons DPM, Griffiths CEM, Ashcroft DM. Global epidemiology of psoriasis: a systematic review of incidence and prevalence. J Invest Dermatol. 2012; https://doi.org/10.1038/jid.2012.339.
2. O'Neill T, Silman AJ. Psoriatic arthritis. Historical background and epidemiology. Baillieres Clin Rheumatol. 1994;8(2):245–61. http://www.ncbi.nlm.nih.gov/pubmed/8076386. Accessed April 15, 2015.
3. Alenius G-M, Stenberg B, Stenlund H, Lundblad M, Dahlqvist SR. Inflammatory joint manifestations are prevalent in psoriasis: prevalence study of joint and axial involvement in psoriatic patients, and evaluation of a psoriatic and arthritic questionnaire. J Rheumatol. 2002;29(12):2577–82. http://www.ncbi.nlm.nih.gov/pubmed/12465155. Accessed April 15, 2015.
4. Harrison BJ, Silman AJ, Barrett EM, Scott DG, Symmons DP. Presence of psoriasis does not influence the presentation or short-term outcome of patients with early inflammatory polyarthritis. J Rheumatol. 1997;24(9):1744–9. http://www.ncbi.

nlm.nih.gov/pubmed/9292798. Accessed April 15, 2015.
5. Shbeeb M, Uramoto KM, Gibson LE, O'Fallon WM, Gabriel SE. The epidemiology of psoriatic arthritis in Olmsted County, Minnesota, USA, 1982-1991. J Rheumatol. 2000;27(5):1247–50. http://www.ncbi.nlm.nih.gov/pubmed/10813295. Accessed April 21, 2015.
6. Gelfand JM, Gladman DD, Mease PJ, et al. Epidemiology of psoriatic arthritis in the population of the United States. J Am Acad Dermatol. 2005;53(4):573. https://doi.org/10.1016/j.jaad.2005.03.046.
7. Setty AR, Choi HK. Psoriatic arthritis epidemiology. Curr Rheumatol Rep. 2007;9(6):449–54. http://www.ncbi.nlm.nih.gov/pubmed/18177597. Accessed April 21, 2015.
8. Chandran V, Raychaudhuri SP. Geoepidemiology and environmental factors of psoriasis and psoriatic arthritis. J Autoimmun. 2010;34(3):J314–21. https://doi.org/10.1016/j.jaut.2009.12.001.
9. Wilson FC, Icen M, Crowson CS, McEvoy MT, Gabriel SE, Kremers HM. Time trends in epidemiology and characteristics of psoriatic arthritis over 3 decades: a population-based study. J Rheumatol. 2009;36(2):361–7. https://doi.org/10.3899/jrheum.080691.
10. Rahman P, Schentag CTGD. Immunogenetic profile of patients with psoriatic arthritis varies according to the age of onset of psoriasis. Arthritis Rheum. 1999;42(4):822–3.
11. Christophers E, Barker J, Griffiths C, et al. The risk of psoriatic arthritis remains constant following initial diagnosis of psoriasis among patients seen in European dermatology clinics. J Eur Acad Dermatol Venereol. 2010;24(5):548–54. https://doi.org/10.1111/j.1468-3083.2009.03463.x.
12. Ibrahim G, Waxman R, Helliwell PS. The prevalence of psoriatic arthritis in people with psoriasis. Arthritis Care Res. 2009;61(10):1373–8. https://doi.org/10.1002/art.24608.
13. Reich K, Krüger K, Mössner R, Augustin M. Epidemiology and clinical pattern of psoriatic arthritis in Germany: a prospective interdisciplinary epidemiological study of 1511 patients with plaque-type psoriasis. Br J Dermatol. 2009;160(5):1040–7. https://doi.org/10.1111/j.1365-2133.2008.09023.x.
14. Moll JMH, Wright V. Psoriatic arthritis. Semin Arthritis Rheum. 1973;3(1):55–78. https://doi.org/10.1016/0049-0172(73)90035-8.
15. Oka A, Mabuchi T, Ozawa A, Inoko H. Current understanding of human genetics and genetic analysis of psoriasis. J Dermatol. https://doi.org/10.1111/j.1346-8138.2012.01504.x.
16. Eppinga H, Konstantinov S, Peppelenbosch M, Thio HB. The microbiome and psoriatic arthritis. Curr Rheumatol Rep. 2014;16(3):407. https://doi.org/10.1007/s11926-013-0407-2.
17. Scher JU, Ubeda C, Artacho A, Attur M, Isaac S, Reddy SM, Marmon S, Neimann A, Brusca S, Patel T, Manasson J, Pamer EG, Littman DRAS. Decreased bacterial diversity characterizes the altered gut microbiota in patients with psoriatic arthritis, resembling dysbiosis in inflammatory bowel disease. Arthritis Rheumatol. 2015;67(1):128–39.
18. Muszer M, Noszczyńska M, Kasperkiewicz K, Skurnik M. Human microbiome: when a friend becomes an enemy. Arch Immunol Ther Exp. 2015; https://doi.org/10.1007/s00005-015-0332-3.
19. Chandran V, Schentag CT, Brockbank JE, et al. Familial aggregation of psoriatic arthritis. Ann Rheum Dis. 2009;68(5):664–7. https://doi.org/10.1136/ard.2008.089367.
20. Gladman DDFV. HLA studies in psoriatic arthritis: current situation and future needs. J Rheumatol. 2003;30(1):4–6.
21. Fitzgerald O, Winchester R. Psoriatic arthritis: from pathogenesis to therapy. Arthritis Res Ther. 2009;11(1):214. https://doi.org/10.1186/ar2580.
22. Winchester R, Minevich G, Steshenko V, et al. HLA associations reveal genetic heterogeneity in psoriatic arthritis and in the psoriasis phenotype. Arthritis Rheum. 2012;64(4):1134–44. https://doi.org/10.1002/art.33415.
23. Winchester R. Genetics of psoriasis and psoriatic arthritis. In: Ritchlin CT, FitzGerald O, editors. Psoriatic and reactive arthritis- a companion to rheumatology. 1st ed. Amsterdam: Elselvier; 2007. p. 65–80.
24. Murdaca G, Gulli R, Spanò F, et al. TNF-α gene polymorphisms: association with disease susceptibility and response to anti-TNF-α treatment in psoriatic arthritis. J Invest Dermatol. 2014;134(10):2503–9. https://doi.org/10.1038/jid.2014.123.
25. Filer C, Ho P, Smith RL, et al. Investigation of association of the IL12B and IL23R genes with psoriatic arthritis. Arthritis Rheum. 2008;58(12):3705–9. https://doi.org/10.1002/art.24128.
26. Scarpa R, Del Puente A, di Girolamo C, Della Valle G, Lubrano E, Oriente P. Interplay between environmental factors, articular involvement, and HLA-B27 in patients with psoriatic arthritis. Ann Rheum Dis. 1992;51(1):78–9. http://www.pubmedcentral.nih.gov/articlerender.fcgi?artid=1004623&tool=pmcentrez&rendertype=abstract. Accessed April 21, 2015.
27. Punzi L, Pianon M, Bertazzolo N, et al. Clinical, laboratory and immunogenetic aspects of post-traumatic psoriatic arthritis: a study of 25 patients. Clin Exp Rheumatol. 16(3):277–81. http://www.ncbi.nlm.nih.gov/pubmed/9631749. Accessed April 21, 2015
28. Lynde CW, Poulin Y, Vender R, Bourcier M, Khalil S. Interleukin 17A: toward a new understanding of psoriasis pathogenesis. J Am Acad Dermatol. 2014; https://doi.org/10.1016/j.jaad.2013.12.036.
29. O'Brien RL, Born WK. Dermal γδ T cells – what have we learned? Cell Immunol. 2015; https://doi.org/10.1016/j.cellimm.2015.01.011.
30. Baliwag J, Barnes DH, Johnston A. Cytokines in psoriasis. Cytokine. 2015; https://doi.org/10.1016/j.cyto.2014.12.014.

31. Haider AS, Lowes MA, Suárez-Fariñas M, et al. Identification of cellular pathways of "type 1," Th17 T cells, and TNF- and inducible nitric oxide synthase-producing dendritic cells in autoimmune inflammation through pharmacogenomic study of cyclosporine A in psoriasis. J Immunol. 2008;180(3):1913–20. http://www.ncbi.nlm.nih.gov/pubmed/18209089. Accessed April 5, 2015.
32. Reece RJ, Canete JD, Parsons WJ, Emery P, Veale DJ. Distinct vascular patterns of early synovitis in psoriatic, reactive, and rheumatoid arthritis. Arthritis Rheum. 1999;42(7):1481–4. https://doi.org/10.1002/1529-0131(199907)42:7<1481::AID-ANR23>3.0.CO;2-E.
33. Sherlock JP, Joyce-Shaikh B, Turner SP, et al. IL-23 induces spondyloarthropathy by acting on ROR-γt+ CD3+CD4-CD8- entheseal resident T cells. Nat Med. 2012;18(7):1069–76. https://doi.org/10.1038/nm.2817.
34. Jandus C, Bioley G, Rivals J-P, Dudler J, Speiser D, Romero P. Increased numbers of circulating polyfunctional Th17 memory cells in patients with seronegative spondylarthritides. Arthritis Rheum. 2008;58(8):2307–17. https://doi.org/10.1002/art.23655.
35. Raychaudhuri SP, Raychaudhuri SK, Genovese MC. IL-17 receptor and its functional significance in psoriatic arthritis. Mol Cell Biochem. 2012;359(1–2):419–29. https://doi.org/10.1007/s11010-011-1036-6.
36. Kirkham BW, Kavanaugh A, Reich K. Interleukin-17A: a unique pathway in immune-mediated diseases: psoriasis, psoriatic arthritis and rheumatoid arthritis. Immunology. 2014;141(2):133–42. https://doi.org/10.1111/imm.12142.
37. Veale DJ. Psoriatic arthritis: recent progress in pathophysiology and drug development. Arthritis Res Ther. 2013;15(6):224. http://www.pubmedcentral.nih.gov/articlerender.fcgi?artid=4061722&tool=pmcentrez&rendertype=abstract. Accessed April 21, 2015
38. Raychaudhuri SK, Maverakis E, Raychaudhuri SP. Diagnosis and classification of psoriasis. Autoimmun Rev. 2014; https://doi.org/10.1016/j.autrev.2014.01.008.
39. Silverberg NB. Update on pediatric psoriasis, part 1: clinical features and demographics. Cutis. 2010;86(3):118–24. http://www.ncbi.nlm.nih.gov/pubmed/21049727. Accessed May 7, 2015.
40. Meier M, Sheth PB. Clinical spectrum and severity of psoriasis. Curr Probl Dermatol. 2009;38:1–20. https://doi.org/10.1159/000232301.
41. Klaassen KMG, van de Kerkhof PCM, Pasch MC. Nail psoriasis: a questionnaire-based survey. Br J Dermatol. 2013;169(2):314–9. https://doi.org/10.1111/bjd.12354.
42. Tan EST, Chong W-S, Tey HL. Nail psoriasis: a review. Am J Clin Dermatol. 2012;13(6):375–88. https://doi.org/10.2165/11597000-000000000-00000.
43. Gladman DD, Shuckett R, Russell ML, Thorne JC, Schachter RK. Psoriatic arthritis (PSA)–an analysis of 220 patients. Q J Med. 1987;62(238):127–41.
44. Cohen MR, Reda DJ, Clegg DO. Baseline relationships between psoriasis and psoriatic arthritis: analysis of 221 patients with active psoriatic arthritis. Department of Veterans Affairs Cooperative Study Group on Seronegative Spondyloarthropathies. J Rheumatol. 1999;26:1752.
45. McHugh NJ, Balachrishnan C, Jones SM. Progression of peripheral joint disease in psoriatic arthritis: a 5-yr prospective study. Rheumatology. 2003;42(6):778–83. https://doi.org/10.1093/rheumatology/keg217.
46. Gladman DD, Stafford-Brady F, Chang CH, Lewandowski K, Russell ML. Longitudinal study of clinical and radiological progression in psoriatic arthritis. J Rheumatol. 1990;17(6):809–12.
47. Gladman DD, Farewell VT, Wong K, Husted J. Mortality studies in psoriatic arthritis: results from a single outpatient center. II. Prognostic indicators for death. Arthritis Rheum. 1998;41(6):1103–10. https://doi.org/10.1002/1529-0131(199806)41:6<1103::AID-ART18>3.0.CO;2-N.
48. Buskila D, Langevitz P, Gladman DD, Urowitz S, Smythe HA. Patients with rheumatoid arthritis are more tender than those with psoriatic arthritis. J Rheumatol. 1992;19(7):1115–9.
49. Deandrade JRCP. A seven day variability study of 499 patients with peripheral rheumatoid arthritis. Arthritis Rheum. 1965;19:302–34.
50. McGonagle D, Lories RJ, Tan AL, et al. The concept of a synovio-entheseal complex and its implications for understanding joint inflammation and damage in psoriatic arthritis and beyond. Arthritis Rheum. 2007;56:2482–91.
51. Balint PV, Kane D, Wilson H, McInnes IB, Sturrock RD. Ultrasonography of entheseal insertions in the lower limb in spondyloarthropathy. Ann Rheum Dis. 2002;61(10):905–10. http://www.pubmedcentral.nih.gov/articlerender.fcgi?artid=1753913&tool=pmcentrez&rendertype=abstract. Accessed March 1, 2015.
52. Healy PJ, Helliwell PS. Measuring clinical enthesitis in psoriatic arthritis: assessment of existing measures and development of an instrument specific to psoriatic arthritis. Arthritis Care Res. 2008;59(5):686–91. https://doi.org/10.1002/art.23568.
53. Brockbank JE, Stein M, Schentag CT, Gladman DD. Dactylitis in psoriatic arthritis: a marker for disease severity? Ann Rheum Dis. 2005;64(2):188–90. https://doi.org/10.1136/ard.2003.018184.
54. Kane D, Greaney T, Bresnihan B, Gibney R, Fitzgerald O. Ultrasonography in the diagnosis and management of psoriatic dactylitis. J Rheumatol. 1999;26(8):1746–51. http://www.ncbi.nlm.nih.gov/pubmed/10451072. Accessed April 21, 2015.
55. Taylor W, Gladman D, Helliwell P, Marchesoni A, Mease P, Mielants H. Classification criteria for psoriatic arthritis: development of new criteria

from a large international study. Arthritis Rheum. 2006;54(8):2665–73. https://doi.org/10.1002/art.21972.
56. Gladman DDRP. Psoriatic arthritis. In: Ruddy S, Harris Jr E, Sledge C, editors. Kelly's textbook of rheumatology. 6th ed. Philadelphia: WB Saunders Company; 2001. p. 1071–9.
57. Daunt AO, Cox NL, Robertson JC, Cawley MI. Indices of disease activity in psoriatic arthritis. J R Soc Med. 1987;80(9):556–8.
58. Helliwell PS, Marchesoni A, Peters M, Platt R, Wright V. Cytidine deaminase activity, C reactive protein, histidine, and erythrocyte sedimentation rate as measures of disease activity in psoriatic arthritis. Ann Rheum Dis. 1991;50(6):362–5. http://www.pubmedcentral.nih.gov/articlerender.fcgi?artid=1004437&tool=pmcentrez&rendertype=abstract. Accessed April 21, 2015.
59. Johnson SR, Schentag CT, Gladman DD. Autoantibodies in biological agent naive patients with psoriatic arthritis. Ann Rheum Dis. 2005;64(5):770–2. https://doi.org/10.1136/ard.2004.031286.
60. Bogliolo L, Alpini C, Caporali R, Scirè CA, Moratti R, Montecucco C. Antibodies to cyclic citrullinated peptides in psoriatic arthritis. J Rheumatol. 2005;32(3):511–5.
61. Vander Cruyssen B, Hoffman IEA, Zmierczak H, et al. Anti-citrullinated peptide antibodies may occur in patients with psoriatic arthritis. Ann Rheum Dis. 2005;64(8):1145–9. https://doi.org/10.1136/ard.2004.032177.
62. Payet J, Goulvestre C, Bialé L, Avouac J, Wipff J, Job-Deslandre C, Batteux F, Dougados M, Kahan AAY. Anticyclic citrullinated peptide antibodies in rheumatoid and nonrheumatoid rheumatic disorders: experience with 1162 patients. J Rheumatol. 2014;41(12):2395–402.
63. Reddy SM, Anandarajah AP, Fisher MC, Mease PJ, Greenberg JD, Kremer JM, Reed G, Chen R, Messing S, Kaukeinen KRC. Comparative analysis of disease activity measures, use of biologic agents, body mass index, radiographic features, and bone density in psoriatic arthritis and rheumatoid arthritis patients followed in a large U.S. disease registry. J Rheumatol. 2010;37(12):2566–72.
64. Siannis F, Farewell VT, Cook RJ, Schentag CT, Gladman DD. Clinical and radiological damage in psoriatic arthritis. Ann Rheum Dis. 2006;65(4):478–81. https://doi.org/10.1136/ard.2005.039826.
65. Williamson L, Dockerty JL, Dalbeth N, McNally E, Ostlere S, Wordsworth BP. Clinical assessment of sacroiliitis and HLA-B27 are poor predictors of sacroiliitis diagnosed by magnetic resonance imaging in psoriatic arthritis. Rheumatology. 2004;43(1):85–8. https://doi.org/10.1093/rheumatology/keg475.
66. Khraishi M, Mong J, Mugford GLI. The electronic Psoriasis and Arthritis Screening Questionnaire (ePASQ): a sensitive and specific tool to diagnose psoriatic arthritis patients. J Cutan Med Surg. 2011;15(3):143–9.
67. Ibrahim GH, Buch MH, Lawson C, Waxman R, Helliwell PS. Evaluation of an existing screening tool for psoriatic arthritis in people with psoriasis and the development of a new instrument: The Psoriasis Epidemiology Screening Tool (PEST) questionnaire. Clin Exp Rheumatol. 2009;27(3):469–74.
68. Husni ME, Meyer KH, Cohen DS, Mody E, Qureshi AA. The PASE questionnaire: pilot-testing a psoriatic arthritis screening and evaluation tool. J Am Acad Dermatol. 2007;57(4):581–7. https://doi.org/10.1016/j.jaad.2007.04.001.
69. Gladman DD, Schentag CT, Tom BDM, et al. Development and initial validation of a screening questionnaire for psoriatic arthritis: the Toronto Psoriatic Arthritis Screen (ToPAS). Ann Rheum Dis. 2009;68(4):497–501. https://doi.org/10.1136/ard.2008.089441.
70. Coates LC, Aslam T, Al Balushi F, et al. Comparison of three screening tools to detect psoriatic arthritis in patients with psoriasis (CONTEST study). Br J Dermatol. 2013;168(4):802–7. https://doi.org/10.1111/bjd.12190.
71. Duffin KC, Krueger GG. Genetic variations in cytokines and cytokine receptors associated with psoriasis found by genome-wide association. J Invest Dermatol. 2009;129(4):827–33. https://doi.org/10.1038/jid.2008.308.
72. Li W-Q, Han J-L, Chan AT, Qureshi A. a. Psoriasis, psoriatic arthritis and increased risk of incident Crohn's disease in US women. Ann Rheum Dis. 2013;72(7):1200–5. https://doi.org/10.1136/annrheumdis-2012-202143.
73. Scarpa R, Manguso F, D'Arienzo A, et al. Microscopic inflammatory changes in colon of patients with both active psoriasis and psoriatic arthritis without bowel symptoms. J Rheumatol. 2000;27(5):1241–6.
74. Michaëlsson G, Gerdén B, Hagforsen E, et al. Psoriasis patients with antibodies to gliadin can be improved by a gluten-free diet. Br J Dermatol. 2000;142(1):44–51. http://www.ncbi.nlm.nih.gov/pubmed/10651693. Accessed March 30, 2015.
75. Bhatia BK, Millsop JW, Debbaneh M, Koo J, Linos E, Liao W. Diet and psoriasis, part II: celiac disease and role of a gluten-free diet. J Am Acad Dermatol. 2014;71(2):350–8. https://doi.org/10.1016/j.jaad.2014.03.017.
76. Campanati A, Neri P, Giuliodori K, et al. Psoriasis beyond the skin surface: a pilot study on the ocular involvement. Int Ophthalmol. 2015;35(3):331–40. https://doi.org/10.1007/s10792-014-9950-8.
77. Lambert JR, Wright V. Eye inflammation in psoriatic arthritis. Ann Rheum Dis. 1976;35(4):354–6. https://doi.org/10.1136/ard.35.4.354.
78. Zeboulon N, Dougados M, Gossec L. Prevalence and characteristics of uveitis in the spondyloarthropathies: a systematic literature review. Ann Rheum

Dis. 2008;67(7):955–9. https://doi.org/10.1136/ard.2007.075754.
79. Poikolainen K, Reunala T, Karvonen J, Lauharanta J, Kärkkäinen P. Alcohol intake: a risk factor for psoriasis in young and middle aged men? BMJ. 1990;300(6727):780–3. http://www.pubmedcentral.nih.gov/articlerender.fcgi?artid=1662565&tool=pmcentrez&rendertype=abstract. Accessed March 27, 2015.
80. Dowlatshahi EA, Wakkee M, Arends LR, Nijsten T. The prevalence and odds of depressive symptoms and clinical depression in psoriasis patients: a systematic review and meta-analysis. J Invest Dermatol. 2014;134(6):1542–51. https://doi.org/10.1038/jid.2013.508.
81. Armstrong AW. Psoriasis and the risk of diabetes mellitus a systematic review and meta-analysis psoriasis and the risk of diabetes mellitus. Arch Dermatol. 2012; https://doi.org/10.1001/2013.jamadermatol.406.
82. Dreiher J, Freud T, Cohen AD. Psoriatic arthritis and diabetes: a population-based cross-sectional study. Dermatol Res Pract. 2013;(2013) https://doi.org/10.1155/2013/580404.
83. Ogdie A, Yu Y, Haynes K, et al. Risk of major cardiovascular events in patients with psoriatic arthritis, psoriasis and rheumatoid arthritis: a population-based cohort study. Ann Rheum Dis. 2015;74(2):326–32. https://doi.org/10.1136/annrheumdis-2014-205675.
84. Pina T, Genre F, Lopez-Mejias R, et al. Relationship of leptin with adiposity and inflammation and Resistin with disease severity in psoriatic patients undergoing anti-TNF-alpha therapy. J Eur Acad Dermatol Venereol. 2015; https://doi.org/10.1111/jdv.13131.
85. Bhole VM, Choi HK, Burns LC, et al. Differences in body mass index among individuals with PsA, psoriasis, RA and the general population. Rheumatology. 2012;51(3):552–6. https://doi.org/10.1093/rheumatology/ker349.
86. Love TJ, Zhu Y, Zhang Y, et al. Obesity and the risk of psoriatic arthritis: a population-based study. Ann Rheum Dis. 2012;71(8):1273–7. https://doi.org/10.1136/annrhcumdis-2012-201299.
87. Li W, Han J, Qureshi AA. Obesity and risk of incident psoriatic arthritis in US women. Ann Rheum Dis. 2012;71(8):1267–72. https://doi.org/10.1136/annrheumdis-2011-201273.
88. Di Minno MND, Peluso R, Iervolino S, Russolillo A, Lupoli R, Scarpa R. Weight loss and achievement of minimal disease activity in patients with psoriatic arthritis starting treatment with tumour necrosis factor α blockers. Ann Rheum Dis. 2014;73(6):1157–62. https://doi.org/10.1136/annrheumdis-2012-202812.
89. Rosenberg P, Urwitz H, Johannesson A, et al. Psoriasis patients with diabetes type 2 are at high risk of developing liver fibrosis during methotrexate treatment. J Hepatol. 2007;46:1111–8. https://doi.org/10.1016/j.jhep.2007.01.024.
90. Puzenat E, Bronsard V, Prey S, et al. What are the best outcome measures for assessing plaque psoriasis severity? A systematic review of the literature. J Eur Acad Dermatol Venereol. 2010;24(Suppl 2):10–6. https://doi.org/10.1111/j.1468-3083.2009.03562.x.
91. Aktan S, Ilknur T, Akin C, Ozkan S. Interobserver reliability of the nail psoriasis severity index. Clin Exp Dermatol. 2007;32(2):141–4. https://doi.org/10.1111/j.1365-2230.2006.02305.x.
92. Felson DT, Anderson JJ, Boers M, et al. American College of Rheumatology preliminary definition of improvement in rheumatoid arthritis. Arthritis Rheum. 1995;38(6):727–35. https://doi.org/10.1002/art.1780380602.
93. Kaltwasser JP, Nash P, Gladman D, et al. Efficacy and safety of leflunomide in the treatment of psoriatic arthritis and psoriasis: a multinational, double-blind, randomized, placebo-controlled clinical trial. Arthritis Rheum. 2004;50(6):1939–50. https://doi.org/10.1002/art.20253.
94. Mease PJ, Kivitz AJ, Burch FX, et al. Etanercept treatment of psoriatic arthritis: safety, efficacy, and effect on disease progression. Arthritis Rheum. 2004;50(7):2264–72. https://doi.org/10.1002/art.20335.
95. Piet LCM, van Gestel AM, Scott DL. EULAR handbook of clinical assessments in rheumatoid arthritis. Alphen Aan Den Rijn: Van Zuiden Communications B.V; 2000.
96. Antoni CE, Kavanaugh A, Kirkham B, et al. Sustained benefits of infliximab therapy for dermatologic and articular manifestations of psoriatic arthritis: results from the infliximab multinational psoriatic arthritis controlled trial (IMPACT). Arthritis Rheum. 2005;52(4):1227–36. https://doi.org/10.1002/art.20967.
97. Clegg DO, Reda DJ, Abdellatif M. Comparison of sulfasalazine and placebo for the treatment of axial and peripheral articular manifestations of the seronegative spondylarthropathies: a Department of Veterans Affairs Cooperative Study. Arthritis Rheum. 1999;42(11):2325–9. https://doi.org/10.1002/1529-0131(199911)42:11<2325::AID-ANR10>3.0.CO;2-C.
98. Helliwell PS, Kavanaugh A. Comparison of composite measures of disease activity in psoriatic arthritis using data from an interventional study with golimumab. Arthritis Care Res. 2014;66(5):749–56. https://doi.org/10.1002/acr.22204.
99. Coates LC, Fransen J, Helliwell PS. Defining minimal disease activity in psoriatic arthritis: a proposed objective target for treatment. Ann Rheum Dis. 2010;69(1):48–53. https://doi.org/10.1136/ard.2008.102053.
100. Coates LC, Helliwell PS. Validation of minimal disease activity criteria for psoriatic arthritis using interventional trial data. Arthritis Care Res. 2010;62(7):965–9. https://doi.org/10.1002/acr.20155.

101. Coates LC, Navarro-Coy N, Brown SR, et al. The TICOPA protocol (TIght COntrol of psoriatic arthritis): a randomised controlled trial to compare intensive management versus standard care in early psoriatic arthritis. BMC Musculoskelet Disord. 2013;14:101. https://doi.org/10.1186/1471-2474-14-101.
102. Coates LC, Moverley AR, McParland L, et al. Results of of a randomised controlled trial comparing tight control of early psoriatic arthritis (TICOPA) with standard care: tight control improves outcomes. Arthritis Rheum. 2013;65(Supp):S346.
103. Debbaneh M, Millsop JW, Bhatia BK, Koo J, Liao W. Diet and psoriasis, part I: impact of weight loss interventions. J Am Acad Dermatol. 2014; https://doi.org/10.1016/j.jaad.2014.02.012.
104. Naldi L, Conti A, Cazzaniga S, et al. Diet and physical exercise in psoriasis: a randomized controlled trial. Br J Dermatol. 2014;170(3):634–42. https://doi.org/10.1111/bjd.12735.
105. Eder L, Thavaneswaran A, Chandran V, Cook RJ, Gladman D. Obesity is associated with a lower probability of achieving sustained minimal disease activity state among patients with psoriatic arthritis. Ann Rheum Dis. 2015;74:813–7.
106. Michaëlsson G, Gustafsson K, Hagforsen E. The psoriasis variant palmoplantar pustulosis can be improved after cessation of smoking. J Am Acad Dermatol. 2006;54(4):737–8. https://doi.org/10.1016/j.jaad.2005.07.024.
107. Mason A, Mason J, Cork M, Hancock H, Dooley G. Topical treatments for chronic plaque psoriasis: an abridged Cochrane systematic review. J Am Acad Dermatol. 2013;69(5):799–807. https://doi.org/10.1016/j.jaad.2013.06.027.
108. van de Kerkhof PCM. An update on topical therapies for mild-moderate psoriasis. Dermatol Clin. 2015;33(1):73–7. https://doi.org/10.1016/j.det.2014.09.006.
109. Chen X, Yang M, Cheng Y, Liu GJ, Zhang M. Narrow-band ultraviolet B phototherapy versus broad-band ultraviolet B or psoralen-ultraviolet a photochemotherapy for psoriasis. Cochrane Database Syst Rev. 2013;10:CD009481. https://doi.org/10.1002/14651858.CD009481.pub2.
110. Menter A, Korman NJ, Elmets CA, et al. Guidelines of care for the management of psoriasis and psoriatic arthritis: section 5. Guidelines of care for the treatment of psoriasis with phototherapy and photochemotherapy. J Am Acad Dermatol. 2010;62(1):114–35. https://doi.org/10.1016/j.jaad.2009.08.026.
111. Sarzi-Puttini P, Santandrea S, Boccassini L, Panni B, Caruso I. The role of NSAIDs in psoriatic arthritis: Evidence from a controlled study with nimesulide. Clin Exp Rheumatol. 2001;19(1 SUPPL. 22):S17.
112. Brenner M, Molin S, Ruebsam K, Weisenseel P, Ruzicka TPJ. Generalized pustular psoriasis induced by systemic glucocorticosteroids: four cases and recommendations for treatment. Br J Dermatol. 2009;161(4):964–6.
113. Eder L, Chandran V, Ueng J, et al. Predictors of response to intra-articular steroid injection in psoriatic arthritis. Rheumatology. 2010;49(7):1367–73. https://doi.org/10.1093/rheumatology/keq102.
114. Tian H, Cronstein BN. Understanding the mechanisms of action of methotrexate: implications for the treatment of rheumatoid arthritis. Bull NYU Hosp Jt Dis. 2007;65(3):168–73.
115. Flytström I, Stenberg B, Svensson A, Bergbrant I-M. Methotrexate vs. ciclosporin in psoriasis: effectiveness, quality of life and safety. A randomized controlled trial. Br J Dermatol. 2008;158(1):116–21. https://doi.org/10.1111/j.1365-2133.2007.08284.x.
116. Ps H, Wj T. Treatment of psoriatic arthritis and rheumatoid arthritis with disease modifying. J Rheumatol. 2008;35:472–6.
117. Soriano ER. The actual role of therapy with traditional disease-modifying antirheumatic drugs in psoriatic arthritis. J Rheumatol. 2012;39:67–70. https://doi.org/10.3899/jrheum.120248.
118. Ceponis A, Kavanaugh A. Use of methotrexate in patients with psoriatic arthritis. Clin Exp Rheumatol. 2010;28(5 SUPPL. 61):S132.
119. Chandran V, Schentag CT, Gladman DD. Reappraisal of the effectiveness of methotrexate in psoriatic arthritis: results from a longitudinal observational cohort. J Rheumatol. 2008;35(3):469–71. doi:07/13/1217 [pii].
120. Kingsley GH, Kowalczyk A, Taylor H, et al. A randomized placebo-controlled trial of methotrexate in psoriatic arthritis. Rheumatology (Oxford). 2012;51(8):1368–77. https://doi.org/10.1093/rheumatology/kes001.
121. Baranauskaite A, Raffayova H, Kungurov N, et al. Infliximab plus methotrexate is superior to methotrexate alone in the treatment of psoriatic arthritis in methotrexate-naive patients: the RESPOND study. Ann Rheum Dis. 2012;71(4):541–8. https://doi.org/10.1136/ard.2011.152223.
122. Singh JA, Guyatt G, Ogdie A, Gladman DD, Deal C, et al. 2018 American College of Rheumatology/National Psoriasis Foundation guideline for the treatment of psoriatic arthritis. Arthritis Care Res. 2019;71:2–29. https://doi.org/10.1002/acr.23789.
123. Mease PG, Gladnman DD, Collier DH, Ritchlin CT, Helliwell PS, Liu L, et al. Etanercept and methotrexate as monotherapy or in combination for psoriatic arthritis: primary results from a randomized, controlled phase III trial. Arthritis Rheumatol. 2019;71:1112–24.
124. Maybury CM, Samarasekera E, Douiri A, Barker JN, Smith CH. Diagnostic accuracy of noninvasive markers of liver fibrosis in patients with psoriasis taking methotrexate: a systematic review and meta-analysis. Br J Dermatol. 2014;170(6):1237–47. https://doi.org/10.1111/bjd.12905.
125. Yélamos O, Puig L. Systemic methotrexate for the treatment of psoriasis. Expert Rev Clin Immunol. 2015:1–11. https://doi.org/10.1586/1744666X.2015.1026894.

126. Nash P, Thaçi D, Behrens F, Falk F, Kaltwasser JP. Leflunomide improves psoriasis in patients with psoriatic arthritis: an in-depth analysis of data from the TOPAS study. Dermatology. 2006;212(3):238–49. https://doi.org/10.1159/000091251.
127. Niu X, Cao W, Ma H, Feng J, Li X, Zhang X. Acitretin exerted a greater influence on T-helper (Th)1 and Th17 than on Th2 cells in treatment of psoriasis vulgaris. J Dermatol. 2012;39(11):916–21. https://doi.org/10.1111/j.1346-8138.2012.01637.x.
128. Gollnick H, Bauer R, Brindley C, et al. Acitretin versus etretinate in psoriasis. Clinical and pharmacokinetic results of a German multicenter study. J Am Acad Dermatol. 1988;19(3):458–68. http://www.ncbi.nlm.nih.gov/pubmed/2971692. Accessed April 4, 2015.
129. Spuls PI, Rozenblit M, Lebwohl M. Retrospective study of the efficacy of narrowband UVB and acitretin. J Dermatolog Treat. 2003;14(Suppl 2):17–20. http://www.ncbi.nlm.nih.gov/pubmed/14578094. Accessed April 4, 2015.
130. Sbidian E, Maza A, Montaudié H, et al. Efficacy and safety of oral retinoids in different psoriasis subtypes: a systematic literature review. J Eur Acad Dermatol Venereol. 2011;25(Suppl 2):28–33. https://doi.org/10.1111/j.1468-3083.2011.03993.x.
131. Menter A, Korman NJ, Elmets CA, et al. Guidelines of care for the management of psoriasis and psoriatic arthritis: section 4. Guidelines of care for the management and treatment of psoriasis with traditional systemic agents. J Am Acad Dermatol. 2009;61(3):451–85. https://doi.org/10.1016/j.jaad.2009.03.027.
132. Foroncewicz B, Mucha K, Lerut J, Majewski S, Krawczyk M, Pączek L. Cyclosporine is superior to tacrolimus in liver transplant recipients with recurrent psoriasis. Ann Transplant. 2014;19:427–33. https://doi.org/10.12659/AOT.890754.
133. Maza A, Montaudié H, Sbidian E, et al. Oral cyclosporin in psoriasis: a systematic review on treatment modalities, risk of kidney toxicity and evidence for use in non-plaque psoriasis. J Eur Acad Dermatol Venereol. 2011;25:19–27. https://doi.org/10.1111/j.1468-3083.2011.03992.x.
134. Papp K, Cather JC, Rosoph L, et al. Efficacy of apremilast in the treatment of moderate to severe psoriasis: a randomised controlled trial. Lancet. 2012;380(9843):738–46. https://doi.org/10.1016/S0140-6736(12)60642-4.
135. Kavanaugh A, Mease PJ, Gomez-Reino JJ, et al. Treatment of psoriatic arthritis in a phase 3 randomised, placebo-controlled trial with apremilast, an oral phosphodiesterase 4 inhibitor. Ann Rheum Dis. 2014;73(6):1020–6. https://doi.org/10.1136/annrheumdis-2013-205056.
136. Kavanaugh A, Mease PJ, Gomez-Reino JJ, et al. Longterm (52-week) results of a phase III randomized, controlled trial of apremilast in patients with psoriatic arthritis. J Rheumatol. 2015;42(3):479–88.
137. Thorlund K, Druyts E, Aviña-Zubieta JA, Mills EJ. Anti-tumor necrosis factor (TNF) drugs for the treatment of psoriatic arthritis: an indirect comparison meta-analysis. Biol Targets Ther. 2012;6:417–27. https://doi.org/10.2147/BTT.S37606.
138. Papp KA, Tyring S, Lahfa M, et al. A global phase III randomized controlled trial of etanercept in psoriasis: safety, efficacy, and effect of dose reduction. Br J Dermatol. 2005;152(6):1304–12. https://doi.org/10.1111/j.1365-2133.2005.06688.x.
139. Bagel J, Lynde C, Tyring S, Kricorian G, Shi Y, Klekotka P. Moderate to severe plaque psoriasis with scalp involvement: a randomized, double-blind, placebo-controlled study of etanercept. J Am Acad Dermatol. 2012;67(1):86–92. https://doi.org/10.1016/j.jaad.2011.07.034.
140. Ortonne JP, Paul C, Berardesca E, et al. A 24-week randomized clinical trial investigating the efficacy and safety of two doses of etanercept in nail psoriasis. Br J Dermatol. 2013;168(5):1080–7. https://doi.org/10.1111/bjd.12060.
141. Paller AS, Siegfried EC, Langley RG, et al. Etanercept treatment for children and adolescents with plaque psoriasis. N Engl J Med. 2008;358(3):241–51. https://doi.org/10.1056/NEJMoa066886.
142. Menter A, Tyring SK, Gordon K, et al. Adalimumab therapy for moderate to severe psoriasis: a randomized, controlled phase III trial. J Am Acad Dermatol. 2008;58(1):106–15. https://doi.org/10.1016/j.jaad.2007.09.010.
143. Saurat J-H, Stingl G, Dubertret L, et al. Efficacy and safety results from the randomized controlled comparative study of adalimumab vs. methotrexate vs. placebo in patients with psoriasis (CHAMPION). Br J Dermatol. 2008;158(3):558–66. https://doi.org/10.1111/j.1365-2133.2007.08315.x.
144. Thaçi D, Unnebrink K, Sundaram M, Sood S, Yamaguchi Y. Adalimumab for the treatment of moderate to severe psoriasis: subanalysis of effects on scalp and nails in the BELIEVE study. J Eur Acad Dermatol Venereol. 2015;29(2):353–60. https://doi.org/10.1111/jdv.12553.
145. Mease PJ, Gladman DD, Ritchlin CT, et al. Adalimumab for the treatment of patients with moderately to severely active psoriatic arthritis: results of a double-blind, randomized, placebo-controlled trial. Arthritis Rheum. 2005;52(10):3279–89. https://doi.org/10.1002/art.21306.
146. Gladman DD, Mease PJ, Ritchlin CT, et al. Adalimumab for long-term treatment of psoriatic arthritis: forty-eight week data from the adalimumab effectiveness in psoriatic arthritis trial. Arthritis Rheum. 2007;56(2):476–88. https://doi.org/10.1002/art.22379.
147. Genovese MC, Mease PJ, Thomson GTD, et al. Safety and efficacy of adalimumab in treatment of patients with psoriatic arthritis who had failed disease modifying antirheumatic drug therapy. J Rheumatol. 2007;34:1040.

148. Oh CJ, Das KM, Gottlieb AB. Treatment with anti-tumor necrosis factor alpha (TNF-alpha) monoclonal antibody dramatically decreases the clinical activity of psoriasis lesions. J Am Acad Dermatol. 2000;42(5 Pt 1):829–30. http://www.ncbi.nlm.nih.gov/pubmed/10775863. Accessed March 27, 2015.
149. Gottlieb AB, Evans R, Li S, et al. Infliximab induction therapy for patients with severe plaque-type psoriasis: a randomized, double-blind, placebo-controlled trial. J Am Acad Dermatol. 2004;51(4):534–42. https://doi.org/10.1016/j.jaad.2004.02.021.
150. de Vries ACQ, Bogaards NA, Hooft L, et al. Interventions for nail psoriasis. Cochrane Database Syst Rev. 2013;1:CD007633. https://doi.org/10.1002/14651858.CD007633.pub2.
151. Antoni C, Krueger GG, de Vlam K, et al. Infliximab improves signs and symptoms of psoriatic arthritis: results of the IMPACT 2 trial. Ann Rheum Dis. 2005;64:1150. https://doi.org/10.1136/ard.2004.032268.
152. Kavanaugh A, Antoni CE, Gladman D, et al. The infliximab multinational psoriatic arthritis controlled trial (IMPACT): results of radiographic analyses after 1 year. Ann Rheum Dis. 2006;65(8):1038–43. https://doi.org/10.1136/ard.2005.045658.
153. Kavanaugh A, McInnes I, Mease P, Krueger GG, Gladman D, Gomez-Reino J, Papp K, Zrubek J, Mudivarthy S, Mack M, Visvanathan SBA. Golimumab, a new human tumor necrosis factor alpha antibody, administered every four weeks as a subcutaneous injection in psoriatic arthritis: twenty-four-week efficacy and safety results of a randomized, placebo-controlled study. Arthritis Rheum. 2010;62(8):2555.
154. Kavanaugh A, Van Der Heijde D, McInnes IB, et al. Golimumab in psoriatic arthritis: one-year clinical efficacy, radiographic, and safety results from a phase III, randomized, placebo-controlled trial. Arthritis Rheum. 2012;64(8):2504–17. https://doi.org/10.1002/art.34436.
155. Kavanaugh A, Husni ME, Harrison DD, Kim L, Lo KH, Leu JH, et al. Safety and efficacy of intravenous golimumab in patients with active psoriatic arthritis: results through week twenty-four of the GO-VIBRANT study. Arthritis Rheumatol. 2017;69(11):2151–61.
156. Kavanaugh A, McInnes I, Mease P, et al. Golimumab, a new human tumor necrosis factor alpha antibody, administered every four weeks as a subcutaneous injection in psoriatic arthritis: twenty-four-week efficacy and safety results of a randomized, placebo-controlled study. Arthritis Rheum. 2009;60(4):976–86. https://doi.org/10.1002/art.24403.
157. Mease PJ, Fleischmann R, Deodhar AA, et al. Effect of certolizumab pegol on signs and symptoms in patients with psoriatic arthritis: 24-week results of a phase 3 double-blind randomised placebo-controlled study (RAPID-PsA). Ann Rheum Dis. 2014;73(1):48–55. https://doi.org/10.1136/annrheumdis-2013-203696.
158. Reich K, Ortonne J-P, Gottlieb AB, et al. Successful treatment of moderate to severe plaque psoriasis with the PEGylated Fab' certolizumab pegol: results of a phase II randomized, placebo-controlled trial with a re-treatment extension. Br J Dermatol. 2012;167(1):180–90. https://doi.org/10.1111/j.1365-2133.2012.10941.x.
159. Gottlieb A, Blauvelt A, Thaçi D, Leonardi CL, Poulin Y, et al. Certolizumabpegol for the treatment of chronic plaque psoriasis: results through 48 weeks from 2 phase 3, multicenter, randomized, double-blinded, placebo-controlled studies (CIMPASI-1 and CIMPASI-2). J Am AcadDermatol. 2018;79(2):302–14.
160. Fagerli KM, Lie E, van der Heijde D, Heiberg MS, Lexberg AS, Rødevand E, Kalstad S, Mikkelsen K, Kvien TK. The role of methotrexate co-medication in TNF-inhibitor treatment in patients with psoriatic arthritis: results from 440 patients included in the NOR-DMARD study. Ann Rheum Dis. 2014 Jan;73(1):132–7.
161. Galloway JB, Hyrich KL, Mercer LK, et al. Anti-TNF therapy is associated with an increased risk of serious infections in patients with rheumatoid arthritis especially in the first 6 months of treatment: updated results from the British Society for Rheumatology Biologics Register with special emph. Rheumatology (Oxford). 2011;50(1):124–31. https://doi.org/10.1093/rheumatology/keq242.
162. Dixon WG, Hyrich KL, Watson KD, et al. Drug-specific risk of tuberculosis in patients with rheumatoid arthritis treated with anti-TNF therapy: results from the British Society for Rheumatology Biologics Register (BSRBR). Ann Rheum Dis. 2010;69(3):522–8. https://doi.org/10.1136/ard.2009.118935.
163. Galloway JB, Mercer LK, Moseley A, et al. Risk of skin and soft tissue infections (including shingles) in patients exposed to anti-tumour necrosis factor therapy: results from the British Society for Rheumatology biologics register. Ann Rheum Dis. 2013;72(2):229–34. https://doi.org/10.1136/annrheumdis-2011-201108.
164. Semble AL, Davis SA, Feldman SR. Safety and tolerability of tumor necrosis factor-α inhibitors in psoriasis: a narrative review. Am J Clin Dermatol. 2014;15(1):37–43. https://doi.org/10.1007/s40257-013-0053-5.
165. Solomon DH, Massarotti E, Garg R, Liu J, Canning C, Schneeweiss S. Association between disease-modifying antirheumatic drugs and diabetes risk in patients with rheumatoid arthritis and psoriasis. JAMA. 2011;305(24):2525–31. https://doi.org/10.1001/jama.2011.878.
166. Wu JJ, Poon K-YT, Channual JC, Shen AY-J. Association between tumor necrosis factor inhibitor therapy and myocardial infarction

risk in patients with psoriasis. Arch Dermatol. 2012;148(11):1244–50. https://doi.org/10.1001/archdermatol.2012.2502.
167. Leonardi CL, Kimball AB, Papp KA, et al. Efficacy and safety of ustekinumab, a human interleukin-12/23 monoclonal antibody, in patients with psoriasis: 76-week results from a randomised, double-blind, placebo-controlled trial (PHOENIX 1). Lancet. 2008;371(9625):1665–74. https://doi.org/10.1016/S0140-6736(08)60725-4.
168. Papp KA, Langley RG, Lebwohl M, et al. Efficacy and safety of ustekinumab, a human interleukin-12/23 monoclonal antibody, in patients with psoriasis: 52-week results from a randomised, double-blind, placebo-controlled trial (PHOENIX 2). Lancet. 2008;371(9625):1675–84. https://doi.org/10.1016/S0140-6736(08)60726-6.
169. Rich P, Bourcier M, Sofen H, et al. Ustekinumab improves nail disease in patients with moderate-to-severe psoriasis: results from PHOENIX 1. Br J Dermatol. 2014;170(2):398–407. https://doi.org/10.1111/bjd.12632.
170. Griffiths CEM, Strober BE, van de Kerkhof P, et al. Comparison of ustekinumab and etanercept for moderate-to-severe psoriasis. N Engl J Med. 2010;362(2):118–28. https://doi.org/10.1056/NEJMoa0810652.
171. McInnes IB, Kavanaugh A, Gottlieb AB, et al. Efficacy and safety of ustekinumab in patients with active psoriatic arthritis: 1 year results of the phase 3, multicentre, double-blind, placebo-controlled PSUMMIT 1 trial. Lancet. 2013;382(9894):780–9. https://doi.org/10.1016/S0140-6736(13)60594-2.
172. Ritchlin C, Rahman P, Kavanaugh A, McInnes IB, Puig L, Li S, Wang Y, Shen YK, Doyle MK, Mendelsohn AMGAP. 2 SG. Efficacy and safety of the anti-IL-12/23 p40 monoclonal antibody, ustekinumab, in patients with active psoriatic arthritis despite conventional non-biological and biological anti-tumour necrosis factor therapy: 6-month and 1-year results of the phase 3, m. Ann Rheum Dis. 2014;73(6):990–9.
173. Kavanaugh A, Ritchlin C, Rahman P, Puig L, Gottlieb AB, Li S, Wang Y, Noonan L, Brodmerkel C, Song M, Mendelsohn AM. MIP-1 and 2 SG. Ustekinumab, an anti-IL-12/23 p40 monoclonal antibody, inhibits radiographic progression in patients with active psoriatic arthritis: results of an integrated analysis of radiographic data from the phase 3, multicentre, randomised, double-blind, placebo-c. Ann Rheum Dis. 2014;73(6):1000–6.
174. NCT02438787. A study to evaluate the efficacy and safety of ustekinumab in the treatment of anti-TNF(alpha) refractory participants with active radiographic axial spondyloarthritis. 2018. "https://clinicaltrials.gov/ct2/show/NCT02438787" https://clinicaltrials.gov/ct2/show/NCT02438787. -NCT02407223. An efficacy and safety study of ustekinumab in participants with active nonradiographic axial spondyloarthritis. 2018. HYPERLINK https://clinicaltrials.gov/ct2/show/NCT02407223 https://clinicaltrials.gov/ct2/show/NCT02407223.
175. Blauvelt A, Papp KA, Griffiths CEM, et al. Efficacy and safety of guselkumab, an anti-interleukin-23 monoclonal antibody, compared with adalimumab for the continuous treatment of patients with moderate to severe psoriasis: results from the phase III, double-blinded, placebo- and active comparator–controlled VOYAGE 1 trial. J Am Acad Dermatol. 2017;76(3):405–17. https://doi.org/10.1016/j.jaad.2016.11.041.
176. Langley RG, Tsai T-F, Flavin S, et al. Efficacy and safety of guselkumab in patients with psoriasis who have an inadequate response to ustekinumab: results of the randomized, double-blind, phase III NAVIGATE trial. Br J Dermatol. 2018;178(1):114–23. https://doi.org/10.1111/bjd.15750.
177. Deodhar A, Gottlieb AB, Boehncke WH, Dong B, Wang Y, Zhuang Y, et al. Efficacy and safety of guselkumab in patients with active psoriatic arthritis: a randomised, double-blind, placebo-controlled, phase 2 study. Lancet. 2020;395(10230):1115–1125. https://doi.org/10.1016/S0140-6736(20)30265-8.
178. Papp KA, Blauvelt A, Bukhalo M, et al. Risankizumab versus Ustekinumab for Moderate-to-Severe Plaque Psoriasis. N Engl J Med. 2017;376(16):1551–60. https://doi.org/10.1056/NEJMoa1607017. Epub 2020 Mar 13.
179. Gordon KB, Strober B, Lebwohl M. Efficacy and safety of risankizumab in moderate-to-severe plaque psoriasis (UltIMMa-1 and UltIMMa-2): results from two double-blind, randomised, placebo-controlled and ustekinumab-controlled phase 3 trials. Lancet. 2018;392:650–61.
180. Reich K, Papp KA, Blauvelt A, et al. Tildrakizumab versus placebo or etanercept for chronic plaque psoriasis (reSURFACE 1 and reSURFACE 2): results from two randomised controlled, phase 3 trials. Lancet. 2017;390(10091):276–88. https://doi.org/10.1016/S0140-6736(17)31279-5.
181. Ryan C, Leonardi CL, Krueger JG, et al. Association between biologic therapies for chronic plaque psoriasis and cardiovascular events: a meta-analysis of randomized controlled trials. JAMA. 2011;306(8):864–71. https://doi.org/10.1001/jama.2011.1211.
182. Langley RG, Papp K, Gottlieb AB, et al. Safety results from a pooled analysis of randomized, controlled phase II and III clinical trials and interim data from an open-label extension trial of the interleukin-12/23 monoclonal antibody, briakinumab, in moderate to severe psoriasis. J Eur Acad Dermatol Venereol. 2013;27(10):1252–61. https://doi.org/10.1111/j.1468-3083.2012.04705.x.
183. Gottlieb AB, Kalb RE, Langley RG, et al. Safety observations in 12095 patients with psoriasis enrolled in an international registry (PSOLAR): experience

with infliximab and other systemic and biologic therapies. J Drugs Dermatol. 2014;13(12):1441–8. http://www.ncbi.nlm.nih.gov/pubmed/25607786. Accessed March 28, 2015.
184. van de Vosse E, Ottenhoff THM. Human host genetic factors in mycobacterial and Salmonella infection: lessons from single gene disorders in IL-12/IL-23-dependent signaling that affect innate and adaptive immunity. Microbes Infect. 2006;8(4):1167–73. https://doi.org/10.1016/j.micinf.2005.10.032.
185. Langley RG, Elewski BE, Lebwohl M, et al. Secukinumab in plaque psoriasis–results of two phase 3 trials. N Engl J Med. 2014;371(4):326–38. https://doi.org/10.1056/NEJMoa1314258.
186. Blauvelt A, Reich K, Tsai T-F, et al. Secukinumab is superior to ustekinumab in clearing skin of subjects with moderate-to-severe plaque psoriasis up to 1 year: Results from the CLEAR study. J Am Acad Dermatol. 2017;76(1):60–69.e9. https://doi.org/10.1016/j.jaad.2016.08.008.
187. McInnes IB, Mease PJ, Kirkham B, et al. Secukinumab, a human anti-interleukin-17A monoclonal antibody, in patients with psoriatic arthritis (FUTURE 2): a randomised, double-blind, placebo-controlled, phase 3 trial. Lancet. 2015;386(9999):1137–46. https://doi.org/10.1016/S0140-6736(15)61134-5.
188. Griffiths CEM, Reich K, Lebwohl M, et al. Comparison of ixekizumab with etanercept or placebo in moderate-to-severe psoriasis (UNCOVER-2 and UNCOVER-3): results from two phase 3 randomised trials. Lancet. 2015; https://doi.org/10.1016/S0140-6736(15)60125-8.
189. Gordon KB, Blauvelt A, Papp KA, et al. Phase 3 trials of Ixekizumab in moderate-to-severe plaque psoriasis. N Engl J Med. 2016;375(4):345–56. https://doi.org/10.1056/NEJMoa1512711.
190. Mease PJ, van der Heijde D, Ritchlin CT, et al. Ixekizumab, an interleukin-17A specific monoclonal antibody, for the treatment of biologic-naive patients with active psoriatic arthritis: results from the 24-week randomised, double-blind, placebo-controlled and active (adalimumab)-controlled period of the phase III trial SPIRIT-P1. Ann Rheum Dis. 2017;76(1):79–87. https://doi.org/10.1136/annrheumdis-2016-209709.
191. Papp KA, Reich K, Paul C, et al. A prospective phase III, randomized, double-blind, placebo-controlled study of brodalumab in patients with moderate-to-severe plaque psoriasis. Br J Dermatol. 2016;175(2):273–86. https://doi.org/10.1111/bjd.14493.
192. Lebwohl M, Strober B, Menter A, et al. Phase 3 studies comparing Brodalumab with Ustekinumab in psoriasis. N Engl J Med. 2015;373(14):1318–28. https://doi.org/10.1056/NEJMoa1503824.
193. Mease PJ, Genovese MC, Greenwald MW, et al. Brodalumab, an anti-IL17RA monoclonal antibody, in psoriatic arthritis. N Engl J Med. 2014;370(24):2295–306. https://doi.org/10.1056/NEJMoa1315231.
194. Leonardi C, Matheson R, Zachariae C, et al. Anti-interleukin-17 monoclonal antibody ixekizumab in chronic plaque psoriasis. N Engl J Med. 2012;366(13):1190–9. https://doi.org/10.1056/NEJMoa1109997.
195. Papp KA, Leonardi C, Menter A, et al. Brodalumab, an anti-interleukin-17-receptor antibody for psoriasis. N Engl J Med. 2012;366(13):1181–9. https://doi.org/10.1056/NEJMoa1109017.
196. Puel A, Cypowyj S, Bustamante J, et al. Chronic mucocutaneous candidiasis in humans with inborn errors of interleukin-17 immunity. Science. 2011;332(6025):65–8. https://doi.org/10.1126/science.1200439.
197. Hueber W, Sands BE, Lewitzky S, et al. Secukinumab, a human anti-IL-17A monoclonal antibody, for moderate to severe Crohn's disease:unexpected results of a randomised, double-blind placebo-controlled trial. Gut. 2012;61:1693–700.
198. Schreiber S, Colombel J-F, Feagan BG, et al. Incidence rates of inflammatory bowel disease in patients with psoriasis, psoriatic arthritis and ankylosing spondylitis treated with secukinumab: a retrospective analysis of pooled data from 21 clinical trials. Ann Rheum Dis. 2019;78:473–9.
199. Mease P, Hall S, FitzGerald O, et al. Tofacitinib or adalimumab versus placebo for psoriatic arthritis. N Engl J Med. 2017;377:1537–1550.
200. Gladman D, Rigby W, Azevedo VF, Behrens F, Blanco R, Kaszuba A, et al. Tofacitinib for psoriatic arthritis in patients with an inadequate response to TNF inhibitors. N Engl J Med. 2017;377(16):1525–36. https://doi.org/10.1056/NEJMoa1615977.
201. Wollenhaupt J, Silverfield J, Lee EB, et al. Safety and efficacy of tofacitinib, an oral janus kinase inhibitor, for the treatment of rheumatoid arthritis in open-label longterm extension studies. J Rheumatol. 2014;41(5):837–52.
202. FDA approves Boxed Warning about increased risk of blood clots and death with higher dose of arthritis and ulcerative colitis medicine tofacitinib (Xeljanz, Xeljanz XR). FDA Drug Safety Communication, 07/26/19. https://www.fda.gov/drugs/drug-safety-and-availability/fda-approves-boxed-warning-about-increased-risk-blood-clots-and-death-higher-dose-arthritis-and.
203. Mease PJ, Gottlieb AB, van der Heijde D, FitzGerald O, Johnsen A, Nys M. Efficacy and safety of abatacept, a T-cell modulator, in a randomised, double-blind, placebo-controlled, phase III study in psoriatic arthritis. Ann Rheum Dis. 2017;76(9):1550–8.
204. Mease P, Genovese MC, Gladstein G, Kivitz AJ, Ritchlin C, Tak PP, et al. Abatacept in the treatment of patients with psoriatic arthri- tis: results of a six-month, multicenter, randomized, double-blind, placebo-controlled, phase II trial. Arthritis Rheum. 2011;63(4):939–48.

205. Lubrano E, Parsons WJ, Perrotta FM. Assessment of response to treatment, remission, and minimal disease activity in axial psoriatic arthritis treated with tumor necrosis factor inhibitors. J Rheumatol. 2016;43(5):918–23.
206. Motaparthi K, Stanisic V, Van Voorhees AS, Lebwohl MG, Hsu S. From the Medical Board of the National Psoriasis Foundation: recommendations for screening for hepatitis B infection prior to initiating anti-tumor necrosis factor-alfa inhibitors or other immunosuppressive agents in patients with psoriasis. J Am Acad Dermatol. 2014;70(1):178–86. https://doi.org/10.1016/j.jaad.2013.08.049.
207. Lebwohl M, Bagel J, Gelfand JM, et al. From the Medical Board of the National Psoriasis Foundation: monitoring and vaccinations in patients treated with biologics for psoriasis. J Am Acad Dermatol. 2008;58(1):94–105. https://doi.org/10.1016/j.jaad.2007.08.030.
208. Gottlieb AB, Langley RG, Strober BE, et al. A randomized, double-blind, placebo-controlled study to evaluate the addition of methotrexate to etanercept in patients with moderate to severe plaque psoriasis. Br J Dermatol. 2012;167(3):649–57. https://doi.org/10.1111/j.1365-2133.2012.11015.x.
209. Lecluse LLA, Driessen RJB, Spuls PI, et al. Extent and clinical consequences of antibody formation against adalimumab in patients with plaque psoriasis. Arch Dermatol. 2010;146(2):127–32. https://doi.org/10.1001/archdermatol.2009.347.
210. Lynde CW, Gupta AK, Guenther L, Poulin Y, Levesque A, Bissonnette R. A randomized study comparing the combination of nbUVB and etanercept to etanercept monotherapy in patients with psoriasis who do not exhibit an excellent response after 12 weeks of etanercept. J Dermatolog Treat. 2012;23(4):261–7. https://doi.org/10.3109/09546634.2011.607795.
211. Wolf P, Weger W, Legat FJ, et al. Treatment with 311-nm ultraviolet B enhanced response of psoriatic lesions in ustekinumab-treated patients: a randomized intraindividual trial. Br J Dermatol. 2012;166(1):147–53. https://doi.org/10.1111/j.1365-2133.2011.10616.x.
212. Schett G, Hu ASR. Oral apremilast is effective with and without concomitant methotrexate therapy in the treatment of subjects with active psoriatic arthritis. Arthritis Rheum. 2011;63(10 Supp):S306.
213. Fagerli KM, Lie E, van der Heijde D, et al. The role of methotrexate co-medication in TNF-inhibitor treatment in patients with psoriatic arthritis: results from 440 patients included in the NOR-DMARD study. Ann Rheum Dis. 2014;73(1):132–7. https://doi.org/10.1136/annrheumdis-2012-202347.
214. Mease PG, Gladnman DD, Collier DH, Ritchlin CT, Helliwell PS, Liu L, et al. Etanercept and methotrexate as monotherapy or in combination for psoriatic arthritis: primary results from a randomized, controlled phase III trial. Arthritis Rheumatol. 2019;71:1112–24.
215. Thibodeaux Q, Ly K, Reddy V, et al. Dual biologic therapy for recalcitrant psoriasis and psoriatic arthritis. JAAD Case Rep. 2019;5:928–30.
216. D'Souza LS, Payette MJ. Estimated cost efficacy of systemic treatments that are approved by the US Food and Drug Administration for the treatment of moderate to severe psoriasis. J Am Acad Dermatol. 2015;72(4):589–98. https://doi.org/10.1016/j.jaad.2014.11.028.

Vasculitis

8

Robert G. Micheletti and Peter A. Merkel

Key Points

- The vasculitides are a group of diseases characterized by inflammatory destruction of blood vessels.
- While skin-limited disease is commonly encountered by the dermatologist, serious organ- and life-threatening complications can occur.
- A systematic approach to diagnosis and evaluation is required to ensure diagnostic accuracy and identify those with systemic disease who are at risk for poor outcomes.
- Inappropriate use and interpretation of laboratory tests may result in confusion and delay and should be avoided.
- Effective coordination of care with other medical providers is an essential part of successful diagnosis and management.

R. G. Micheletti (✉)
Department of Dermatology, University of Pennsylvania, Philadelphia, PA, USA
e-mail: robert.micheletti@uphs.upenn.edu

P. A. Merkel
Division of Rheumatology, University of Pennsylvania, Philadelphia, PA, USA
e-mail: pmerkel@upenn.edu

Interdisciplinary Introduction

"Vasculitis" refers to inflammation and destruction of blood vessels, which results in tissue damage. The vasculitides are a rare and heterogeneous group of diseases. Diagnosis of any particular type of vasculitis can be made based on characteristic clinical findings and histology, with careful clinicopathologic correlation. Cutaneous eruptions are frequently encountered in many types of vasculitis. The cutaneous eruption, which is highly visible and accessible for biopsy, may be the presenting sign of systemic disease and as such represents an important opportunity for diagnosis and treatment. The eruption itself is also a significant source of morbidity.

This chapter will achieve the following: (i) review the classification of vasculitis; (ii) outline the cardinal features of the major vasculitides; (iii) focus on the diagnosis and management of small-vessel vasculitis, which is encountered frequently by dermatologists, rheumatologists, and other physicians; and (iv) discuss the diagnostic approach and systemic evaluation in cases in which vasculitis is a consideration, all with the goal of improving diagnosis and management for this complex group of diseases.

A. Garg et al. (eds.), *Interdisciplinary Approaches to Overlap Disorders in Dermatology & Rheumatology*,
https://doi.org/10.1007/978-3-319-18446-3_8

Nomenclature and Classification of Vasculitis

The 2012 revised International Chapel Hill Consensus Conference nomenclature (Table 8.1) names a limited set of vasculitides described according to size of the affected blood vessels affected, which often correlates with clinical morphology [1]. Importantly, however, the Chapel Hill nomenclature is not the same as classification schema, as it does not contain diagnostic criteria. The 1990 American College of Rheumatology Classification Criteria, by contrast, include sets of clinical features (criteria) that are sensitive and specific for the most common forms of vasculitis; it remains the standard system used in research [2]. However, this schema was created before antineutrophil cytoplasmic antibody (ANCA) testing and some forms of diagnostic imaging were in widespread use, and it is currently undergoing revision [3].

While nomenclature and classification schemes have limitations, it is indeed helpful to correlate clinical manifestations of vasculitis with size of the vessels affected. It is also important to recognize that "leukocytoclastic vasculitis" is not a specific disease or diagnosis but rather one of the possible pathologic findings in vasculitis.

Pathophysiology and Clinical Features

Small-Vessel Vasculitis

Small-vessel vasculitis of the skin is commonly mediated by immune complex deposition. Circulating antigens (whether triggered by medications, infections, connective tissue disease, or neoplasia) are bound by antibodies, forming immune complexes [4]. These complexes become lodged within small vessels of the superficial dermis (which are analogous to the small branches at the top of a tree), often in dependent areas, such as the legs, or in areas of pressure. These complexes activate complement, inducing an inflammatory response that leads to vessel destruction and extravasation of red blood cells.

The lesions in small-vessel vasculitis are small, superficial, and localized to the area fed by the affected vessels. Classically, they present as crops of purpuric, round, 1-to-5 mm papules (so-called "palpable purpura"). The complement cascade and inflammation account for the palpability as well as associated symptoms, such as burn or itch. Red blood cell extravasation, meanwhile, results in purpura.

Additionally, urticarial papules, pustules, vesicles, petechiae, and erythema multiforme-like lesions may appear. When several small lesions

Table 8.1 Classification of vasculitis by vessel size

Affected vessels	Classification	Subclassification
Small	Cutaneous small vessel (leukocytoclastic) vasculitis	Idiopathic Infectious Medication exposure Inflammatory (CTD)
	Small vessel vasculitis—special types	IgA Vasculitis (Henoch-Schönlein purpura) Urticarial vasculitis Acute hemorrhagic edema of infancy Erythema elevatum diutinum
Small and medium	Cryoglobulinemic	Types II and III
	ANCA-associated	EGPA (Churg-Strauss), Microscopic Polyangiitis, GPA (Wegener)
Medium	Polyarteritis nodosa (PAN)	Benign cutaneous form Systemic form
Large	Temporal arteritis Takayasu arteritis (TAK)	

ANCA antineutrophilic cytoplasmic antibodies, *CTD* connective tissue disease, *EGPA* eosinophilic granulomatosis with polyangiitis, *GPA* granulomatosis with polyangiitis

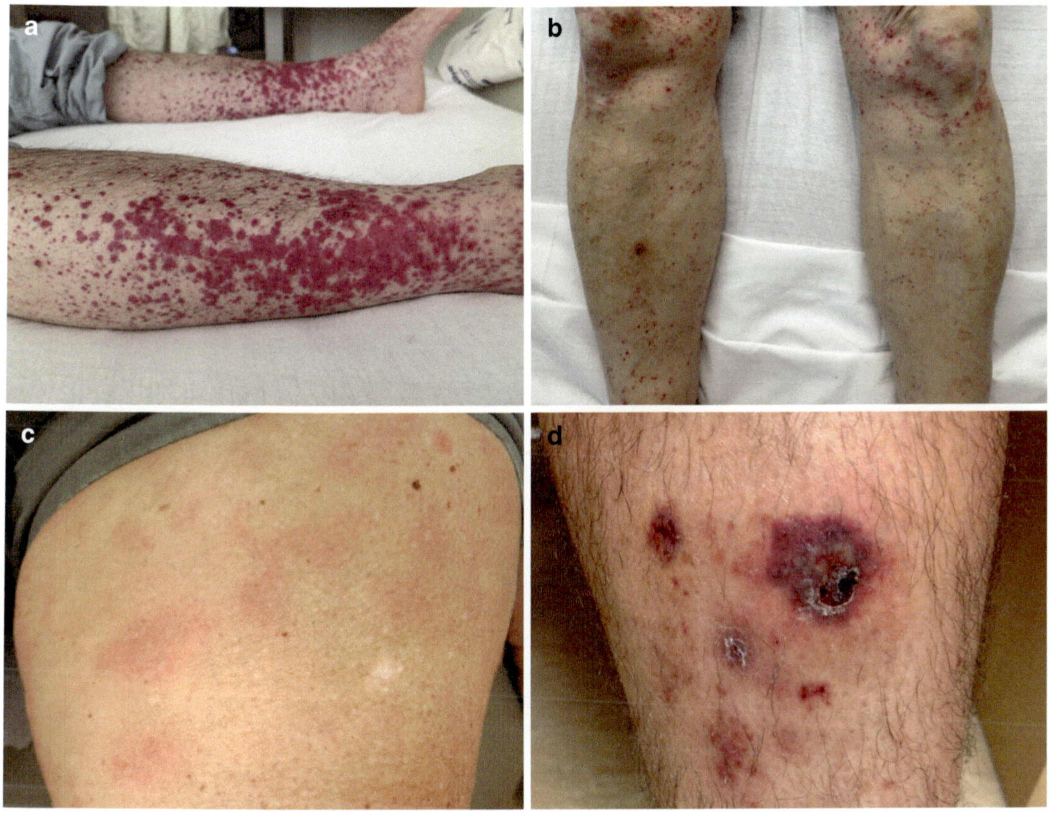

Fig. 8.1 Clinical manifestations of vasculitis involving small vessels. (**a**) Coalescing purpuric macules and papules; (**b**) Scattered purpuric macules and petechiae; (**c**) Urticarial papules; and (**d**) Rounded ulceration formed by coalescing purpuric papules

coalesce, rounded purpuric patches, plaques, or ulcers may form (Fig. 8.1). If such lesions are seen in isolation, the differential diagnosis includes cutaneous small-vessel vasculitis, IgA vasculitis (Henoch-Schönlein purpura), and urticarial vasculitis.

Medium-Vessel Vasculitis

The affected vessels in medium-vessel vasculitis are located in the deep dermis or subcutis and are analogous to the trunk of a tree. The resulting affected area includes all downstream vessels (analogous to overlying tree branches) and the tissue they supply. Cases of medium-vessel vasculitis usually involve both small- and medium-sized arteries.

Medium-vessel vasculitis of the skin manifests with lesions of larger size and more destructive potential than those seen in small-vessel vasculitis. Characteristic findings include livedo reticularis, subcutaneous nodules, retiform (or "stellate") purpura, hemorrhagic bullae, ulceration and necrosis (Fig. 8.2). Livedo reticularis is a net-like, mottled or reticulated, pink or red-blue discoloration of the skin, resulting from reduced blood flow and oxygen tension in the venous plexus of the skin. Hemorrhagic bullae, ulceration and necrosis occur due to devitalization of tissue; if necrosis or purpura occur in the livedoid areas, the terms retiform or stellate purpura may apply.

The morphologies of both livedo reticularis and retiform purpura derive from the size of the vessel involved; a single involved "trunk" may

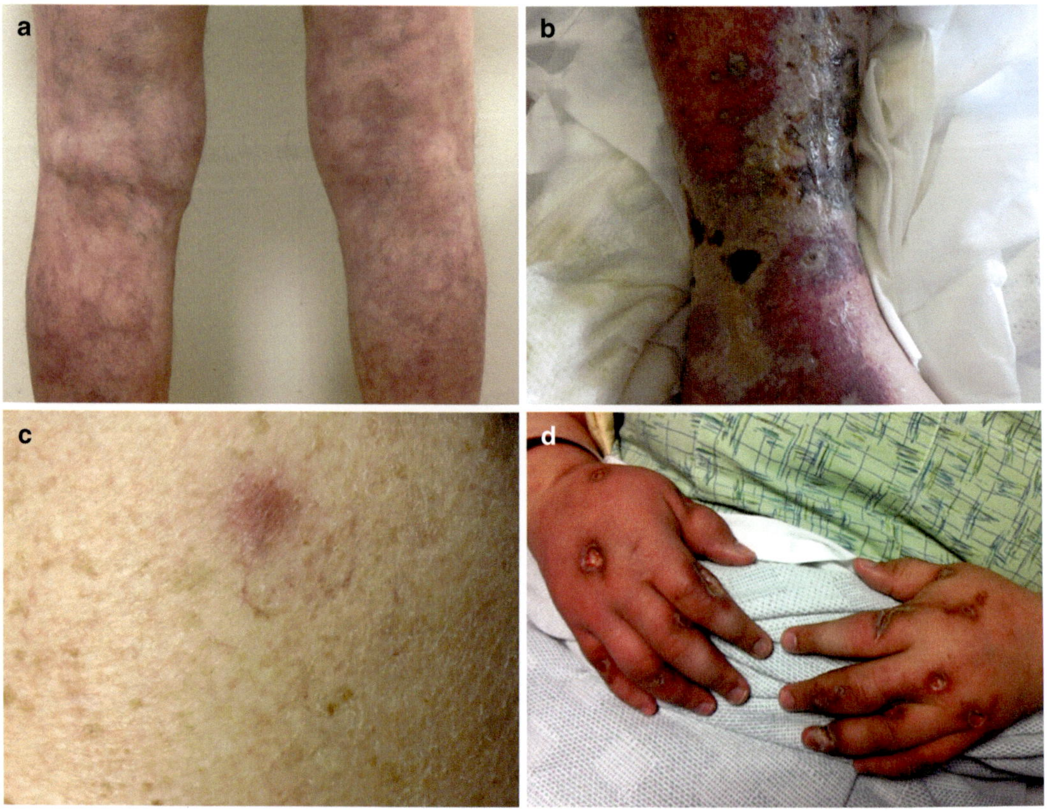

Fig. 8.2 Clinical manifestations of vasculitis involving medium-sized vessels. (**a**) Extensive livedo reticularis in a patient with eosinophilic granulomatosis with polyangiitis (Churg-Strauss); (**b**) Retiform purpura and ulceration in a patient with cryoglobulinemic vasculitis; (**c**) A tender nodule on the leg of a patient with polyarteritis nodosa (PAN); and (**d**) Digital ulceration and infarct in a patient with PAN. (*Photo courtesy of Antoine Sreih, MD*)

affect a large number of overlying branches, while the presence of nearby "trees" with branches feeding adjacent and intervening areas of skin accounts for the uneven, netlike, jagged, or retiform appearance of the lesions. The jagged or netlike shape seen in livedo reticularis and retiform purpura is an important diagnostic clue that can help distinguish medium-vessel vasculitis from small-vessel vasculitis, which has a more rounded shape, as discussed above.

When findings of medium-vessel vasculitis are seen in the skin, the differential diagnosis includes cutaneous or systemic polyarteritis nodosa (PAN). If these findings are seen together with an eruption suggestive of small-vessel vasculitis (e.g., palpable purpura), the differential diagnosis broadens to include ANCA-associated vasculitis or cryoglobulinemic vasculitis, each of which may have overlapping small- and medium-vessel manifestations.

Extracutaneous Manifestations

Just as the size and morphology of cutaneous lesions are predictive of the type of underlying vasculitis, extracutaneous manifestations can offer important clues to the size of vessel affected. Both small- and medium-vessel vasculitis can affect the kidney, for example, but with different manifestations. Small-vessel vasculitis affects the glomerulus, disrupting the kidney's filtering function and leading to hematuria and proteinuria. Medium-vessel vasculitis, by contrast, results in characteristic aneurysmal dilation and narrowing of renal arteries, manifesting as renovascular hypertension or renal infarction.

Another important distinction can be made based on the presence or absence of neurologic manifestations. Small-vessel vasculitis does not typically affect the nerves. Medium-vessel vasculitis, by contrast, can result in a motor neuropathy ("mononeuritis multiplex").

Types of Vasculitis with Skin Involvement

Cutaneous Small-Vessel Vasculitis/Small-Vessel Vasculitis of the Skin

Small-vessel vasculitis of the skin is most commonly immune complex-mediated, self-limited, and confined to the skin. It may be idiopathic or triggered by infection, drug, connective tissue disease, or neoplasia. Care should be taken to differentiate single-organ vasculitis of the skin from other types of vasculitis or systemic disease.

Cutaneous Manifestations

Palpable purpura is the classic presentation of small-vessel vasculitis of the skin, but purpuric macules, petechiae, urticarial papules, and erythema multiforme-like lesions may be seen. Rounded small ulcers may occur from coalescing palpable purpura. The eruption favors dependent areas, such as the lower extremities, as well as areas of pressure.

Systemic Findings

Arthralgias are fairly common during flares. The presence of frank arthritis, constitutional symptoms, abdominal pain, melena, hematuria, or cough suggests the presence of systemic disease [5].

IgA Vasculitis

IgA vasculitis (Henoch-Schönlein purpura) is a small-vessel vasculitis mediated by IgA immune complexes. The initial presentation is often indistinguishable from that of other forms of cutaneous small-vessel vasculitis.

Cutaneous Manifestations

Patients present with palpable purpura and other small-vessel lesions. There is a preference for dependent areas, as lesions result from immune complex deposition.

Systemic Findings

Abdominal pain or gastrointestinal bleeding occur in 65% of patients, arthralgias or arthritis in 63%, and glomerulonephritis in 40% [6]. Symptoms of an antecedent infectious trigger may be present or recently resolved.

Urticarial Vasculitis

As many as 5–10% of patients with chronic urticarial eruptions actually have urticarial vasculitis [7]. This type of small-vessel vasculitis may be skin-limited or, particularly when associated with low complement levels, involve internal organs, with patients sometimes meeting criteria for systemic lupus erythematosus.

Cutaneous Manifestations

Patients present with hive-like eruptions. Unlike in true urticaria, individual lesions last greater than 24 hours, classically burn instead of itch, may evolve into ecchymoses, and typically do not respond to antihistamines. Other manifestations of small-vessel vasculitis, such as palpable purpura, may be present.

Systemic Findings

Clues to a diagnosis of urticarial vasculitis include the presence of fever or other constitutional symptoms as well as arthralgias.

Cryoglobulinemic Vasculitis

Cryoglobulinemic vasculitis is an immune-complex mediated vasculitis that results from B-cell stimulation, most commonly by chronic infection with hepatitis C virus. Cryoglobulinemic vasculitis not associated with hepatitis C virus infection is rare but can occur in association with lupus, Sjögren syndrome, hepatitis B virus or human immunodeficiency virus, or as an idiopathic disorder. A monoclonal gammopathy (Type I cryoglobulins) with cryoglobulinemic characteristics can occur with some B cell lymphomas or plasma cell disorders.

Cutaneous Manifestations

The eruption includes manifestations of both small- and medium- vessel disease, including palpable purpura but also livedo reticularis, retiform purpura, and ulceration. There is a predilection for the lower extremities as well as cold-exposed sites, such as the feet, hands, and ears.

Systemic Findings

Arthralgias and peripheral neuropathy are the most common extracutaneous manifestations. Disease follows a benign course in about half of patients, but one-third develop severe glomerulonephritis or other visceral complications. Patients with cryoglobulinemic vasculitis associated with the systemic disorders reviewed above may also present with the usual signs and symptoms of those diseases.

Granulomatosis with Polyangiitis (Wegner's)

Granulomatosis with polyangiitis (GPA) is an ANCA-associated vasculitis characterized by necrotizing granulomatous vasculitis of the upper and lower respiratory tract, necrotizing glomerulonephritis, and small and medium vessel vasculitis of other organs. GPA is frequently an organ- and life-threatening disease.

Cutaneous Manifestations

Cutaneous manifestations of GPA occur in about 50% of patients [8]. Morphologically, these include a mix of small- and medium-vessel manifestations, including palpable purpura but also subcutaneous nodules and ulcers (also called "malignant pyoderma") [9]. Flesh-colored papules with central necrosis on the extensor surfaces of the elbows are typical of GPA and represent palisaded and neutrophilic granulomatous dermatitis histologically.

Systemic Findings

Upper airway symptoms such as rhinorrhea, severe sinusitis, nasal ulcerations, epistaxis, and upper airway nodules are ubiquitous in patients with GPA, present in 90%. Renal (85%), pulmonary (70%), and ophthalmic (60%) manifestations are also common [10].

Microscopic Polyangiitis

Microscopic polyangiitis (MPA) is an ANCA-associated vasculitis that, unlike GPA, lacks upper respiratory tract involvement and granulomatous inflammation.

Cutaneous Manifestations

The skin is involved in 44% of patients with MPA, showing a mix of small- and medium-vessel involvement. Purpuric papules and macules are most common. Livedo reticularis, retiform purpura, cutaneous ulcers, and digital infarcts are also seen [11].

Systemic Findings

Constitutional symptoms, including fever and flu-like symptoms, are common. Glomerulonephritis occurs in 80–90% and pulmonary capillaritis in 25–65%. Peripheral neuropathy, including mononeuritis multiplex, is a prominent and characteristic feature (58%) [12].

Eosinophilic Granulomatosis with Polyangiitis (Churg-Strauss)

EGPA is an ANCA-associated vasculitis that presents with eosinophilia, asthma, and eosinophil-associated disease manifestations.

Cutaneous Manifestations

A cutaneous eruption is seen in two-thirds of patients with EGPA. These include non-specific, allergic-type lesions such as urticarial, pruritus, and non-specific rash, as well as manifestations of vasculitis such as palpable purpura (50%) and livedo reticularis. Nodules on the extensor elbows are also common (30%) [13].

Systemic Findings

Most patients have asthma, sometimes long-standing and sometimes adult-onset, before the onset of vasculitis. Atopy, nasal polyps, and eosinophilic pulmonary infiltrates are common, unlike in GPA. Peripheral neuropathy is frequent, and, unlike in GPA, cardiomyopathy is relatively common.

Polyarteritis Nodosa

PAN is characterized by necrotizing vasculitis of medium-sized vessels. PAN may be either skin-limited (so-called cutaneous PAN, 10% of patients) or systemic (90%). Patients with cutaneous PAN must be followed closely due to the potential for systemic complications to develop over time [14].

Cutaneous Manifestations

An eruption is seen in 60% of patients with systemic PAN. They consist of medium-vessel manifestations, such as retiform purpura, ulcers, digital necrosis, livedo reticularis, and subcutaneous nodules distributed along blood vessels [15]. The legs are most commonly affected, followed by the arms and trunk. Skin-limited PAN presents with similar cutaneous findings.

Systemic Findings

Systemic symptoms of PAN include fever and weight loss (90%), arthralgia or arthritis (75%), and peripheral neuritis (75%). Approximately 50% of patients have renal involvement, which may present with hypertension. Some 40% have gastrointestinal involvement, presenting with abdominal pain and gastrointestinal bleeding. Other manifestations may include stroke, myocardial infarction, and bowel infarction. The lungs are spared [16]. Regardless of organ system, the characteristic abnormality in PAN is stenosis or aneurysm of medium-sized arteries.

Giant Cell Arteritis and Takayasu Arteritis

Giant cell arteritis (temporal arteritis, GCA) and Takayasu arteritis (TAK) are vasculitides affecting large arteries (the aorta and its primary branches). Cutaneous manifestations of these diseases are rare.

GCA commonly involves branches of the carotid artery and exclusively affects adults over age 50 years. Headache, jaw claudication, and constitutional symptoms are common. Blindness can occur if untreated. GCA is frequently associated with polymyalgia rheumatica, and diagnosis is made on the basis of temporal artery biopsy. Ultrasound of the temporal artery and other imaging techniques (3-Tesla MRI and positron emission tomography) are gaining acceptance as a diagnostic approach to GCA.

In GCA, the temporal arteries can be nodular and tender. The overlying scalp may appear red or cyanotic. Frank necrosis of the scalp or tongue are extremely rare signs of GCA.

TAK affects the aorta and its major branches. Most patients are young women. TAK may present with limb claudication, pulselessness, and abnormal blood pressure readings; constitutional symptoms; and dizziness, angina, or bowel ischemia. Characteristic angiographic changes are diagnostic.

Rare cutaneous eruptions of TAK may resemble erythema nodosum or pyoderma gangrenosum. Histologically, a necrotizing vasculitis may be present [17].

Initial Evaluation of Patients with Possible Vasculitis

The eruption of vasculitis should initially be considered a symptom of disease rather than a distinct entity, for two reasons. First, identical lesions may be produced in a variety of other disease states, including infection and coagulopathy/vasculopathy, which must be ruled out. Second, when cutaneous vasculitis is confirmed, it is crucially important to establish whether systemic manifestations of vasculitis (e.g., renal, joint, gastrointestinal) or underlying causes or disease associations (e.g., infection, medication reaction, connective tissue disease) are present, as such associations affect management and prognosis. Patients with evidence of systemic vasculitis need urgent medical treatment and referral to colleagues in rheumatology, nephrology, and other specialties.

When a patient presents with an eruption suspicious for vasculitis, initial evaluation should attempt to answer three basic questions:

1. Is the eruption due to vasculitis?
2. Are other organ systems involved?
3. Are there findings that help establish a particular diagnosis or etiology?

The answer to the first question can often be established via a skin biopsy, which should be performed in nearly all circumstances. To answer the second question, a thorough review of systems, physical exam, and basic set of laboratory tests should be performed in a timely fashion. Answering the third question may necessitate a more targeted and specialized "second-level" set of testing. Here we review the available modalities for evaluation of patients with vasculitis, followed by a suggested workup by specific type of vasculitis.

Table 8.2 Partial differential diagnosis of purpuric macules and papules

Skin-limited, small-vessel vasculitis
IgA vasculitis (Henoch-Schönlein purpura)
Cryoglobulinemic vasculitis
ANCA-associated vasculitis
Polyarteritis nodosa (PAN)
Bacteremia
Arthropod bites
Macular purpura due to trauma, skin fragility, or anticoagulation
Platelet dysfunction or deficiency
Pigmented purpuric dermatosis
Cholesterol emboli
Septic emboli
Livedoid vasculopathy

Skin Biopsy

Biopsy Selection and Performance

A skin biopsy should be performed whenever possible to confirm the diagnosis of vasculitis and guide further management. Even the most experienced clinician can be fooled by conditions that mimic vasculitis (Table 8.2).

The type of biopsy performed is dictated by lesion morphology, which suggests where the pathology may be located. For cutaneous manifestations of small-vessel vasculitis, such as palpable purpura, a 4 mm punch biopsy should be sufficient to sample the entire dermis. For "deeper" manifestations of medium- or small-to-medium vessel vasculitis, such as subcutaneous nodules or retiform purpura, sampling of the deep dermis and subcutis is required. This may be accomplished using an incisional biopsy or deep or "telescoping" punch biopsy (e.g., 6 mm punch followed by 4 mm punch) to ensure an adequate amount of fat is sampled.

Because of the natural progression of vasculitis lesions, the timing and selection of the biopsy site is critical. A biopsy performed too early or too late in the development of a lesion may be nondiagnostic. Ideally, a representative, well-established, but not old, lesion (1–2 days old) should be biopsied. For this reason, if new lesions are present, every effort should be made to perform a biopsy the same day the patient is seen.

Whenever relevant and possible, a second biopsy should be performed for direct immunofluorescence studies, as detection of immune complex deposition may have diagnostic and prognostic significance [18]. Proper selection of the biopsy site is even more critical for immunofluorescence studies than for routine biopsy, as immune complexes are most likely to be seen in "fresh" lesions, or those that are between 8 and 24 hours old. Because the subsequent inflammatory cascade destroys deposited immune complexes, older lesions may be falsely negative. Biopsies for direct immunofluorescence should be taken from lesional skin, and the specimen should be placed in Michel's medium or normal saline (not formalin) for processing. Alternatively, a single biopsy can be obtained and cut in half to be sent for both standard processing and direct immunofluorescence.

Histologic Findings in Cutaneous Vasculitis

Characteristic histologic features of leukocytoclastic vasculitis include a neutrophilic inflammatory infiltrate involving dermal blood vessels, granulocytic debris and nuclear dust (leukocytoclasis), fibrinoid necrosis and disruption of vessel walls, and extravasation of red blood cells into the surrounding skin (Fig. 8.3) [19]. Differentiation between small- and medium-sized blood vessels can be somewhat subjective, but small vessels are typically located in the superficial and mid dermis, while medium-sized vessels are located in the deep dermis and subcutaneous fat. The severity of the histologic changes and the depth of the inflammatory infiltrate may predict disease severity or even underlying malignancy [20].

Several other histopathological findings are suggestive of specific etiologies. The presence of tissue eosinophilia may suggest drug-induced vasculitis [21]. The presence of extravascular granulomas with vasculitis is suggestive of GPA or EGPA, especially if eosinophils are also present. The presence of IgA deposits in vessel walls on direct immunofluorescence studies suggests a diagnosis of IgA vasculitis [1] and increases the likelihood of the renal, joint, and gastrointestinal symptoms seen commonly in that syndrome. The presence of IgM may correlate with renal involvement [22] or cryoglobulinemia [23]. A continuous band of C3 or IgG at the dermoepidermal junction (sometimes called a positive lupus band test, though this name has been applied to different findings), may suggest hypocomplementemic urticarial vasculitis and underlying systemic lupus erythematosus.

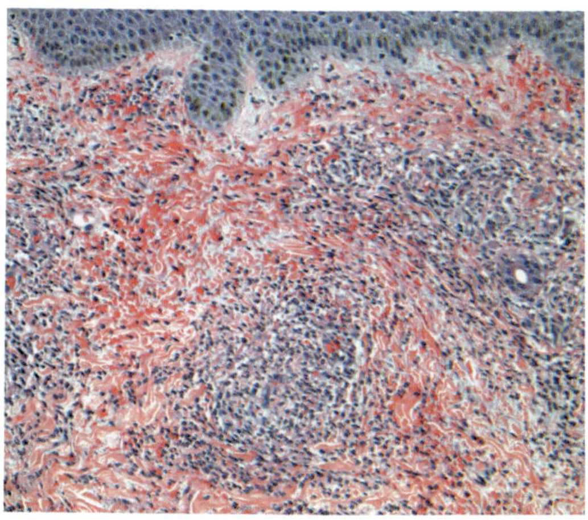

Fig. 8.3 Small vessel vasculitis of the skin showing neutrophilic infiltration of superficial and mid dermal blood vessels, leukocytoclasis, fibrinoid necrosis of vessel walls, and extravasation of red blood cells

Common Pitfalls in Using Skin Pathology to Evaluate Possible Vasculitis

The term "leukocytoclastic vasculitis" is sometimes used improperly on histology reports to describe isolated perivascular neutrophilic inflammation or leukocytoclasis without true fibrinoid necrosis of vessel walls. Although such findings are suggestive and may represent early vasculitis, they are not diagnostic of the condition and may lead to confusion. It is, therefore, important to read the pathology report in its entirety, including direct immunofluorescence, if done, and not rely solely on the summary text.

Similarly, the simple presence of leukocytoclastic vasculitis in a biopsy specimen does nothing to establish its etiology. It is important to understand that "leukocytoclastic vasculitis" is *not* a specific disease entity but a pathologic term and a common finding in the skin in patients with vasculitis. It is important to consider mimickers, such as arthropod bites, ulcers, and neutrophilic dermatoses, in which a secondary vasculitis can be seen, but no clinical syndrome of idiopathic vasculitis is present (Fig. 8.4). Careful clinicopathologic correlation is required.

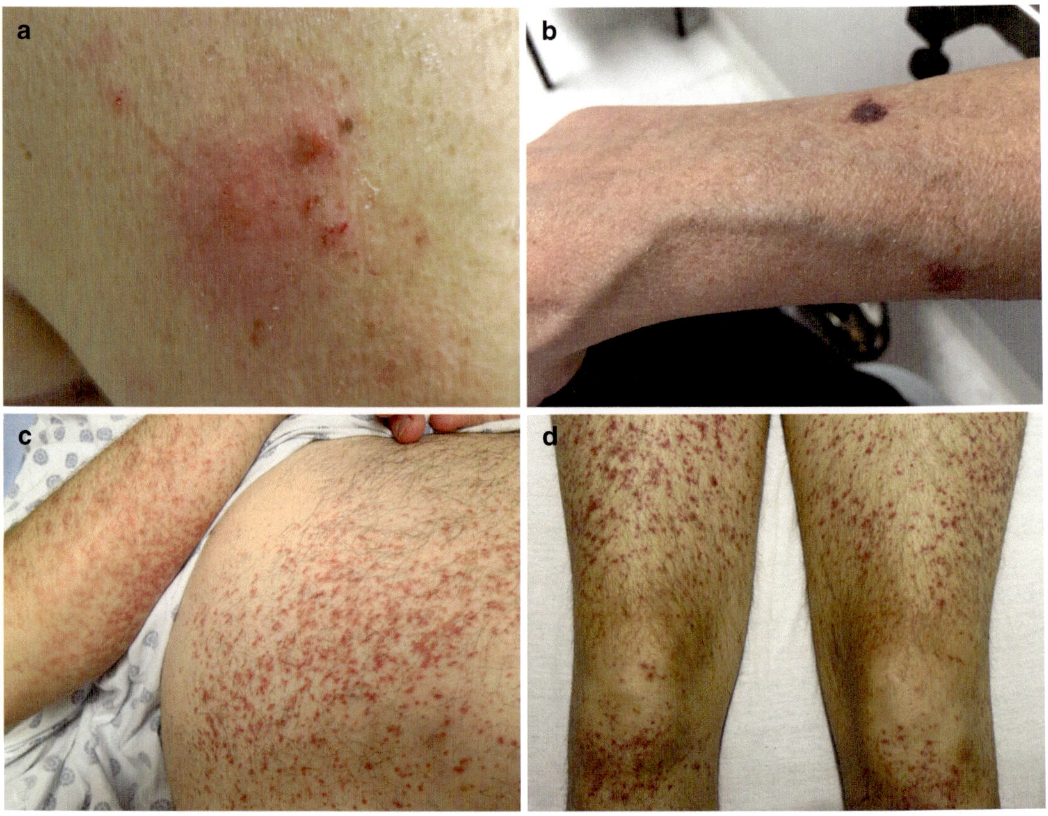

Fig. 8.4 Various "mimickers" that may be mistaken for vasculitis clinically or histologically. (**a**) Arthropod bites and (**b**) Actinic purpura that showed leukocytoclastic vasculitis on biopsy; (**c**) Extensive pigmented purpuric dermatosis clinically mimicking small vessel vasculitis; and (**d**) Viral eruption mimicking palpable purpura but with no histologic evidence of vasculitis

Review of Systems and Medical History

A thorough history and review of systems is essential for separating patients with skin-limited vasculitis from those with systemic involvement or underlying disease. In skin-limited vasculitis, extracutaneous organ manifestations are lacking, although fever and fatigue may occur [5].Review of systems should include fever, weight loss, or other constitutional symptoms; arthralgias or arthritis; myalgias; abdominal pain, melena, or hematochezia; cough, hemoptysis, or dyspnea; hematuria; sinusitis or rhinitis; paresthesias, weakness, or foot drop (Table 8.3); and any other symptom suggestive of additional organ-system involvement with vasculitis. Pertinent positives can direct further targeted workup. Additionally, because disease processes may develop over time, and patients with or without extra-cutaneous manifestations of vasculitis may have identical skin findings on initial presentation, the review of systems should be repeated at subsequent visits.

In addition, a thorough history of the timing and onset of the eruption and other symptoms should be obtained. Questions should review potential triggers, including preceding infectious symptoms, ingestion of prescribed and non-prescribed drugs, and comorbid medical conditions.

Table 8.3 Possible signs and symptoms of systemic vasculitis with corresponding laboratory evaluation

Organ System	Symptoms	Signs	Work-up
Constitutional	Fever, chills, sweats, weight loss, fatigue	Fever	CBC, ESR, CRP, ANA
HEENT	Hair loss, dry eyes/mouth, eye pain, oral/nasal ulcers, sinusitis, epistaxis	Iritis, sinus tenderness, otitis, lymphadenopathy	ANCA, ophthalmologic exam, laryngoscopy
Cardiovascular	CP, orthopnea, dyspnea	Gallop, rub, edema	ECG, echocardiogram
Pulmonary	SOB, cough, hemoptysis, wheeze	Crackles, wheeze, rhonchi	Chest x-ray
Gastrointestinal	Abdominal pain, melena nausea/vomting	Abd tenderness, hepatosplenomegaly	Fecal occult blood, liver function tests
Musculoskeletal	Joint pains, muscle aches	Joint swelling	X-ray, ultrasound
Renal	Hematuria, frothy urine	Hypertension,lower extremity edema	BMP, urinalysis, urine sediment, UProt/Cr
Neuro	Paresthesias, numbness, weakness	Foot/wrist drop, reflexes, sensation, proprioception	Nerve conduction studies

*Signs, symptoms, and laboratory evaluation **highlighted in red** are suggested essential elements of initial basic screening

ANA antinuclear antibodies, *ANCA* antineutrophilic cytoplasmic antibodies, *BMP* basic metabolic panel, *CBC* complete blood count, *CP* chest pain, *CRP* C-reactive protein, *ECG* electrocardiogram, *ESR* erythrocyte sedimentation rate, *SOB* shortness of breath, *UProt/Cr* urine protein to creatinine ratio

Laboratory Studies

No standard protocol for laboratory studies exists in cutaneous vasculitis. Rather, laboratory evaluation should be guided by clinical signs and symptoms, with the goal of identifying the underlying cause and extent of systemic organ involvement. Not every test needs to be ordered in every patient. False positive or irrelevant results can be confusing. Here we review the utility of certain laboratory tests in vasculitis to help guide clinicians in ordering.

Basic Tests That Should Be Ordered in All Patients

Initial tests that should be ordered in all patients include urinalysis with microscopic examination, serum creatinine, and complete blood count (CBC). When the presentation is straightforward and typical of cutaneous small-vessel vasculitis, there is a recent medication or infectious trigger, and the review of systems is unremarkable, no further laboratory testing may be required.

Urinalysis with Microscopic Examination

Urinalysis is the single most important laboratory test for evaluating a patient with suspected vasculitis, because renal disease is seen in many vasculitides, and its presence is likely to change management. Though common and potentially devastating, renal vasculitis rarely results in signs or symptoms until end-stage renal failure occurs. Therefore, urinalysis (including microscopic examination) should be performed in all patients with suspected vasculitis, and it should be repeated periodically as long as active vasculitis is present in another organ system, such as the skin.

If any blood is present on routine urinalysis, the urine should be evaluated for the presence of red blood cell casts and dysmorphic red blood cells by someone trained to do so (usually a nephrologist). Note that this is not a routine test performed by laboratory technicians.

The presence of protein on urinalysis can be more fully evaluated using a spot urine protein / creatinine ratio or a 24-hour urine protein study. Any significant amount of protein should prompt referral to a nephrologist and initiation of steroids or other systemic therapy.

While small-vessel vasculitis affecting the glomeruli produces hematuria and proteinuria, urinalysis may be normal in patients with vasculitis of medium-sized renal vessels (PAN). Instead, they may present with hypertension, creatinine elevation, and abnormal angiographic findings (see below).

Basic Metabolic Panel

Serum creatinine and estimated glomerular filtration rate (GFR), both measured in the basic metabolic panel (BMP), are other important measures of renal function. Serum creatinine must always be interpreted in relation to the patient's baseline creatinine, if known, as well as in the context of patient age, sex, ethnicity, and habitus. Creatinine may fall within the normal range yet be abnormal for the patient in question. A small change in creatinine may in fact represent a large decrease in GFR; for example, a change from 0.4 mg/dL to 0.8 mg/dL is a 50% decrease in GFR.

Complete Blood Count

A CBC should be ordered in all patients. Anemia or thrombocytosis consistent with systemic inflammation may suggest vasculitis not limited to the skin. Significant anemia can result from gastrointestinal vasculitis with bleeding. An elevated eosinophil count may suggest untreated EGPA (Churg-Strauss).

Other Laboratory Tests Useful in Select Cases

Liver Function Tests

Vasculitis can involve the liver, but significant hepatic dysfunction is rare. Baseline values are useful in preparation for administration of treatments that may be hepatotoxic.

Acute Phase Reactants

Measurement of acute phase reactants are of limited value in the evaluation and management of vasculitis affecting the skin. Erythrocyte sedimentation rate (ESR) and C-reactive protein (CRP) levels are elevated in most patients with vasculitis, but these tests are neither sensitive nor specific for the diagnosis of vasculitis. Inflammatory markers are frequently elevated in conditions which mimic vasculitis, and elevation (or absence thereof) is not necessarily predictive of systemic involvement or disease activity. There is variable correlation between the levels of acute phase reactants and disease activity.

Serologic Tests of Autoimmunity

"Autoimmune serologies" can play an important role in the diagnosis of vasculitis, but they require interpretation and by themselves are not diagnostic. All positive and negative results should be interpreted in the context of clinical signs and symptoms as well as biopsy results. Inappropriate ordering of these tests can be a source of confusion and misdiagnosis.

Antineutrophilic Cytoplasmic Antibodies (ANCAs)

ANCA testing is an essential component of evaluating patients for ANCA-associated vasculitides. However, it can also be a source of confusion. ANCA testing involves two laboratory methods: i) immunofluorescence testing, which results in staining patterns interpreted by a technician as cytoplasmic (C-ANCA), perinuclear (P-ANCA), or atypical; and ii) ELISA testing for two specific autoantigens, proteinase-3 (PR3) or myeloperoxidase (MPO). To interpret ANCA testing properly, clinicians must understand the test characteristics of both the immunofluorescence and ELISA testing.

Immunofluorescence testing is less specific than ELISA testing for ANCA-associated vasculitis, and the combination of the two tests provides the highest diagnostic utility. Although the C-ANCA pattern is fairly specific for granulomatosis with polyangiitis (Wegener's, GPA) and MPA, it can be seen in patients without vasculitis. The P-ANCA immunofluorescence pattern is much less specific, and positive tests can be seen in all forms of ANCA-associated vasculitis, as well as in a series of other autoimmune diseases or drug exposures. Atypical ANCA patterns have no specific diagnostic significance.

ELISA testing for ANCA, by contrast, provides a considerably higher degree of diagnostic specificity for vasculitis. Anti-PR3 ANCA, especially in combination with C-ANCA positivity by immunofluorescence, is extremely specific for ANCA-associated vasculitis. The combination of positive tests for P-ANCA and anti-MPO antibodies is also fairly specific for ANCA-associated vasculitis. Importantly, positive tests for ANCA, including by ELISA, can be seen in situations not involving vasculitis, such as bacteremia (anti-PR3) and certain drug exposures (anti-MPO). Patients presenting with dual positivity (both C-ANCA and P-ANCA positive) should be suspected of having a drug-induced vasculitis (e.g., levamisole-induced vasculitis / vasculopathy with cocaine use).

The current standard of care when ANCA testing is desired in the evaluation of vasculitis is to test for ANCA by both immunofluorescence and ELISA; the combination of C-ANCA with anti-PR3 or P-ANCA with anti-MPO is considered a positive result. Ultimately, ANCA testing confirmed with ELISA is most useful in the appropriate clinical context, where signs and symptoms are suggestive and histology shows vasculitis. It is reasonable to order such testing in patients presenting with skin vasculitis, especially in those with chronic or recurrent lesions or concerning systemic symptoms with no obvious cause.

Anti-Nuclear Antibodies

Testing for anti-nuclear antibodies (ANA) and related antibodies is warranted in evaluation of vasculitis if there is suspicion for systemic lupus or Sjögren syndrome as an underlying cause. In both conditions, the vasculitis typically affects small vessels. As in the case of ANCA, ANA testing has its limitations; while extremely sensitive, it is not specific for lupus, and a positive result must be interpreted in the context of relevant signs and symptoms. A low-titer test for ANA (e.g., 1:80 or 1:160) is often a false positive or clinically irrelevant. Other than testing for ANA and anti-SSA, testing for antibodies to additional nuclear antigens such as double-stranded DNA and Smith/RNP should only be performed if the ANA is positive and systemic lupus remains a consideration.

Rheumatoid Factor

In nations with access to modern therapies for rheumatoid arthritis, rheumatoid vasculitis has become an extremely rare manifestation of this disease, as it is usually associated with long-standing, severe rheumatoid arthritis. Such patients may have small-medium vessel manifestations, such as digital infarcts, ulcers, and mononeuritis multiplex. Since rheumatoid factor (RF) is positive in >95% of patients with rheumatoid vasculitis [24], the absence of a positive RF is useful to exclude this form of vasculitis in patients with arthritis. However, the presence of RF is not specific for any form of vasculitis.

RF testing is sometimes useful as a screening tool for mixed cryoglobulins and cryoglobulinemic vasculitis. Routine testing for RF measures the IgM version of RF, which is one of the types of cryoglobulins present in most cases of Type II and III, mixed cryoglobulinemia [25]. Because testing for cryoglobulins can be difficult and unreliable (see below) and typically takes a few days to complete, testing for RF may be a useful first step in patients in whom cryoglobulinemic vasculitis is suspected.

Complement Levels

C3 and C4 serum complement levels measured during a flare may be low in certain types of vasculitis, such as urticarial vasculitis, cryoglobulinemic vasculitis, or rheumatoid vasculitis, and may signal more significant systemic involvement. Complement levels are also commonly low in the setting of systemic lupus erythematosus.

Complement testing is particularly important in the setting of suspected urticarial vasculitis, to differentiate hypocomplementemic from normocomplementemic urticarial vasculitis. Low complement levels in patients with urticarial vasculitis increase the likelihood of systemic lupus and extra-cutaneous manifestations of disease.

Cryoglobulins

Cryoglobulins are cold-precipitable circulating immunoglobulins that form immune complexes that can deposit in vessels and damage end organs, resulting in cutaneous and systemic manifestations of vasculitis. Testing for cryoglobulins is best performed during vasculitis flares. The blood sample should be kept warm (37 °C) and transported to the lab immediately after being drawn. The test is limited by a high false-negative rate due to improper collection and processing techniques; therefore, repeated testing should be performed (along with RF testing) when suspicion for cryoglobulinemic vasculitis is high. Patients with suspected cryoglobulinemic vasculitis should also be tested for hepatitis C virus, hepatitis B virus, and human immunodeficiency virus, and for the presence of paraproteins by serum and urine protein electrophoresis and/or immunofixation.

Serum Protein Electrophoresis (SPEP) and Immunofixation

A monoclonal gammopathy or lymphoproliferative disorder can rarely cause small-vessel vasculitis, including IgA vasculitis, cryoglobulinemic vasculitis, or non-specific small-vessel vasculitis. In such cases, identification of a clinically significant monoclonal disease is crucial to establish the correct diagnosis and treatment plan. SPEP can be used to look for evidence of a paraprotein. Immunofixation is a more comprehensive screen for clonal immunoglobulins that may be performed if suspicion is high. Other abnormalities may be noted on CBC or blood smear.

Serologic Tests for Infections

Hepatitis C virus is strongly associated with cryoglobulinemic vasculitis, as are, to a lesser extent, other persistent viral infections, such as HIV and hepatitis B. Prior to widespread introduction of vaccination against hepatitis B virus, this infection was cause of the majority of cases of PAN and still must be considered in patients who live in or have emigrated from countries without comprehensive vaccination programs. It is also reasonable to test for hepatitis B and C infection in patients presenting with skin vasculitis of otherwise unclear etiology as well as prior to starting many immunosuppressive agents.

Cases of small-vessel vasculitis and IgA vasculitis may be secondary to infection with *Streptococcus* and a host of other bacterial and viral infections. When there is history of an exposure or symptoms of current or past infection, targeted testing (e.g., ASO titer) may be indicated.

Urine Drug Screen

Exposure to certain illegal recreational drugs may cause vasculitis, presenting with isolated palpable purpura, retiform purpura, necrosis, and ulceration. Levamisole, an additive currently found in much of the "street" cocaine sold in the United States and some other countries, may cause a fairly unique vasculitis and vasculopathy leading to necrotic lesions on the extremities (often non-distal areas), ears, cheeks, and nose. Levamisole-associated vasculopathy is also frequently associated with positive tests for both anti-PR3 and anti-MPO ANCA (dual positivity in the same patient), as well as cytopenias. Because its half-life is only 5.6 hours, confirming the presence of levamisole in urine samples can be difficult, but its use is currently so widespread that its presence in cocaine can be assumed in most cases [26].

Cocaine itself is not clearly associated with vasculitis but can lead to severe midline nasal destructive lesions (due to inhalation) as well as positive tests for ANCA, thereby mimicking granulomatosis with polyangiitis (Wegener's). Methamphetamines are also a well-established, but rare, cause of vasculitis.

Diagnostic Imaging Studies in the Evaluation of Possible Vasculitis

Chest Imaging

Data are lacking to guide imaging in the evaluation of vasculitis. However, in our experience, chest x-ray is not typically a useful screening test in patients with vasculitis who do not have pulmonary symptoms. If a patient has cough, dyspnea, or other pulmonary symptoms, however, a computed tomography (CT) scan is indicated to detect subtle but important changes, such as nodules or cavities, which may be evidence of pulmonary vasculitis. Patients with suspected or known GPA, MPA, or EGPA, should undergo baseline screening CT scan even if asymptomatic. Intravenous iodinated contrast is usually not needed for chest CT imaging in case of suspected vasculitis and is sometimes contraindicated (e.g., in vasculitis with renal involvement). The exception is when evaluating for pulmonary embolus, a potential complication of ANCA-associated vasculitis.

Sinus and Upper Airway Imaging

Sinus and upper airway involvement are common complications of GPA and EGPA. CT of the sinuses and neck are valuable in these conditions and can complement direct examination by an otolaryngologist. Head CT or MRI can be used to study not only the sinuses but also the mastoid air spaces and the orbits, both areas of involvement in ANCA-associated vasculitis.

Catheter-Based Angiography, MR Angiography, and CT Angiography

Angiography is an important diagnostic tool in cases of suspected medium- or large-vessel vasculitis. In the proper setting, angiography demonstrating aneurysmal dilation and stenosis of abdominal or renal vessels is pathognomonic of systemic polyarteritis. Angiography of extremities may also reveal the presence of stenosis associated with gangrenous lesions. The choice of modality for angiography may depend on the availability and expertise at a given medical center. However, the use of catheter-based studies is becoming increasingly uncommon, as the resolution of CT or MR angiography continues to increase, including for distal extremity vessels. MR angiography has the advantage of avoiding radiation exposure and use of iodinated contrast. These advantages may compound when serial imaging is needed.

Nerve Conduction Studies and Electromyography

These studies may provide objective evidence of neuropathy and are appropriate in patients with neurological signs and symptoms consistent with a vasculitis affecting medium-sized vessels, such as wrist or foot drop (i.e., mononeuritis multiplex).

Workup and Treatment of Specific Vasculitides with Skin Involvement

Cutaneous Small-Vessel Vasculitis/ Small-Vessel Vasculitis of the Skin

Diagnostic Evaluation

Punch biopsies of lesional skin should be performed for H&E and direct immunofluorescence to confirm the diagnosis. In most cases, the vasculitis is skin-limited, but systemic vasculitis and important underlying disease states should be ruled out. A thorough review of systems and physical exam should be performed. Basic labs are indicated, including CBC, BMP, and (most importantly) urinalysis with microscopic examination. Ordering of additional studies should be guided by signs or symptoms of systemic disease or when vasculitis is recurrent or refractory with unknown cause.

Treatment

Skin-limited small-vessel vasculitis is typically self-limited. Systemic therapy is indicated for severe, intractable, or recurrent disease (8–10% of such cases become chronic and recurrent [27]). There is a dearth of high-quality data to direct management. Colchicine, dapsone, and azathioprine are commonly used. Additional medications, including methotrexate, leflunomide, biologics, and other agents can be considered for refractory disease. Use of these drugs for this indication is supported only by case series and expert opinion [28].

IgA Vasculitis

Diagnostic Evaluation

The approach to diagnosis and evaluation is initially the same as in any other patient presenting with palpable purpura. Biopsies for H&E and direct immunofluorescence should be performed to help confirm the diagnosis. A thorough review of systems and exam are paramount given the high rate of systemic involvement, with particular attention to the gastrointestinal and renal systems. Urinalysis and blood pressure should be monitored weekly while the rash is present, then monthly for up to 6 months, as late glomerulonephritis can occur [29]. Serum creatinine should also be monitored over time. Most patients with nephritis will develop urinary abnormalities within 4 weeks [30].

Treatment

The treatment of IgA vasculitis remains challenging, with no drug, including systemic glucocorticoids, found to change the course of disease or prevent organ damage. Many cases of IgA vasculitis can be treated with observation alone, especially for skin-limited disease. A Cochrane review did not find evidence of benefit from prophylactic use of glucocorticoids to prevent systemic complications, but some experts advise the use of glucocorticoids when severe skin, gastrointestinal, or renal disease occurs [31]. Glucocorticoid-sparing forms of immunosuppression have been attempted, but there is no evidence that these agents are effective. Fortunately, most cases of IgA vasculitis are self-limited, and long-term renal complications are uncommon. However, some (mostly adult) patients develop recurrent bouts of skin disease over months to years, associated with progressive decline in renal function.

Urticarial Vasculitis

Diagnostic Evaluation

Patients with a hive-like eruption that follows an atypical course, as above, or patients with "red flag" symptoms such as fever or arthralgias, should undergo skin biopsy [32]. In urticarial vasculitis, skin biopsy reveals vasculitis involving small vessels. Evaluation should include a thorough review of systems and physical exam, as well as basic labs, urinalysis with microscopy, and other studies dictated by the findings on presentation.

C3 and C4 levels (ordered during a flare) are critical. Patients with normal complement levels usually have an idiopathic small-vessel vasculitis that is skin-limited and self-resolving, best considered a subset of cutaneous small-vessel vasculitis. Those with low C3 and C4 (hypocomplementemic urticarial vasculitis syndrome) are more likely to have systemic lupus (50%), arthritis, obstructive pulmonary disease, gastrointestinal symptoms, and glomerulonephritis [33].

Treatment

Treatment depends on severity and symptoms. Colchicine, dapsone, pentoxifylline, hydroxychloroquine, and immunosuppressive agents such as prednisone, mycophenolate, azathioprine, and rituximab have all been used, but data from controlled clinical trials are not available [34, 35].

Cryoglobulinemic Vasculitis

Diagnostic Evaluation

RF is a good surrogate marker for the presence of cryoglobulins, positive in the vast majority of those with cryoglobulinemic vasculitis, often at extremely high levels. Cryoglobulins should be drawn during a flare and kept at 37 ° C from the time of collection through delivery to the testing lab. The test should be repeated if negative when clinical suspicion is high. Complement levels are usually low. Tests for hepatitis C virus, hepatitis B virus, human immunodeficiency virus, and SPEP should be checked to look for possible triggers. Testing and evaluation for lupus, Sjögren syndrome, or lymphoma should be pursued, as appropriate.

Treatment

It is important to address underlying hepatitis C infection or another disease process, if identified. Idiopathic, refractory, or severe disease should be treated with systemic agents such as high-dose glucocorticoids and rituximab [36, 37]. Acute, severe disease may be treated with glucocorticoids and plasma exchange.

Granulomatosis with Polyangiitis (Wegener's)

Diagnostic Evaluation

GPA is associated with a positive test for ANCA in 90% of cases, typically C-ANCA/anti-PR3 but sometimes P-ANCA/anti-MPO. ANCA-negative GPA is relatively uncommon but does occur and can be quite severe [38]. Diagnosis of GPA requires careful clinicopathologic correlation. A biopsy showing leukocytoclastic vasculitis with extravascular granulomas is classic but not always present. In the right clinical context, skin vasculitis in combination with a positive test for ANCA may be diagnostic for GPA.

Treatment

Most cases of GPA are treated by inducing remission with a combination of high-dose glucocorticoids and either cyclophosphamide or rituximab [38], followed by maintenance therapy with methotrexate, azathioprine, or rituximab. Less severe disease can be treated with glucocorticoids and methotrexate. Disease relapse is common. Targeted agents, including the oral C5a receptor inhibitor avacopan, as well as lower dose glucocorticoid regimens, are under investigation [39].

Microscopic Polyangiitis

Diagnostic Evaluation

MPA is most frequently associated with positive tests for P-ANCA/anti-MPO, but patients may be positive for C-ANCA/anti-PR3. Lesional skin biopsy reveals necrotizing leukocytoclastic vasculitis in the reticular dermis. MPA lacks the granulomatous inflammation and upper respiratory tract involvement of GPA and the eosinophilia of EGPA. However, it is important to understand that cases that appear to be MPA may progress to include additional manifestations that lead to reclassifying patients with GPA.

Treatment

Treatment of MPA is similar to that of GPA. Relapses are common, though less so than in GPA.

Eosinophilic Granulomatosis with Polyangiitis (Churg-Strauss)

Diagnostic Evaluation

Peripheral eosinophilia is characteristic. Approximately 40% of EGPA patients are ANCA positive, most frequently (75%) P-ANCA / MPO. Necrotizing granulomatous vasculitis with eosinophils may be seen on biopsy.

Treatment

Treatment of non-severe EGPA may include glucocorticoids alone. However, cyclophosphamide is usually added in the setting of neuropathy, refractory glomerulonephritis, myocardial disease, severe gastrointestinal disease, or CNS involvement—the manifestations that make up the "five-factor score" that signify poor prognosis. A case series indicated that rituximab may be a useful agent for EGPA, particularly for patients who test positive for ANCA [40]. Mepolizumab, an anti-IL-5 antibody, showed efficacy in a randomized trial and is now approved by the US Food and Drug Administration for treatment of EGPA [41].

Polyarteritis Nodosa

Diagnostic Evaluation

Biopsies are crucial for diagnosis and reveal fibrinoid necrosis of medium-sized vessels, as well as surrounding small vessels, with thrombosis and neutrophilic inflammation. Skin biopsies must be deep enough to sample the subcutaneous tissue where medium-sized vessels reside. Computed tomography (CT) or conventional angiography can reveal characteristic microaneurysms along the renal, gastrointestinal, and other vessels of the viscera [42]. Patients with PAN are ANCA-negative. Until recently, most cases of PAN were considered secondary to infection with hepatitis B virus. With the widespread adoption of vaccination for hepatitis B virus, the prevalence of PAN has been markedly reduced. Testing for hepatitis B and C virus infection should be done in all suspected cases of PAN.

Treatment

Hepatitis B or C infection should be treated, if present. Early diagnosis and treatment are important to avoid mortality. High-dose glucocorticoids are the mainstay of therapy of PAN. Cyclophosphamide may be added for patients with serious systemic involvement. Maintenance therapy or treatment of less severe disease may be accomplished with methotrexate or azathioprine. Skin-limited disease (cutaneous PAN) may respond to alternative therapies such as dapsone or colchicine.

Referral and Coordination of Care

Given the wide variety of potential systemic manifestations, appropriately partnering with colleagues in multiple specialties is an essential part of the diagnosis and management of vasculitis. Biopsy of an affected organ can provide diagnostic confirmation in the right clinical context. Because the skin often is the most easily accessible affected organ, dermatologists should make every effort to accommodate referrals for possible vasculitis while active skin disease is present.

Conversely, if evidence of serious systemic disease is present, patients should be referred to a clinician (usually a rheumatologist) experienced in the management of vasculitis with systemic immunosuppressive therapies. Additional expert care of individual organ systems by nephrologists, pulmonologists, and other providers can be essential. Effective communication among members of the care team is vital to ensure timely diagnosis and treatment.

Summary

The cutaneous eruption may be the first and most visible manifestations of vasculitis. The size and morphology of lesions help predict the clinical syndrome, but a suspected diagnosis of vasculitis should always be confirmed with biopsy and close clinicopathologic correlation. Once the diagnosis of vasculitis is confirmed, important systemic manifestations or underlying associated disease states must be identified quickly to limit morbidity and mortality. Inappropriate use and interpretation of laboratory tests may result in confusion and delay. A systematic and sensible approach to evaluation begins with a thorough review of systems and physical exam, followed by important basic labs (CBC, BMP, UA with microscopic examination) and other selected testing dictated by the review of systems and exam. A familiarity with disease presentations and test characteristics may improve diagnostic accuracy and enable timely initiation of appropriate therapy. Coordination of care between dermatology, rheumatology, nephrology, and other experts is an essential component of successful diagnosis and management of vasculitis.

References

1. Jennette JC, et al. 2012 revised international Chapel Hill consensus conference nomenclature of vasculitides. Arthritis Rheum. 2013;65(1):1–11.
2. Hunder GG, et al. The American College of Rheumatology 1990 criteria for the classification of vasculitis. Introduction. Arthritis Rheum. 1990;33(8):1065–7.
3. Luqmani RA, et al. Nomenclature and classification of vasculitis - update on the ACR/EULAR diagnosis and classification of vasculitis study (DCVAS). Clin Exp Immunol. 2011;164(Suppl 1):11–3.
4. Mackel SE, Jordon RE. Leukocytoclastic vasculitis. A cutaneous expression of immune complex disease. Arch Dermatol. 1982;118(5):296–301.
5. Russell JP, Gibson LE. Primary cutaneous small vessel vasculitis: approach to diagnosis and treatment. Int J Dermatol. 2006;45(1):3–13.
6. Calvo-Rio V, et al. Henoch-Schonlein purpura in northern Spain: clinical spectrum of the disease in 417 patients from a single center. Medicine (Baltimore). 2014;93(2):106–13.
7. Peroni A, et al. Urticarial lesions: if not urticaria, what else? The differential diagnosis of urticaria: part II. Systemic diseases. J Am Acad Dermatol. 2010;62(4):557–70; quiz 571–2
8. Daoud MS, et al. Cutaneous Wegener's granulomatosis: clinical, histopathologic, and immunopathologic features of thirty patients. J Am Acad Dermatol. 1994;31(4):605–12.
9. Tashtoush B, et al. Large pyoderma gangrenosum-like ulcers: a rare presentation of granulomatosis with polyangiitis. Case Rep Rheumatol. 2014;2014:850364.
10. Hoffman GS, et al. Wegener granulomatosis: an analysis of 158 patients. Ann Intern Med. 1992;116(6):488–98.
11. Niiyama S, et al. Dermatological manifestations associated with microscopic polyangiitis. Rheumatol Int. 2008;28(6):593–5.
12. Guillevin L, et al. Microscopic polyangiitis: clinical and laboratory findings in eighty-five patients. Arthritis Rheum. 1999;42(3):421–30.
13. Guillevin L, et al. Churg-Strauss syndrome. Clinical study and long-term follow-up of 96 patients. Medicine (Baltimore). 1999;78(1):26–37.
14. Chen KR. Cutaneous polyarteritis nodosa: a clinical and histopathological study of 20 cases. J Dermatol. 1989;16(6):429–42.
15. Pagnoux C, et al. Clinical features and outcomes in 348 patients with polyarteritis nodosa: a systematic retrospective study of patients diagnosed between 1963 and 2005 and entered into the French Vasculitis study group database. Arthritis Rheum. 2010;62(2):616–26.
16. Hernandez-Rodriguez J, et al. Diagnosis and classification of polyarteritis nodosa. J Autoimmun. 2014;48-49:84–9.
17. Pascual-Lopez M, et al. Takayasu's disease with cutaneous involvement. Dermatology. 2004;208(1):10–5.
18. Minz RW, et al. Direct immunofluorescence of skin biopsy: perspective of an immunopathologist. Indian J Dermatol Venereol Leprol. 2010;76(2):150–7.
19. Carlson JA. The histological assessment of cutaneous vasculitis. Histopathology. 2010;56(1):3–23.
20. Podjasek JO, et al. Histopathological findings in cutaneous small-vessel vasculitis associated with solid-organ malignancy. Br J Dermatol. 2014;171(6):1397–401.
21. Bahrami S, et al. Tissue eosinophilia as an indicator of drug-induced cutaneous small-vessel vasculitis. Arch Dermatol. 2006;142(2):155–61.
22. Takeuchi S, Soma Y, Kawakami T. IgM in lesional skin of adults with Henoch-Schonlein purpura is an indication of renal involvement. J Am Acad Dermatol. 2010;63(6):1026–9.
23. Gibson LE. Cutaneous vasculitis update. Dermatol Clin. 2001;19(4):603–15, vii

24. Voskuyl AE, et al. Diagnostic strategy for the assessment of rheumatoid vasculitis. Ann Rheum Dis. 2003;62(5):407–13.
25. Ferri C, et al. Mixed cryoglobulinemia: demographic, clinical, and serologic features and survival in 231 patients. Semin Arthritis Rheum. 2004;33(6):355–74.
26. Gross RL, et al. A novel cutaneous vasculitis syndrome induced by levamisole-contaminated cocaine. Clin Rheumatol. 2011;30(10):1385–92.
27. Loricera J, et al. Single-organ cutaneous small-vessel vasculitis according to the 2012 revised international Chapel Hill consensus conference nomenclature of vasculitides: a study of 60 patients from a series of 766 cutaneous vasculitis cases. Rheumatology (Oxford). 2015;54(1):77–82.
28. Micheletti RG, Werth VP. Small vessel vasculitis of the skin. Rheum Dis Clin N Am. 2015;41(1):21–32, vii
29. Jauhola O, et al. Renal manifestations of Henoch-Schonlein purpura in a 6-month prospective study of 223 children. Arch Dis Child. 2010;95(11):877–82.
30. Saulsbury FT. Clinical update: Henoch-Schonlein purpura. Lancet. 2007;369(9566):976–8.
31. Hahn D, et al. Interventions for preventing and treating kidney disease in Henoch-Schonlein Purpura (HSP). Cochrane Database Syst Rev. 2015;(8):Cd005128.
32. Micheletti R, Rosenbach M. An approach to the hospitalized patient with urticaria and fever. Dermatol Ther. 2011;24(2):187–95.
33. Jara LJ, et al. Hypocomplementemic urticarial vasculitis syndrome. Curr Rheumatol Rep. 2009;11(6):410–5.
34. Lopez LR, et al. The hypocomplementemic urticarial-vasculitis syndrome: therapeutic response to hydroxychloroquine. J Allergy Clin Immunol. 1984;73(5 Pt 1):600–3.
35. Nurnberg W, Grabbe J, Czarnetzki BM. Urticarial vasculitis syndrome effectively treated with dapsone and pentoxifylline. Acta Derm Venereol. 1995;75(1):54–6.
36. De Vita S, et al. A randomized controlled trial of rituximab for the treatment of severe cryoglobulinemic vasculitis. Arthritis Rheum. 2012;64(3):843–53.
37. Sneller MC, Hu Z, Langford CA. A randomized controlled trial of rituximab following failure of antiviral therapy for hepatitis C virus-associated cryoglobulinemic vasculitis. Arthritis Rheum. 2012;64(3):835–42.
38. Finkielman JD, et al. ANCA are detectable in nearly all patients with active severe Wegener's granulomatosis. Am J Med. 2007;120(7):643.e9–14.
39. Jayne DRW, et al. Avacopan for the treatment of ANCA-associated vasculitis. N Engl J Med. 2021;384(7):599–609.
40. Mohammad AJ, et al. Rituximab for the treatment of eosinophilic granulomatosis with polyangiitis (Churg-Strauss). Ann Rheum Dis. 2016;75(2):396–401.
41. Wechsler ME, et al. Mepolizumab or placebo for eosinophilic granulomatosis with polyangiitis. N Engl J Med. 2017;376(20):1921–32.
42. Das CJ, Pangtey GS. Images in clinical medicine. Arterial microaneurysms in polyarteritis nodosa. N Engl J Med. 2006;355(24):2574.

9 Sarcoidosis

Misha Rosenbach and Robert P. Baughman

Key Points

- Sarcoidosis is a multisystem, granulomatous inflammatory disorder which commonly involves the skin.
- African Americans are disproportionately affected in the United States
- Etiology and proposed triggering antigens are unknown.
- Sarcoidosis is one of the "great imitators" and can present with nearly any clinical morphologic lesion type.
- The nose, particularly the nasal alar rim, as well as the periorbital and perioral areas, scars, and tattoos are frequent sites of cutaneous involvement.
- Non-caseating epithelioid granulomas are the hallmark pathologic sign of sarcoidosis.
- Patients with cutaneous sarcoidosis require thorough evaluation for the extent of systemic disease.
- Treatment of cutaneous sarcoidosis requires a stepwise approach which includes topical, intralesional and systemic therapies.

M. Rosenbach (✉)
Dermatology & Internal Medicine, Cutaneous Sarcoidosis Clinic, University of Pennsylvania, Philadelphia, PA, USA
e-mail: Misha.Rosenbach@pennmedicine.upenn.edu

R. P. Baughman
University of Cincinnati Medical Center, Department of Internal Medicine, Cincinnati, OH, USA

Interdisciplinary Introduction

Sarcoidosis is a multisystem, inflammatory disorder of unknown etiology that can affect every organ system in the body [1, 2]. The disease is characterized by the development of non-caseating granulomas, which can cause disease through either active inflammation or scarring and fibrosis. Sarcoidosis occurs worldwide and can affect patients of any race, ethnic group, or age [3]. Patients likely inherit a genetic predisposition for developing the disease, which, coupled with an environmental, infectious, or antigenic exposure, triggers an immune cascade, leading to granulomatous inflammation, which may spontaneously remit, persist, or lead to subsequent fibrosis.

Patients with sarcoidosis nearly always have lung involvement, which can range from incidental hilar adenopathy identified on routine chest radiography to devastating lung disease requiring transplantation. The skin is the second most commonly affected organ, with 30% of sarcoidosis patients displaying signs of cutaneous inflammation due to the disease [4, 5]. The eyes, joints, and lymph nodes are also frequently affected, and many patients develop disease-related fatigue. Patients can also develop granulomas in the heart, nervous system, liver, kidneys, or bone marrow, while the metabolic effects of the disease can lead to significant complications, morbidity or mortality.

A. Garg et al. (eds.), *Interdisciplinary Approaches to Overlap Disorders in Dermatology & Rheumatology*,
https://doi.org/10.1007/978-3-319-18446-3_9

Sarcoidosis is classically defined by evidence of granulomatous inflammation in more than one organ system, highlighting the multidisciplinary nature of this disease [6, 7]. Cooperation between patients' primary doctors (frequently pulmonologists or rheumatologists) and dermatology is essential in both the diagnosis and management of sarcoidosis.

While there are characteristic clinical, laboratory, and radiographic features that can be suggestive of the disease, pathologic confirmation is generally recommended to make the diagnosis. Superficial and easily accessible, the skin is the organ of choice for biopsy if skin lesions are present. Cutaneous sarcoidosis is a protean disease, one of the "great imitators," and can present with almost any primary lesion morphology; diagnosis requires evaluation by an experienced dermatologist and a low threshold to biopsy [8].

Once a diagnosis is established, patients with sarcoidosis require thorough evaluation for the extent of disease, with treatment depending on the most severely affected organ system. While certain therapeutic options will broadly treat all sarcoidal inflammation, in some cases each affected organ system may respond differently. Whether in diagnosis, management of cutaneous involvement, or alleviation of treatment-related cutaneous side effects, the dermatologist has an essential role to play in the treatment of patients with sarcoidosis [9].

Epidemiology & Risk Factors

Sarcoidosis occurs in patients of all races, and ethnic backgrounds, and has been described in all age groups. The overall rates vary, with the incidence highest in Sweden (64 per 100,000) and the UK (20 per 100,000) and the lowest in Spain and Japan (both 1.4 per 100,000) [10, 11]. In the United States, the highest-risk group is African Americans, with an incidence of 35–64 per 100,000 [12]; African American women have a 2–3% lifetime risk of developing sarcoidosis and tend to develop more severe disease [13]. Fewer than 5% of patients will die from sarcoidosis, usually due to advanced lung disease and fibrosis or from severe cardiac involvement [2, 14].

Overall the disease exhibits a bimodal age distribution, with incidence peaks in the mid-twenties to thirties and, in women, another small peak from 45–65 in some countries [15]. The disease is less common in children, teenagers and patients older than 70, but it has been rarely reported in infants. There exist conflicting reports regarding potential seasonal variation in disease presentation and diagnosis [16–18].

Beyond racial and age variations in incidence [19], there is evidence for clustering of disease among family members, including twins [20]. Monozygotic twins are at an 80-fold increased risk of developing sarcoidosis, while dizygotic twins are at a 7-fold increased risk [21]. The largest epidemiologic study to date, A Case Control Etiologic Study of Sarcoidosis (ACCESS), documented a relative risk for developing sarcoidosis of 4.7 in patients with an affected first or second degree relative, with an excess risk among siblings [22].

Occupational exposures and environmental factors may play a role in disease development as well. Sarcoidosis closely resembles chronic berylliosis clinically, radiographically, and histopathologically. Sarcoid-like granulomatous reactions can also occur at sites of foreign bodies, such as sutures, asphalt or remote debris injury, and in response to certain tattoo pigments that contain metallic components. Clusters of sarcoidosis cases have been reported in patients with certain occupational exposures, such as US Navy shipyard personnel [23] and firefighters [24], who may be exposed to inhalation of dusts or metals; the rates in New York City firefighters increased after the terrorist attacks on the World Trade Center on September 11, 2001 [25]. The ACCESS study identified "high microbial" environments as potential risk factors, including exposure to insecticides, molds, and mildew [26].

It is often difficult to separate the effects of environment from those of genetics; one study found 40% of patients with sarcoidosis had exposure to a patient with the disease (versus 1–2% of controls). Cases occurred within households but also in friendships and neighborhoods. This study also identified an increased rate of disease among nurses [27, 28]. Further complicating the picture, certain environmental exposures may be more likely to induce disease in patients of specific backgrounds or with certain human leukocyte antigen (HLA) haplotypes. Caucasian patients show an increased risk with exposure to industrial organic dusts, but not with metal exposure. African Americans have an increased risk with metal exposure or employment in the transportation industry [29]. Patients with HLA DRB1*1101 have an increased risk of disease with occupational insecticide exposure [29].

Sarcoidosis is not due to a single gene mutation but rather represents a complex, polygenic disease with several potential variants. Certain HLA alleles may confer risk for developing the disease in some patients, though the prevalence and impact of those alleles varies by racial/ethnic group. HLA DRB1*03, DRB1*11, DRB1*12, DRB1*14, and DRB1*15 appear to confer risk for disease overall, although HLA-DQB1 genes may be more important in African Americans [30].

HLA-B8/DR3 has been associated with increased risk for developing an acute form of sarcoidosis, Lofgren syndrome, that is characterized by hilar adenopathy, fever, arthritis, and erythema nodosum (EN) and carries an overall good prognosis with low risk for chronic disease. Similarly, patients with DRB1*03 alleles appear to have a good prognosis with protection against chronic disease [30].

Specific mutations including polymorphisms in genes encoding inflammatory cytokines (such as the *TNF* gene and the *IL23 receptor* gene) and genes involved in apoptosis and immune cell activation (such as *ANXA11* and *BTNL2)* [31, 32] have been identified as increasing sarcoidosis risk in some populations [33]. It is likely that genetic polymorphisms and HLA alleles confer risk for development of an abnormal immune response to an inciting antigenic exposure—one that is either too vigorous or cannot cease appropriately.

Pathogenesis

Sarcoidosis is a multisystem disorder characterized by granuloma formation in affected organs. In some patients it will spontaneously remit, while others will experience either chronic, active inflammation, or fibrosis and scarring. The disease phenotype may vary somewhat by race/ethnicity, country, and genetic background. As reviewed, patients inherit susceptibility risk for development of the disease, and, when exposed to an antigen, develop granulomatous inflammation. There exists substantial debate over the triggering antigen, with some experts postulating that in the future this entity will be known as "the sarcoidoses" rather than "sarcoidosis," based on different patterns of granulomatous response to different triggering antigens [34].

The development of an epithelioid granuloma, which is nearly always non-caseating, is the hallmark pathologic sign of sarcoidosis. Overall, sarcoidosis is considered a Th1-predominant disease, although the innate and Th17 arms of the immune system likely also play a role [35]. Initial granuloma formation likely involves innate phagocytic cells that engulf the disease-specific antigen. Innate immune signals such as Toll-like receptor-2 and nucleotide-binding oligomerization domain 1 appear, and tumor necrosis factor (TNF) and other inflammatory cytokines are produced [36]. Monocytes with MHC II molecules upregulate CD4+ Th1 T-helper cells after antigen regulation, leading to a Th1 cytokine predominance, with increased expression of interferon-gamma (IFNγ) as a key inflammatory mediator, along with upregulation of interleukin-2 (IL2) and IL18 [37, 38]. Macrophages and some CD8+ T-cells elaborate TNFα, leading to persistent Th1 activity, IFNγ elevation, macrophage signaling and accumulation, and subsequent B-cell stimulation and hypergammaglobulinemia. Recent research suggested the Th17 response may also play a role in sarcoidal granuloma formation [39]. TNFα and GMCSF lead to macrophage fusion and the formation of characteristic multinucleated giant cells within the granulomatous inflammation. Chemokines are also upregulated, including monocyte chemotactic factor, which draws monocytes into the affected tissue. Patients may develop lymphopenia, and patients with sarcoidosis tend to display anergic responses, with reduced delayed-type hypersensitivity. Th1 cytokine production is present for the duration of active disease, with some authors suggesting that markers of those cytokines (such as the serum IL-12 receptor level) may be used to follow disease activity, though this approach is not widely used [40].

The determinants of the course that an individual patient's sarcoidosis will ultimately take – either spontaneous improvement (seen in 60% within 2–3 years [41]), chronic active granulomatous inflammation, or a fibrotic phenotype – is as yet unknown.

Some have suggested that persistent sarcoidal inflammation is due to abnormal T-regulatory cells or overall abnormal T-cell function [35, 42, 43].

Beyond the genetic risks and inflammatory pathways involved, much of the active research in sarcoidosis focuses on determining the triggering agent for the disease. In the Kveim-Siltzbach skin test, ground spleen from patients with sarcoidosis is injected intradermally, eliciting a granulomatous reaction 4–6 weeks later in patients with sarcoidosis; this finding provides some evidence for a transmissible antigen [44]. Patients have developed sarcoidosis following organ transplantation [35, 45]. Growing evidence suggests that the etiologic antigen is either a microbial infective agent, inert environmental element or compound, or autologous self-antigen, such as a misfolded protein.

Due to the clinical, radiographic, and histologic overlap between sarcoidosis and mycobacterial infections (particularly tuberculosis), a mycobacterial agent has long been hypothesized as a trigger for sarcoidosis. Mycobacteria are fastidious and can be challenging to culture, but acid-fast staining generally also fails to reveal organisms on routine testing in sarcoidosis. Additionally, despite treatment with broadly immunosuppressive agents, patients with sarcoidosis do not typically experience disseminated or reactivated mycobacterial infections.

As diagnostic techniques have advanced, however, mycobacteria have been detected with greater frequency in sarcoidal specimens. With the advent of PCR, approximately one quarter of evaluated specimens in a large meta-analysis were found to have evidence of mycobacterial genetic material, 10–20 times more frequent than in controls [46]. Proteomic testing identified the presence of mycobacterial protein catalase-peroxidase (mKatG) in sarcoidosis tissues in approximately one half of cases [47]. Additional advanced diagnostic techniques such as mass spectrometry, protein immunoblot, and deep sequencing have identified other mycobacterial compounds (heath shock proteins, ESAT6, and others) in sarcoidal specimens [35, 48, 49]. These mycobacterial antigens may trigger a Th1 cytokine response in genetically predisposed patients, leading to the observed clinical phenotypes.

It is possible that patients with sarcoidosis exhibit an abnormal immune response to a transiently present or rapidly killed mycobacterial agent, leading to robust granulomatous inflammation, and then due to genetic and immunologic factors, the granulomatous cascade continues unabated, even once the inciting agent is cleared. No studies have confirmed a mycobacterial agent as the definitive trigger of sarcoidosis, however.

Besides mycobacteria, other infectious agents have been evaluated for a possible role in inducing sarcoidosis. Numerous studies, primarily out of Japan, have shown high rates of Propionibacterium acnes in sarcoidosis tissue samples [50]. This agent has been detected by both culture and DNA identification; investigators have also demonstrated abnormal responses to *P. acnes* proteins in patients with sarcoidosis [51, 52]. TLR-2, which is involved in the host response to *P. acnes* and in acne pathogenesis, is also hypothesized to play a role in innate immune signaling in early granuloma formation. However, *P. acnes* is a common bacterium that has also been detected in tissue specimens from control patients, and its role as a potential inciting pathogen remains unclear. It is plausible that *P. acnes* may play a role in triggering sarcoidosis in specific geographic locations, countries, or in specific racial/ethnic groups, but not in all patients.

Other infectious agents identified as potential triggers of sarcoidosis include fungi (particularly cryptococcus) and viruses, including a variety of human herpes viruses (EBV, CMV, HHV6, HHV7) as well as HIV and HTLV1 [35]. Other suggested triggers include spirochetes, Borrelial species, *T. whipplei,* rickettsia, and chlamydia; however none of these organisms have been substantiated as triggers in controlled trials or epidemiologic studies [53].

Some authors have suggested that the intensely polarized Th1 cytokine skew in sarcoidosis may lead to immunologic control of an infection but failure to clear the triggering antigen, thereby causing additional granuloma formation to trap microbial antigens and triggering a relentless cycle of Th1 inflammation [35]. Based on the properties of the Kveim reagent, one group suggested that the requirements of a sarcoid-triggering antigen should be: poor solubility, resistance to heat, and resistance to chemical degradation; they identified the amyloid precursor protein serum amyloid A (SAA) as a potential pathogenic agent [54]. The same group demonstrated abundant SAA within sarcoidosis tissues and localized to the epithelioid granulomas, with lower rates seen in other granulomatous diseases [55]. Lastly, the same group demonstrated that SAA could trigger Th1 granulomatous inflammation and identified elevated SAA in sarcoidosis bronchoalveolar lavage specimens, with levels correlating to severity of pulmonary disease [35, 54, 55].

Beyond host proteins or infectious agents, other exogenous materials have been suspected as potential antigenic triggers of sarcoidosis. Among the culprits hypothesized are: pine pollen; wood burning or dust; dust of zirconium, nickel, silica, or talc, and others [56–59]. Notably, some of these elements may induce non-sarcoidal hypersensitivity pneumonitis with granulomatous inflammation, similar to chronic beryllium disease, but without the multiorgan phenotype of true sarcoidosis [53, 60–62].

There may be one antigen that triggers all of sarcoidosis, with patients displaying certain disease phenotypes based on their genetic background. Alternatively, numerous antigenic triggers may exist, and the interplay between inciting agent and the host immune response may be what determines the individual disease course.

Clinical Features

Sarcoidosis can present with a wide variety of phenotypes. The disease is classically defined by clinicoradiologic evidence of inflammation in more than one organ system, with histology demonstrating noncaseating epithelioid cell granulomas [1]. While there may exist isolated, single-organ forms of sarcoidosis or sarcoid-like disease [7], all patients with suspected sarcoidosis require a thorough evaluation of numerous organs to assess extent of disease. Sarcoidosis remains a diagnosis of exclusion, with no gold-standard confirmatory diagnostic test, and other causes of granulomatous inflammation must be excluded before a diagnosis of sarcoidosis is rendered.

The vast majority of patients with sarcoidosis have lung involvement (90%), with skin involvement (25–30%), eye involvement (25%), and involvement of other organs occurring somewhat less frequently (Table 9.1). Organ involvement may be asymptomatic at onset and can remain so throughout the course of the disease. Approximately a third of sarcoidosis patients will

Table 9.1 Organ involvement in 393 consecutive patients seen in one sarcoidosis clinic as measured by the WASOG criteria [112]

Organ system involvement or metabolic derangement	Percent (%) of patients
Pulmonary	88
Ocular	32.4
Cutaneous	27.7
Neurologic	14.4
Non-thoracic lymph node	14.2
Calcium Abnormalities	14.1
Hepatic	10.9
Splenic	6.7
Cardiac	6
Renal	1.1
Other (Marrow, Bone/Joint, ENT, Salivary/Parotid)	11.2

Adapted from Zhou, 2021 [176]

experience nonspecific symptoms, such as low-grade fevers, fatigue, malaise, or weight loss; the frequency of these symptoms may vary by ethnic group. Certain specific disease phenotypes, such as Lofgren syndrome (see below), are more likely to have significant fever [63].

The disease course in sarcoidosis may be quite variable. Disease activity can wax and wane, sometimes spontaneously, and 60% of patients may experience spontaneous remission, including complete, durable resolution of all disease signs and symptoms [1]. Patients with chronic and/or progressive disease often require persistent treatment. Some 10–20% of patients with sarcoidosis will experience longstanding, permanent sequelae from the disease, and 1–5% of patients can die of sarcoidosis, usually from severe, progressive pulmonary involvement or neuro- or cardiac sarcoidosis [1, 64–68]. The pattern of organ involvement and chronicity may vary by racial/ethnic background and geography: for example, African American patients are more likely to have skin involvement and a chronic disease course, while Northern Europeans more likely to present with Lofgren syndrome, and Japanese patients are markedly more likely to have cardiac involvement [69].

Pulmonary Sarcoidosis

The most common pulmonary symptoms in sarcoidosis patients are cough, dyspnea, and chest pan. The cough is often persistent, dry, and nonproductive. Dyspnea may occur with or without wheezing but does not routinely respond to bronchodilators. Atypical chest pain is often present but usually does not correspond to abnormalities seen on chest imaging, such as adenopathy or parenchymal lung disease. Up to half of patients are diagnosed with pulmonary sarcoidosis as an incidental finding on chest radiography when they have no or minimal symptoms [4, 70]. Physical exam is usually unrevealing; a subset of patients will have audible crackles or wheezes, however, particularly if bronchiectasis is present. In end-stage pulmonary disease, patients may exhibit distal fingertip clubbing [63].

Chest imaging is recommended for all patients with sarcoidosis. Chest x-ray findings were classified by Scadding into four stages: stage 1, adenopathy alone; stage 2, adenopathy plus infiltrates; stage 3, infiltrates alone; and stage 4, fibrosis. Over 90% of pulmonary sarcoidosis can be classified using this schema. Additionally, the chest x-ray stage can predict the outcome of the pulmonary involvement: 90% of stage 1 patients have a normal chest x-ray after 2–5 years, while only 30% of patients with stage 3 disease will experience resolution of their chest x-ray. However, resolution of the chest x-ray does not predict resolution of involvement in other organs. A patient can have a clearing of their adenopathy but persistent skin lesions or other extrapulmonary involvement.

CT scanning is more sensitive than chest x-ray for both adenopathy and parenchymal disease in pulmonary sarcoidosis. Routine CT scanning is not recommended in the assessment of sarcoidosis patients, but it may be helpful in categorizing chest radiographic findings or evaluating patients with atypical, persistent, resistant, or challenging-to-treat disease. Characteristic features seen on CT include significant adenopathy, bronchovascular thickening, micronodular disease and upper lobe infiltrates. Nodules are the most common feature of pulmonary sarcoidosis, seen in 80–100% of patients; these represent areas of granulomatous inflammation [71, 72]. Lung parenchymal involvement tends to be bilateral and symmetrical, with central and upper lung regions involved most frequently [71, 73]. In severe or progressive pulmonary disease, fibrosis may become more prominent. For a patient who presents with granulomatous skin lesions, a CT scan of chest showing symmetrical adenopathy and/or parenchymal disease is highly supportive of the diagnosis of sarcoidosis.

Cutaneous Sarcoidosis

Cutaneous sarcoidosis is one of the "great imitators" and can present with nearly any clinical morphologic lesion type. Cutaneous involvement is divided into "specific lesions" (those that demonstrate granulomas histologically) and "nonspecific lesions" (reactive cutaneous phenomena that do not display granulomas upon biopsy, with EN as the classic example). Cutaneous sarcoidosis tends to be clinically asymptomatic. Lesions in certain anatomic locations and ulcerative lesions may be painful, and patients with cutaneous sarcoidosis will sometimes complain of itch. However, the clinical appearance of the lesions is generally what prompts patients to seek diagnosis and treatment.

While the specific lesions of sarcoidosis are quite varied, certain cutaneous manifestations are more common than others. Sarcoidosis tends to affect the nose (Fig. 9.1), particularly the nasal alar rim (Fig. 9.2), as well as the periorbital and perioral areas, scars, and tattoos. Common morphologies include violaceous macules, papules or plaques (Fig. 9.3), some of which may be annular in shape (Fig. 9.4); another common presentation is indurated nodules and plaques of the nose and

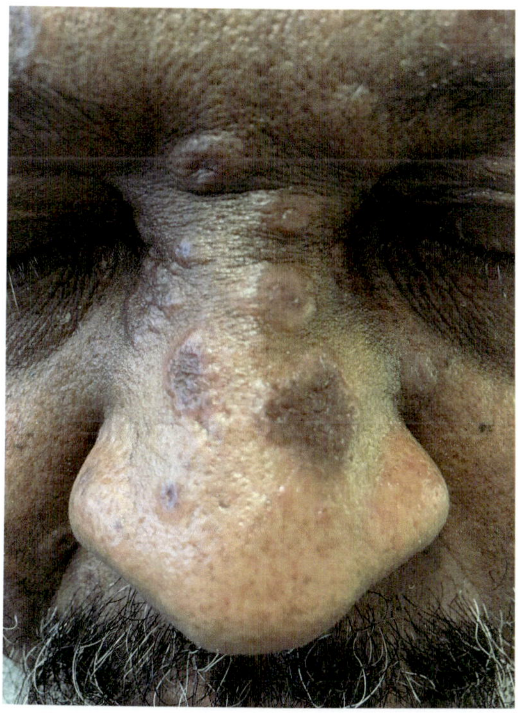

Fig. 9.1 Cutaneous sarcoidosis: plaques across the nasal bridge. This patient has no subcutaneous component to his disease, and these flat papules or small plaques, while occurring on the nose, are generally not described as lupus pernio – instead, as flat papules or plaques on the nose. Lupus pernio lesions should be more extensive and have a subcutaneous component

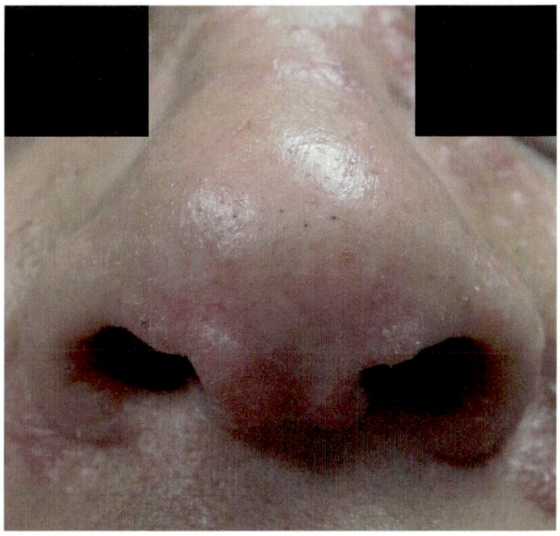

Fig. 9.2 Lupus pernio-like papules. By the strictest definition, papules on the nasal alar rim are not truly lupus pernio. However, patients with extensive papules and scaling, with some distortion of the columella, such as this patient, likely have deeper involvement, as is also the case with lupus pernio. These patients often exhibit a chronic, recalcitrant course, and the technical distinction between lupus pernio requiring plaques or nodules versus smaller lesions such as these may be irrelevant in clinical practice

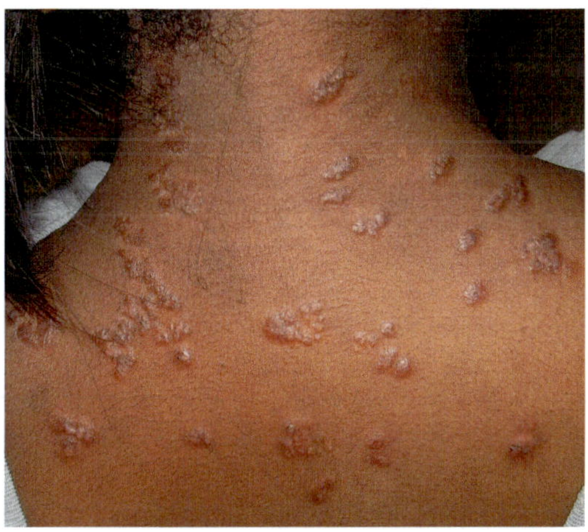

Fig. 9.3 Sarcoidosis papules. These small, raised, palpable areas of granulomatous inflammation can be red, pink, purple, or flesh-colored and may have variable scale. Neck involvement is common, but lesions can occur anywhere

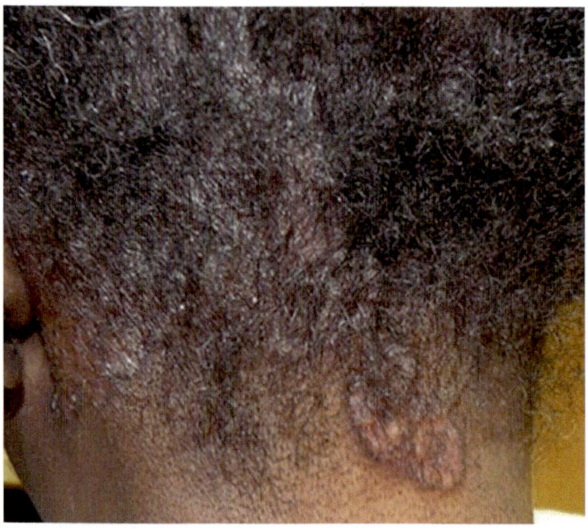

Fig. 9.4 Annular sarcoidosis. This patient has scalp involvement extending down onto the neck. The lesions are circular or annular (in rings), which is a common pattern seen in cutaneous sarcoidosis. The color can vary from the middle to the outer edge of the lesions, and they may develop scale

Table 9.2 Cutaneous sarcoidosis lesion types

Frequency	Morphology
Common	Macules/Papules
	Plaque
	Lupus pernio
	Subcutaneous
	Lesions involving scar/tattoo
Uncommon	Psoriasiform
	Lichenoid
	Verrucous
	Ichthyosiform
	Atrophic
	Ulcerative
	Hypopigmented
Rare	Erythroderma
	Photodistributed
	Alopecia (scarring or non-scarring)
	Nails
	Mucosal
	Genital
Non-specific lesions	Erythema nodosum (EN)
	Calcinosis cutis
	Digital clubbing

Adapted from Wanat and Rosenbach [74]

central face, known as lupus pernio. Flesh-colored subcutaneous nodules or plaques and papules within scars or tattoos are also common presentations. Less common morphologies include psoriasiform lesions, lichenoid papules, verrucous hyperkeratotic lesions, acquired ichthyosis, atrophic or ulcerative lesions, hypopigmented macules or patches, erythroderma, and alopecia (scarring or non-scarring). (Table 9.2) [74].

Macular sarcoidosis can be red-brown/orange, flesh-colored, or hypopigmented (Fig. 9.5); it generally presents with numerous lesions concentrated on the face or in areas of trauma. Papular sarcoidosis can present similarly, although it tends to favor sites of repetitive friction, rubbing, or trauma (such as the elbows and knees). These lesions often resolve without scarring, but postinflammatory changes may persist [75–79]. Plaques are commonly found on the face, back, and extensor surfaces; they are more likely than macular or popular lesions to be seen in patients with a chronic disease course. When treated, plaques are also more likely to leave dyspigmentation and scarring [4, 78, 80].

The term "lupus pernio" is a source of some confusion, as non-dermatologists may sometimes use it to refer to any chronic cutaneous

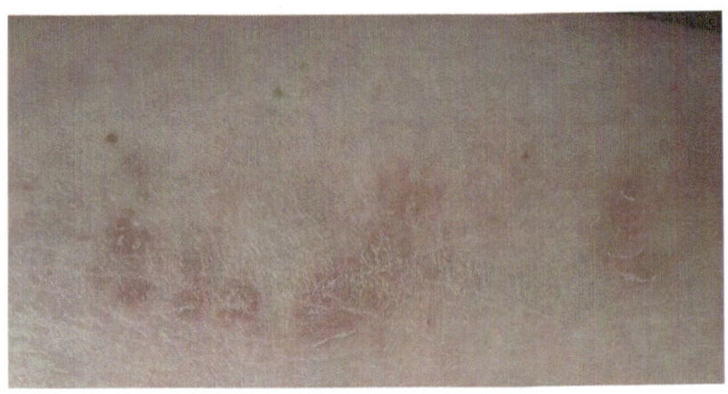

Fig. 9.5 Sarcoidosis macules: these flat, slightly red-brown lesions indicate cutaneous granulomatous inflammation due to sarcoidosis. This case exhibits fine scale, which, when extensive, can lead to acquired ichthyosis and itchyosiform sarcoidosis

lesion of sarcoidosis. By the strictest definition, however, lupus pernio refers to red-to-violaceous subcutaneous plaques or nodules, often with superficial scale, on the nose (Fig. 9.6a, b), cheeks, or central face. This morphologic variant portends a chronic, recalcitrant course and will often leave significant discoloration and sometimes scarring behind even with adequate treatment. Lupus pernio is more common in African Americans, particularly female patients. Lupus pernio is sugges-

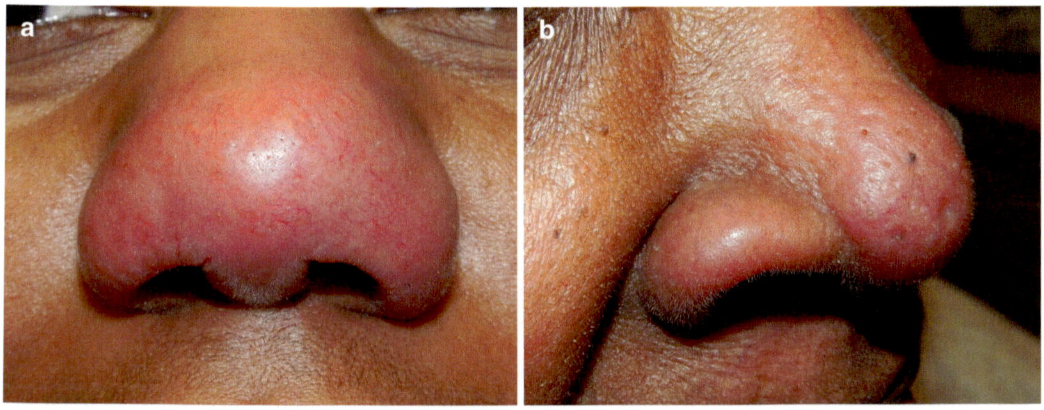

Fig. 9.6 (**a**, **b**) Lupus pernio. (**a**) violaceous, subcutaneous plaque throughout the entire nasal tip. (**b**) violaceous, slightly crusted nodule on the distal nasal tip

tive of sinus, oropharyngeal, and upper airway sarcoidosis involvement and may also be associated with arthritis, bone cysts, pulmonary fibrosis, and uveitis [81–86].

There is debate over whether all chronic facial sarcoidosis lesions represent lupus pernio. Purists argue that papular lesions on the face are a distinct entity and do not carry the same prognostic significance. In truth, the data supporting this distinction are not robust, and many patients with facial sarcoid lesions, including papular disease, can exhibit a course similar to that seen in patients with the deeper plaques and nodules of true lupus pernio.

Subcutaneous sarcoidosis, also known as "Darier-Roussy" disease, affects the deep dermis and subcutaneous tissue, including the fat (Fig. 9.7). Clinically, this entity presents as ill-defined, flesh-colored, subcutaneous plaques and nodules, which can be quite extensive. It is important to distinguish subcutaneous sarcoidosis, characterized by typical non-caseating epithelioid granulomas throughout the deep dermis and subcutis, from EN. The latter presents with red-brown, tender, inflamed nodules, typically on the anterior shins, and is characterized by a predominantly septal panniculitis on histology. Subcutaneous sarcoidosis is more common on the arms, and the lesions are neither clinically inflammatory nor painful [87–92].

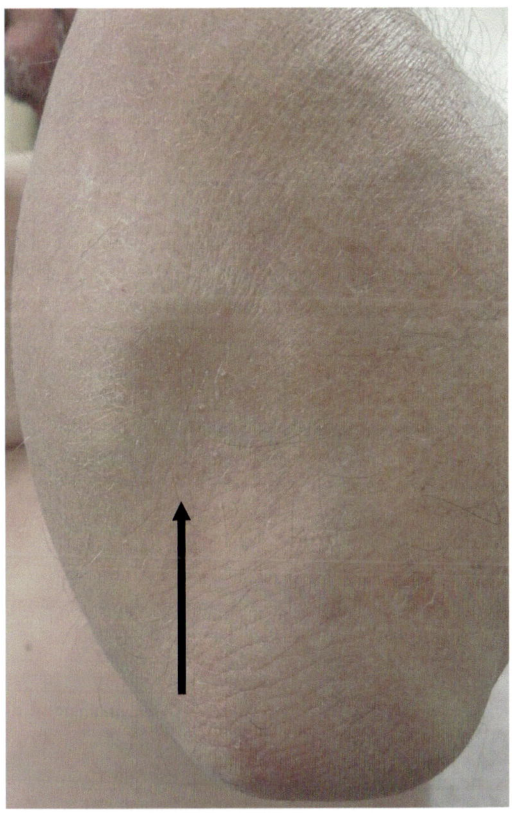

Fig. 9.7 Subcutaneous sarcoidosis: This form of sarcoidosis may be clinically subtle and only appreciable on careful palpation in some patients. The lesions will feel firmer than underlying/surrounding fat and may have a slight give to them

Sarcoidosis frequently affects scars, sites of remote trauma, and areas of foreign body deposition, including tattoos (Fig. 9.8a, b), remote traumatic injuries with debris implantation, and sites

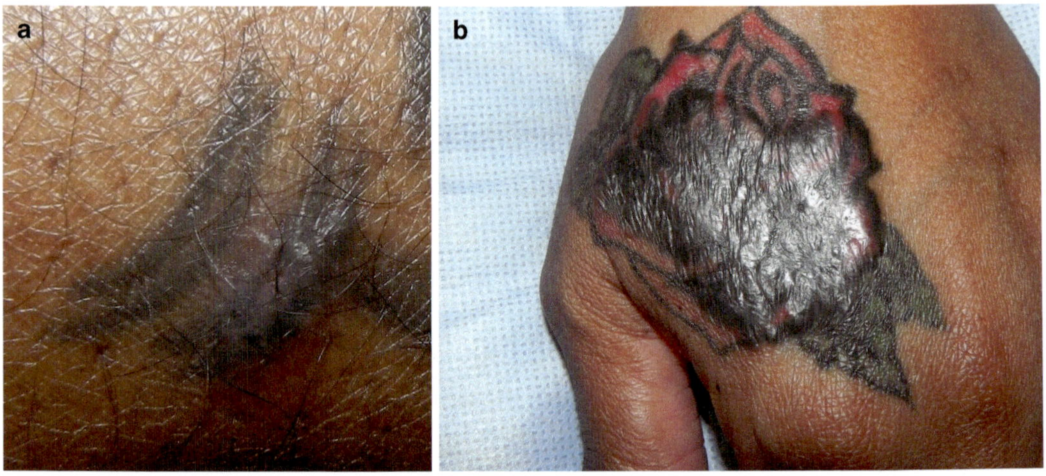

Fig. 9.8 (**a**, **b**) Tattoo sarcoidosis. (**a**) focal involvement of one portion of a larger tattoo. It is essential to completely examine all patients' tattoos, as tattoo sarcoidosis can be subtle but is a reasonable target for biopsy to demonstrate characteristic granulomatous inflammation. Skin biopsy can sometimes spare patients more invasive testing. (**b**) more extensive tattoo involvement, with a large plaque cutting across multiple colors of the tattoo. Tattoo pigment can elicit a granulomatous response; in patients with sarcoidosis, however, when the disease affects tattoos it will often cause lesions in more than one color of the tattoo

of injection (either medicinal or cosmetic). Scar sarcoidosis tends to present with red-to-violaceous papules, nodules, plaques, or subcutaneous swelling, within and immediately around scars [93]. Granulomas within tattoos warrant special consideration. The differential diagnosis can include mycobacterial infection, particularly in freshly placed tattoos, if the granulomas are confined to "shaded" areas, wherein the pigment was diluted with tap water, or if there are pustules present. The differential diagnosis also includes isolated granulomatous hypersensitivity reaction to tattoo pigment; a systemic workup to exclude extracutaneous involvement is always indicated [74].

Sarcoidosis of the digit may affect any compartment, from the bone, to the joint/tendon structure, to the skin and subcutis (Fig. 9.9). It may be clinically challenging to distinguish skin involvement from bone involvement. Hand radiographs will reveal honeycombing and bone cysts if the bone is involved.

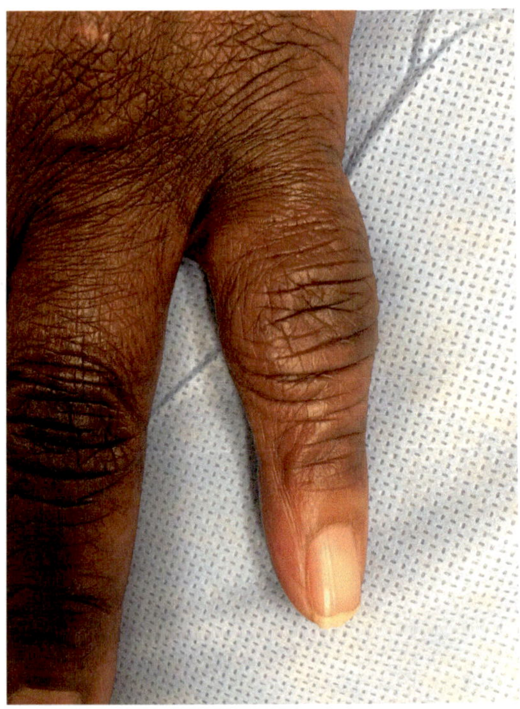

Fig. 9.9 Sarcoidosis of the digit. Sarcoid can affect any compartment of the digit, from the bone, to the joint/tendon structure, to the skin and subcutis; it may be clinically challenging to distinguish skin involvement from bone involvement. Hand radiographs will reveal honeycombing and bone cysts if the bone is involved

The less common clinical presentations of cutaneous sarcoidosis are quite varied, and less is known about associations with internal organ involvement, prognostic implications, or disease course. Patients may present with psoriasiform sarcoidosis [94] characterized by erythematous plaques with overlying silvery scale (Fig. 9.10); this entity may need to be distinguished from coexistent sarcoidosis and psoriasis [95], which have also been reported and demonstrated in one epidemiological study [96]. Lichenoid sarcoidosis is characterized by small, flat-topped, skin-colored to violaceous papules; lesions lack the characteristic "Wickham striae" seen in true lichen planus [97]. Verrucous or hyperkeratotic sarcoidosis has been described on the legs of African-American patients and may be mistaken for warts or other hyperkeratotic skin lesions [98]. Notably some patients with this form of sarcoidosis may be misdiagnosed as having early squamous cell carcinomas on superficial shave biopsies of the skin [99]. Ichthyosiform sarcoidosis looks like classic lower extremity acquired ichthyosis, with polygonal patches of dry, flaky skin resembling dried out mudflats (or fish scales); biopsy shows classic histologic findings of sarcoidosis with characteristic granulomas [100]. Ulcerative sarcoidosis is uncommon and can closely resemble necrobiosis lipoidica both clinically and histopathologically (Fig. 9.11). Typical lesions are single or grouped atrophic plaques that ulcerate and may display yellow-orange discoloration [101, 102]. Hypopigmented sarcoidosis can occur de novo as well-defined, circular or oval macules or patches; lesions often contain a palpable granulomatous component that may subtly demonstrate the characteristic violaceous hue of the disease [103]. Sarcoidosis can rarely cause erythroderma, defined as >80% body surface area erythema, often with fine scale [104].

Scalp sarcoidosis (Fig. 9.12) can present with variable clinical signs, ranging from pauci-inflammatory disease to thick scale and violaceous inflammation. It can also cause both scarring and a non-scarring alopecia [105].

Nail involvement in sarcoidosis is uncommon, but manifestations may include pitting, onycholysis, trachyonychia, or complete loss of the nail plate. Nail sarcoidosis is strongly associated with bone involvement and a chronic disease course [106].

Mucosal sarcoidosis is uncommon but can affect the buccal mucosa, gingiva, lips, and/or tongue; lesions may include papules, bland erythema, or ulcerations [107]. Genital sarcoidosis is also rare and can present with plaques, nodules, or ill-defined masses or swelling. Granulomatous lesions affecting the vulva, vagina, scrotum, penis or testicles are more likely a manifestation of underlying inflammatory bowel disease rather than sarcoidosis [74].

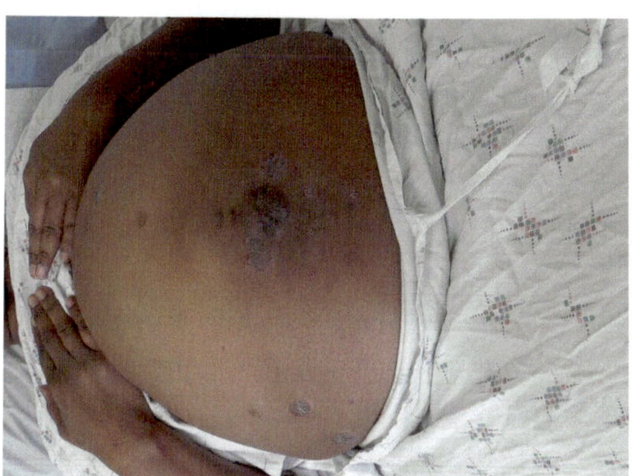

Fig. 9.10 Sarcoidosis plaques. These purple, flat, larger lesions have scale and may resemble psoriasis

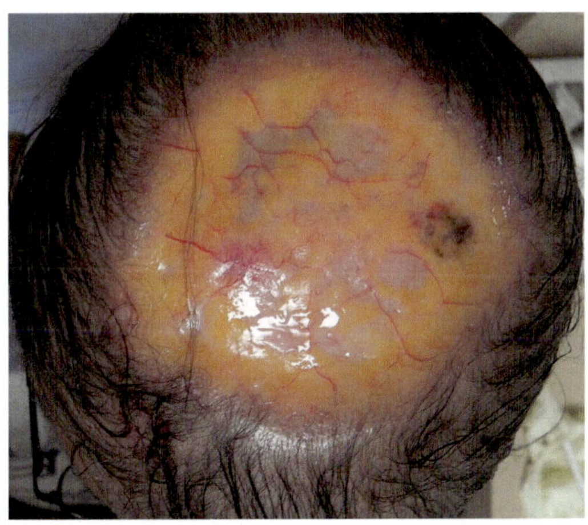

Fig. 9.11 Ulcerative sarcoidosis. This form of sarcoid can be challenging to diagnosis, as the presence of granulomatous inflammation within an ulcer may be a sign of infection, such as mycobacterial infection, and sarcoidosis is a diagnosis of exclusion. Multisystem involvement can be helpful, as in this case, where the patient had uveitis and hilar adenopathy. Ulcerative sarcoidosis will closely resemble necrobiosis lipoidica clinically and sometimes histologically

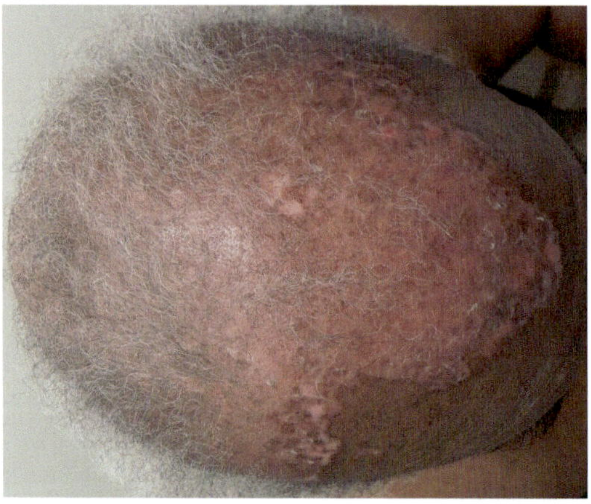

Fig. 9.12 Scalp sarcoidosis. Involvement of the scalp is relatively common in cutaneous sarcoidosis, but lesion morphology can be quite varied. Some lesions may resemble the orange, atrophic patches of necrobiosis lipoidica; others may be psoriasiform, as in this case. Patients with scalp sarcoidosis can develop either a scarring or a non-scarring alopecia

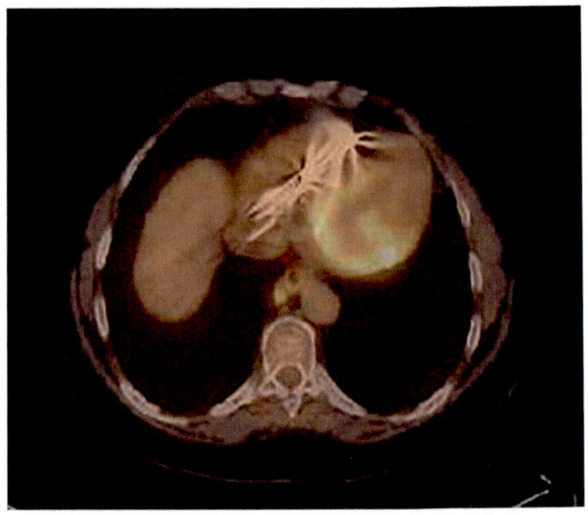

Fig. 9.13 PET CT demonstrating cardiac sarcoidosis that was not apparent on echocardiogram or cardiac MRI

Other Organ Involvement

Although the pulmonary and cutaneous presentations are the primary focus of this chapter, sarcoidosis can manifest in any organ system. Cardiac sarcoidosis warrants particular attention. Most literature cites a rate of approximately 5% among sarcoidosis patients [108]; however, autopsy studies suggest the rate is much higher, and analysis of patients who die of unexplained cardiac causes not uncommonly reveals occult cardiac sarcoidosis (Fig. 9.13). Cardiac sarcoidosis may be clinically silent in more than one quarter of patients. When it does cause signs or symptoms, the main manifestations are conduction abnormalities, ventricular arrhythmias, and heart failure [109].

Neurosarcoidosis occurs in 5–10% of cases and usually presents close to disease onset [110]. Clinically, patients can develop disease in any part of the nervous system, including cranial neuropathies (particularly facial neuropathy, optic neuropathy, or hearing loss), leptomeningeal disease (which can present with headache or more severe symptoms, such as seizures), parenchymal disease, cord involvement, or peripheral nerve involvement [110].

Ocular sarcoidosis is common, although the precise incidence is unclear and may vary by ethnicity and geography, with ranges of 13–80% reported. Most studies suggest the overall rate is approximately 25–30% [111]. The most common clinical features include uveitis, dry eyes, and conjunctival nodules.

Many patients with sarcoidosis will have granulomatous involvement of the lymph nodes, liver, or spleen; however, these findings are not clinically relevant in the majority of patients and rarely drive therapy. Lymph node involvement in sarcoidosis most commonly presents with bilateral hilar adenopathy; all sarcoid lymphadenopathy tends to be bilateral and symmetrical. Patients with active sarcoidosis may also develop metabolic abnormalities, particularly hypercalcemia, which, if persistent, can lead to symptoms, as well as potentially hypercalciuria and the development of renal stones. In a subset of patients, this will lead to renal dysfunction.

Specific Sarcoidosis Phenotypes

Lofgren noted in the 1940s that some of his patients with EN had symmetrical hilar adenopathy on chest x-ray. Approximately one third had iritis. These patients were treated with bed rest and high dose aspirin. Most experienced resolution of symptoms within weeks. Peri-articular arthritis has also been noted in this group of patients, whose presentation is now termed Lofgren syndrome.

In one study from Sweden, over 70% of patients with Lofgren syndrome were positive for HLA type DQB1*0201/DRB1*0301. Of these, disease resolution within two years was seen in over 95% of cases. By contrast, approximately half of the patients who were DQB1*0201/DRB1*0301 negative developed chronic disease. In the United States, the role of DQB1*0201/DRB1*0301 in predicting prognosis is less clear. It is also important to note that, in contrast to the typical definition of Lofgren syndrome, the patients in the Swedish cohort presented with peri-articular arthritis and hilar adenopathy, but not EN, which is a classic feature of the syndrome.

Heerfordt syndrome, also known uveoparotid fever, is another specific sarcoidosis phenotype, characterized by parotid gland enlargement, facial nerve palsy, uveitis, and fever. In both Lofgren syndrome and Heerfordt syndrome, the clinical presentation is generally sufficient for diagnosis in the absence of biopsy findings. However, histopathologic demonstration of typical granulomatous inflammation can help confirm the clinical suspicion.

Diagnostic Considerations

Sarcoidosis is a diagnosis of exclusion, with no gold-standard confirmatory test. Patients may be presumed to have the disease when they exhibit clinical, laboratory, and/or radiographic signs of multiorgan inflammation, with at least one biopsy demonstrating characteristic "naked" epithelioid granulomas. Certain clinical features may be helpful in raising the pre-test probability of sarcoidosis (Table 9.3). In areas where there are high rates of tuberculosis or leprosy, rendering a diagnosis of sarcoidosis can be challenging, and clinicians should maintain a high index of suspicion for alternative etiologies of granulomatous inflammation.

All patients should undergo a thorough history and review of systems to identify potentially symptomatic organ systems and allow for targeted diagnostic evaluation. Certain clinicoradiographic features may be very suggestive of sarcoidosis. Researchers have suggested classifying organ involvement as either "definitive," "highly probable," "probable," or "possible," based on organ-specific features [112, 113]. Organ involvement is typically definitive if there is histopathologic confirmation of granulomatous inflammation and other potential etiologies are excluded.

Table 9.3 Clinical features affecting the probability of sarcoidosis

More likely sarcoidosis	Less likely sarcoidosis
African-American or Northern European	Age < 15 or < 60
Female	History of smoking
Asymptomatic	Exposure to metal dusts, aerosols, organic antigens
Family history of sarcoidosis	History of tuberculosis
Multiorgan disease	History of recurrent infections
Suggestive laboratory findings: Lymphopenia Hypergammaglobulinemia Elevated serum calcium Elevated biomarkers (ACE, sIL2R, Vitamin D 1,25)	Systemic diseases capable of causing granulomatous inflammation Malignancy Inflammatory bowel disease Immunodeficiency Vasculitidites

Adapted from Culver [174]

Severe presentations may not require tissue confirmation. In cases of Lofgren syndrome, Heerfodt syndrome, asymptomatic bilateral hilar adenopathy, or bilateral hilar adenopathy coexisting with uveitis, sarcoidosis is highly likely [63, 114].

In nearly all other clinical scenarios, tissue confirmation of non-caseating epithelioid granulomas is advised. Factors unique to each patient may alter the risk-benefit analysis for biopsy, including severity of disease, likelihood of alternative diagnoses, organ or anatomic site affected, and need for treatment [1, 63]. Biopsy should be performed from the safest location with the highest yield; in many cases, the skin is preferable, with alternatives including superficial lymph nodes or easily-accessible ocular lesions. Due to the protean nature of the disease, clinicians should have a high index of suspicion and low threshold to sample cutaneous lesions, as skin biopsy is one of the diagnostic options with highest yield and lowest risk.

Histopathologically, the hallmark of sarcoidosis is the presence of extensive superficial and deep dermal epithelioid cell granulomas devoid or with a sparse rim of lymphocytes and/or plasma cells. Necrosis or caseation is usually absent, and extensive necrosis should prompt consideration for alternative etiologies, including infection or malignancy. Giant cells are variably present, and tend to be of the Langhans type, with nuclei arrayed in a peripheral arc. Asteroid bodies (eosinophilic stellate inclusions) and Schaumann bodies (calcific basophilic inclusions) are variably present and not specific for sarcoidosis. One quarter of cutaneous sarcoidosis biopsies will display polarizable foreign material, which does not exclude sarcoidosis [115–117]. Special stains for microorganisms (AFB, Fite) should invariably be negative, and tissue cultures should be performed if there is any suspicion for infection. Sarcoidosis remains a diagnosis of exclusion even with supportive pathology (Table 9.4).

Existing biomarkers (including angiotensin converting enzyme levels, vitamin D levels or ratios, and serum interleukin receptor levels) are nonspecific and do not offer sufficient sensitivity or specificity to warrant routine use. Emerging data in limited studies suggest there may be a role for novel markers such as chitotriosidase, but these findings have not been replicated in the clinical arena.

A thorough multisystem evaluation is essential in all patients with sarcoidosis (Table 9.5). Pulmonary involvement is seen in most patients with sarcoidosis. Imaging is important to evaluate the extent of pulmonic involvement and is abnormal in more than 90% of patients [71]. Chest radiography can demonstrate mediastinal nodal or lung parenchymal involvement and is used to determine the Scadding classification, as reviewed: stage 0 (normal; 8–16% of patients at presentation), stage 1 (bilateral hilar lymphadenopathy; 25–65%), stage 2 (hilar adenopathy and pulmonary infiltrates; 14–49%), stage 3 (pulmonary infiltrates without adenopathy; 10%), stage 4 (pulmonary fibrosis; 5% at presentation) [118, 119].

High resolution chest CT is the diagnostic test of choice for evaluating interstitial lung disease but is not routinely required in patients with sarcoidosis. CT is indicated if there are atypical clinical or chest radiography findings, a normal chest x-ray but persistent suspicion for sarcoid-

Table 9.4 Differential diagnosis of sarcoidosis biopsies

Lung	Skin	Other
Tuberculosis	Granuloma annulare	Brucellosis
Atypical mycobacteria	Necrobiosis lipoidica	Toxoplasmosis
Cryptococcosis	Necrobiotic xanthogranuloma	Kikuchi's disease
Aspergillosis	Cutaneous Crohn disease	Cat-scratch disease
Histoplasmosis	Rheumatoid nodule	Schistosomiasis
Coccidioidomycosis	Foreign body reaction: Tattoo, Paraffin/silicone/cosmetics	Sarcoid-like granulomatous reaction in lymph nodes associated with malignancy
Blastomycosis	Tuberculosis	Lymphoma (Hodgkin's, Non-Hodgkin's)
Pneumocystis jirovecii	Atypical mycobacteria	Inflammatory bowel disease
Mycoplasma	Deep fungal infection	Giant cell myocarditis
Hypersensensitivity pneumonitis	Malignancy: Granulomatous lymphoma	Viral infection
Pneumoconiosis: Beryllium, other	Granulomatosis with polyangiitis	Drug reaction
Drug reactions	Pyoderma gangrenosum	
Aspiration of foreign material		
Granulomatosis with polyangiitis		
Chronic interstitial pneumonia		

Adapted from Statement on Sarcoidosis [1]

Table 9.5 Suggested Systemic Work-Up in Patient with Sarcoidosis

Detailed history (family history, environmental/occupational exposures [beryllium, pine tree, microbe-rich, heavy metals,] …)
Symptomatology (dyspnea, cough, palpitations, fatigue/malaise/low grade fevers, …)
Physical examination
Chest X-ray (posterior–anterior and lateral)
Pulmonary function tests (including DLCO)
Routine ophthalmologic examination
Complete blood count
Comprehensive serum chemistries (including calcium, liver function tests, creatinine)
[a]If history of nephrolithiasis, then urinalysis with urine calcium)
Electrocardiogram
[a]If palpitations or abnormalities on EKG, consider Holter monitor and additional cardiac imaging
Tuberculin skin test or interferon-gamma release assay
Thyroid function testing
Biomarkers: serum ACE, Vitamin D25/Vitamin D1,25, …

Adapted from Wanat and Rosenbach [74]
[a]*DLCO* diffusion capacity for carbon monoxide, *ACE* angiotensin-converting enzyme

osis, or complications from pulmonary involvement [1, 71, 120]. However, CT is incomplete and unreliable in distinguishing areas of active granulomatous inflammation from areas of damage, fibrosis, and scarring.

Standard pulmonary function testing (PFT), including spirometry and diffusion of carbon monoxide, is suggested in patients with sarcoidosis. Diffusion of carbon monoxide is a useful test for detection of early interstitial lung disease [120]. PFTs can be used to evaluate for restrictive or obstructive lung disease. Most sarcoidosis is restrictive, but one third of patients will have obstructive patterns. PFTs provide information about the forced vital capacity (FVC) and forced expiratory volume in 1 second (FEV1), both of which will be abnormal in the presence of obstructive disease. FVC will be reduced in restrictive lung disease. PFTs correlate only modestly with chest imaging but may be useful in tracking disease activity and monitoring for functional improvement or deterioration as the disease progresses [120].

PET scanning is increasingly utilized to assess active disease in sarcoidosis patients. While not routinely performed, it is often used when malignancy is suspected. It can detect ongoing inflammation in both lymph nodes and parenchymal infiltrates. In sarcoidosis patients, PET scanning may detect activity in multiple organs, including the bones, spleen, and liver, even in an asymptomatic patient.

MRI, especially with gadolinium enhancement, can detect sarcoidal lesions in the brain, heart, and bone. Again, the disease visualized on imaging can be more extensive than suspected clinically. MRI and PET scanning should be employed in patients with symptoms suggesting cardiac sarcoidosis, such as palpitations or evidence of congestive heart failure. Some endobronchial lesions may be amenable to endoscopic biopsies, while peripheral lesions may be accessible to CT-guided biopsy. Mediastinoscopy and surgical lung biopsies are rarely required [63].

Beyond the cutaneous and pulmonary assessment, patients should be asked about palpitations or syncope to screen for cardiac involvement, and all patients should undergo screening with an ECG. Symptomatic patients may require further testing, including echocardiogram; patients with echocardiographic abnormalities may benefit from cardiac MRI or FDG-PET imaging [109]. Depending on findings, Holter monitor screening for arrhythmias may be indicated as well.

Neurosarcoidosis is often clinically apparent; evaluation depends on the clinical symptomatology, and referral to an experienced neurologist may be beneficial. MRI with gadolinium is the primary diagnostic modality, though some patients will require CSF analysis, or EMG for suspected peripheral nerve involvement [110].

Given the high rates of ocular involvement in patients with sarcoidosis, all sarcoid patients should be evaluated by an ophthalmologist at the time of diagnosis and should be screened annually or evaluated if new symptoms develop.

It is rarely necessary to evaluate patients for hepatic or splenic sarcoidal involvement, and sarcoidosis in the marrow is relatively rare. Significant abnormalities in these organ systems should be apparent on routine lab work and physical exam.

All sarcoidosis patients should undergo measurement of serum calcium (corrected for albumin), as hypercalcemia can be a significant problem in sarcoidosis. Patients with a history of nephrolithiasis warrant evaluation for hypercalciuria. Persistent hypercalcemia and hypercalciuria can result in renal dysfunction.

Disease and Comorbidity Assessment

Sarcoidosis is by definition a multiorgan disease, and patients with the disease tend to be followed closely by multiple physicians, each monitoring their target organ and working together to manage the patient. Even so, patients with sarcoidosis require evaluation for potential comorbid conditions.

First, patients with sarcoidosis require close monitoring for treatment-related adverse events (see below, "principles of management" section). Systemic corticosteroids are the mainstay of treatment for most patients with sarcoidosis, and these can have a range of acute and chronic side effects that require monitoring and mitigation.

Additionally, more than half of patients with sarcoidosis suffer from a comorbid disease, most commonly hypertension, diabetes, thyroid disease, and obesity [121]. Several small studies have suggested an increased risk of malignancy in patients with sarcoidosis, and sarcoidal granulomas can be found in biopsies in patients with malignancies [122]. One meta-analysis of 16 cohort and case-control studies demonstrated a moderate association of sarcoidosis with malignancy [123]. The risk appears to be greatest for lymphoma and lymphoproliferative diseases. New symptoms or radiologic findings in patients with sarcoidosis should not automatically be attributed to the underlying disease and warrant appropriate evaluation in all cases, including tissue sampling, if necessary [124, 125].

Importantly for dermatologists, patients with sarcoidosis may be at two-fold higher risk of developing both melanoma and nonmelanoma skin cancers [123, 126]. This is true for African-American patients in addition to those of other races, although it should be noted that incomplete sampling of verrucous or hyperkeratotic sarcoidosis may lead to a false pathologic impression of a superficial squamous cell carcinoma. The association between sarcoidosis and malignancy may be due to inherent sarcoidosis-related immune dysregulation, sarcoid-like reactions due to malignancies, sarcoid-like reactions due to chemotherapeutic agents, or sarcoid treatment-related/immunosuppression-related malignancy development [124].

Sarcoidosis may also occur in association with diseases other than malignancy, potentially due to shared genetic risk factors or the immune/inflammatory milieu of the disease state. Sarcoidosis and psoriasis, both Th1- and Th17-mediated diseases, appear to co-occur more frequently than would be expected by chance alone [95, 96]. Patients with sarcoidosis appear to be at increased risk for thyroid disease, an association demonstrated in case-control studies and replicated in a database study [127–131]. As both entities may present with non-specific constitutional symptoms, it is important that physicians keep this potential association in mind. Case reports have suggested other Th1-associatd diseases, such as alopecia areata and vitiligo, may occur more than expected in patients with sarcoidosis [132].

Principles of Management

The most important principle of managing sarcoidosis is that treatment should be tailored to the specific patient and clinical phenotype, depending largely on the organs involved. Many patients present with asymptomatic or minimally symptomatic disease and can safely be monitored for disease progression. Approximately half of patients will experience spontaneous improvement and resolution within the first 2 years of diagnosis. Outside this group, the goals of treatment should be to improve symptomatology and prevent morbidity, balancing the risks of the treatment with the potential therapeutic benefits.

While many treatments for sarcoidosis will affect, and improve, all aspects of disease-related inflammation, several therapeutic options (particularly localized treatments, such as eye drops, topical skin-directed therapy, or inhalers) will treat only the targeted organ. Treatments may take 2–3 months to take effect, and both patients and treating physicians should exercise patience before deeming a therapeutic trial a failure.

There is a relative lack of high-quality evidence or comparative-effectiveness data for sarcoidosis treatment, and no treatments are currently FDA approved for this indication. Historically, it has been a challenge to conduct clinical trials for sarcoidosis due to difficulty in distinguishing active inflammation from disease-related damage, as well as the subjectivity or effort-dependence of a number of endpoints. Recently validated instruments to measure cutaneous disease hold promise for future trials [133, 134]. The most widely used clinical assessment tool is the Sarcoidosis Activity and Severity Index (SASI), which can accurately and reliably capture the extent of cutaneous disease activity; several studies have demonstrated its ability to document change in skin lesions over time in response to therapy [134].

Another cutaneous sarcoidosis assessment tool, the Cutaneous Sarcoidosis Activity and Morphology Instrument, was developed to capture sarcoidosis morphology-specific information; it was subsequently validated and demonstrated excellent reliability and correlation with patient-reported outcomes measures [133, 135].

A third instrument, the Sarcoidosis Assessment Tool, was developed and validated as a sarcoidosis-specific patient-reported outcome instrument that can reliably document the impact of sarcoidosis on patient quality of life and has demonstrated sensitivity to change and clinically significant differences that correlate to disease severity [136, 137]. Taken together, these scoring systems provide the tools necessary to conduct clinical trials with a focus on responsiveness of skin disease to therapeutic intervention.

Importantly, treatment agents used in sarcoidosis may affect different organ systems at different rates. For hydroxychloroquine and methotrexate, for example, studies have found a higher rate of response for skin lesions than pulmonary disease. Neurologic and cardiac disease can be even more refractory. It can also be challenging to assess response in extracutaneous disease: one advantage of monitoring skin lesions is the ability to differentiate between active inflammation and scarring, but this can be more difficult for other organs.

Treatment of cutaneous and pulmonary sarcoidosis is reviewed in detail below. Individual treatment stratagems may vary from those described here, particularly for patients with severe cardiac or neurologic involvement, who often require combination treatment with multiple agents. Patients with suspected cardiac sarcoidosis should undergo a full evaluation with an experienced cardiologist as described above, ideally prior to initiating aggressive treatment, which can sometimes precipitate arrhythmias.

Treatment for Cutaneous Sarcoidosis

Treatment of cutaneous sarcoidosis requires a stepwise approach [141] (Fig. 9.14 and Table 9.6). Skin-directed therapeutics may be used in patients with mild disease or to treat limited recalcitrant lesions in those with moderate to severe disease. Topical treatment options include corticosteroids (applied to the skin or injected intralesionally). High-potency topical steroids can lead to resolution of isolated or sparse skin lesions, whereas intralesional injections can ameliorate thicker plaques or subcutaneous nodules [142–144]. Steroid-sparing skin-directed options include topical tacrolimus, phototherapy, photodynamic therapy, and laser therapy [74, 141]. Photodynamic therapy tends to be helpful only while treatment is maintained. Lasers can help select features of sarcoidosis, but they can also induce new lesions or exacerbations and are best used by experienced clinicians.

Systemic therapy for cutaneous sarcoidosis can be divided broadly into immunomodulatory therapies and immunosuppressive therapies. As with topical therapy, most immunomodulatory

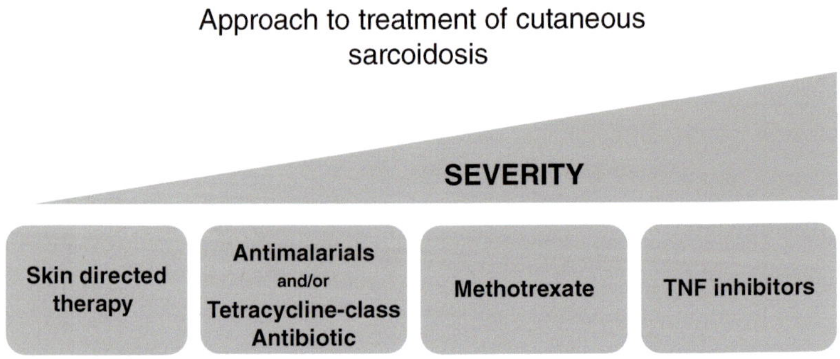

Fig. 9.14 Treatment of cutaneous sarcoidosis algorithm. (Adapted from Wanat and Rosenbach [141])

Table 9.6 Therapeutic options for cutaneous sarcoidosis

	Medication
Topical therapy	Topical corticosteroids (strength depending on anatomic site)
	Tacrolimus
Intralesional	Triamcinolone (10–40 mg/kg)
Physical	Phototherapy (UVA)
	Photodynamic therapy
	Laser[a] (Pulsed-dye, CO2, ruby, KTP)
	Surgical excision
Immunomodulatory	Hydroxychloroquine/Chloroquine
	Chloroquine
	Minocycline/doxycycline
	Pentoxifylline
	Apremilast
	Systemic Retinoids
	Thalidomide
Immunosuppressants	Prednisone
	Methotrexate
TNF inhibitors	Adalimumab
	Infliximab
JAK-inhibitors	Tofacitinib [177]

Adapted from Wanat and Rosenbach [74]
[a]Lasers should be used with caution as they can induce or worsen disease

therapies used for cutaneous sarcoidosis have little impact on extracutaneous disease. If significant extracutaneous disease is present, it is generally advisable to tailor treatment to control the extracutaneous disease, and then supplement with added skin-directed therapy as needed.

Antimalarial agents are among the medications whose use in cutaneous sarcoidosis is supported by the most evidence and experience. Two-thirds to three-quarters of patients improve on these agents [74, 145–148]. Potential adverse effects include hair loss, mild, generally self-limited gastrointestinal disturbances, and, rarely, a lichenoid skin eruption. Ocular toxicity from antimalarials is generally less common than assumed, developing only in approximately 5% of patients after more than 5 years of cumulative use. The risk of ocular toxicity increases with dose, duration, renal or hepatic impairment, and age.

Tetracycline class antibiotics, particularly minocycline, can be beneficial in treating most forms of cutaneous sarcoidosis [149, 150]. These agents are particularly helpful in cases where infectious causes of granulomatous inflammation cannot be completely excluded.

Recently, a novel regimen of concomitant levofloxacin, ethambutol, azithromycin, and rifampin has been described for the treatment of chronic cutaneous sarcoidosis with improvements in SASI scoring [151]. Possible mechanisms of action include immunomodulation and, in cases where there is an infectious causative antigen, direct antimicrobial action [151].

Additional non-immunosuppressive systemic therapeutic options for treating cutaneous sarcoidosis include pentoxifylline, apremilast (documented SASI improvement [140]), and systemic retinoids [74, 152–154].

Systemic immunosuppressive therapies used for cutaneous sarcoidosis tend to be effective for extracutaneous disease as well. These are good options in patients who fail the above treatments, or those who have moderate-to-severe skin sarcoidosis along with mild extracutaneous disease [141].

Traditional systemic agents used in sarcoidosis include corticosteroids, methotrexate, and thalidomide. Prednisone can be helpful in obtaining quick disease control, which may be necessary in patients with rapidly progressive, disfiguring, or ulcerative cutaneous sarcoidosis. Doses should start at 20–40 mg/day with slow tapering [141, 155–157].

Methotrexate is generally the first-line systemic immunosuppressive agent used for widespread cutaneous sarcoidosis that fails to respond to antimalarials. Methotrexate is also commonly used as the first-line non-corticosteroid agent for systemic sarcoidosis; benefit is generally seen in 60–75% of patients. Usual doses range from 15 to 25 mg weekly, tapered slowly to the lowest dose able to maintain disease control. Methotrexate can take three months to start working and six months to fully take effect; patients should therefore be counseled to expect a slow response to therapy [158–161].

Azathioprine and mycophenolate mofetil are sometimes used for pulmonary, neuro-, or cardiac sarcoidosis. However, these agents are minimally effective in treating cutaneous disease in most cases.

Thalidomide has traditionally been used for recalcitrant cutaneous sarcoidosis. However, it carries a high frequency of neuropathy and risk of venous thrombosis; additionally, the federally regulated registry that exists to minimize the risk associated with its teratogenicity makes prescribing a challenge. Additionally, a recent blinded study showed a lack of efficacy of thalidomide compared to placebo in sarcoidosis [162]. While this agent may still be beneficial in a subset of patients, newer agents hold more promise and are generally the next-line drugs in patients who fail to respond to methotrexate.

Tumor necrosis factor alpha inhibitors, particularly infliximab and, to a lesser degree, adalimumab, are highly effective agents that can clear even chronic, recalcitrant skin sarcoidosis, including lupus pernio. Infliximab (3–7 mg/kg at 0, 2, and 6 weeks and then every 4–6 weeks) can lead to rapid improvement of refractory skin lesions [74, 163–168] and SASI [138] score. Adalimumab (80 mg loading dose, 40 mg weekly) has also been shown to improve refractory skin disease [169–171]; notably both agents need to be used at higher doses than dermatologists normally utilize for skin disease (such as psoriasis). Etanercept, perhaps because of its wide use, has been more associated than other agents with TNF-induced sarcoid-like granulomatous disease, and a trial evaluating etanercept in sarcoidosis was discontinued due to lack of efficacy and increased adverse events [172]. Golimumab showed a non-significant trend towards improvement in skin disease by SASI score in one randomized trial [139], whereas ustekinumab was ineffective (Table 9.7).

Treatment of Pulmonary Sarcoidosis

Pulmonary sarcoidosis is generally responsive to systemic corticosteroids, and most treatment guidelines suggest initial dosing between 20–40 mg daily, with a rapid taper to the lowest possible dose; most clinicians attempt to taper to 10 mg daily or lower [173] (Fig. 9.15). Inhaled corticosteroids may be helpful in managing cough or a reactive airway component of the disease.

Cytotoxic medications are often utilized as steroid sparing agents or in patients for whom corticosteroids are contraindicated; these agents may take months to demonstrate efficacy in many cases. Methotrexate is the most widely used and

Table 9.7 Therapeutic trials in sarcoidosis

	Study design	Photo comparisons	SASI	PGA
Infliximab [138]	DBPC	NR	Significantly different from placebo	Significantly different from placebo
Infliximab [83]	Case series	Superior to other treatments	NR	NR
Golimumab [139]	DBPC	NR	Trend towards improvement, not significantly different from placebo	NR
Ustekinumab [139]	DBPC	NR	No improvement	NR
Aprelimast [140]	OLPS	Significant improvement	Significant improvement	NR
CLEAR [140]	SMPC	NR	Significant improvement	NR

DBPC double blind, placebo controlled, *OLPS* open label prospective series, *SMPC* single masked placebo controlled, *CLEAR* concomitant levofloxacin, ethambutol, azithromycin, and rifampin, *SASI* Sarcoidosis Activity and Severity Index, *PGA* Physicians Global Assessment

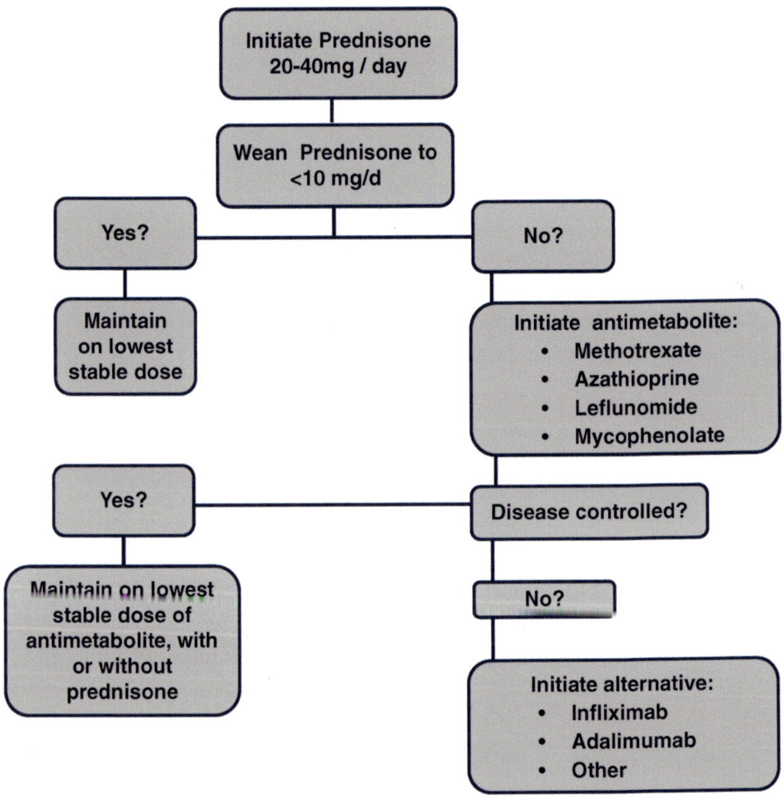

Fig. 9.15 Treatment of symptomatic pulmonary sarcoidosis. (Adapted from Baughman and Lower [175])

has the highest quality supportive evidence. It is typically dosed at 10–20 mg weekly, with supplemental folic acid. Azathioprine and mycophenolate mofetil may also be used in as steroid sparing agents. Leflunomide is typically given at 20 mg daily, and patients have approximately 50% response rate. TNF-inhibitors are often used as third line agents for pulmonary sarcoidosis but may be efficacious in many cases [173].

Summary

Sarcoidosis is by its very nature a multiorgan, multidisciplinary disease. Genetically susceptible patients are exposed to an environmental (or autologous) antigens, setting off a cascade of Th1-predominant immune inflammation, which can present with a variety of signs and symptoms and may follow numerous disease courses. Some patients present with predominantly single-organ disease, whereas multiple sites are affected in other patients. A significant subset of patients may experience clinically asymptomatic disease. Approximately half of patients will spontaneously resolve their disease, while a significant minority of patients will experience chronic inflammation, sometimes with fibrosis, scarring, and permanent morbidity – as well as, in some cases, mortality.

All patients with sarcoidosis require initial extensive evaluation to determine the extent of disease and most affected organs. Patients must be followed closely for asymptomatic sarcoidosis-related inflammation of other organs and require close monitoring even if untreated, as the disease can wax and wane. Formal evaluation with organ-specific testing at regular intervals is indicated, as patients may be minimally symptomatic from chronic, progressive disease, which, if unrecognized, can lead to significant long-term organ dysfunction.

Treatment requires balancing the disease activity and morbidity with treatment-related risks and side effects and should be individualized. Often one treatment for sarcoidosis will improve all sites of inflammation, but organ-specific targeted therapies exist, and selection of the appropriate treatment should involve multidisciplinary discussion and close collaboration between treating physicians.

References

1. Statement on sarcoidosis. Joint Statement of the American Thoracic Society (ATS), the European Respiratory Society (ERS) and the World Association of Sarcoidosis and Other Granulomatous Disorders (WASOG) adopted by the ATS Board of Directors and by the ERS Executive Committee, February 1999. Am J Respir Crit Care Med. 1999;160(2):736–55.
2. Costabel U, Hunninghake GW. ATS/ERS/WASOG statement on sarcoidosis. Sarcoidosis Statement Committee. American Thoracic Society. European Respiratory Society. World Association for sarcoidosis and other granulomatous disorders. Eur Respir J. 1999;14(4):735–7.
3. Siltzbach LE, et al. Course and prognosis of sarcoidosis around the world. Am J Med. 1974;57(6):847–52.
4. Baughman RP, et al. Clinical characteristics of patients in a case control study of sarcoidosis. Am J Respir Crit Care Med. 2001;164(10 Pt 1):1885–9.
5. Mana J, Marcoval J. Skin manifestations of sarcoidosis. Presse Med. 2012;41(6 Pt 2):e355–74.
6. Judson MA. The diagnosis of sarcoidosis. Clin Chest Med. 2008;29(3):415–27, viii.
7. Judson MA, Baughman RP. How many organs need to be involved to diagnose sarcoidosis? An unanswered question that, hopefully, will become irrelevant. Sarcoidosis Vasc Diffuse Lung Dis. 2014;31:6–7.
8. Hanno R, Callen JP. Sarcoidosis: a disorder with prominent cutaneous features and their interrelationship with systemic disease. Med Clin North Am. 1980;64(5):847–66.
9. Hanno R, et al. Cutaneous sarcoidal granulomas and the development of systemic sarcoidosis. Arch Dermatol. 1981;117(4):203–7.
10. Rybicki B, et al. Racial differences in sarcoidosis incidence: a 5-year study in a health maintenance organization. 1997;145:234–41.
11. Rybicki BA, et al. Epidemiology, demographics, and genetics of sarcoidosis. Semin Respir Infect. 1998;13(3):166–73.
12. Reich JM. A critical analysis of sarcoidosis incidence assessment. Multidiscip Respir Med. 2013;8(1):57.
13. Mirsaeidi M, et al. Racial difference in sarcoidosis mortality in the United States. Chest. 2015;147(2):438–49.
14. Deng JC, Baughman RP, Lynch JP 3rd. Cardiac involvement in sarcoidosis. Semin Respir Crit Care Med. 2002;23(6):513–27.
15. Hosoda Y, Sasagawa S, Yasuda N. Epidemiology of sarcoidosis: new frontiers to explore. Curr Opin Pulm Med. 2002;8:424–8.
16. Demirkok SS, Basaranoglu M, Akbilgic O. Seasonal variation of the onset of presentations in stage 1 sarcoidosis. Int J Clin Pract. 2006;60(11):1443–50.
17. Gerke AK, et al. An analysis of seasonality of sarcoidosis in the United States veteran population: 2000–2007. Sarcoidosis Vasc Diffuse Lung Dis. 2012;29(2):155–8.
18. Gupta D, Agarwal R, Aggarwal AN. Seasonality of sarcoidosis: the 'heat' is on. Sarcoidosis Vasc Diffuse Lung Dis. 2013;30(3):241–3.
19. Adrianto I, et al. Genome-wide association study of African and European Americans implicates multiple shared and ethnic specific loci in sarcoidosis susceptibility. PLoS One. 2012;7(8):e43907.
20. McGrath DS, et al. Epidemiology of familial sarcoidosis in the UK. Thorax. 2000;55(9):751–4.
21. Sverrild A, Backer V, Kyvik KO, et al. Heredity in sarcoidosis: a registry based twin study. Thorax. 2008;63:894–6.
22. Rossman MD, Kreider ME. Lesson learned from ACCESS (a case controlled etiologic study of sarcoidosis). Proc Am Thorac Soc. 2007;4(5):453–6.

23. Centers for Disease Control and Prevention (CDC). Sarcoidosis among U.S. Navy enlisted men, 1965–1993. Morb Mortal Wkly Rep. 1997;46:539–43.
24. Prezant DJ, Dhala A, Goldstein A, et al. The incidence and severity of sarcoidosis in New York City Firefighters. Chest. 1999;116:1183–93.
25. Izbicki G, et al. World Trade Center "sarcoid-like" granulomatous pulmonary disease in New York City Fire Department rescue workers. Chest. 2007;131(5):1414–23.
26. Barnard J, Rose C, Newman L, et al. Job and industry classification associated with sarcoidosis in a case control etiologic study of sarcoidosis. J Occup Environ Med. 2005;47:226–34.
27. Parkes SA, et al. Epidemiology of sarcoidosis in the Isle of Man--1: a case controlled study. Thorax. 1987;42(6):420–6.
28. Hills SE, Parkes SA, Baker SB. Epidemiology of sarcoidosis in the Isle of Man--2: evidence for space-time clustering. Thorax. 1987;42(6):427–30.
29. Grunewald J, et al. Different HLA-DRB1 allele distributions in distinct clinical subgroups of sarcoidosis patients. Respir Res. 2010;11:25.
30. Fischer A, et al. Genetics of sarcoidosis. Semin Respir Crit Care Med. 2014;35(3):296–306.
31. Valentonyte R, et al. Sarcoidosis is associated with a truncating splice site mutation in BTNL2. Nat Genet. 2005;37(4):357–64.
32. Feng X, et al. Annexin A11 (ANXA11) gene polymorphisms are associated with sarcoidosis in a Han Chinese population: a case-control study. BMJ Open. 2014;4(7):–e004466.
33. Fischer A, Rybicki BA. Granuloma genes in sarcoidosis: what is new? Curr Opin Pulm Med. 2015;21(5):510–6.
34. Newman KL, Newman LS. Occupational causes of sarcoidosis. Curr Opin Allergy Clin Immunol. 2012;12(2):145–50.
35. Chen ES, Moller DR. Etiologies of sarcoidosis. Clin Rev Allergy Immunol. 2015;49(1):6–18.
36. Clay H, et al. Dichotomous role of the macrophage in early Mycobacterium marinum infection of the zebrafish. Cell Host Microbe. 2007;2(1):29–39.
37. Moller DR, et al. Enhanced expression of IL-12 associated with Th1 cytokine profiles in active pulmonary sarcoidosis. J Immunol. 1996;156(12):4952–60.
38. Shigehara K, et al. IL-12 and IL-18 are increased and stimulate IFN-gamma production in sarcoid lungs. J Immunol. 2001;166(1):642–9.
39. Facco M, et al. Sarcoidosis is a Th1/Th17 multisystem disorder. Thorax. 2011;66(2):144–50.
40. Shigehara K, et al. Increased circulating interleukin-12 (IL-12) p40 in pulmonary sarcoidosis. Clin Exp Immunol. 2003;132(1):152–7.
41. Sones M, Israel HL. Course and prognosis of sarcoidosis. Am J Med. 1960;29(1):84–93.
42. Miyara M, et al. The immune paradox of sarcoidosis and regulatory T cells. J Exp Med. 2006;203(2):359–70.
43. Lee N-S, et al. Low levels of NF-κB/p65 mark anergic CD4+ T cells and correlate with disease severity in sarcoidosis. Clin Vaccine Immunol CVI. 2011;18(2):223–34.
44. Munro CS, Mitchell DN. The K veim response: still useful, still a puzzle. Thorax. 1987;42(5):321–31.
45. Morita R, et al. Donor cell-derived sarcoidosis after allogeneic BMT. Bone Marrow Transplant. 2009;43(6):507–8.
46. Gupta D, et al. Molecular evidence for the role of mycobacteria in sarcoidosis: a meta-analysis. Eur Respir J. 2007;30(3):508–16.
47. Chen ES, et al. T cell responses to mycobacterial catalase-peroxidase profile a pathogenic antigen in systemic sarcoidosis. J Immunol (Baltimore, Md : 1950). 2008;181(12):8784–96.
48. Hanngren A, et al. Tuberculostearic acid in lymph nodes from patients with sarcoidosis. Sarcoidosis. 1987;4(2):101–4.
49. Dubaniewicz A, et al. Mycobacterium tuberculosis complex and mycobacterial heat shock proteins in lymph node tissue from patients with pulmonary sarcoidosis. J Clin Microbiol. 2006;44(9):3448–51.
50. Homma JY, et al. Bacteriological investigation on biopsy specimens from patients with sarcoidosis. Jpn J Exp Med. 1978;48(3):251–5.
51. Eishi Y, et al. Quantitative analysis of mycobacterial and propionibacterial DNA in lymph nodes of Japanese and European patients with sarcoidosis. J Clin Microbiol. 2002;40(1):198–204.
52. Ebe Y, et al. Proliferative response of peripheral blood mononuclear cells and levels of antibody to recombinant protein from Propionibacterium acnes DNA expression library in Japanese patients with sarcoidosis. Sarcoidosis Vasc Diffuse Lung Dis. 2000;17(3):256–65.
53. Chen ES, Moller DR. Etiology of sarcoidosis. Clin Chest Med. 2008;29(3):365–77, vii.
54. Chen ES, et al. Serum amyloid A regulates granulomatous inflammation in sarcoidosis through Toll-like receptor-2. Am J Respir Crit Care Med. 2010;181(4):360–73.
55. Bargagli E, et al. Analysis of serum amyloid A in sarcoidosis patients. Respir Med. 2011;105(5):775–80.
56. Rafnsson V, et al. Association between exposure to crystalline silica and risk of sarcoidosis. Occup Environ Med. 1998;55(10):657–60.
57. Werfel U, et al. Sarcoid granulomatosis after zirconium exposure with multiple organ involvement. Eur Respir J. 1998;12(3):750.
58. Cummings MM, Hudgins PC. Chemical constituents of pine pollen and their possible relationship to sarcoidosis. Am J Med Sci. 1958;236(3):311–7.
59. Cummings MM. An evaluation of the possible relationship of pine pollen to sarcoidosis. Acta Med Scand. 2009;176:48–50.
60. Tukiainen P, et al. Pulmonary granulomatous reaction: talc pneumoconiosis or chronic sarcoidosis? Br J Ind Med. 1984;41(1):84–7.

61. Farber HW, Fairman RP, Glauser FL. Talc granulomatosis: laboratory findings similar to sarcoidosis. Am Rev Respir Dis. 1982;125(2):258–61.
62. James DG. A clinicopathological classification of granulomatous disorders. Postgrad Med J. 2000;76(898):457–65.
63. Valeyre D, et al. Clinical presentation of sarcoidosis and diagnostic work-up. Semin Respir Crit Care Med. 2014;35(3):336–51.
64. Hillerdal G, et al. Sarcoidosis: epidemiology and prognosis. A 15-year European study. Am Rev Respir Dis. 1984;130(1):29–32.
65. Johns CJ, et al. Longitudinal study of chronic sarcoidosis with low-dose maintenance corticosteroid therapy. Outcome and complications. Ann N Y Acad Sci. 1986;465:702–12.
66. Gideon NM, Mannino DM. Sarcoidosis mortality in the United States 1979–1991: an analysis of multiple-cause mortality data. Am J Med. 1996;100(4):423–7.
67. Perry A, Vuitch F. Causes of death in patients with sarcoidosis. A morphologic study of 38 autopsies with clinicopathologic correlations. Arch Pathol Lab Med. 1995;119(2):167–72.
68. Takada K, et al. The clinical course and prognosis of patients with severe, moderate or mild sarcoidosis. J Clin Epidemiol. 1993;46(4):359–66.
69. Iwai K, et al. Racial difference in cardiac sarcoidosis incidence observed at autopsy. Sarcoidosis. 1994;11(1):26–31.
70. Reich JM, Johnson RE. Course and prognosis of sarcoidosis in a nonreferral setting. Analysis of 86 patients observed for 10 years. Am J Med. 1985;78(1):61–7.
71. Nunes H, et al. Imaging in sarcoidosis. Semin Respir Crit Care Med. 2007;28(1):102–20.
72. Nishimura K, et al. Pulmonary sarcoidosis: correlation of CT and histopathologic findings. Radiology. 1993;189(1):105–9.
73. Lynch JP 3rd, Kazerooni EA, Gay SE. Pulmonary sarcoidosis. Clin Chest Med. 1997;18(4):755–85.
74. Wanat KA, Rosenbach M. Cutaneous sarcoidosis. Clin Chest Med. 2015;36(4):685–702.
75. Elgart ML. Cutaneous sarcoidosis: definitions and types of lesions. Clin Dermatol. 1986;4(4):35–45.
76. Marcoval J, Moreno A, Mana J. Papular sarcoidosis of the knees: a clue for the diagnosis of erythema nodosum-associated sarcoidosis. J Am Acad Dermatol. 2003;49(1):75–8.
77. Elgart ML. Cutaneous lesions of sarcoidosis. Prim Care. 1978;5(2):249–62.
78. Marcoval J, Mana J, Rubio M. Specific cutaneous lesions in patients with systemic sarcoidosis: relationship to severity and chronicity of disease. Clin Exp Dermatol. 2011;36(7):739–44.
79. Mana J, et al. Granulomatous cutaneous sarcoidosis: diagnosis, relationship to systemic disease, prognosis and treatment. Sarcoidosis Vasc Diffuse Lung Dis. 2013;30(4):268–81.
80. Ishak R, et al. Cutaneous sarcoidosis: clinicopathologic study of 76 patients from Lebanon. Int J Dermatol. 2015;54(1):33–41.
81. Sharma OP, Papanikolaou IC. Lupus pernio: a tale of four characters in search of a malady. Sarcoidosis Vasc Diffuse Lung Dis. 2009;26(2):167–71.
82. Spiteri MA, et al. Lupus pernio: a clinico-radiological study of thirty-five cases. Br J Dermatol. 1985;112(3):315–22.
83. Stagaki E, et al. The treatment of lupus pernio: results of 116 treatment courses in 54 patients. Chest. 2009;135(2):468–76.
84. Yanardag H, Pamuk ON, Pamuk GE. Lupus pernio in sarcoidosis: clinical features and treatment outcomes of 14 patients. J Clin Rheumatol. 2003;9(2):72–6.
85. Efthimiou P, Kukar M. Lupus pernio: sarcoid-specific cutaneous manifestation associated with chronic sarcoid arthropathy. J Clin Rheumatol. 2011;17(6):343.
86. Neville E, et al. Sarcoidosis of the upper respiratory tract and its association with lupus pernio. Thorax. 1976;31(6):660–4.
87. Ahmed I, Harshad SR. Subcutaneous sarcoidosis: is it a specific subset of cutaneous sarcoidosis frequently associated with systemic disease? J Am Acad Dermatol. 2006;54(1):55–60.
88. Dalle Vedove C, Colato C, Girolomoni G. Subcutaneous sarcoidosis: report of two cases and review of the literature. Clin Rheumatol. 2011;30(8):1123–8.
89. El Sayed F, Dhaybi R, Ammoury A. Subcutaneous nodular sarcoidosis and systemic involvement successfully treated with doxycycline. 2006;54:42–4.
90. Higgins EM, Salisbury JR, Du Vivier AW. Subcutaneous sarcoidosis. Clin Exp Dermatol. 1993;18(1):65–6.
91. Marcoval J, et al. Subcutaneous sarcoidosis--clinicopathological study of 10 cases. Br J Dermatol. 2005;153(4):790–4.
92. Marcoval J, et al. Subcutaneous sarcoidosis. Dermatol Clin. 2008;26(4):553–6, ix.
93. Marchell RM, Judson MA. Cutaneous sarcoidosis. Semin Respir Crit Care Med. 2010;31(4):442–51.
94. Burgoyne JS, Wood MG. Psoriasiform sarcoidosis. Arch Dermatol. 1972;106(6):896–8.
95. Wanat KA, et al. Sarcoidosis and psoriasis: a case series and review of the literature exploring co-incidence vs coincidence. JAMA Dermatol. 2013;149(7):848–52.
96. Khalid U, Gislason GH, Hansen PR. Sarcoidosis in patients with psoriasis: a population-based cohort study. PLoS One. 2014;9(10):e109632.
97. Nishizawa A, et al. Diffuse disseminated lichenoid-type cutaneous sarcoidosis mimicking erythroderma. Int J Dermatol. 2014;53(8):e369–70.
98. Stockman DL, et al. Verrucous cutaneous sarcoidosis: case report and review of this unusual variant of cutaneous sarcoidosis. Am J Dermatopathol. 2013;35(2):273–6.

99. Pezzetta S, et al. Verrucous sarcoidosis of the skin simulating squamous cell carcinoma. Sarcoidosis Vasc Diffuse Lung Dis. 2013;30(1):70–2.
100. Kelley BP, et al. Ichthyosiform sarcoidosis: a case report and review of the literature. Dermatol Online J. 2010;16(8):5.
101. Yoo SS, et al. Clinicopathologic features of ulcerative-atrophic sarcoidosis. Int J Dermatol. 2004;43(2):108–12.
102. Albertini JG, Tyler W, Miller OF 3rd. Ulcerative sarcoidosis. Case report and review of the literature. Arch Dermatol. 1997;133(2):215–9.
103. Hall RS, Floro JF, King LE Jr. Hypopigmented lesions in sarcoidosis. J Am Acad Dermatol. 1984;11(6):1163–4.
104. Yoon CH, Lee C. Erythrodermic form of cutaneous sarcoidosis. Clin Exp Dermatol. 2003;28:575–6.
105. House NS, Welsh JP, English JC 3rd. Sarcoidosis-induced alopecia. Dermatol Online J. 2012;18(8):4.
106. Santoro F, Sloan SB. Nail dystrophy and bony involvement in chronic sarcoidosis. J Am Acad Dermatol. 2009;60(6):1050–2.
107. Motswaledi MH, et al. Oral sarcoidosis: a case report and review of the literature. Aust Dent J. 2014;59(3):389–94.
108. Ayyala US, Nair AP, Padilla ML. Cardiac sarcoidosis. Clin Chest Med. 2008;29(3):493–508, ix.
109. Birnie D, et al. Cardiac sarcoidosis. Clin Chest Med. 2015;36(4):657–68.
110. Tavee JO, Stern BJ. Neurosarcoidosis. Clin Chest Med. 2015;36(4):643–56.
111. Pasadhika S, Rosenbaum JT. Ocular sarcoidosis. Clin Chest Med. 2015;36(4):669–83.
112. Judson MA, et al. Defining organ involvement in sarcoidosis: the ACCESS proposed instrument. ACCESS Research Group. A Case Control Etiologic Study of Sarcoidosis. Sarcoidosis Vasc Diffuse Lung Dis. 1999;16(1):75–86.
113. Judson MA, et al. The WASOG sarcoidosis organ assessment instrument: an update of a previous clinical tool. Sarcoidosis Vasc Diffuse Lung Dis. 2014;31(1):19–27.
114. Winterbauer RH, Belic N, Moores KD. Clinical interpretation of bilateral hilar adenopathy. Ann Intern Med. 1973;78(1):65–71.
115. Ball NJ, Kho GT, Martinka M. The histologic spectrum of cutaneous sarcoidosis: a study of twenty-eight cases. J Cutan Pathol. 2004;31(2):160–8.
116. Cardoso JC, et al. Cutaneous sarcoidosis: a histopathological study. J Eur Acad Dermatol Venereol. 2009;23(6):678–82.
117. Mangas C, et al. Clinical spectrum and histological analysis of 32 cases of specific cutaneous sarcoidosis. J Cutan Pathol. 2006;33(12):772–7.
118. Scadding JG. Prognosis of intrathoracic sarcoidosis in England. A review of 136 cases after five years' observation. Br Med J. 1961;2(5261):1165–72.
119. Nunes H, Soler P, Valeyre D. Pulmonary sarcoidosis. Allergy. 2005;60(5):565–82.
120. Costabel U, Guzman J, Baughman RP. Systemic evaluation of a potential cutaneous sarcoidosis patient. Clin Dermatol. 2007;25(3):303–11.
121. Martusewicz-Boros MM, et al. What comorbidities accompany sarcoidosis? A large cohort (n=1779) patients analysis. Sarcoidosis Vasc Diffuse Lung Dis. 2015;32(2):115–20.
122. Kiess AP, et al. Sarcoid in cancer patients: clinical characteristics and associated disease status. Sarcoidosis Vasc Diffuse Lung Dis. 2015;32(3):200–7.
123. Bonifazi M, et al. Sarcoidosis and cancer risk: systematic review and meta-analysis of observational studies. Chest. 2015;147(3):778–91.
124. Chopra A, Judson MA. How are cancer and connective tissue diseases related to sarcoidosis? Curr Opin Pulm Med. 2015;21(5):517–24.
125. Chalayer E, et al. Sarcoidosis and lymphoma: a comparative study. QJM. 2015;108(11):871–8.
126. Westers-Attema A, et al. Multiple cutaneous squamous cell carcinoma in cutaneous sarcoidosis. J Dermatol. 2015;42(8):845–6.
127. Papadopoulos KI, et al. High frequency of endocrine autoimmunity in patients with sarcoidosis. Eur J Endocrinol. 1996;134(3):331–6.
128. Nakamura H, et al. High incidence of positive autoantibodies against thyroid peroxidase and thyroglobulin in patients with sarcoidosis. Clin Endocrinol (Oxf). 1997;46(4):467–72.
129. Anolik RB, et al. Thyroid dysfunction and cutaneous sarcoidosis. J Am Acad Dermatol. 2012;66(1):167–8.
130. Antonelli A, et al. Prevalence of hypothyroidism and Graves disease in sarcoidosis. Chest. 2006;130(2):526–32.
131. Rajoriya N, et al. Immune-mediated and chronic inflammatory disease in people with sarcoidosis: disease associations in a large UK database. Postgrad Med J. 2009;85(1003):233–7.
132. Melnick L, et al. Coexistent sarcoidosis and alopecia areata or vitiligo: a case series and review of the literature. J Clin Exp Derm Res. 2014;149(5):236.
133. Rosenbach M, et al. Reliability and convergent validity of the cutaneous sarcoidosis activity and morphology instrument for assessing cutaneous sarcoidosis. JAMA Dermatol. 2013;149(5):550–6.
134. Baughman RP, et al. Chronic facial sarcoidosis including lupus pernio: clinical description and proposed scoring systems. Am J Clin Dermatol. 2008;9(3):155–61.
135. Yeung H, et al. Reliability and validity of cutaneous sarcoidosis outcome instruments among dermatologists, pulmonologists, and rheumatologists. JAMA Dermatol. 2015;151(12):1317–22.
136. Judson MA, et al. Validation and important differences for the Sarcoidosis Assessment Tool. A new patient-reported outcome measure. Am J Respir Crit Care Med. 2015;191(7):786–95.
137. Victorson DE, et al. A conceptual model of health-related quality of life in sarcoidosis. Qual Life Res. 2014;23(1):89–101.
138. Baughman RP, et al. Infliximab therapy in patients with chronic sarcoidosis and pulmonary involvement. Am J Respir Crit Care Med. 2006;174(7):795–802.

139. Judson MA, et al. Safety and efficacy of ustekinumab or golimumab in patients with chronic sarcoidosis. Eur Respir J. 2014;44(5):1296–307.
140. Baughman RP, et al. Efficacy and safety of apremilast in chronic cutaneous sarcoidosis. Arch Dermatol. 2012;148(2):262–4.
141. Wanat KA, Rosenbach M. A practical approach to cutaneous sarcoidosis. Am J Clin Dermatol. 2014;15(4):283–97.
142. Khatri KA, Chotzen VA, Burrall BA. Lupus pernio: successful treatment with a potent topical corticosteroid. Arch Dermatol. 1995;131(5):617–8.
143. Wise RD. Clinical resolution of facial cutaneous sarcoidosis with systemic colchicine and a topical corticosteroid ointment. Compr Ther. 2008;34(2):105–10.
144. Singh SK, Singh S, Pandey SS. Cutaneous sarcoidosis without systemic involvement : response to intralesional corticosteroid. Indian J Dermatol Venereol Leprol. 1996;62(4):273–4.
145. Marchetti M, Baker MG, Noland MM. Treatment of subcutaneous sarcoidosis with hydroxychloroquine: report of 2 cases. Dermatol Online J. 2014;20:21250.
146. Jones E, Callen JP. Hydroxychloroquine is effective therapy for control of cutaneous sarcoidal granulomas. J Am Acad Dermatol. 1990;23(3 Pt 1):487–9.
147. Modi S, Rosen T. Micropapular cutaneous sarcoidosis: case series successfully managed with hydroxychloroquine sulfate. Cutis. 2008;81(4):351–4.
148. Zic JA, et al. Treatment of cutaneous sarcoidosis with chloroquine. Review of the literature. Arch Dermatol. 1991;127(7):1034–40.
149. Miyazaki E, et al. Minocycline for the treatment of sarcoidosis: is the mechanism of action immunomodulating or antimicrobial effect? Clin Rheumatol. 2008;27(9):1195–7.
150. Steen T, English JC. Oral minocycline in treatment of cutaneous sarcoidosis. JAMA Dermatol. 2013;149(6):758–60.
151. Drake WP, et al. Oral antimycobacterial therapy in chronic cutaneous sarcoidosis: a randomized, single-masked, placebo-controlled study. JAMA Dermatol. 2013;149(9):1040–9.
152. Baughman RP, Judson MA, Ingledue R, et al. Efficacy and safety of apremilast in chronic cutaneous sarcoidosis. Arch Dermatol. 2012;148:262–4.
153. Zabel P, et al. Pentoxifylline in treatment of sarcoidosis. Am J Respir Crit Care Med. 1997;155(5):1665–9.
154. Georgiou S, et al. Cutaneous sarcoidosis: complete remission after oral isotretinoin therapy. Acta Derm Venereol. 1998;78(6):457–9.
155. Baughman RP, Lower EE. Evidence-based therapy for cutaneous sarcoidosis. Clin Dermatol. 2007;25(3):334–40.
156. Doherty CB, Rosen T. Evidence-based therapy for cutaneous sarcoidosis. Drugs. 2008;68(10):1361–83.
157. Mosam A, Morar N. Recalcitrant cutaneous sarcoidosis: an evidence-based sequential approach. J Dermatolog Treat. 2004;15(6):353–9
158. Veien NK, Brodthagen H. Cutaneous sarcoidosis treated with methotrexate. Br J Dermatol. 1977;97(2):213–6.
159. Vorselaars ADM, et al. Methotrexate vs azathioprine in second-line therapy of sarcoidosis. Chest. 2013;144(3):805–12.
160. Webster GF, et al. Methotrexate therapy in cutaneous sarcoidosis. Ann Intern Med. 1989;111(6):538–9.
161. Webster GF, et al. Weekly low-dose methotrexate therapy for cutaneous sarcoidosis. J Am Acad Dermatol. 1991;24(3):451–4.
162. Droitcourt C, et al. A randomized, investigator-masked, double-blind, placebo-controlled trial on thalidomide in severe cutaneous sarcoidosis. Chest. 2014;146(4):1046–54.
163. Heffernan MP, Anadkat MJ. Recalcitrant cutaneous sarcoidosis responding to infliximab. Arch Dermatol. 2005;141(7):910–1.
164. Meyerle JH, Shorr A. The use of infliximab in cutaneous sarcoidosis. J Drugs Dermatol. 2003;2(4):413–4.
165. Sené T, et al. Infliximab as a steroid-sparing agent in refractory cutaneous sarcoidosis: single-center retrospective study of 9 patients. J Am Acad Dermatol. 2012;66(2):328–32.
166. Tuchinda P, Bremmer M, Gaspari AA. A case series of refractory cutaneous sarcoidosis successfully treated with infliximab. Dermatol Ther. 2012;2(1):11.
167. Wanat KA, Rosenbach M. Case series demonstrating improvement in chronic cutaneous sarcoidosis following treatment with TNF inhibitors. Arch Dermatol. 2012;148(9):1097–100.
168. Rosen T, Doherty C. Successful long-term management of refractory cutaneous and upper airway sarcoidosis with periodic infliximab infusion. Dermatol Online J. 2007;13(3):14.
169. Field S, et al. Recalcitrant cutaneous sarcoidosis responding to adalimumab but not to etanercept. Clin Exp Dermatol. 2010;35(7):795–6.
170. Heffernan MP, Smith DI. Adalimumab for treatment of cutaneous sarcoidosis. Arch Dermatol. 2006;142(1):17 9.
171. Pariser RJ, et al. A double-blind, randomized, placebo-controlled trial of adalimumab in the treatment of cutaneous sarcoidosis. J Am Acad Dermatol. 2013;68(5):765–73.
172. Utz JP, et al. Etanercept for the treatment of stage II and III progressive pulmonary sarcoidosis. Chest. 2003;124(1):177–85.
173. Wijsenbeek MS, Culver DA. Treatment of sarcoidosis. Clin Chest Med. 2015;36(4):751–67.
174. Culver DA. Diagnosing sarcoidosis. Curr Opin Pulm Med. 2015;21(5):499–509.
175. Baughman RP, Lower EE. Treatment of sarcoidosis. Clin Rev Allergy Immunol. 2015;49(1):79–92.
176. Zhou Y. Organ involvement in 393 consecutive patients seen in one sarcoidosis clinic as measured by the WASOG criteria. Unpublished table in presentation delivered at the American Thoracic Society meeting; 2016.
177. https://www.medrxiv.org/content/10.1101/2021.07.01.21259700v1.full.pdf

Reactive Erythemas and Panniculitides in Connective Tissue Disease

10

Daniel R. Mazori and Alisa N. Femia

Key Points

- Reactive erythemas are cutaneous eruptions that generally develop in response to a systemic trigger
- Associated conditions include autoimmune diseases, inflammatory bowel disease (IBD), malignancy, and infection
- Reactive erythemas often require systemic immunomodulatory therapy that may influence the underlying disease state, and they may also respond to therapy directed towards the underlying disease association
- An interdisciplinary approach to management and surveillance in patients with reactive erythemas is imperative

Interdisciplinary Introduction

Reactive erythemas are inflammatory dermatoses that often have extracutaneous manifestations. These conditions include several types of panniculitis, as well as pyoderma gangrenosum (PG), Sweet syndrome, palisaded neutrophilic granulomatous dermatitis (PNGD), interstitial granulomatous dermatitis (IGD), and interstitial granulomatous drug reaction (IGDR). Although their pathogenesis is largely uncertain, reactive erythemas generally occur as a response to a systemic trigger or underlying disorder, such as connective tissue diseases, inflammatory bowel disease (IBD), malignancy, infections, systemic vasculitides, medication use, and pregnancy.

The cutaneous manifestations of the various reactive erythemas differ according to the specific disease, but lesions are typically pink to violaceous during the active phase of inflammation. Musculoskeletal symptoms are common in patients with reactive erythemas. These symptoms may be related either to the underlying condition or to the reactive process itself, may parallel or be independent of the cutaneous manifestations, and vary according to the cutaneous association. For example, seronegative, non-erosive, monoarticular arthritis is the most common arthritis in PG, whereas in PNGD and IGD, rheumatoid arthritis (RA) is the most common association. Musculoskeletal manifestations of Sweet syndrome may include arthritis as well as myositis, fasciitis, tendinitis, and/or tenosynovitis. Arthralgias in the absence of arthritis are also common in patients with reactive erythemas, occurring in up to half of patients with EN, as well as in patients with PG. The arthralgias of IGD tend to be symmetric, polyarticular, and favor peripheral

D. R. Mazori · A. N. Femia (✉)
Ronald O. Perelman Department of Dermatology, NYU Grossman School of Medicine, New York, NY, USA
e-mail: daniel.mazori@nyulangone.org

A. Garg et al. (eds.), *Interdisciplinary Approaches to Overlap Disorders in Dermatology & Rheumatology*, https://doi.org/10.1007/978-3-319-18446-3_10

joints, while 10% of patients with IGDR have an underlying arthropathy.

While some reactive erythemas may occur in the absence of a systemic association, reactive erythemas often serve as a clue to an underlying internal disease. For example, PNGD and IGD are often associated with autoimmune disease or malignancy. PG is frequently associated with IBD, and both PG and Sweet syndrome are commonly associated with hematologic malignancies. Furthermore, both PG and an IGD-like eruption [1] have been reported as coinciding with the transformation of myelodysplastic syndrome (MDS) into acute myeloid leukemia, and the development of panniculitis in patients with systemic sclerosis (SSc) may be a portent of pulmonary hypertension. Given the frequency of internal disease associations with the reactive erythemas, interdisciplinary management, including long-term monitoring and surveillance for internal disease in patients with reactive erythemas, is imperative.

Erythema Nodosum, Erythema Induratum, and Connective Tissue Panniculitides

The subcutaneous fat, or panniculus, is composed of fat lobules (collections of adipocytes) and septae (interlobular connective tissue). Inflammation occurring within the subcutaneous fat is known as panniculitis. Clinical distinction between the panniculitides can be difficult, as all forms typically present with tender, erythematous subcutaneous nodules; however, the location on the body can often serve as a clinical clue, as we review in detail below.

Due to the large degree of clinical overlap between the panniculitides, classification is primarily based on histology. The most important distinction is whether the panniculitis predominantly affects the septae or the fat lobules (although a degree of overlap is present in almost all cases), or whether the infiltrate is mixed (see Table 10.1). For example, EN is, as a rule, a septal panniculitis, whereas lupus erythematosus panniculitis (LEP) affects the fat lobules; this classification has implications for disease course and sequelae. Once the distinction between a septal or lobular panniculitis has been made, the histologic presence of vasculitis may also help further subclassify the panniculitides.

Erythema nodosum is the prototypical septal panniculitis. In septal panniculitides, the fat lobules are relatively spared, and thus healing occurs without atrophy. In contrast, lobular or mixed panniculitides, such as erythema induratum/nodular vasculitis (EI/NV) and those associated with connective tissue diseases, can obliterate the fat lobules. The resulting sequelae include disfiguring and irreversible contour change (see Fig. 10.1), and, in severe or long-standing lesions, ulcerations and calcinosis, which are painful and cause functional impairment.

Of note, the term Weber-Christian disease, or nodular panniculitis, was used in older literature to describe an idiopathic, relapsing syndrome of fever, lobular panniculitis, and variable internal organ involvement. Many such cases have since been reclassified as other diseases, and therefore in the authors' experience and the literature at large, the terminology has mostly been abandoned in favor of more specific diagnoses [2, 3].

Erythema Nodosum

Key Summary Capsule Bullets

- Prototypical septal panniculitis; thus, heals without permanent sequelae
- Presents with acute onset of erythematous, tender subcutaneous nodules and/or plaques in crops on bilateral pretibial surfaces, often with associated arthralgias
- Etiologies vary regionally, but idiopathic and post-streptococcal are most common
- Diagnosed clinically, with skin biopsies generally reserved for atypical cases
- Treatment is directed towards underlying cause and is otherwise supportive and aimed at alleviating symptoms
- Spontaneous resolution is expected within several weeks in the majority of patients

Table 10.1 Classification of the panniculitides

–	Clinical features	Main site(s) of involvement	Type of panniculitis	Vasculitis	Other characteristic histologic features
Erythema nodosum	Acute-onset, tender, erythematous subcutaneous nodules	Bilateral shins	Septal	No	Miescher granulomas
Erythema induratum/ nodular vasculitis (EI/NV)	Erythematous subcutaneous nodules that ulcerate	Bilateral calves	Lobular or mixed, granulomatous	Yes	–
Lupus erythematosus panniculitis (LEP)	Tender, erythematous subcutaneous nodules and/or plaques, some with overlying discoid lupus erythematosus (DLE)	Fatty areas of face (especially cheeks), proximal limbs, trunk (including breasts)	Lobular	Usually no	Mucin, hyaline fact necrosis, lymphoid follicles with germinal centers, overlying DLE
Dermatomyositis-associated panniculitis (DAP)	Tender, erythematous subcutaneous nodules and/or plaques	Buttocks, thighs, arms	Lobular	Usually yes	Vacuolar interface dermatitis, dermal mucin, calcification
Panniculitis of sclerosing disorders (morphea, systemic sclerosis/SSc)	Morphea: indurated, sclerotic plaques SSc: well-circumscribed, indurated, painful, hyperpigmented plaques	Morphea: extremities, trunk Systemic sclerosis: shin	Morphea: septal SSc: mixed	No	Morphea: thickened, hyalinized collagen SSc: lipophagic fat necrosis, lipomembranous change
Pancreatic panniculitis (PP)	Erythematous, edematous subcutaneous nodules that ulcerate and drain oily material; associated with various pancreatic disorders	Legs > trunk, upper extremities, buttocks, scalp	Lobular or mixed (septal only early in course)	No	"Ghost cells" (anucleate adipocytes)
Lipodermatosclerosis (LDS)	Tender, erythematous plaques (acute); sclerotic plaques with "inverted champagne bottle" appearance (chronic); associated with chronic venous insufficiency	One or both lower extremities, often above medial malleoli	Mixed	No	Lobular necrosis, hemosiderin deposition (acute); lipomembranous change, septal sclerosis (chronic)
Infectious panniculitis	Subcutaneous nodules and abscesses that may be inflamed and fluctuant	Legs, feet	Mixed, neutrophilic	No	Positive cultures and special stains
Alpha-1 antitrypsin deficiency panniculitis	Erythematous, subcutaneous nodules and/or plaques that ulcerate and drain oily material; associated with alpha-1 antitrypsin, deficiency	Trunk, proximal extremities	Mixed	Yes	"Splaying" of neutrophils between dermal collagen bundles, liquefactive necrosis with "skip areas" of normal fat

(continued)

Table 10.1 (continued)

–	Clinical features	Main site(s) of involvement	Type of panniculitis	Vasculitis	Other characteristic histologic features
Sclerema neonatorum	Woody induration of skin in preterm neonates	Diffuse; spares, palms, soles, genitalia	Minimal	No	Needle-shaped clefts within adipocytes and giant cells
Subcutaneous fat necrosis of the newborn	Indurated, subcutaneous nodules and/or plaques in full- and post-term neonates	Bilateral extremities, buttocks, back	Lobular, granulomatous	No	Needle-shaped clefts within adipocytes and giant cells
Post-steroid panniculitis	Erythematous, indurated, subcutaneous nodules and/or plaques after abrupt cessation of systemic corticosteroids	Cheeks	Lobular, granulomatous	No	Needle-shaped clefts within adipocytes and giant cells
Traumatic panniculitis	Tender subcutaneous nodules	Any site of blunt trauma	Mixed	No	–
Cold panniculitis	Acute-onset, erythematous, subcutaneous nodules and/or plaques	Cold-exposed areas (chin, cheeks, thighs)	Lobular or mixed	No	–
Factitial panniculitis	Tender, erythematous nodules; potential presence of geometric ulcers and/or abscesses	Buttocks, thighs (areas accessible for self-injection)	Lobular, neutrophilic	No	Fat necrosis, foreign (sometimes birefringent) material

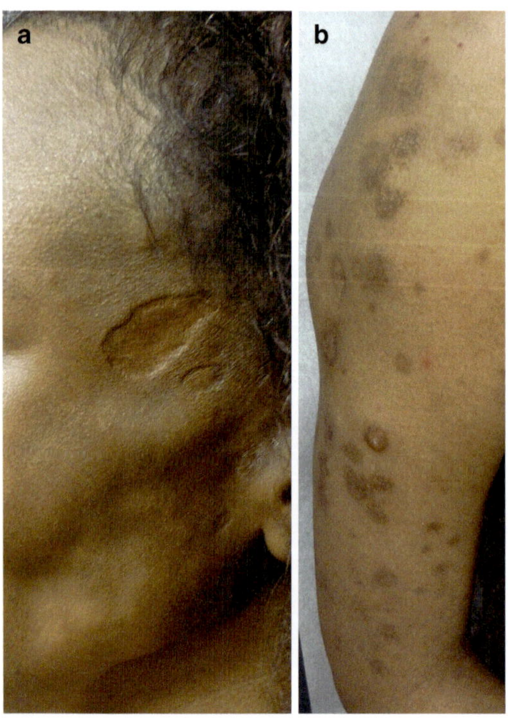

Fig. 10.1 Lupus erythematosus panniculitis (LEP): contour changes on the (**a**) face and (**b**) proximal upper extremity due to atrophy of the pannus with longstanding disease

Classification and Epidemiology

Erythema nodosum is the most common panniculitis and the prototypical septal panniculitis. Its incidence has been estimated as 2–5 per 100,000 people per year [4, 5]. It predominates in women of childbearing age, with the largest case series reporting a female-to-male ratio of 5:1 [6, 7]. Erythema nodosum has been linked to various underlying triggers, and the relative ranking of etiologies varies geographically. For example, the most common association is group A streptococcal tonsillopharyngitis in Israel, France, and Turkey; sarcoidosis in Spain and Greece; and primary tuberculosis in Thailand [8].

Pathogenesis

The pathogenesis of EN is poorly understood, but the disorder is generally regarded as a delayed hypersensitivity reaction to antigens associated with various systemic conditions or medications. Type 1 helper (Th1) cells are believed to play a role, and the Th1 cytokines interleukin-2 (IL-2) and interferon-γ (IFN-γ) have been found to be overexpressed in the skin and peripheral blood of patients with EN as compared with healthy controls [9]. Further supporting the role of Th1 cells in EN pathogenesis is the finding that lymphocytes from a patient with estradiol-induced EN produced more IFN-γ when re-exposed to estradiol than did lymphocytes from a healthy control [10]. Other potential mediators of EN include neutrophils [11, 12] and tumor necrosis factor-α (TNF-α) [13].

Clinical Features

In the vast majority of patients, EN presents acutely with crops of erythematous, tender subcutaneous nodules and/or plaques on the pretibial regions of the bilateral lower extremities (see Fig. 10.2). Less commonly, EN may also involve the knees, thighs, upper extremities, and trunk. The nodules heal in approximately 3–6 weeks without scarring, ulceration, atrophy, or other permanent sequelae. This lack of scarring is attributed to the fact that the underlying inflammatory process targets the subcutaneous septae, with relative sparing of the fat lobules, which remain intact.

Erythema nodosum may be associated with several underlying conditions; this list is vast and varies according to the geographic region. Group A streptococcal tonsillopharyngitis in the 1–3 weeks prior to onset is the most common identifiable cause (6–44% of patients) [4–7, 14]. Most other etiologies involve either the pulmonary system (4–30% of patients) or gastrointestinal system (2–9%) [4–8, 14].

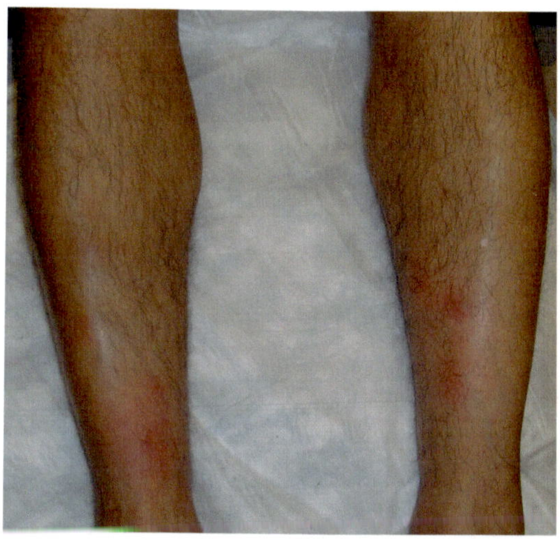

Fig. 10.2 Erythema nodosum: erythematous nodules on the bilateral pretibial surfaces

EN-associated diseases with pulmonary manifestations include granulomatous conditions, such as sarcoidosis, primary tuberculosis, and fungal infections (e.g. coccidioidomycosis, histoplasmosis, blastomycosis). Bacterial infections, namely *Chlamydophila pneumoniae* or *psittaci* may also present with pulmonary symptoms; yersiniosis presenting with pulmonary but not gastrointestinal symptoms has also been described [15]. Hodgkin lymphoma may also involve the lungs, often presenting with lymphadenopathy.

Etiologies associated with gastrointestinal findings include Behçet disease, IBD (Crohn disease more so than ulcerative colitis [16]), and bacterial gastroenteritis (e.g. due to *Yersinia enterocolitica*, Salmonella, Campylobacter). Other triggers of EN include medication use in the 1–2 weeks prior to onset (classically penicillins, sulphonamides, halides, or oral contraceptive pills; 0–10% of patients) and pregnancy (0–6%) [4–8, 14].

Extracutaneous clinical features of EN vary depending on the underlying systemic association. A large prospective study found that the presence of cough, sore throat, diarrhea, arthritis, and pulmonary pathology were predictors of secondary EN [8]. Other clinical features, such as fever, leukocytosis, and elevated inflammatory markers (e.g., C-reactive protein [CRP], erythrocyte sedimentation rate [ESR]), are significantly more common in patients with secondary EN than idiopathic EN. By contrast, in a large prospective study, recurrence of EN predicted an idiopathic etiology [8]. Up to 50% of patients with EN have arthralgias [6–8].

Histopathology

Histopathologically, EN is typified by a septal panniculitis without vasculitis. The inflammatory cells within the septae characteristically aggregate around a banana- or stellate-shaped cleft, forming structures known as Miescher granulomas, which are relatively specific for erythema nodosum. The septal infiltrate variably extends into the periphery of adjacent fat lobules and may be accompanied by a lymphocytic perivascular dermal infiltrate.

As lesions age, the predominant cell type in the septal infiltrate and Miescher granulomas changes from neutrophils to histiocytes to multinucleated giant cells. Miescher granulomas also decrease in number as lesions evolve. Early lesions also feature septal edema and hemorrhage, which are replaced by septal fibrosis in late lesions [17]. Although the endothelium of small vessels may be necrotic, true vasculitis is characteristically absent [18]. The exception to this is EN associated with Behçet disease, in which vasculitis is common [19].

Diagnostic Considerations

Histologically, several conditions other than EN may involve the fat septae, but these are not considered primary panniculitides (see Table 10.2). The clinical differential diagnosis of EN includes other conditions that can cause tender, erythematous subcutaneous nodules and/or plaques on the legs, which we review below.

Like EN, EI/NV affects predominantly young to middle-aged women and may be idiopathic or precipitated by infection (classically tuberculosis) or medications. However, unlike EN, EI/NV favors the calves, may ulcerate and drain, and heals with scarring (see Fig. 10.3). Furthermore, EI/NV is readily differentiated from EN histologically by its characteristic lobular or mixed panniculitis and usual presence of vasculitis.

Pancreatic panniculitis (PP) is an uncommon manifestation of various pancreatic disorders, including acute and chronic pancreatitis and pancreatic carcinoma. PP may mimic EN, as it frequently arises on the legs and early histology demonstrates a septal panniculitis. Factors that distinguish PP include its predilection for sites other than the legs (i.e., chest, upper extremities, buttocks, scalp), potential for ulceration and drainage of oily material, and association with elevated serum amylase and lipase. In addition, the histology of PP is typically lobular or mixed, with septal involvement seen only early in the course. Characteristic "ghost cells" (anucleate adipocytes) due to fat necrosis also help to distinguish PP histologically.

Lipodermatosclerosis (LDS) is a panniculitis associated with chronic venous insufficiency. Although the tender, erythematous plaques of the acute phase of LDS may be confused for EN, clinical features more suggestive of LDS include a background of venous insufficiency (i.e., varicose veins, chronic lower extremity edema, hemosiderin discoloration) and predilection for the area of the leg above the medial malleolus.

Table 10.2 Conditions that are not primary panniculitides but histologically involve the fat septae

Condition	Vasculitis present histologically?
Rheumatoid nodule	No
Subcutaneous granuloma annulare	No
Necrobiosis lipoidica diabeticorum	No
Superficial thrombophlebitis	Yes
Cutaneous polyarteritis nodosa	Yes
Necrobiotic xanthogranuloma	No

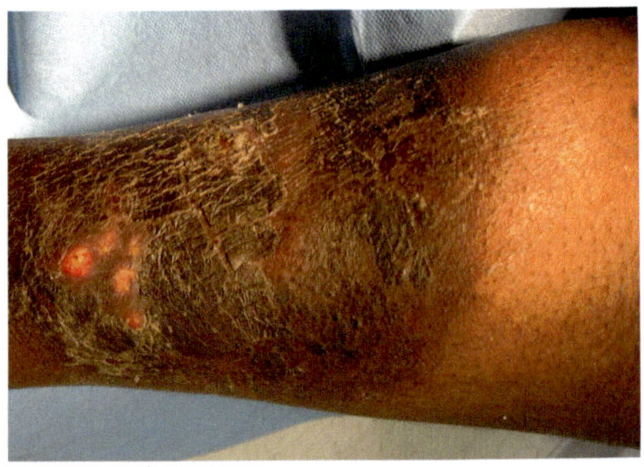

Fig. 10.3 Erythema induratum/nodular vasculitis (EI/NV): hyperpigmented plaques with ulcerations overlying tender subcutaneous nodules on the calf

Moreover, unlike EN, early LDS histologically demonstrates a mixed panniculitis, ischemic fat necrosis, and septal fibrosis. As LDS progresses, the clinical picture is characterized by indurated skin with an "inverted champagne bottle" appearance.

Infectious panniculitis (i.e., bacterial, fungal, or atypical mycobacterial) usually occurs in immunosuppressed patients. The diagnosis is favored when the histology demonstrates a mixed neutrophilic panniculitis, vascular proliferation, cellular necrosis including necrosis of sweat glands, and discrete abscesses. Furthermore, microorganisms can often be identified via special stains and cultures [20], although in some cases, repeated stains and cultures may be necessary prior to identifying an infectious cause.

Subcutaneous panniculitis-like T-cell lymphoma (SPTCL) is a rare cutaneous lymphoma in which neoplastic cytotoxic T-cells infiltrate the subcutaneous fat lobules, resulting in a predominantly lobular panniculitis. The diagnosis of SPTCL should be considered in patients with presumed EN who follow an atypical course or those with systemic B symptoms (e.g., night sweats and weight loss). The diagnosis can be confirmed with immunohistochemical identification of a monoclonal T-cell receptor gene rearrangement.

Unlike EN, subcutaneous Sweet syndrome is a predominantly lobular panniculitis. Cellulitis and erysipelas usually affect the lower extremities unilaterally, in contrast to EN, which is typically bilateral. The tender, erythematous lesions of superficial thrombophlebitis are distinguished by their distribution along a superficial vein and presence of a palpable cord. The cutaneous nodules of polyarteritis nodosa may be differentiated from EN both clinically (as they may ulcerate and co-occur with livedo racemosa) and histologically (as they display a necrotizing vasculitis of medium-sized arteries in the septae). In subcutaneous sarcoidosis, nodules favor the upper extremities, are generally asymptomatic to slightly tender, and demonstrate noncaseating granulomas. Lastly, the nodules of subcutaneous granuloma annulare (GA) tend to be painless, occur in children, and feature histiocytic palisades surrounding degenerated collagen and mucin in the septae.

Disease and Comorbidity Assessment

The evaluation of patients with EN generally begins with an evaluation for potential underlying causes, through history (including a medication review and travel history), review of systems (focusing on articular, respiratory, and gastrointestinal symptoms), and physical examination. Further testing is driven by the patient's associated symptoms and the region's most frequent etiologic factors, but workup generally includes a complete blood count (CBC) with differential, complete metabolic panel, anti-streptolysin O titer (at the time of diagnosis and again 2–4 weeks later), throat culture, tuberculin skin test, pregnancy test in women, and chest radiograph. However, the etiology of EN remains unidentifiable in 32–72% of patients [4–7, 14]. Additional studies, such as a colonoscopy, are considered on a case-by-case basis.

Skin biopsies are generally reserved for persistent or refractory cases of EN, or for atypical cases in which mimickers of EN are suspected as reviewed above. In these cases, a deep incisional biopsy is preferred over a punch biopsy, to ensure adequate sampling of the subcutaneous fat. Depending on the clinical suspicion, tissue should be sent for culture, special stains, immunohistochemistry, and/or T-cell receptor gene rearrangement studies. Biopsy is not generally recommended in straightforward cases, particularly because the morbidity associated with a deep incisional biopsy on the lower leg, which may take months to heal and will certainly scar, may exceed the morbidity from EN itself, which typically heals within weeks without atrophy or scarring.

Principles of Management

Therapy in EN is supportive and directed at the underlying cause, as the skin lesions themselves are typically self-limited and resolve without scarring. In patients with idiopathic EN or those desiring treatment for symptomatic relief, several medical therapies may be considered. A prospective study of 100 patients with EN found that bed rest and non-steroidal anti-inflammatory drugs (NSAIDs) resulted in clinical improvement in 95% of patients (93/98), generally within 7 days. Among the five patients who were NSAID-resistant, oral potassium iodide was used with similar efficacy [8]. For resistant or recurrent disease, colchicine as well as oral dapsone have been reported [21].

Management of pregnant patients with EN should be done in conjunction with the patient's obstetrician, particularly because NSAIDs and potassium iodide are relatively contraindicated in pregnancy [22]. In addition, any patient being managed with potassium iodide should have close monitoring of thyroid function, as thyroid abnormalities may develop with this therapy. The use of systemic corticosteroids is generally not necessary, and a risk-benefit analysis prior to considering corticosteroid use should include the possibility of an underlying infectious cause.

In addition to symptom management, if the underlying cause of EN can be identified, it should be treated. For the treatment of EN related to Behçet disease, two double-blinded trials found that colchicine was superior to placebo [23, 24]. Expert clinical opinion and one case report support the use of infliximab for IBD-related EN, with lesions improving soon after the first infusion and nearly resolving after the second to third dose [25, 26]. In cases of drug-induced EN, the offending medication should be discontinued.

An important exception to the need to treat the underlying cause is streptococcal-associated EN: in patients with evidence of an antecedent streptococcal infection, but without streptococcal-related symptoms, treatment with antibiotics may not be necessary. In such cases, EN is indicative of an immune response, not active infection, and many cases have been reported to resolve without antibiotic use [5].

Lastly, patients should be provided with anticipatory guidance regarding the risk of recurrence, which is more likely in idiopathic EN within the first year of onset [5, 8].

Erythema Induratum/Nodular Vasculitis

Key Summary Capsule Bullets

- Lobular or mixed (septal and lobular) panniculitis; thus, may ulcerate, drain, and scar
- Presents with crops of erythematous, tender, subcutaneous nodules and/or plaques on bilateral calves
- Associated with *Mycobacterium tuberculosis* infection (EI) or other systemic conditions, medications, or idiopathic etiology (NV)
- Differentiated from EN by typical location on bilateral calves, rather than pretibial surfaces, and potential for permanent sequelae

Classification

EI, or NV, is a lobular panniculitis that predominantly affects women and most often occurs on the lower extremities, although involvement of other body surfaces areas may be seen. When lesions occur in association with a *Mycobacterium tuberculosis* infection, the term EI is applied. Otherwise, the term NV is used.

Clinical Features

Clinically, EI/NV resembles EN in several ways: both conditions predominate in women of childbearing age, manifest as crops of tender, erythematous, subcutaneous nodules and/or plaques, predominantly involving the legs, and may be idiopathic or precipitated by systemic conditions or medications. However, there are several important ways the two conditions can be distinguished. First, in contrast to EN, which typically affects the pretibial surfaces, EI/NV generally affects the calves (see Fig. 10.3). Moreover, EI/NV is characterized by a lobular or mixed panniculitis and vasculitis, whereas EN is a predominantly septal panniculitis without vasculitis. Only EI/NV has a substantial lobular component and, thus, the potential to ulcerate, drain, and scar [27].

Although vasculitis (chiefly of small lobular venules) is found in most cases of EI/NV, its requirement for the histopathologic diagnosis is controversial [28].

Principles of Management

Treatment of EI centers on antimicrobial treatment of the underlying tuberculosis infection. Treatment of NV is similar to that of EN, primarily consisting of bed rest, NSAIDs, or potassium iodide. Systemic corticosteroids or Mycophenolate mofetil (MMF) may be used in severe cases [27].

Lupus Erythematosus Panniculitis

Key Summary Capsule Bullets

- Uncommon subtype of chronic cutaneous lupus erythematosus (LE)
- Presents with tender, erythematous, subcutaneous nodules and/or plaques on fatty areas of face (especially cheeks), proximal limbs, and trunk (including unilateral breast involvement)
- More often associated with DLE (33–67% of patients, "lupus profundus") than SLE (10–41%)
- Lobular panniculitis; thus, may scar, ulcerate, and develop calcinosis
- Antimalarials and photoprotection are considered first-line therapy

Classification and Epidemiology

LEP, or lupus panniculitis, represents 2–3% of all cases of cutaneous lupus [29]. It is classified as a type of chronic cutaneous lupus, a category that also includes discoid lupus erythematosus (DLE) [30]. When LEP has overlying clinical and/or histologic features of DLE, the term lupus profundus is used.

Like lupus erythematosus (LE) in general, LEP is more common in women, with the largest case series reporting a female-to-male ratio of 4:1 to 4.5:1 [31, 32]. The disease may occur at any age, but patients tend to be in their late 30s or early 40s [31, 32].

Pathogenesis

The basis of LEP is poorly understood, but it is believed to mirror that of other forms of cutaneous lupus. One case series suggests a role for plasmacytoid dendritic cells, which produce type 1 interferons that can recruit CXCR3+ cytotoxic T cells to the subcutaneous fat [33]. In addition, the finding of partial C4 deficiency in one patient with LEP suggests that decreased opsonization of immune complexes may be an underlying mechanism [34]. Although the pathogenesis is unclear, trauma has also been reported to trigger the onset of lupus panniculitis [35].

Clinical Features

The tender, erythematous subcutaneous nodules and/or plaques of LEP favor fatty areas of the face (especially the cheeks), proximal limbs, and trunk. When LEP affects the breasts (usually unilaterally), the term lupus mastitis (LM) is applied. Involvement of the distal legs is unusual and should prompt consideration of other panniculitides. Lesions may arise at one or multiple sites. About one-third of patients have clinically evident DLE overlying their LEP; in these cases, the term lupus profundus is applied [32].

Because LEP is a predominantly lobular panniculitis, without treatment, the fat lobules are destroyed, and patients develop permanent atrophic contour change that is often disfiguring (see Fig. 10.1). Ulcerations and calcinosis may also occur in longstanding lesions and can be detected mammographically in patients with LM [31, 32], often mimicking breast malignancy.

Most patients with LEP (59–90%, depending on the series) do not have systemic lupus erythematosus (SLE) [31, 32]. In the remaining minority, the two conditions either develop simultaneously or LEP develops after the onset of SLE, typically when the systemic disease is quiescent. Rarely, LEP precedes the diagnosis of SLE by several years [31]. When patients with LEP have SLE, manifestations of SLE tend to be relatively non-severe, with involvement mainly of the skin (photosensitivity, discoid lupus, malar rash) and joints (arthritis) [36].

There is some evidence that the LM subset of LEP may be more strongly associated with systemic lupus. One review of 31 patients with LM found that the majority had a preceding diagnosis of SLE (59% of patients) or DLE (23%), although reporting bias may be responsible for this association [37].

Lupus panniculitis has also been described in the setting of other autoimmune conditions, including SSc, dermatomyositis, Sjögren syndrome, mixed connective tissue disease, Hashimoto's thyroiditis, *autoimmune hemolytic anemia*, and immune thrombocytopenia [31, 32]. The clinical features of LEP do not appear to differ between patients with and without systemic disease [31].

Histopathologic findings of LEP include a primarily lobular panniculitis, mucin between fat lobules, hyaline fact necrosis, lymphoid follicles with germinal centers (rarely seen in other panniculitides), nuclear dust, and calcification [38]. Approximately 67% of patients have histopathologic features of overlying DLE, including epidermal atrophy, a dermal lymphocytic infiltrate, follicular plugging, a thickened basement membrane, and dermal mucin [31, 39]. Direct immunofluorescence tends to be positive at the dermal-epidermal junction and within dermal blood vessel walls, regardless of whether patients also have systemic lupus [31].

Diagnostic Considerations

The differential diagnosis of LEP includes other lobular panniculitides, most importantly infectious panniculitis, dermatomyositis-associated panniculitis (DAP), and SPTCL. These conditions may be clinically indistinguishable from lupus panniculitis; therefore, clinicopathologic correlation is required for diagnosis. Whereas the subcutaneous infiltrate of LEP is predominantly lobular and lymphocytic, the infiltrate seen in infectious panniculitis is more evenly mixed (both septal and lobular) and mainly neutrophilic [20]. Lupus panniculitis and DAP are histologically identical in many cases, but the former is favored when overlying features of DLE are present. In addition, histology featuring lymphoid follicles with germinal centers and hyaline necrosis of lobules is fairly characteristic of lupus panniculitis [40].

SPTCL is the most challenging entity to distinguish from lupus panniculitis. Clinically speaking, SPTCL is favored in the setting of systemic B symptoms (fever, chills, night sweats, and/or weight loss), as LEP only uncommonly manifests as part of an SLE flare; however, up to 50% of patients with SPTCL lack constitutional symptoms [40]. A history of SLE or even DLE is not necessarily evidence in favor of the diagnosis of LEP over SPTCL: about 19% of patients with SPTCL have an associated autoimmune disease, most commonly SLE [41], and also including DLE [42, 43].

Lupus panniculitis and SPTCL may also overlap histologically, with some cases of LEP featuring atypical lymphocytes rimming adipocytes (once considered typical of SPTCL [38]) and some cases of SPTCL demonstrating a vacuolar interface dermatitis and dermal mucin [44]. Histologically, the findings most specific for LEP are a positive lupus band test, lymphoid follicles with reactive germinal centers (which have never been observed in SPTCL [38]), relative lack of CD8+ T cells, polyclonal T-cell receptor gene rearrangement (in contrast to the monoclonal population in SPTCL), and the presence of plasma cells [38]. In addition to such histologic findings, an elevated ferritin level may favor the diagnosis of SPTCL over lupus panniculitis.

Given this potential for clinical and histologic overlap, SPTCL should be considered in patients who present atypically with LEP or do not respond to traditional LEP therapies [44]. In such cases, repeated, deep incisional biopsies may be necessary to establish the diagnosis of SPTCL. Biopsies that do not include an adequate sample of the subcutaneous fat may be misrepresentative and prolong time to accurate diagnosis.

For LM specifically, the differential diagnosis includes breast malignancy, chronic granulomatous mastitis (CGM), and diabetic mastopathy. As is the case in breast malignancy, the overlying skin in LM may be erythematous, dimpled, indurated, and/or ulcerated. There can be nipple retraction and discharge [45, 46], as well as significant breast atrophy and disfigurement [47, 48]. LM may also mimic malignancy radiologically, as over half of mammograms in LM show either calcifications alone or an irregular, ill-defined mass with or without calcifications [37]. However, unlike in breast cancer, where surgical excision is a mainstay of therapy, in LM, there is a theoretical risk of disease activation with trauma, and LM should not be excised. Biopsy for accurate diagnosis is therefore essential.

CGM is an idiopathic, chronic inflammatory condition that often presents with tender, erythematous nodules on the breast that may ulcerate and drain; thus, it may mimic both LM and breast malignancy. However, unlike LM or breast malignancy, CGM features noncaseating granulomas histologically. Diabetic mastopathy is a rare condition that may mimic LM but typically occurs in patients with longstanding type 1 diabetes mellitus. Histopathologically, diabetic mastopathy demonstrates a circumscribed, lymphocytic, lobular, periductal, or perivascular infiltrate, whereas the lymphocytic infiltrate of LM is less circumscribed and mainly lobular. An additional differentiating feature is that, unlike LM, diabetic mastopathy features dense fibrosis and epithelioid fibroblasts [37, 49, 50].

Disease and Comorbidity Assessment

Unlike in EN, a skin biopsy is often required to diagnose LEP, especially when certain clinical clues, such as overlying DLE, are absent. A deep incisional biopsy is preferred over a punch biopsy in order to ensure adequate sampling of the subcutaneous fat. Depending on the clinical suspicion, tissue should be sent for culture, special stains, immunohistochemistry, and T-cell receptor gene rearrangement studies to rule out infectious panniculitis and/or SPTCL.

Once LEP or lupus profundus is diagnosed, patients who have never undergone evaluation for SLE should do so, via a thorough review of systems, CBC with differential, urinalysis, and antinuclear antibodies. Additional autoimmune serologies may be sent on a case-by-case basis. Antinuclear antibodies are elevated in 65–95% of patients with LEP; the titer usually ranges from 1:40 to 1:80 in patients without systemic lupus and is greater in those with systemic disease [31, 32]. Patients without evidence of SLE at the time of diagnosis should be monitored clinically for the development of systemic disease.

Principles of Management

Lupus panniculitis is generally a chronic disease characterized by flares and remissions. One retrospective review of 40 patients found disease duration to be an average of 6 years; however, this range is broad (in the same review, 0–38 years), and relapses can continue to occur over decades [32]. Thus, patients often require a prolonged treatment course, especially given the potential for disfiguring scarring as a result of uncontrolled disease activity. The mainstays of treatment during the inflammatory phase are systemic agents, as topical therapies insufficiently penetrate the subcutaneous fat, while intralesional corticosteroid injections may result in atrophy that can be difficult to distinguish from the primary disease process.

Antimalarials are often considered first-line agents in LEP, with one series reporting improvement in 70% of patients [32]. Other therapeutic options include methotrexate (MTX) [51], thalidomide [34, 52, 53], dapsone [54], intravenous immunoglobulin (IVIG) [55], cyclosporine [56–58], and rituximab [59]. Methotrexate is often used as the next agent when antimalarials fail.

MMF, which is traditionally used in the treatment of lupus nephritis, has not been reported in the literature specifically as a treatment for LEP; anecdotally, however, it has been used successfuly. In addition, strict photoprotection should be recommended, especially in patients with coexistent DLE or SLE, although the exact role of ultraviolet radiation in triggering lupus panniculitis is unknown.

Importantly, medical therapies for LEP can halt progression but lack the ability to restore fat that has already been lost. The use of nonpermanent fillers, including hyaluronic acid and poly-L-lactic acid [60] as well as polymethylmethacrylate, a permanent dermal filler [61], has been reported for soft tissue augmentation and volume restoration in patients with quiescent lupus panniculitis. However, prior to considering filler therapy, it is imperative to ensure disease quiescence for a prolonged period, generally 1–2 years, in order to minimize the theoretical risk of reactivation by the filler. In one report, magnetic resonance imaging was used as an adjunctive tool to confirm the absence of subclinical disease activity [60].

Dermatomyositis-Associated Panniculitis

Key Summary Capsule Bullets

- Rare manifestation of DM
- Presents with tender, erythematous subcutaneous nodules and/or plaques often affecting buttocks, thighs, and arms
- Usually parallels classic features of DM; development prior to DM onset (less common) necessitates monitoring for DM
- Lobular panniculitis; thus, may scar, ulcerate, and develop calcinosis

Classification and Epidemiology

Panniculitis is generally regarded as a rare manifestation of classic [62], drug-induced [63], or amyopathic dermatomyositis (DM) [64–66], although some small studies have found clinical and/or histologic evidence of panniculitis in 9–20% of DM patients [67, 68].

Patients with DM who develop panniculitis are demographically similar to the broader cohort of all patients with dermatomyositis, with a male-to-female ratio of 1:2.4 and mean age of 36 years (range 2–80 years) [62].

Pathogenesis

The etiology of panniculitis in DM is unknown. It has been postulated that the cause is "spill-over" of inflammatory cells from muscle into adjacent fat [68]. Supporting this hypothesis is the observation that panniculitis often follows the same course as the muscular features of dermatomyositis [62]. However, the finding, in some patients, of clinical and/or histopathologic panniculitis without myositis suggests that additional or alternative mechanisms are involved [64–66, 68]. Furthermore, panniculitis can occur prior to, concomitant with, or after the onset of typical symptoms of dermatomyositis [62].

Clinical Features

The tender, erythematous subcutaneous nodules and/or plaques of DAP favor the buttocks, thighs, and arms, and compared with LEP, less commonly involve the trunk or face [62, 69]. In exceptional cases, the lesions may migrate [70] or vesiculate [64]. As in LEP and other lobular panniculitides, DAP has the potential to damage the fat lobules and result in ulceration; painful calcinosis causing functional impairment; and irreversible, disfiguring contour changes [71–73]. These sequelae have also been reported to arise insidiously when the preceding panniculitis is not clinically evident [69, 72].

Disease activity in DAP usually tracks in parallel with the classic cutaneous and/or muscular features of DM, manifesting either during a flare of previously diagnosed DM (in 50% of patients) or among the presenting signs of the disease (in 20%). Less frequently (29%), panniculitis occurs as an isolated manifestation weeks to years before the diagnosis of dermatomyositis [62].

Histopathologically, DAP is characterized by a lymphoplasmacytic lobular infiltrate. Vacuolar interface dermatitis, dermal mucin, calcification, and vasculitis may be seen [62, 74, 75]. Calcinosis and membranocystic changes in an arabesque pattern [76] (believed to represent degenerated adipocyte or macrophage membranes) have been reported in association with treatment resistance [62].

Diagnostic Considerations

The differential diagnosis of DAP includes other lobular panniculitides including LEP, infection (including infectious panniculitis, cellulitis, and erysipelas), and SPTCL. Clinicopathologic correlation helps to distinguish DAP from LEP [77]. Infectious panniculitis and SPTCL, by contrast, may be clinically indistinguishable from DAP [78–80]. However, infectious panniculitis may be distinguished from DAP by positive cultures and special stains, as well as histologic features including neutrophilic panniculitis, vascular proliferation, and coagulation necrosis of vessels and sweat glands (as opposed to fibrinoid necrosis in dermatomyositis) [20, 62]. Unlike cellulitis or erysipelas, DAP is usually bilateral and multifocal.

In one reported case, a patient with subcutaneous fat loss on the face due to DAP developed paradoxical fat hypertrophy of her right arm. Although rare, this phenomenon may be worth considering in patients with DM who develop limb asymmetry, as, in the reported case, fat hypertrophy of one limb could be mistaken for muscle wasting of the contralateral extremity [69].

Disease and Comorbidity Assessment

The treatment of DAP often involves the initiation or escalation of immunosuppressive therapy; therefore, skin biopsies with tissue culture and special stains for microorganisms should be considered in the diagnostic workup. As with the other panniculitides, a deep incisional biopsy is preferred to ensure adequate sampling of the subcutaneous fat. T-cell receptor gene rearrangement studies may be performed on the initial biopsy if SPTCL is suspected, or future biopsies in patients who do not respond to standard therapies for DAP. Although a skin biopsy is the gold standard in the diagnosis of DAP, magnetic resonance imaging has been reported in one case to be an effective adjunct for both diagnosis and assessment of treatment response [81].

Although patients with DM who develop panniculitis were initially believed to be at lower risk for malignancy [82], there have been three reported cases of new or recurrent malignancy (rhabdomyosarcoma, rectal carcinoma, and ovarian adenocarcinoma) in patients with DM and panniculitis [75, 79, 83]. Thus, the same malignancy screening guidelines apply to all patients with DM regardless of whether panniculitis is present.

In patients with a lobular panniculitis in whom the underlying etiology is not identifiable, long-term monitoring for the development of a connective tissue disease such as DM is warranted, as panniculitis has been reported to precede the diagnosis of DM by 2 years [62].

Principles of Management

DAP does not resolve spontaneously [62] and typically results in lipoatrophy, which can be severely disfiguring. Ulceration and calcinosis, which may be painful, can also occur [71–73]. Thus, early and aggressive treatment during the inflammatory stage of the disease is essential. Fortunately, the largest review of 24 patients with DAP found that the disease is generally responsive to the initiation or escalation of immunosuppressive treatment for the underlying DM, most often with systemic corticosteroids (prednisone or pulse methylprednisolone) [62].

Although antimalarials are often considered first-line for cutaneous dermatomyositis, these medications are insufficient to control cutaneous disease in the majority of patients, and the limited reports evaluating their efficacy in DAP showed mixed results. In addition to antimalarials, MTX, azathioprine (AZA), and/or thalidomide have been used successfully in conjunction with systemic corticosteroids in DAP [67, 74, 82, 84], and although not reported specifically for DAP, MMF may be effective for cutaneous dermatomyositis. MTX [75] and cyclosporine [74, 82] have also been reported as effective corticosteroid-sparing treatments for this condition.

IVIG has been found to be effective for both the cutaneous [85] and muscular manifestations [86] of recalcitrant DM; similarly, patients with DAP refractory to systemic therapies, including systemic corticosteroids, MTX, and AZA, have improved dramatically with IVIG [87, 88]. MTX, MMF, and IVIG are often considered preferred therapies for cutaneous DM, and they may be used with or without systemic corticosteroids for DM-associated panniculitis.

In addition to the above therapies, photoprotection is recommended for patients with DAP, as DM is a photo-exacerbated condition, and DAP usually flares in parallel with the disease's classic manifestations. Treatment of panniculitis in drug-induced dermatomyositis involves withdrawal of the causative agent [63]. In patients with associated malignancy, therapeutic decisions should be made in collaboration with the patient's oncologist.

Volume restoration with inert dermal fillers has not been reported specifically in DAP but has been performed successfully in LEP [60] and may be considered after a period of clinical remission (at least 1 year) to minimize the risk of filler-induced disease reactivation.

Panniculitis of Sclerosing Disorders

Key Summary Capsule Bullets

- Rare manifestation of morphea and SSc
- In morphea, presents with indurated sclerotic plaques due to principal subcutaneous involvement or subcutaneous extension
- First-line treatment in morphea subtype includes MTX and ultraviolet A1 phototherapy
- In SSc, panniculitis is rare; typically presents as well-circumscribed, indurated, painful, hyperpigmented plaques on pretibial area
- May be related to venous hypertension and signify impending pulmonary hypertension in SSc

Classification

Morphea and systemic sclerosis (SSc, or scleroderma) are two fibrosing connective tissue disorders in which inflammation of the subcutaneous fat can occur. Although the term localized scleroderma has been applied to describe morphea, it is important to differentiate this condition from SSc, because in morphea the fibrosis is generally limited to the dermis and subcutaneous tissue, but in SSc it can involve both the skin and the connective tissue of internal organs. Thus, systemic involvement is typical in SSc, whereas in morphea, internal organ manifestations are generally absent. In both disorders, panniculitis can occur but is a rare manifestation.

Clinical Features

While classification schemes in morphea are controversial, a deep variant, known as morphea profunda, is widely recognized, involving at least the subcutaneous fat and potentially extending to muscle and bone. Patients present with bound-down, sclerotic plaques that are better felt than seen, and may be localized or generalized (see Fig. 10.4).

Histopathologically, morphea profunda is characterized by thickened, hyalinized collagen in the deep dermis and subcutaneous septae, as well as a perivascular and interstitial lymphocyte-predominant infiltrate. The presence of mucin has also been reported [89]. In addition to morphea profunda, subcutaneous extension may occur in other types of morphea, such as deep circumscribed morphea, pansclerotic morphea, generalized morphea, and linear morphea.

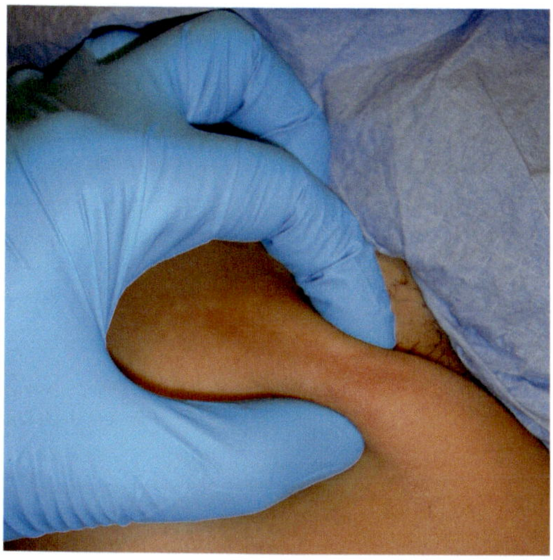

Fig. 10.4 Morphea profunda: indurated, sclerotic, hyperpigmented plauqe on the anterior thigh

Panniculitis rarely occurs in patients with SSc, but in patients who develop this complication, the typical presentation is well-circumscribed, indurated, painful, hyperpigmented plaques on the pretibial area [90]. Involvement of the arm, lateral thighs, gluteal region, and abdomen has also been described [91, 92]. The histopathology of these lesions is significant for a mixed septal-lobular panniculitis. The lobular features range from mild lipophagic fat necrosis to extensive lipomembranous change, characterized by membranous fat necrosis and resultant fat microcysts with luminal projections [91, 92].

Importantly, unlike LEP and DAP, panniculitis related to SSc has not been reported to develop in the absence of other manifestations of the disease. One retrospective study of 128 patients with diffuse or limited cutaneous SSc found that 10 (8%) had panniculitis. Significantly, the patients with panniculitis were more likely to have pulmonary hypertension as well as ventilation/perfusion lung scan defects, suggesting that pulmonary infarction was the major cause of pulmonary hypertension. Given the clinicopathologic overlap between these patients' SSc-associated panniculitis and LDS, a type of panniculitis associated with chronic venous insufficiency, the authors hypothesized that venous hypertension of the legs was responsible for both the panniculitis and (as a result of venous thrombosis and pulmonary infarction) the pulmonary hypertension [90]. Whether panniculitis truly presages pulmonary hypertension in SSc remains to be elucidated.

Principles of Management

Aggressive therapy is often necessary for morphea extending to the fat, as morphea is a fibrosing condition with the potential for permanent, irreversible sequelae, including joint contractures and limb-length discrepancies. First-line therapies for deep morphea include ultraviolet A1 phototherapy and MTX, in combination with systemic corticosteroids if progression is rapid or if the skin overlying a joint is involved [93, 94]. MMF [95], cyclosporine [96–99], extracorporeal photopheresis [1, 100, 101], abatacept [102], bosentan [103], and anti-thymocyte globulin [104] have also been reported with success. Although volume restoration with inert dermal fillers has not been reported in morphea profunda, it has been used successfully to re-contour the sequelae of linear morphea [105]. As with other autoimmune diseases, filler therapy should only be considered once disease is quiescent.

Treatment of panniculitis in SSc is likely to mirror that of the disorder's classic cutaneous manifestations, as the former has never been reported to occur in the absence of the latter.

Pyoderma Gangrenosum

Key Summary Capsule Bullets

- Four clinical variants: ulcerative/classic, bullous/atypical, pustular, vegetative
- Morphology, location, and disease associations differ with each variant
- Diagnosis of exclusion with no pathognomonic features and several disease mimickers
- Benefits of skin biopsy outweigh risk of biopsy-induced pathergy
- Ideal biopsy is elliptical incision that includes both lesion edge and ulcer base

- Treatment includes wound care measures, pain control, and topical and/or systemic therapy

Classification and Epidemiology

PG is an inflammatory skin condition that is associated with systemic disease—most often IBD, arthritis (usually seronegative monoarticular arthritis), or a hematologic disorder—in a reported 52–67% of cases [106, 107]. Alternatively, PG may occur as part of the rare genetic condition PAPA (pyogenic arthritis, PG, and acne) syndrome. In addition, rare familial cases not associated with PAPA syndrome have been reported [108]. Despite its name, PG is neither infectious nor gangrenous. Rather, PG is considered a neutrophilic dermatosis, due to the dense neutrophilic infiltrate that is characteristically seen on histology.

PG is rare. According to the only population-based PG study, the estimated incidence is six cases per million people per year [109]. Although PG is frequently associated with IBD, the prevalence of PG in IBD patients is low, ranging in the literature from 0.5% to 5% [110]. PG is slightly more common in women and peaks between the second and sixth decades of life, although any age group, including children, may be affected [106, 107, 109, 111].

Pathogenesis

The pathogenic basis of PG is uncertain, but an aberrant immune response mediated by neutrophils and T-cells directed against an unknown self-antigen is thought to be responsible [112].

Evidence for the role of neutrophils is derived from case reports that describe abnormal neutrophil chemotaxis in PG [113]; overexpression [114–116] and induction [115] of the neutrophil chemokine interleukin-8 (IL-8) in PG lesions; and correlation of improvement of PG with a reduction in serum IL-8 [114, 116, 117]. In addition, TNF-α and IL-1 have been implicated in PG pathogenesis, and both induce IL-8 expression [118, 119]. Notably, TNF-α inhibitors such as infliximab and the IL-1 inhibitors anakinra and gevokizumab (currently in phase III clinical trials for PG) have been successfully reported in the treatment of PG [120, 121] and PAPA syndrome [122].

The role of aberrant T-cells in PG pathogenesis is supported by the presence of expanded T-cell clones in PG lesions and in the peripheral blood of patients with PG [123]. In addition, the well-documented response of PG to cyclosporine, a suppressor of Th cells, supports the role of T-cells in PG pathogenesis [124]. Recent reports of PG responsive to the IL-23 inhibitor ustekinumab also implicate T-cells in PG pathogenesis, as IL-23 is essential for the differentiation of Th17 cells [125–128].

In PAPA syndrome, the *PSTPIP1/CD2BP1* gene on chromosome 15q, which encodes proline-serine-threonine phosphatase-interacting protein 1 (PSTPIP1, also known as CD2 antigen-binding protein 1), is mutated, and this mutation is thought to promote inflammation. No genetic mutation has been identified in the rare cases of familial PG distinct from PAPA syndrome [108].

Clinical Features

PG has four clinically distinct variants with different prevalence, morphology, location, and systemic disease associations. Ulcerative (classic) PG is the most common variant, while the bullous (atypical), pustular, and vegetative variants are less frequently encountered. In all variants other than vegetative PG, rapid progression is typical, and pain is often out of proportion to what may be expected based upon physical examination. Disease in any one individual is typically limited to only one variant. PG may follow an acute, relapsing, or chronic course, with relapsing or chronic being more likely when PG is associated with systemic disease.

Ulcerative PG generally begins as one or multiple severely painful pustules or nodules on the lower extremities, especially the pretibial region.

Over the course of days, the lesions ulcerate centrally and expand peripherally (see Fig. 10.5). The resulting ulcer features a typically violaceous, undermined border, which is a characteristic feature and a sign of disease activity (see Fig. 10.6). Clinically, the undermined border appears as PG expands centrifugally, presenting as erosion underneath a border of necrotic skin. The ulcer base often appears purulent and/or necrotic. When ulceration extends through the subcutaneous fat and muscular fascia, underlying structures, such as tendons and ligaments, may be exposed. Lesions typically express an exudate, which may be purulent, hemorrhagic, and/or malodorous. Healing results in a typical pattern of cribriform scarring (see Fig. 10.7), which may serve as a diagnostic clue in patients with undiagnosed recurrent PG or with multiple lesions in various stages of development.

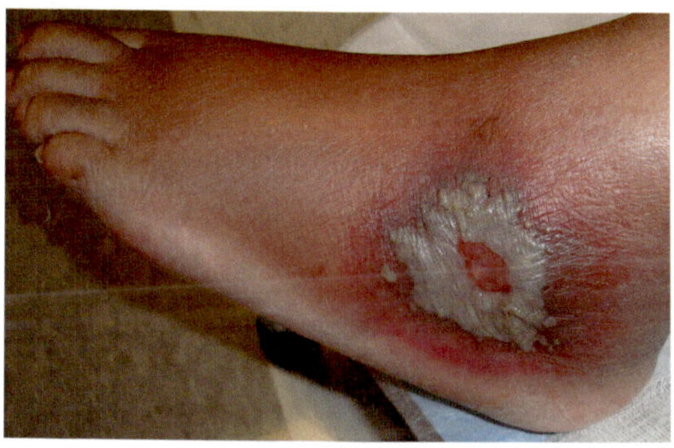

Fig. 10.5 Ulcerative pyoderma gangrenosum (PG): hemorrhagic pustule that ulcerated centrally and developed a violaceous, undermined border over the course of days

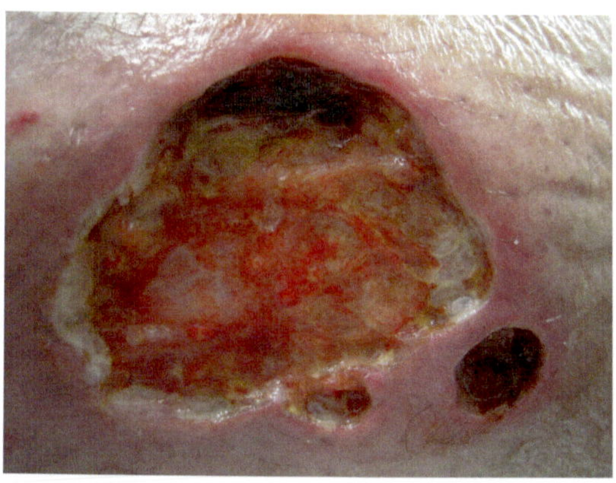

Fig. 10.6 Ulcerative PG: central ulcer surrounded by an undermined border with a violaceous to erythematous rim

Although the pretibial region is the most commonly involved site in ulcerative PG, any skin surface may be affected. For example, peristomal PG is often seen in patients with an underlying IBD. In rare cases, PG of the genitals may occur; this presentation may be more common in newborns [129].

Ulcerative PG is associated with systemic disease in the majority of patients: IBD (ulcerative colitis or Crohn disease, 27–36% of patients), arthritis (usually seronegative, non-erosive arthritis of a large joint, 19–37%), or a hematologic disorder (most often IgA monoclonal gammopathy, 11%) [106, 107]. Rarely, PG has been associated with solid organ malignancies, and this possibility should be considered in patients with a history of malignancy or with PG of unknown etiology [130]. In cases in which no underlying disorder is identified, the presence of leukocyte adhesion deficiency-1, an autosomal recessive disorder characterized by recurrent bacterial infections, persistent neutrophilia, and poor wound healing, should be considered, as this disorder has been associated with PG-like lesions in several cases [131].

Bullous PG typically manifests as painful, blue-grey, hemorrhagic vesicles on the face and upper extremities, especially the dorsal hands.

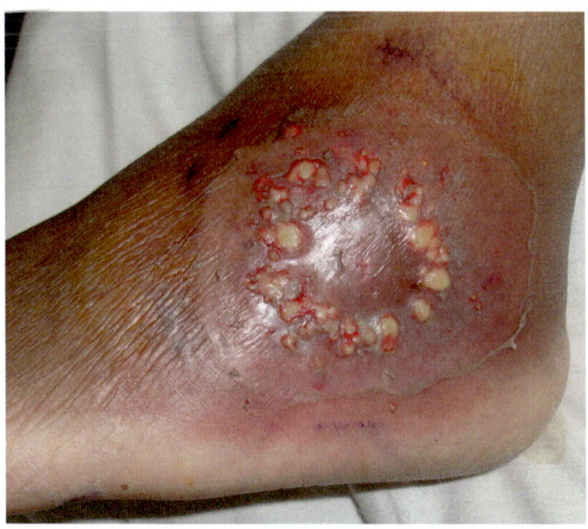

Fig. 10.7 Uulcerative PG: healing of an ulcer in a cribriform pattern with loss of the undermined border

The vesicles expand rapidly and centrifugally into bullae and then rupture, leaving behind deep erosions or superficial ulcers that may lack the undermined border of ulcerative PG. Bullous PG is more likely to be associated with a hematologic disorder (66% of patients) than with IBD (11%) or arthritis (3–18%) [106, 132]. The most common hematologic disorder associated with bullous PG is acute myelogenous leukemia (AML), followed by chronic myelogenous leukemia, and less frequently, MDS, multiple myeloma, and myeloid metaplasia [132]. The development of bullous PG may coincide with transformation of the underlying hematologic disorder (e.g., MDS into AML) [132]. Furthermore, the development of bullous PG in patients with AML portends a poor prognosis; therefore, swift recognition of a potential underlying hematologic disorder in patients with bullous PG is imperative.

Vegetative PG (also referred to as superficial granulomatous pyoderma) is characterized by a superficial and sometimes verrucous ulcer, plaque, or nodule. Unlike ulcerative PG, vegetative PG develops slowly and is typically painless. According to the largest review of vegetative PG, including 46 patients, the lesion favors the trunk in 52% of cases, the extremities in 31%, and the head or groin in the minority. Compared with other variants, vegetative PG is less aggressive and lacks a clear association with systemic disease [133].

In pustular PG, painful pustules surrounded by erythema are symmetrically distributed on the extensor surfaces of the lower extremities and upper trunk. Pustular PG occurs almost exclusively in association with IBD, often during flares; thus, concomitant fever, arthralgias, and myalgias are common. Pyostomatitis vegetans, which presents with oropharyngeal pustules and snail track-like erosions, is generally considered a mucosal variant of pustular PG.

Rarely, patients with PG develop sterile neutrophilic infiltrates in the lungs (the most common extramucocutaneous site), heart, muscles, bones, central nervous system, spleen, liver, lymph nodes, gastrointestinal tract, or cornea [134].

The potential for pathergy, or the development or worsening of lesions in areas of skin trauma, should be considered in all patients with PG. However, while pathergy has long been considered a key trigger of PG, one of the largest retrospective cohort studies on PG, including 103 patients, found a pathergic response was present in only 31% of patients [111]. These findings have important implications in the management of patients with PG. For example, while gentle wound care and avoidance of aggressive debridement is essential to prevent a pathergic response, the potential for pathergy should not hinder the use of biopsy in establishing proper diagnosis.

The presence of a leukemoid reaction may be seen in patients with PG, as has been reported in two cases [135]. In such cases, patients may be febrile, and the white blood cell count is highly elevated (>50,000/μL), sometimes with neutrophil precursors present in the serum. Exclusion of infectious etiologies in such cases is imperative.

There are no pathognomonic features of PG seen histologically. Typically, a heavy neutrophilic infiltrate is expected; however, one retrospective review of 103 patients with PG found that only 8 of 67 histopathology reports documented "typical neutrophilic infiltrate and early abscess formation" [111], and therefore the lack of this finding on histopathology could not be used to exclude the diagnosis of PG.

Histopathologic findings in PG also differ depending upon the area of the lesion sampled. For example, the base of the ulcer will typically demonstrate an intradermal abscess (collections of neutrophils), while the undermined border classically features early abscess formation and a mixed neutrophilic and lymphocytic infiltrate, and the erythematous rim may demonstrate lymphocytic vasculitis [136].

Additional features can differ depending upon PG subtype. For example, subcorneal neutrophils are often seen in ulcerative and pustular PG, and subepidermal bullae in bullous PG, whereas in vegetative PG, pseudoepitheliomatous hyperplasia, sinus tracts, and "three-layered granulomas" (made of an inner layer of neutrophilic abscesses, middle layer of histiocytes and giant cells, and outer layer of plasma cells and eosinophils) can be seen [133].

Histopathology may also differ based on the underlying systemic association; for example, in the setting of hematologic malignancy, atypical lymphocytes may be present. Despite the highly variable findings on histopathology of PG, skin biopsy is essential for excluding mimicking conditions, and for this reason should be considered in all patients.

Diagnostic Considerations

Pathognomonic clinical, laboratory, or histologic features of PG are lacking. As such, PG is considered a diagnosis of exclusion, requiring the presence of consistent clinical features as well as the elimination of several disease mimickers as possibilities (see Table 10.3). Consideration of skin biopsy evaluated with infectious stains, as well as tissue culture for bacteria, mycobacteria, and fungus, is important in establishing the diagnosis of PG, especially given that treatment for PG is often immunosuppressive in nature, and, thus, likely to exacerbate any infectious etiology.

One retrospective cohort study and literature review from a tertiary referral center emphasized the need to exclude alternative diagnoses in patients with potential PG [137]. In this study, 64 of 95 patients (67%) with ulcerations resembling PG received PG-directed therapy prior to the establishment of a correct, alternative diagnosis. Of these patients, 23% were refractory to PG-directed therapy, 12% experienced an exacerbation of the underlying condition, and 23% had a further delay in proper diagnosis. Ultimate diagnoses were delayed on average by 10 months, and misdiagnoses included malignancies, vasculopathies, vasculitis, infectious etiologies, and drug-induced or exogenous tissue injury [137]. These findings underscore the importance of careful exclusion of alternative etiologies to prevent unnecessary morbidity and mortality in patients with suspected PG. For example, correct diagnosis of PG in a patient with a suspected infectious etiology may prevent unnecessary wound debridement that has the potential to exacerbate PG. Alternatively, correct diagnosis of an infectious etiology mimicking PG may protect a patient from undergoing immunosuppressive therapy that may worsen the underlying infection.

Given the importance of considering all etiologies, exclusion of alternative diagnoses is considered one of the two major diagnostic criteria for PG that have been proposed [138] and adapted [134], though not validated. According to these guidelines, two major and two minor criteria are required for a diagnosis of PG (see Table 10.4).

Table 10.3 Differential diagnosis of pyoderma gangrenosum (PG)

Vasculopathy (e.g. antiphospholipid antibody syndrome, venous stasis ulcer, livedoid vasculopathy)
Vasculitis (e.g. granulomatosis with polyangiitis, polyarteritis nodosa, cryoglobulinemic vasculitis)
Neuropathic etiologies (e.g. diabetic ulcer, Charcot-Marie-Tooth disease)
Malignancy (e.g. basal cell carcinoma, squamous cell carcinoma, cutaneous T-cell lymphoma, leukemia cutis)
Infection (e.g. bacterial, myocobacterial, fungal)
Other neutrophilic dermatoses (e.g. Sweet syndrome)
Metastatic Crohn disease
Exogenous tissue injury (e.g. arthropod/spider bites, factitious dermatitis)

Disease and Comorbidity Assessment

In the assessment of suspected PG, two primary objectives are most relevant: (1) the exclusion of disease mimickers, and (2) the determination of whether an underlying systemic disease is present. To this end, a complete history and physical examination should be performed with an emphasis on symptoms and signs suggestive of gastrointestinal, rheumatologic, hematologic, and vascular disorders.

In addition, as reviewed, a skin biopsy is essential for ruling out mimickers of PG. Given the relative infrequency of pathergy among PG patients [111], as well as the morbidity and mortality associated with misdiagnosis and mistreatment [137], most experts concur that the benefits

Table 10.4 Diagnostic criteria for PG [135]

Major criteria
1. Rapid[a] progression of a painful[b] necrolytic cutaneous ulcer[c] with an irregular, violaceous, and undermined border
2. Exclusion of other causes of cutaneous ulceration
Minor criteria
1. History suggestive of pathergy[d] or clinical finding of cribriform scarring
2. Systemic diseases associated with PG[e]
3. Histopathologic findings (sterile dermal neutrophilia ± mixed inflammation ± lymphocytic vasculitis)
4. Treatment response (rapid response to systemic glucocorticoid treatment)[f]

[a]Characteristic margin expansion of 1–2 cm/d, or a 50% increase in ulcer size within 1 month
[b]Pain is usually out of proportion to the size of the ulceration
[c]Typically preceded by a papule, pustule, or bulla
[d]Ulcer development at sites of minor cutaneous injury
[e]Inflammatory bowel disease, polyarthritis, myelocytic leukemia, or preleukemia
[f]Generally responds to a dosage of 1–2 mg/kg/d, with a 50% decrease in size within 1 month

of a skin biopsy outweigh the risk of biopsy-induced pathergy.

An elliptical incision with adequate subcutaneous fat sampling is ideal for histopathologic analysis in PG. However, in some cases, particularly in superficial lesions, a punch biopsy may provide adequate depth for analysis, and this technique further minimizes the relatively low risk of pathergy. In cases in which an elliptical incision cannot be performed but sampling of a deeper lesion is required, the "double-punch" technique may be utilized. In this technique, a second punch biopsy is performed within the ulcer created by the first punch biopsy in order to obtain a deeper sample. All biopsies should aim to include sampling of both the edge of the lesion as well as of the ulcer base, if an ulcer is present. In general, in addition to the sample sent for routine hematoxylin and eosin (H&E) analysis, a second biopsy should also be performed and sent for bacterial, mycobacterial, and fungal cultures. In addition, stains infectious etiologies should be requested on the sample sent for H&E. It is ideal for biopsies to be interpreted by a dermatopathologist, as histopathologic analysis can be challenging given the lack of pathognomonic features for PG and the need to exclude the many disease mimickers, as reviewed above.

Although no guidelines for a formal workup in PG exist, experts concur that a search for an underlying condition and testing to exclude alternative diagnoses are warranted. A thorough history, review of systems, and physical examination are essential and help to guide further workup. Among other entities, eliciting signs or symptoms of an underlying IBD or hematologic disorder is important, given that these conditions occur commonly in patients with PG.

Particular attention should also be given to the musculoskeletal system, as up to 37% of patients with PG have arthritis. Most commonly, as reviewed, arthritis in PG manifests as a seronegative, non-erosive arthritis of a large joint (knee, ankle, or elbow). However, RA, ankylosing spondylitis, and osteoarthritis have been reported as well [106, 107, 132]. Of note, the severity of the arthritis does not usually correlate with the severity of PG [138].

Workup generally includes, at minimum, a CBC with differential, complete metabolic panel, and urinalysis. Fecal occult blood test, sigmoidoscopy, or colonoscopy is often useful, particularly in patients with gastrointestinal symptoms or with ulcerative or pustular PG. A peripheral blood smear, serum and urine immunofixation and electrophoresis, and/or bone marrow aspirate or biopsy should also be considered, especially in patients with constitutional symptoms or abnormalities on CBC, or those with the bullous subtype of PG. Hepatitis B and C panels may also be useful, particularly in high-risk populations, and serologic and/or radiographic examination may be helpful in patients with an accompanying arthritis.

Depending upon an individual patient's comorbidities and disease manifestations, additional workup to rule out alternative diagnoses may include: antinuclear antibody, antineutrophilic cytoplasmic antibodies, hypercoagulability studies (especially antiphospholipid antibody), rheumatoid factor, cryoglobulins, HIV testing, rapid plasma reagin, and a chest radiograph. In addition, a Doppler ultrasound may help identify an underlying vasculopathy, and X-ray or magnetic resonance imaging may help exclude underlying osteomyelitis.

If there is a systemic disease associated with PG, as there is in most cases, it may or may not parallel the course of the cutaneous disease (with the exception of pustular PG, which usually flares along with the underlying IBD). Systemic conditions often precede the development of PG; however, associated conditions may also develop after the onset of PG, and therefore, a high index of suspicion for an underlying condition should be maintained in the follow-up of all patients with PG.

Principles of Management

The primary goal in the management of PG is to promote wound healing through inhibition of the underlying aberrant immune reaction. Given the rarity of PG and the lack of validated outcome measures, evidence for treatment is mostly derived from small case series and case reports, and there is no gold standard therapy. Ideally, treatment should include wound care measures along with topical and/or systemic therapy. Goals of therapy are to promote wound healing, control pain, and control inflammation. The algorithm chosen for any given patient depends upon the severity of the PG (considering depth, size, number of lesions, and location) as well as the presence of an underlying systemic condition.

The major goal of wound care in PG is to prevent superinfection without provoking pathergy, as wound care itself appears to have little impact on re-epithelialization [124, 139]. As in the management of other wounds, the choice of dressing is directed by lesion characteristics. For example, absorbent dressings are recommended over occlusive dressings for exudative lesions or peristomal PG [139, 140]. Wet-to-dry dressings should be categorically avoided because the mechanical debridement that occurs during dressing changes may pathergize lesions. Barrier creams or ointments should be used to help prevent skin breakdown and infection at wound edges [140].

Pain control should be addressed as soon as the diagnosis of PG is established, especially given that PG is often refractory to treatment, requiring multiple therapeutic trials before an effective therapy can be found. NSAIDs can be helpful for pain, as can opiates when appropriate. In patients with persistent pain, consultation with a pain specialist may be helpful. As effective therapy is established, pain will begin to resolve, often prior to the appearance of substantial visible improvement.

Once the diagnosis of PG is established, topical treatment may be sufficient for superficial disease that lacks a systemic association, as is the case in vegetative PG [133]. Topical therapy is also helpful adjunctively in severe PG, particularly at the inflamed borders. Options include potent topical or intralesional corticosteroids, topical tacrolimus or pimecrolimus, topical cyclosporine (ophthalmic preparation), and topical dapsone (an anti-neutrophilic agent). Topical tacrolimus was somewhat more effective than clobetasol in a comparison study [141]; however, topical tacrolimus must be used with caution given the potential for a large degree of systemic absorption. In one reported case, topical application of crushed dapsone tablets led to sustained resolution of peristomal PG without systemic side effects [142]. A branded topical formulation of dapsone is now available, and may be useful, particularly in superficial PG. Other topical medications that have been used successfully in isolated cases include: 5-aminosalicylic acid, becaplermin (a platelet-derived growth factor), sodium cromoglycate, and topical nitrogen mustard [140].

The majority of patients with PG require a combination of systemic and topical therapy [111]. Initial treatment should be directed towards the underlying disease if one is present, as this frequently results in improvement or complete remission [124]. For example, infliximab is considered first-line for IBD-associated PG. In the only randomized, double-blinded, placebo-controlled trial for PG, 46% of patients treated with 1 infusion of infliximab improved after 2 weeks, compared with 6% in the placebo group ($p = 0.025$). By the fourth and sixth weeks, 69% of infliximab-treated patients (including those treated in an open-label fashion) had improved, 21% of whom had achieved complete remission [121].

Minocycline and other tetracyclines may be helpful in the treatment of PG, particularly while awaiting the results of cultures taken to exclude an infectious etiology. Minocycline has both anti-inflammatory and antimicrobial properties, including activity against some atypical mycobacteria. In a series of four patients with PG, minocycline proved effective within weeks when used at doses of 200–300 mg/day [143].

Other therapies that may be initiated while infection is being ruled out include IVIG, oral dapsone, and colchicine, which, like dapsone, has anti-neutrophilic properties. These medications are generally used in conjunction with immunosuppressive agents, which may be added once infection has been excluded. IVIG, for example, resulted in complete or nearly complete remission in 12 of 13 patients when used primarily as adjunctive therapy at 2 g/kg [144]. In another series, oral dapsone at 100–200 mg/day caused or contributed to resolution of recalcitrant PG in two of three patients [145].

Medium- to high-dose systemic corticosteroids and/or cyclosporine may be useful for PG refractory to topical treatment or treatment of an associated disease, PG that extends into underlying structures (i.e., muscles, tendons, ligaments), and extracutaneous PG [124]. A randomized, single-blinded trial of 121 patients with PG found that prednisolone and cyclosporine were equally effective, with each agent resulting in healing in about half of patients within 6 months [146]. Corticosteroids are generally initiated at 0.5–1 mg/kg/day of methylprednisolone or 1 g/day for 1–5 days if given as pulsed doses, and cyclosporine is typically started at 5 mg/kg/day [124]. Importantly, persistence of a lesion does not necessarily indicate treatment failure, as wounds may take time to heal despite successful immunosuppression. Signs of treatment response include loss of the undermined border and a halt in lesion growth (see Fig. 10.7).

For patients who require maintenance therapy or whose PG is refractory to the agents reviewed, monotherapy may be considered with other TNF-α inhibitors, granulocyte apheresis, or thalidomide. Alternatively, the following agents may be used as corticosteroid-sparing adjuncts: MTX, MMF, cyclophosphamide, IVIG, dapsone, and AZA [140, 147].

Recently, the successful use of platelet-rich plasma, or autologous plasma that is centrifuged to contain a high concentration of platelets, has been documented in PG. Platelet-rich plasma is thought to enhance wound healing due to the many growth factors it contains, which help promote the cell recruitment and proliferation necessary for proper wound healing [148]. Apremilast, a phosphodiesterase-4 inhibitor, has yet to be studied in PG, but it may be a potential therapeutic option given its inhibition of TNF-α [149] and its efficacy in a randomized, double-blinded, placebo-controlled phase II trial for Behçet disease, which, like PG, is a neutrophilic dermatosis [150].

Given the potential for pathergy, the role of surgery in the management of PG is controversial. Although the removal of necrotic tissue may help prevent superinfection, there are several case reports of worsening of PG following debridement [151], with sequelae ranging from disfiguring scars [152] to large tissue defects [153–155] to digital amputations [156]. Of note, PG was active at the time of debridement in each of these patients as none were treated with systemic immunotherapy either prior to debridement or concurrently. On the other hand, improvement with gentle debridement and/or grafting has been described in patients simultaneously being treated with systemic agents [154, 157–160]. These data suggest that the decision to pursue surgery for PG should be made with careful consideration of the risks and benefits, and that, if performed, surgical interventions should be limited to periods of disease quiescence or remission and pharmacologic immunosuppression. If patients with a history of PG need to undergo surgery for other reasons, these procedures should be performed with caution, and perioperative systemic corticosteroids and/or cyclosporine should be considered to minimize the risk of pathergy [161].

Sweet Syndrome

Key Summary Capsule Bullets

- Presents with acute onset of fever, leukocytosis, and neutrophil-rich skin lesions, although fever and/or leukocytosis may be absent in the minority
- Lesions are brightly erythematous to violaceous, edematous or "juicy," tender papules, plaques, and/or nodules
- Three variants: classic/idiopathic, malignancy-associated, drug-induced
- Workup focuses on identifying underlying associations, including infection, medication, pregnancy, IBD, or malignancy
- Systemic corticosteroids are mainstay of therapy

Classification and Epidemiology

Sweet syndrome, or acute febrile neutrophilic dermatosis, is a rare inflammatory disorder with cutaneous and systemic manifestations. Classically, patients present with a tender, erythematous, edematous eruption, fever, and leukocytosis.

Sweet syndrome is one of the neutrophilic dermatoses, a group of inflammatory conditions that includes PG (see above), erythema elevatum diutinum (EED), and subcorneal pustular dermatosis (Sneddon-Wilkinson disease). These conditions are characterized by sterile, neutrophilic, cutaneous and extracutaneous infiltrates, as well as an association with systemic conditions (such as hematologic disorders and IBD). Other neutrophilic dermatoses include palmoplantar pustulosis, neutrophilic dermatosis of the dorsal hands, amicrobial pustulosis of the folds, Behçet disease, bowel-associated dermatosis-arthritis syndrome, and rheumatoid neutrophilic dermatitis. Although the classic features of these diseases are distinct from each other, many consider the neutrophilic dermatoses to exist along a spectrum, and there are several reports of multiple of these conditions coexisting in the same patient [162–172].

Sweet syndrome is generally divided into three categories: classic/idiopathic (associated with infection, vaccination, IBD, or pregnancy), malignancy-associated (hematologic or solid malignancies), or drug-induced. In a review of 77 patients with Sweet syndrome, 53% were affected by the classic subtype, 35% had malignancy-associated disease, and 12% had drug-induced Sweet syndrome [173]. Most commonly, adult women are affected, except in hematologic malignancy-associated cases, in which there is an equal sex distribution [174]. Patients with classic or drug-induced Sweet syndrome tend to be younger (with median ages of 46 and 45, respectively) than those with the malignancy-associated subtype (median age 71 years) [173]. Rarely, Sweet syndrome occurs in the pediatric population. In children under 3 years, the disorder is twice as common in males and is not associated with malignancy. In contrast, there is no sex predilection amongst children over 3 years, but a strong association with hematologic malignancy has been demonstrated [175].

Pathogenesis

The pathogenesis of Sweet syndrome is poorly understood. Currently, the most compelling hypothesis is that this condition represents a neutrophil-predominant inflammatory reaction, mediated in part by granulocyte-colony stimulating factor (G-CSF), a pro-neutrophil cytokine. Evidence for the role of G-CSF includes the finding that patients with active Sweet syndrome have significantly higher serum G-CSF than patients with inactive disease or healthy controls [176]. Moreover, G-CSF may represent the link between the heterogeneous conditions and states associated with Sweet syndrome, as the cytokine is elevated in infection [177, 178], pregnancy [179, 180], and ulcerative colitis [181], may be produced by Sweet syndrome-associated malignancies [182], and is the most common cause of drug-induced Sweet syndrome [183]. Hypersensitivity reactions to antigens from bacteria, viruses, or tumors as well as genetic susceptibilities involving the MEFV gene, HLA-B54, and chromosome 3q have also been implicated in pathogenesis.

Clinical Features

Acute febrile neutrophilic dermatosis, the non-eponymous name for Sweet syndrome, reflects the disease's typical presentation with the acute onset of fever and neutrophil-rich skin lesions. The lesions are typically one or multiple, brightly erythematous to violaceous, tender papules, plaques, and/or nodules (see Fig. 10.8). The lesions characteristically appear edematous, or "juicy," due to significant interstitial edema in the upper dermis. Lesions typically present asymmetrically on the upper extremities but may also involve the head, neck, trunk, and (less likely in the classic subtype) lower extremities. Due to pathergy, the involved sites may correspond to areas of trauma. Mucosal involvement can occur and is variable, favoring the eyes in classic Sweet syndrome and oropharynx in the malignancy-associated subtype [174].

Patients with Sweet syndrome tend to appear ill, as fever usually accompanies the cutaneous manifestations or precedes the eruption by days to weeks. Fever, however, is not universal, and may spare roughly 10–20% of patients with the classic or malignancy-associated variants. Other constitutional symptoms, such as malaise, arthralgias, myalgias, and/or headache, may be present [174].

The morphology of Sweet syndrome may vary. An annular, arcuate, or target-like configuration may develop over time, as smaller lesions coalesce or central clearing develops. The malignancy-associated subtype may be vesiculobullous at first and then ulcerate (see Fig. 10.9). A subcutaneous variant presents as deep dermal to subcutaneous nodules that favor the lower extremities [169]. When a Sweet syndrome-like eruption including pustules occurs on the dorsal

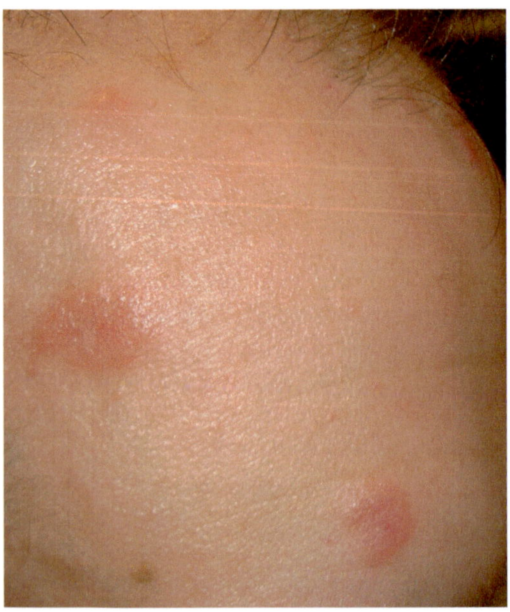

Fig. 10.8 Histiocytoid Sweet syndrome: erythematous and edematous papules and plaques on the forehead

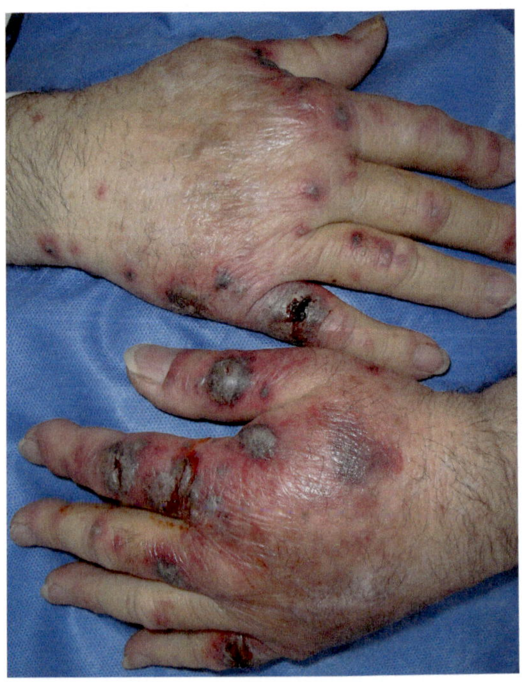

Fig. 10.9 Sweet syndrome: hemorrhagic vesicles and bullae, some of which have ruptured with resulting ulcerations, on the bilateral dorsal hands

hands, it is often termed neutrophilic dermatosis of the dorsal hands, but many consider it a variant of Sweet syndrome.

Extracutaneous manifestations of Sweet syndrome may occur in virtually any organ. Musculoskeletal involvement is common and may manifest as arthralgias, acute sterile arthritis, pigmented villonodular synovitis, myositis, fasciitis, tendinitis, or tenosynovitis. The eyes are also frequently affected, with manifestations including conjunctivitis, episcleritis, glaucoma, peripheral ulcerative keratitis, and iritis; ophthalmologic evaluation in patients suspected to have Sweet syndrome is essential. Uncommonly, central nervous system involvement may manifest as encephalitis or aseptic meningitis. Patients may also develop sterile osteomyelitis or involvement of the ears, kidneys, intestines, liver, heart, lungs, or spleen [174]. Sweet syndrome may also be uncommonly associated with the systemic inflammatory response syndrome (SIRS), and such cases have even been reported to be fatal [184, 185].

The histopathologic features of Sweet syndrome include papillary dermal edema and a neutrophil-predominant dermal infiltrate in a perivascular to nodular and diffuse distribution. Although the absence of leukocytoclastic vasculitis (LCV) is a traditional diagnostic criterion of Sweet syndrome, evidence suggests that its presence should not rule out the diagnosis [186]. In fact, evidence of vasculitis may be seen in up to 29% of histopathology specimens in Sweet syndrome and is thought to be a secondary phenomenon due to the dense neutrophilic infiltrate [187]. Eosinophils may be present in classic or drug-induced Sweet syndrome [174]. New lesions of Sweet syndrome occasionally demonstrate a "histiocytoid" pattern characterized by a superficial to mid-dermal infiltrate predominated by histiocyte-like immature myeloid cells [188]. In subcutaneous Sweet syndrome, neutrophils predominate in the subcutaneous fat lobules, with minimal dermal involvement [189]. Lastly, in unusual cases of "necrotizing" Sweet syndrome, the neutrophil-predominant infiltrate extends into the fascia and skeletal muscle, with resultant fat necrosis and myonecrosis [190].

About 80% of patients with classic Sweet syndrome have peripheral leukocytosis with neutrophilia, compared with 47–60% with the malignancy-associated subtype and 38% with the drug-induced subtype [174]. Thus, the absence of neutrophilia does not exclude Sweet syndrome. In fact, patients with an underlying hematologic malignancy may develop Sweet syndrome despite being neutropenic [191].

Diagnostic Considerations

Diagnostic criteria for classic and malignancy-associated Sweet syndrome have been proposed [192] and revised [193]; the presence of both major criteria and two of four minor criteria are required for diagnosis (see Table 10.5). Guidelines also exist for the diagnosis of drug-induced Sweet syndrome, with five of five criteria required for diagnosis (see Table 10.6) [72].

Because Sweet syndrome classically presents with fever and leukocytosis, cutaneous and systemic infections are an important consideration in the differential diagnosis. Sweet syndrome may resemble bacterial (e.g., cellulitis, erysipelas, *carbunculosis*), fungal (e.g., coccidioidomy-

Table 10.5 Diagnostic criteria for classic and malignancy-associated Sweet syndrome [195]

Major criteria (both required)
Abrupt onset of tender or painful erythematous plaques or nodules occasionally with vesicles, pustules, or bullae
Predominantly neutrophilic infiltration in the dermis without leukocytoclastic vasculitis (LCV)
Minor criteria (2 of 4 required)
Preceded by a nonspecific respiratory or gastrointestinal tract infection, vaccination, or associated with inflammatory diseases such as chronic autoimmune disorders, infections, hemoproliferative disorders or solid malignant tumors, or pregnancy
Accompanied by periods of general malaise and fever (>38 °C)
3 of 4 of the following laboratory values during onset: ESR >20 mm; positive C-reactive protein; >70% neutrophils and bands in the peripheral blood smear; >8000 leukocytes
Excellent response to treatment with systemic corticosteroids or potassium iodide

Table 10.6 Diagnostic criteria for drug-induced Sweet syndrome (all required) [196]

1. Abrupt onset of painful erythematous plaques or nodules
2. Histopathologic evidence of a dense neutrophilic infiltrate without evidence of leukocytoclastic vasculitis (LCV)
3. Pyrexia >38 °C
4. Temporal relationship between drug ingestion and clinical presentation, or temporally related recurrence after oral challenge
5. Temporally related resolution of lesions after drug withdrawal or treatment with systemic corticosteroids

cosis, sporotrichosis), or atypical mycobacterial infections. Necrotizing Sweet syndrome may also mimic necrotizing fasciitis and should be considered in patients with clinicopathologic features consistent with necrotizing fasciitis as well as risk factors for Sweet syndrome. The distinction between the two disorders is crucial because surgical debridement, the mainstay of treatment for necrotizing fasciitis, can exacerbate Sweet syndrome due to pathergy. The presence of myonecrosis, which is usually present in necrotizing Sweet syndrome but absent until the final stages of necrotizing fasciitis, may help differentiate the two conditions [190].

When the lesions of Sweet syndrome are target-like, the clinical differential diagnosis may include erythema multiforme [194]. Features favoring erythema multiforme include oral mucosal involvement and the absence of fever, flu-like symptoms, leukocytosis, or highly elevated inflammatory markers. Moreover, Sweet syndrome and erythema multiforme are histopathologically distinct.

Both Sweet syndrome and neutrophilic eccrine hidradenitis occur in patients with AML and have a similar clinical presentation, but only in the latter does the neutrophilic infiltrate surround eccrine glands. EED is distinguished from Sweet syndrome by its asymptomatic, firm lesions with a predilection for extensor surfaces and histopathology predominated by LCV or dermal fibrosis and mucin. The abrupt-onset, erythematous plaques of Wells' syndrome are differentiated by their symmetric, widespread distribution, their association with peripheral eosinophilia, and the histopathologic finding of "flame figures" (masses of collagen and eosinophils).

Malignancy-associated Sweet syndrome may be vesiculobullous and ulcerate (see Fig. 10.9), thus, mimicking bullous PG. Leukemia cutis presents with firm papules, plaques, and nodules and can be distinguished histologically from Sweet syndrome; immunophenotyping enables differentiation of the histiocytes of leukemia cutis and the histiocyte-like immature myeloid cells of histiocytoid Sweet syndrome [188, 195]. The nodules of subcutaneous sarcoidosis, unlike those of subcutaneous Sweet syndrome, favor the upper extremities and histopathologically feature noncaseating granulomas. When subcutaneous Sweet syndrome occurs on the shins, it may be indistinguishable from EN; however, the neutrophilic infiltrate is predominantly lobular in subcutaneous Sweet syndrome but septal in EN. Moreover, EN is characterized by Miescher granulomas (small, nodular aggregates of histiocytes around a central stellate cleft), while this feature is absent or rare in subcutaneous Sweet syndrome [189].

Disease and Comorbidity Assessment

The evaluation of patients with suspected Sweet syndrome includes a history, physical examination, and laboratory studies, including a skin biopsy, to confirm the diagnosis and identify any underlying association.

In classic Sweet syndrome, patients may report an infection in the 1–3 weeks prior to onset, usually of the upper respiratory tract (streptococcosis) or gastrointestinal tract (salmonellosis or yersiniosis). Alternatively, classic Sweet syndrome can develop in the setting of vaccination, pregnancy, or known or new IBD (Crohn disease or ulcerative colitis). A possible association exists between Sweet syndrome and Behçet disease, EN, relapsing polychondritis, RA, sarcoidosis, Grave's disease, and

Hashimoto's thyroiditis. In addition, over 30 cases have been reported of Sweet syndrome associated with LE, including SLE, subacute cutaneous lupus, neonatal lupus, and drug-induced lupus [174]. In one review of 30 such patients, 9 carried a diagnosis of lupus preceding the onset of Sweet syndrome, and 21 were diagnosed concomitantly. In these patients, a higher male-to-female ratio was seen (1:2) as compared with SLE and Sweet syndrome alone [196].

Malignancy-associated Sweet syndrome typically reflects an underlying hematologic malignancy (especially AML), but solid malignancies (most often genitourinary, breast, and gastrointestinal carcinomas) have also been reported [197]. In a review of 77 patients with Sweet syndrome, 78% of malignancy-associated cases were due to hematologic malignancies or myelodysplastic/myeloproliferative disorders, while the remainder were associated with solid tumors [173]. Subcutaneous Sweet syndrome may be particularly associated with hematologic disorders [169]. Sweet syndrome may signify a new or recurrent malignancy and is the presenting sign of malignancy in roughly two-thirds of patients [198].

Drug-induced Sweet syndrome has been attributed to several medications, but a systematic review determined that there is sufficient evidence for only G-CSF and tretinoin to be implicated as causes [183]. Use of these agents generally precedes the onset of Sweet syndrome by 1–2 weeks [183].

The initial physical examination for patients with Sweet syndrome involves the measurement of vital signs (to evaluate for fever and exclude SIRS or sepsis), as well as examination of the skin, mucosal surfaces, lymph nodes (to evaluate for lymphadenopathy suggestive of a hematologic malignancy), and other organ systems as directed by a patient's symptoms (to evaluate for extracutaneous disease).

Skin biopsy is obtained in almost all cases to confirm the diagnosis. If infectious etiologies are considered likely in the differential, skin biopsies for bacterial, fungal, and mycobacterial cultures may be obtained. Incisional biopsies are preferred if subcutaneous or necrotizing Sweet syndrome is suspected, in order to ensure adequate sampling of the subcutaneous tissue.

A CBC with differential is recommended in all patients to screen for hematologic disorders, and if abnormal, consideration should be given to a bone marrow biopsy. Patients with anemia identified on CBC are more likely to have a malignancy. Other initial laboratory studies include antistreptococcal antibodies and throat culture, as well as a pregnancy test in women. Erythrocyte sedimentation rate and CRP serum levels are generally also obtained; ESR is elevated in the large majority of patients. Chest radiograph should be obtained in any patient with pulmonary symptoms, as lung involvement may occur in Sweet syndrome and is responsive to therapy.

Depending on the initial workup, further assessment for IBD or malignancy may be warranted. As there are no established guidelines for malignancy screening in patients with Sweet syndrome, one option is to begin with age-appropriate screening. Some have proposed that the malignancy workup include the following: digital rectal examination (including prostate examination in men); thyroid examination; breast and pelvic exam (including cervical cancer screening) in women; testicular exam in men; carcinoembryonic antigen level; complete metabolic panel; urinalysis and cytology; chest radiograph; sigmoidoscopy in patients over 50 years; and endometrial biopsy in menopausal women or those with a history of abnormal uterine bleeding, estrogen therapy, infertility, or obesity [197]. In addition, positron emission tomography (PET) and PET-computed tomography (PET-CT) have been used to screen for malignancies in patients with Sweet syndrome and are particularly helpful in the evaluation of hematologic disorders [199, 200].

In patients in whom an underlying condition is not apparent after screening, and particularly in young women, the diagnosis of SLE should be considered. A recent literature review including 47 patients with both SLE and neutrophilic dermatoses found that the neutrophilic dermatosis was the initial presentation in 15 patients (32%) [201].

If, after extensive workup, no underlying cause is identified for Sweet syndrome, a CBC with differential may be repeated annually or twice yearly, as hematologic malignancies have developed as late as 11 years after initial presentation of Sweet syndrome. On the other hand, a solid malignancy is unlikely to develop if one has not been detected within the first year after the onset of Sweet syndrome [197].

Principles of Management

Systemic corticosteroids are the mainstay of therapy for Sweet syndrome. Oral prednisone is generally initiated at 1 mg/kg/day, results in remission within 2–5 days, and is tapered over 4–6 weeks. Recurrences are common, and some patients may require a corticosteroid taper over 2–3 months or repeated pulses of intravenous methylprednisolone (up to 1 g/day for 3–5 days) [174].

For patients with multiple recurrences requiring long-term therapy, several corticosteroid-sparing agents may be used. Colchicine has been shown to be beneficial, likely due to its anti-neutrophilic effect. In a retrospective study, colchicine (1.5 mg/day for 10–21 days) was found to lead to resolution of classic Sweet syndrome in 18 of 20 patients. Defervescence occurred within 1–3 days, and cutaneous lesions and arthralgias began to improve within 2–5 days. There was no evidence of recurrence during a median follow-up of 8.5 years [202]. Potassium iodide has also been reported as effective; when used at 900 mg/day in a prospective study, 7 of 8 patients had resolution of fever, lesional tenderness, and arthralgias within 1–2 days, and resolution of cutaneous lesions within 3–4 days. The five patients who were treated for 2 weeks did not subsequently relapse [203].

Other potential therapies include indomethacin, clofazimine, cyclosporine, and dapsone. In an open-trial of indomethacin (150 mg/day for 1 week, then 100 mg/day for 2 weeks) for classic or malignancy-associated Sweet syndrome, 18 of 19 adults had resolution of fever and arthralgias within 2 days and resolution of cutaneous disease within 1–2 weeks. None relapsed during a mean follow-up of 20.1 months [204]. In a series including six patients with classic or malignancy-associated Sweet syndrome who flared upon discontinuation of methylprednisolone, clofazimine (200 mg/day for 4 weeks, then 100 mg/day for 4 weeks) resulted in "almost complete remission" without the need for subsequent systemic therapy [193]. Cyclosporine (2–10 mg/kg/day) or dapsone (100–200 mg/day) therapy may also be successful, but evidence is limited to case reports [174].

Pregnant patients with Sweet syndrome are generally treated with systemic corticosteroids [205–207]. Avoidance of potassium iodide and indomethacin at or after 30 weeks of gestation is important, as both are category D medications. Decisions regarding treatment in pregnant patients should be made in conjunction with an obstetrics specialist.

In addition to the above therapies, the treatment of drug-induced Sweet syndrome involves discontinuation of the suspected triggering agent. Recurrence upon rechallenge has been reported in 67% of patients [174]. When readministration of the drug is necessary, premedication with oral prednisone (0.5 mg/kg/day for 5 days) has been reported to prevent the recurrence of Sweet-like lesions, but this approach has not been formally evaluated in Sweet syndrome [208].

The skin lesions of Sweet syndrome heal without scarring. Malignancy-associated Sweet syndrome recurs at a rate similar to that of the drug-induced subtype (69%), usually in association with hematologic relapse. Recurrences of Sweet syndrome occur in 41% of patients whose disease is associated with solid malignancy, often due to recurrence of the malignancy itself (41%) [174]. Recurrence may be seen in up to 30% of patients with the classic subtype, often upon tapering of corticosteroids [174].

Palisaded Neutrophilic Granulomatous Dermatitis and Interstitial Granulomatous Dermatitis

PNGD and interstitial granulomatous dermatitis (IGD) are two granulomatous conditions that often present in patients with underlying autoimmune disease. RA is the most commonly reported autoimmune association with PNGD and IGD; however, SLE and other connective tissue diseases have been associated with these conditions as well. Medications, particularly TNF-α inhibitors, have also been associated with an IGD-like eruption, and when this occurs, the term IGDR is applied. While PNGD and IGD have been traditionally classified as distinct clinical and histological entities, and each is known to have its own characteristic features [209–214], the two conditions feature many similarities and, in many cases, there is a large degree of clinical and histologic overlap. Furthermore, the two entities share similar disease associations and therapeutic algorithms. In this section, we have described PNGD and IGD separately in order to fully encompass disease characteristics and associations. Nevertheless, we recognize the potential for overlap between these entities, and like many others, regard these entities as existing along a spectrum [215, 216].

Palisaded Neutrophilic Granulomatous Dermatitis

Key Summary Capsule Bullets

- Presents with skin-colored to red-violet umbilicated papules and/or nodules symmetrically on extensor elbows and fingers, but cutaneous findings may vary considerably
- Almost always associated with a systemic condition, most often RA, SLE, and ANCA-positive vasculitides, which may be active or quiescent
- Histopathology shows pan-dermal LCV, dense neutrophils, and degenerated collagen (early lesions) or palisading granulomas surrounding degenerated collagen and mucin (late lesions)
- May be challenging to differentiate from IGD due to clinicopathologic overlap

Classification and Epidemiology

PNGD is a cutaneous manifestation of RA, SLE, and other immune complex-mediated systemic diseases. Before the term PNGD was described, the condition was referred to by names such as rheumatoid papules, Churg-Strauss granuloma, cutaneous extravascular necrotizing granuloma, and superficial ulcerating rheumatoid necrobiosis [217].

Although PNGD is considered rare, the prevalence was found to be 6.5% in one study of 215 patients with RA [218]. Adult women are most frequently affected [219], which likely reflects the age and sex predilection of the systemic conditions often associated with PNGD.

Pathogenesis

The pathogenesis of PNGD is poorly understood, but it is thought to be related to the underlying systemic disease. Supporting this theory is the finding that patients with RA and PNGD have higher Disease Activity Score 28 (DAS28) scores than those without PNGD [218], suggesting that in some patients, PNGD and the underlying systemic disease may run a parallel course. Specifically, the underlying disease is believed to generate large immune complexes which, due to their size, deposit within dermal vessel walls, inciting a LCV [217]. This hypothesis is supported by the presence, in some patients, of immunoreactants within the vasculature of lesional skin [217, 220–223]. Ischemic tissue injury to the dermis is thought to occur from LCV, resulting in degenerated collagen, which may trigger a granulomatous reaction that ultimately resolves with fibrosis [217].

Clinical Features

PNGD was originally described as multiple, skin-colored to red-violet papules and/or nodules symmetrically distributed on the extensor surfaces of the elbows and fingers (see Fig. 10.10). Early in the course, lesions may be erythematous or urticarial-like annular plaques, and as the disease evolves, an infiltrative or waxy quality with a violaceous hue may develop. Umbilication due to a central ulcer and/or crust is characteristic of the papules (see Fig. 10.10) [217, 220, 223]. Despite this characterization, PNGD may vary considerably in terms of color (e.g. yellow-red [224], red-brown [225]), shape (e.g. macules, patches, plaques, pustules [226], vesicles [225]), secondary skin features (e.g. edema [227]), and symptoms (e.g. none, pain, pruritus). Moreover, PNGD can occur on virtually any skin surface, although the upper extremities are the most common site, followed by the lower extremities, trunk, and head and neck [219]. Lesions in atypical areas should prompt examination of the extensor surfaces, which, if affected symmetrically, may aid in the diagnosis [226, 228, 229].

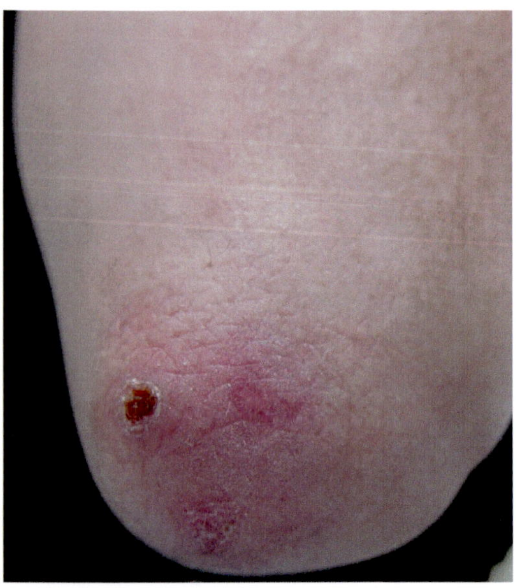

Fig. 10.10 Palisaded neutrophilic granulomatous dermatitis (PNGD): violaceous papules on the elbow, one with a central hemorrhagic crust

The histopathology of PNGD varies with lesion age, with gradual resolution of the initial LCV and neutrophilic infiltrate and organization of histiocytes into granulomas [217, 223, 226]. Early (i.e., days to weeks old) lesions classically demonstrate LCV, a dense neutrophilic infiltrate, and basophilic degenerated collagen throughout the dermis [217, 226]. Interstitial histiocytes may also be present throughout the dermis [217, 222, 226, 228, 230–233]. Fully developed (i.e., weeks to months old) lesions are characterized by histiocytes organized into granulomas and palisaded around fibrin, degenerated collagen, and mucin. Leukocytoclasia with or without vasculitis may be present [217, 226]. Finally, in resolving lesions, palisaded granulomas have little leukocytoclasia, lack mucin, and are separated by dermal fibrosis [217].

Diagnostic Considerations

An important consideration in the differential diagnosis of PNGD is IGD. Unlike PNGD, IGD classically presents with indurated cords or annular plaques. Histologically, IGD is concentrated in the mid to deep dermis ("bottom heavy") as compared with PNGD, which tends to be more superficial. Moreover, the histopathology of IGD is not classically thought to evolve over time [211]. Nevertheless, differentiating PNGD from IGD may be challenging if lesions are clinically consistent with PNGD but histologically consistent with IGD [210, 234, 235] or vice versa [236–238]. In some cases, the histopathology combines features of IGD (e.g. "bottom heavy" histiocytic infiltrate) and PNGD (e.g. pan-dermal mucin [230] or leukocytoclasia [226, 239]). Thus, the differentiation between PNGD and IGD may be difficult both clinically and histopathologically.

The clinical differential diagnosis of PNGD also includes papular eruptions that favor the bilateral elbows, knees, and other extensor surfaces. Rheumatoid neutrophilic dermatitis is a rare condition that, like PNGD, classically presents with erythematous, umbilicated papules or annular plaques that may affect the extensor surfaces. However, unlike PNGD, rheumatoid neutrophilic dermatitis typically lacks LCV or granulomas on skin biopsy. Rheumatoid nodules are granulomatous nodules that typically affect extensor surfaces; however, these nodules are situated deep in the subcutis, as compared with the dermal location of PNGD. EED is a rare form of vasculitis that presents with papules and nodules primarily overlying extensor surfaces. In contrast to PNGD, the lesions of EED typically darken over time, from yellow-pink to red, brown, or purple, and typically heal with extensive dermal fibrosis, resulting in firm papules overlying extensor surfaces even once the inflammation is quiescent. Histologically, EED lesions lack palisaded granulomas. Xanthoma tuberosum is another cause of subcutaneous nodules on the extensor surfaces; however, this entity is distinguished by its pink-yellow color, usual association with a personal or family history of hyperlipidemia, and histopathologic evidence of foamy macrophages and cholesterol clefts. Lastly, tendinous xanthomas are subcutaneous, while PNGD is a dermal process.

The histopathologic differential diagnosis of PNGD depends upon lesion age. In early PNGD, the histology may resemble that of cutaneous LCV; however, the two may be differentiated by the greater amount of extravasated erythrocytes and lack of an interstitial neutrophilic infiltrate or degenerated collagen in LCV [217]. Moreover, cutaneous LCV is characterized on exam by petechiae and/or palpable purpura in dependent areas such as the lower legs, which are typically absent in PNGD.

The histopathologic differential diagnosis of later stage PNGD (i.e., fully developed or resolving lesions) includes other conditions characterized by palisading granulomas. GA is distinguished by more mucin, less vasculitis, thinner bundles of degenerated collagen, and fewer neutrophils and fibrin [220]. Moreover, GA most commonly presents as asymptomatic, skin-colored or erythematous, annular or arciform plaques on the wrist, ankle, or dorsal hand or foot, without overlying scale. In eosinophilic granulomatosis with polyangiitis, granulomas surround eosinophils, not neutrophils [217]. Furthermore, granulomatosis with polyangiitis most commonly presents as palpable purpura. Finally, the degenerated collagen and palisading granulomas of necrobiosis lipoidica are differentiated from PNGD by a "layered cake" pattern that extends into the subcutaneous fat septae. Plasma cells are typically seen, while neutrophils and mucin are absent. Moreover, necrobiosis lipoidica is clinically distinct from PNGD, as it is typified by yellow-brown, atrophic plaques with central telangiectasias on the bilateral shins.

Disease and Comorbidity Assessment

The diagnosis of PNGD generally requires clinicopathologic correlation with one or multiple biopsies, given the potential for variable and overlapping clinical and histopathologic features. The workup should aim to identify an underlying cause, as the vast majority of reported cases have an associated systemic condition that precedes, occurs with, or follows the diagnosis of PNGD [219, 220, 223]. The most common association is RA, followed by SLE. ANCA-positive vasculitides are also often reported as associated with PNGD [219]. Other reported underlying diseases include other systemic vasculitides, malignancy (particularly immunoproliferative disorders), IBD, other connective tissue diseases, and infectious diseases (see Table 10.7).

In exceptional cases, patients with PNGD lack an underlying association [240] or have extracutaneous features (e.g. fatigue, fever, diffuse polyarthralgia, reactive lymphadenopathy, abnormal

Table 10.7 Systemic conditions associated with palisaded neutrophilic granulomatous dermatitis (PNGD)

Arthritides	Rheumatoid arthritis (RA) [226, 227, 232, 248] Ankylosing spondylitis [248]
Connective tissue diseases	Systemic lupus erythematosus (SLE) [225, 233, 237, 249, 251] Systemic sclerosis (SSc) [222] Mixed connective tissue disease [236] Undifferentiated connective tissue disease [220, 227]
Systemic Vasculitides	Eosinophilic granulomatosis with polyangiitis [226] Granulomatosis with polyangiitis [226, 252] Behçet's disease [240] Takayasu arteritis [226, 253] Polyarteritis nodosa [223] Microscopic polyangiitis [229] Unclassified vasculitis [223]
Immunoproliferative disorders	Myelodysplastic syndrome (MDS) [226] Leukemia [223, 226] Lymphoma [223] Multiple myeloma [223]
Infectious diseases	Cellulitis [249] Subacute bacterial endocarditis [223] Hepatitis [223] Streptococcal infection [226] Acquired immunodeficiency syndrome [222]
Other	Sjögren's syndrome [228] Polymyalgia rheumatica [254] Adult-onset Still's disease [232] Sarcoidosis [235, 255, 256] Ulcerative colitis [223, 242] Type 1 diabetes mellitus [257] Celiac disease [257] Mixed cryoglobulinemia [226] Metastatic prostate adenocarcinoma [226] Multiple sclerosis [226] Thrombotic thrombocytopenic purpura/hemolytic uremic syndrome [226]

liver chemistries) that cannot be accounted for by another condition. These extracutaneous manifestations follow the course of cutaneous disease in PNGD, resolving spontaneously or in response to the same treatment [234, 241]. Additionally, PNGD has been attributed to medications, such as penicillin [223], allopurinol [242], MTX [229], and adalimumab [231, 243]. However, these rare reports may be confounded by the fact that the patients were often taking these medications (with the possible exception of allopurinol) for underlying systemic diseases known to be associated with PNGD. Furthermore, although lesions resolved with discontinuation of the suspected medication, immunosuppressive therapy directed at the underlying condition was often initiated at the same time, which may have affected PNGD activity. There are no reported cases in which re-challenge of a medication thought to provoke PNGD has been attempted.

Given the strong association between PNGD and systemic disease, screening for underlying conditions should be performed in conjunction with the patient's primary pare condition and relevant specialists. Evaluation should include a thorough history (including medication review), review of systems, physical examination, and basic laboratory panels including CBC and complete metabolic panel. In patients with arthralgias or arthritis, joint radiographs as well as serum rheumatoid factor and anti-citrullinated protein antibodies should be considered. Age- and sex-appropriate malignancy screening is important in all patients.

If an underlying condition is not readily identified, additional tests to consider include serum anti-nuclear antibody titers and additional autoimmune serologies, serum and urine protein electrophoresis and immunofixation, and a chest radiograph. A computed tomography (CT) scan of the chest, abdomen, and pelvis should also be considered to screen for underlying malignancy.

If, despite this expanded workup, an underlying condition cannot be identified, long-term, symptom-directed screening is warranted, as PNGD may predate the onset of systemic disease by several years [220]. It is important to note that PNGD may manifest during flares [220, 222, 226, 237, 244] or periods of quiescence of the underlying disorder [219, 221, 234, 239, 245].

Principles of Management

Data on the treatment of PNGD are limited to case reports and case series and confounded by the occurrence of spontaneous resolution in about 20% of patients [219]. In the remaining 80%, PNGD generally responds to systemic treatment of the underlying disease [219], most often with the initiation [223, 246] or continuation of systemic corticosteroids [217, 220, 223, 228, 232, 234, 242]. Dapsone [65, 222, 224, 226, 239, 241, 247], MMF [236], hydroxychloroquine (HCQ) [220], colchicine [237], or cyclophosphamide [230] have been used in combination with corticosteroids or as monotherapy, with some success. MTX is often used for granulomatous conditions and may be attempted; however, to date, the only two cases in the literature on MTX for PNGD report no to partial efficacy [225, 241]. Recurrence has been reported after tapering corticosteroids [224] or dapsone [226, 239]. Other treatment options include AZA [236], TNF-α inhibitors [228, 244], antimicrobials for an associated infection [234, 248], and insulin replacement therapy for diabetes mellitus [249]. Intralesional corticosteroids may be useful as adjunctive therapy for localized disease [223, 226, 247, 250]. Topical corticosteroids yield mixed results as they are unlikely to sufficiently penetrate the dermis [65, 223, 228, 229, 231, 239, 244, 246].

Interstitial Granulomatous Dermatitis and Interstitial Granulomatous Drug Reaction

Key Summary Capsule Bullets

- Two clinical variants of IGD: plaque-variant (most patients) and cutaneous cord-variant
- IGD is associated with arthritis or arthralgias in more than half of patients; also associated with various autoimmune conditions and in some cases, malignancy
- IGDR is caused by chronic use of TNF-α inhibitors, calcium channel blockers, and other medications
- Mainstay of treatment is systemic immunosuppressive agents in IGD and drug withdrawal in IGDR

Classification and Epidemiology

IGD is a disorder with cutaneous and often articular manifestations that may be associated with an underlying systemic disease. IGD is also known as interstitial granulomatous dermatitis with arthritis (IGDA) or Ackerman's syndrome. When IGD occurs in the setting of exposure to medications, such as TNF-α inhibitors, the term IGDR is applied.

IGD predominates in women by a ratio of 3:1 [212]. IGDR has been reported only in adults, which may reflect the tendency of the implicated medications to be used in this age group.

Pathogenesis

IGD has been posited but not proven to be initiated by circulating immune complexes that are small enough to diffuse into the interstitial dermis, where they deposit and incite a granulomatous reaction [217]. The formation of these immune complexes may be related to an underlying systemic disease. In IGDR, the antigenic trigger is unknown but may be the triggering medication itself or another molecule that becomes immunogenic as a result of exposure to the medication [213].

Clinical Features

Interstitial Granulomatous Dermatitis

IGD has two major clinical variants: IGD with plaques and IGD with cutaneous cords. Approximately 90% of patients with IGD have the plaque variant [212], which classically manifests with multiple, skin-colored to tan or erythematous, waxy, papules and plaques. As IGD is a dermal process, there is no associated scale. The lesions may be annular and are usually asymptomatic but may be minimally pruritic or painful [212]. Typical sites of involvement include the lateral trunk and proximal, medial extremities in a symmetric distribution [212]. Uncommon sites include the face [251], breasts [252], and palms [253]. Widespread involvement may occur [254].

The remaining 10% of patients with IGD have the variant with cutaneous cords. In this variant, the clinical picture is characterized by linear or arciform, erythematous, indurated cords on the lateral trunk, which correspond to the so-called "rope sign." This "rope sign" has traditionally been considered pathognomonic of IGD [212].

In more than half of patients, the cutaneous lesions of IGD are associated with prior, concurrent, or subsequent arthritis or arthralgias [212]. Characteristically, the arthritis manifests as either RA or a symmetric, seronegative, non-erosive, oligo- to polyarthritis of small and/or large joints. Similarly, the arthralgias are symmetric, polyarticular, favor peripheral over central joints, and may be migratory [212, 255–257]. These articular symptoms generally respond to treatment of the cutaneous disease [255, 257]. Antinuclear antibody titers are positive in about half of patients with IGD [212].

Both clinical variants of IGD share the same histopathologic features: interstitial and palisading histiocytes diffusely throughout the dermis, small foci of degenerated collagen ("piecemeal fragmentation") that are surrounded by an empty space, and, thus, appear "free floating" ("floating sign"), and perivascular and interstitial lymphocytes. The histiocytic infiltrate may be concentrated in the mid to deep reticular dermis ("bottom heavy"), and extension into the subcutaneous tissue occurs in about 30% of patients. Mucin, vasculitis, neutrophils, and eosinophils tend to be sparse or absent [212].

Interstitial Granulomatous Drug Reaction

IGDR presents similarly to IGD but may be distinguished by its predilection for intertriginous areas and a weaker association with constitutional and articular symptoms and autoantibodies. For example, the original series of patients with IGDR, which remains the largest to date, found that 10% of patients had an underlying arthropathy [213], compared with more than half of patients with IGD [212]. The lesions of IGDR may be pruritic [213]or tender [258–260]. Variations in morphology (e.g., papules [213] and nodules [260]) and configuration (e.g. livedoid [213]) have been reported.

Like PNGD and IGD, IGDR may atypically manifest on virtually any skin surface (e.g. trunk, lower extremities [213], palms and soles [259, 261], head [258, 262], neck [263]). In one reported case, IGDR presented with erythroderma [264].

The medications most commonly associated with IGDR are TNF-α inhibitors and calcium channel blockers, although several other medications have also been reported (see Table 10.8). TNF-α inhibitors have caused IGDR in patients being treated for both RA and psoriatic arthritis [265–267]. The eruption most often occurs years after the initiation of the causative medication but may occur as soon as weeks or months into therapy. IGDR tends to resolve after discontinuation of the triggering medication [213].

Histopathologically, IGDR shares the diffuse, interstitial lymphohistiocytic infiltrate of IGD, and the two entities cannot be definitively distinguished based on histopathology alone. Features favoring IGDR include a vacuolar interface

Table 10.8 Agents implicated in interstitial granulomatous drug reaction (number of cases)

TNF-α inhibitors: infliximab (2), adalimumab (2), etanercept (2), thalidomide (1), lenalidomide (1) [271, 274–276]
Calcium channel blockers: diltiazem (4), verapamil (2), nifedipine (1) [216]
Angiotensin converting enzyme inhibitors: enalapril (5), lisinopril (1) [216, 273, 283]
HMG-CoA reductase inhibitors: atorvastatin (1), simvastatin (1), lovastatin (1), pravastatin (1) [216, 279]
H1- and H2-receptor antagonists: ranitidine (1), famotidine (1), cimetidine (1), brompheniramine (1) [216]
Furosemide (3) [216, 283]
Beta-blockers: propranolol (1), atenolol (1) [216]
Herbal supplements including Panax notoginseng (3) [277, 284, 285]
Candesartan (1) [283]
Carbamazepine (1) [216]
Bupropion (1) [216]
Diazepam (1) [216]
Gemfibrozil (1) [216]
Febuxostat (1) [278]
Ganciclovir (1) [269]
Trastuzumab (1) [267]
Sorafenib (1) [268]
Darifenacin (1) [272]
Fluindione (1) [283]
Anakinra (1) [286]
Sennoside (1) [270]
Strontium ranelate (1) [280]

dermatitis, atypical lymphocytes, and abundant eosinophils [213]. However, the histiocytes may be palisaded [264], and lymphocyte atypia [213] and interface dermatitis [267–271] may be absent. Of note, three cases have been reported in which patients presented with clinical features of drug-induced hypersensitivity syndrome, but histopathology consistent with IGDR [272, 273].

Diagnostic Considerations

IGD and IGDR may be distinguished by factors elicited on history (with exposure to a known medication trigger suggestive of IGDR and constitutional or articular symptoms more likely in IGD); physical examination (IGDR has a tendency to occur in intertriginous zones); histopathology (IGD lacks a vacuolar interface dermatitis and lymphoid atypia and has more completely degenerated collagen); and serology (IGD is more likely to be associated with autoantibodies). However, differentiation may be challenging in cases in which IGDR lacks characteristic clinical and histopathologic features [260], especially as patients may take drugs implicated in IGDR for conditions associated with IGD, given that IGDR can occur years after initiation of the offending medication. In uncertain cases, a trial off a potentially triggering medication may be warranted. Whether patients with IGDR due to TNF-α inhibitors may tolerate other medications in the same class has yet to be documented in the literature.

The differential diagnosis of IGD and IGDR includes interstitial GA and PNGD. Although it is characterized by annular plaques, interstitial GA favors the wrists, ankles, and dorsal hands and feet, and it is not associated with articular symptoms and autoantibodies (as in IGD) or medication exposure (as in IGDR). Histopathologically, interstitial GA features more mucin than IGD or IGDR, as well as histiocytes concentrated in the upper to mid dermis ("top heavy"). Neutrophils, vacuolar interface dermatitis, and atypical lymphocytes are generally absent.

Both IGD and IGDR typically lack the LCV, leukocytoclasia, and predominant neutrophils seen in early PNGD as well as the palisaded granulomas and neutrophilic debris seen in late PNGD [213]. Moreover, unlike PNGD, neither IGD nor IGDR are thought to evolve histopathologically over time [211].

The clinical differential diagnosis of IGD with cutaneous cords also includes superficial thrombophlebitis of the breast (Mondor disease), which typically follows breast trauma or surgery. The plaques of cutaneous larva migrans, which is caused by the hookworms *Ancylostoma braziliense* or *Ancylostoma caninum*, may resemble the cutaneous cords seen in IGD., but they are characteristically serpiginous, and, unlike IGD, they favor the feet, are pruritic, and occur after travel to a tropical or subtropical country. Granulomatous mycosis fungoides and its variant granulomatous slack skin present with violaceous, intertriginous plaques; this condition can be distinguished from IGD with cutaneous cords on skin biopsy.

The differential diagnosis of IGD with plaques includes rheumatoid neutrophilic dermatitis, which is histopathologically distinguished by its dense neutrophilic dermal infiltrate and abundant leukocytoclasia.

The diagnosis of IGDR requires clinicopathologic correlation as well as a history of generally chronic exposure to one or multiple medications identified as triggers for this condition. If the cutaneous eruption does not resolve within months of medication discontinuation, consideration should be given to a workup directed at excluding cutaneous T-cell lymphoma [213].

Disease and Comorbidity Assessment

The evaluation of patients with suspected IGD begins with a thorough history (with careful attention to medications), review of systems, physical examination, and routine laboratory studies.

As described above, more than half of patients with IGD have arthritis (rheumatoid or non-erosive and seronegative) or polyarthralgias that can predate, manifest with, or follow the cutaneous disease [212]. In addition to RA, other autoimmune conditions have been reported as associated with IGD, most commonly autoimmune thyroiditis [253, 257, 274] and SLE [257, 275–278], and less frequently undifferentiated connective tissue disease [279], antiphospholipid antibody syndrome [280], autoimmune hepatitis [235], vitiligo [257], hemolytic anemia [257], and autoimmune thrombocytopenia [212]. Other underlying conditions include hematologic dyscrasias (e.g., monoclonal gammopathy of undetermined significance [212, 251], MDS [254], acute *myeloid leukemia* [254, 281]) and solid malignancies (e.g. bronchial [282] and hypopharyngeal [212] squamous cell carcinomas, and breast cancer [212]).

Antinuclear antibody titers are positive in about half of IGD patients [212]. Thus, the workup should generally include autoimmune serologic testing in addition to thyroid function studies, age- and sex-appropriate malignancy screening, and serum and urine protein electrophoresis and immunofixation. Consideration may be given to a CT scan of the chest, abdomen, and pelvis and/or additional "blind" malignancy screening in patients in whom an underlying condition is not readily identified.

Principles of Management

In the majority of reported cases, IGD completely remits after a mean of 8.8 months [212]. In the remaining patients, IGD tends to follow a chronic, relapsing course [212]. Progression of IGD to localized acquired cutis laxa despite systemic treatment was reported in one patient with a chronic, relapsing course in whom the initial IGD biopsy showed elastophagocytosis [283]. Treatment for IGD may not be required if symptoms are absent or mild and the extent of involvement is limited.

When treatment is desirable, data from case reports suggest that the cutaneous and/or articular manifestations of IGD may be treated with systemic corticosteroids [235, 255, 275, 277, 284], TNF-α inhibitors (infliximab [252], adalimumab [285]), HCQ [279], MTX [279, 286], and narrow-band ultraviolet B phototherapy [287]. Recalcitrant IGD has been successfully treated with IVIG [251], tocilizumab [288], lenalidomide [254], cyclosporine [289], and combination therapy (MTX and etanercept [290]; systemic corticosteroids, MTX, and AZA [283]). For localized disease, resolution has been reported with intralesional triamcinolone [276], but topical corticosteroids have not been consistently reported to be effective [284, 285, 291, 292]. When associated with autoimmune thyroiditis, IGD did not improve despite normalization of thyroid function [253].

The mainstay of treatment of IGDR is discontinuation of the offending agent(s), with resolution occurring in most patients within weeks to months. Reintroduction of the same medication or substitution with another in the same class generally leads to recurrence [213].

Summary

The evaluation of patients with reactive erythemas requires an interdisciplinary approach, relying on collaboration between dermatologists, rheumatologists, and other specialists. The main goals of this evaluation are generally twofold: (1) to exclude disease mimickers, and (2) to identify an underlying systemic disease, if one is present. Given the rarity of the reactive erythemas, no formal guidelines exist to direct the assessment of patients who develop them. However, the tenets of evaluation are a thorough history, review of systems, and physical examination of the skin, mucosal surfaces, lymph nodes, and other organ systems. Comprehensive laboratory and radiologic evaluations should be directed towards any identified abnormalities and further testing based upon the specific disease associations of the reactive erythema in question. A skin biopsy is often a key diagnostic component; however, in some cases, such as in classic EN, a skin biopsy may not be necessary.

Given that a reactive erythema may precede the clinical onset of an underlying disease, ongoing surveillance for associated conditions should be performed in patients in whom an underlying condition is not initially identified. For example, in a patient with LEP, but not SLE, clinical monitoring for the subsequent development of SLE is warranted, although SLE will develop only in the minority. Similarly, an increased index of suspicion for an underlying condition should be maintained in the follow-up of all patients with PG, Sweet syndrome, PNGD, and IGD.

Management of reactive erythemas may include supportive care, targeted treatment of the underlying disorder, and/or systemic immunomodulatory therapy directed towards the skin disease. Because reactive erythemas generally involve the dermis and/or subcutaneous tissues, topical therapies are unlikely to sufficiently penetrate the skin, and, thus, systemic therapies are often required. In cases where extracutaneous manifestations are present, these symptoms may respond to treatment of the cutaneous disease. If a drug etiology is suspected, the causative agent should be discontinued. Importantly, if patients are pregnant or have an underlying disorder such as RA, IBD, or a malignancy, treatment of the cutaneous disease should be performed in collaboration with the specialists managing the pregnancy or underlying condition. Overall, recognition of the interdisciplinary nature of the reactive erythemas is imperative for proper management and long-term care.

References

1. Cornejo KM, et al. A cutaneous interstitial granulomatous dermatitis-like eruption arising in myelodysplasia with leukemic progression. Am J Dermatopathol. 2013;35(2):e26–29.
2. Panush RS, et al. Weber-Christian disease. Analysis of 15 cases and review of the literature. Medicine (Baltimore). 1985;64(3 SRC - BaiduScholar):181–91.
3. White JW Jr, Winkelmann RK. Weber-Christian panniculitis: a review of 30 cases with this diagnosis. J Am Acad Dermatol. 1998;39(1 SRC BaiduScholar):56–62.
4. Erez A, et al. Erythema nodosum in the Negev area-a survey of 50 patients. Isr J Med Sci. 1987;23(12 SRC - BaiduScholar):1228–31.
5. Garcia-Porrua C, Gonzalez-Gay MA, Vazquez-Caruncho M. Erythema nodosum: etiologic and predictive factors in a defined population. Arthritis Rheum. 2000;43(3 SRC - BaiduScholar):584–92.
6. Cribier B, et al. Erythema nodosum and associated diseases. A study of 129 cases. Int J Dermatol. 1998;37(9 SRC - BaiduScholar):667–72.
7. Psychos DN, et al. Erythema nodosum: the underlying conditions. Clin Rheumatol. 2000;19(3 SRC - BaiduScholar):212–6.
8. Mert A, Kumbasar H, Ozaras R. Erythema nodosum: an evaluation of 100 cases. Clin Exp Rheumatol. 2007;25(4):563–70.
9. Llorente L, et al. Elevated Th1 cytokine mRNA in skin biopsies and peripheral circulation in patients with erythema nodosum. Eur Cytokine Netw. 1997;8(1):67–71.
10. Halevy S, et al. In vitro interferon-gamma release test in the diagnosis of drug-induced erythema nodosum. Isr Med Assoc. 2004;6(1 SRC - BaiduScholar):59–60.
11. Kunz M, Beutel S, Brocker E. Leucocyte activation in erythema nodosum. Clin Exp Dermatol. 1999;24(5 SRC - BaiduScholar):396–401.
12. Nomiyama J, et al. Erythema nodosum caused by the administration of granulocyte colony-stimulating factor in a patient with refractory anemia. Am J Hematol. 1994;47(4 SRC - BaiduScholar):333.
13. Petkovic TR, Pejcic T, Videnovic-Ivanov J. Tumor necrosis factor alpha gene polymorphism in serbian patients with sarcoidosis. Srp Arh Celok Lek. 2013;141:169–72. p. 3–4 SRC - BaiduScholar.

14. Puavilai S, et al. Etiology of erythema nodosum. Assoc Thai. 1995;78(2 SRC - BaiduScholar):72–5.
15. Baert F, Knockaert D, Bobbaers H. Bilateral hilar lymphadenopathy associated with Yersinia enterocolitica infection. Clin Infect Dis. 1994;19(1):197–8.
16. Veloso FT, et al. Immune-related systemic manifestations of inflammatory bowel disease. A prospective study of 792 patients. J Clin Gastroenterol. 1996;23(1 SRC - BaiduScholar):29–34.
17. Sánchez Yus E, Sanz Vico MD, de Diego V, et al. Miescher's radial granuloma. A characteristic marker of erythema nodosum. Am J Dermatopathol. 1989;11(5 SRC - BaiduScholar):434–42.
18. Honma T, et al. Ultrastructure of endothelial cell necrosis in classical erythema nodosum. Hum Pathol. 1993;24(4):384–90.
19. Kim B, LeBoit PE. Histopathologic features of erythema nodosum-like lesions in Behcet disease: a comparison with erythema nodosum focusing on the role of vasculitis. Am J Dermatopathol. 2000;22(5 SRC - BaiduScholar):379–90.
20. Patterson JW, et al. Infection-induced panniculitis. J Cutan Pathol. 1989;16(4 SRC - BaiduScholar):183–93.
21. Song JS, Halim K, Vleugels RA, Merola JF. Dapsone for treatment of erythema nodosum. Dermatol Online J. 2016;22(2):13030/qt8z782742. PMID: 27267197.
22. Acosta KA, et al. Etiology and therapeutic management of erythema nodosum during pregnancy: an update. Am J Clin Dermatol. 2013;14(3 SRC - BaiduScholar):215–22.
23. Yurdakul S, Mat C, Tuzun Y. A double-blind trial of colchicine in Behcet's syndrome. Arthritis Rheum. 2001;44(11 SRC - BaiduScholar):2686–92.
24. Davatchi F, Sadeghi Abdollahi B, Tehrani Banihashemi A. Colchicine versus placebo in Behcet's disease: randomized, double-blind, controlled crossover trial. Mod Rheumatol. 2009;19(5):542–9.
25. Siemanowski B, Regueiro M. Efficacy of infliximab for extraintestinal manifestations of inflammatory bowel disease. Curr Treat Options Gastroenterol. 2007;10(3 SRC - BaiduScholar):178–84.
26. Kugathasan S, et al. Dermatologic manifestations of Crohn disease in children: response to infliximab. J Pediatr Gastroenterol Nutr. 2003;37(2 SRC - BaiduScholar):150–4.
27. Gilchrist H, Patterson JW. Erythema nodosum and erythema induratum (nodular vasculitis): diagnosis and management. Dermatol Ther. 2010;23(4):320–7.
28. Segura S, et al. Vasculitis in erythema induratum of Bazin: a histopathologic study of 101 biopsy specimens from 86 patients. J Am Acad Dermatol. 2008;59(5 SRC - BaiduScholar):839–51.
29. Jarukitsopa S, Hoganson DD, Crowson CS. Epidemiology of systemic lupus erythematosus and cutaneous lupus in a predominantly white population in the United States. Arthritis Care Res (Hoboken). 2015;67(6):817–28.
30. Petri M, Orbai AM, Alarcón GS. Derivation and validation of the Systemic Lupus International Collaborating Clinics classification criteria for systemic lupus erythematosus. Arthritis Rheum. 2012;64(8 SRC - BaiduScholar):2677–86.
31. Arai S, Katsuoka K. Clinical entity of Lupus erythematosus panniculitis/lupus erythematosus profundus. Autoimmun Rev. 2009;8(6):449–52.
32. Martens PB, et al. Lupus panniculitis: clinical perspectives from a case series. J Rheumatol. 1999;26(1 SRC - BaiduScholar):68–72.
33. Wenzel J, et al. CXCR3-mediated recruitment of cytotoxic lymphocytes in lupus erythematosus profundus. J Am Acad Dermatol. 2007;56(4 SRC - BaiduScholar):648–50.
34. Burrows NP, et al. Lupus erythematosus profundus with partial C4 deficiency responding to thalidomide. Br J Dermatol. 1991;125(1 SRC - BaiduScholar):62–7.
35. Tuffanelli DL. Lupus erythematosus panniculitis (profundus): clinical and immunologic studies. Arch Dermatol. 1971;103(3 SRC - BaiduScholar): 231–42.
36. Watanabe T, Tsuchida T. Lupus erythematosus profundus: a cutaneous marker for a distinct clinical subset? Br J Dermatol. 1996;134(1 SRC - BaiduScholar):123–5.
37. Warne RR, et al. Lupus mastitis: a mimicker of breast carcinoma. BMJ Case Rep. 2011;2011:bcr115066. SRC - BaiduScholar.
38. Massone C, et al. Lupus erythematosus panniculitis (lupus profundus): clinical, histopathological, and molecular analysis of nine cases. J Cutan Pathol. 2005;32(6 SRC - BaiduScholar):396–404.
39. Ng PP, et al. Lupus erythematosus panniculitis: a clinicopathologic study. Int J Dermatol. 2002;41(8 SRC - BaiduScholar):488–90.
40. Arps DP, Patel RM. Lupus profundus (panniculitis): a potential mimic of subcutaneous panniculitis-like T-cell lymphoma. Arch Pathol Lab Med. 2013;137(9):1211–5.
41. Willemze R, et al. Subcutaneous panniculitis-like T-cell lymphoma: definition, classification, and prognostic factors: an Lymphoma Group Study of 83 cases. Blood. 2008;111(2):838–45.
42. Velez NF, et al. Full facial edema: a novel presentation of subcutaneous panniculitis-like T-cell lymphoma. J Clin Oncol. 2012;30(25 SRC - BaiduScholar):e233–6.
43. Li JY, et al. Subcutaneous panniculitis-like T-cell lymphoma accompanied with discoid lupus erythematosus. Chin Med J. 2013;126(18 SRC - BaiduScholar):3590.
44. Cassis TB, et al. Subcutaneous panniculitis-like T-cell lymphoma with vacuolar interface dermatitis resembling lupus erythematosus panniculitis. J Am Acad Dermatol. 2004;50(3 SRC - BaiduScholar):465–9.
45. Dandinoglu, et al. Can lupus mastitis be treated surgically? Orthop Muscul Syst. 2014;3(1):148–9.

46. Cernea SS, et al. Lupus mastitis. J Am Acad Dermatol. 1993;29(2 Pt 2 SRC - BaiduScholar):343–6.
47. Fernandez-Torres R, et al. Lupus mastitis, a mimicker of erysipelatoides breast carcinoma. J Am Acad Dermatol. 2009;60(6 SRC - BaiduScholar):1074–6.
48. Whitaker-Worth DL, et al. Dermatologic diseases of the breast and nipple. J Am Acad Dermatol. 2000;43(5 Pt 1 SRC - BaiduScholar):733–51; quiz 752734.
49. Mosier AD, et al. Serial MR findings and comprehensive review of bilateral lupus mastitis with an additional case report. J Radiol Case Rep. 2013;7(1 SRC - BaiduScholar):48–58.
50. Kinonen C, et al. Lupus mastitis: an uncommon complication of systemic or discoid lupus. Am Pathol. 2010;34(6 SRC - BaiduScholar):901–6.
51. Grossberg E, Scherschun L, Fivenson DP. Lupus profundus: not a benign disease. Lupus. 2001;10(7):514–6.
52. Wienert S, et al. Facets of lupus erythematosus: panniculitis responding to thalidomide. J Dtsch Dermatol Ges. 2008;6(3 SRC - BaiduScholar):214–6.
53. Ordi-Ros J, et al. Thalidomide in the treatment of cutaneous lupus refractory to conventional therapy. J Rheumatol. 2000;27(6 SRC - BaiduScholar):1429–33.
54. Ujiie H, et al. Lupus erythematosus profundus successfully treated with dapsone: review of the literature. Arch Dermatol. 2006;142(3 SRC - BaiduScholar):399–401.
55. Santo J, Gomes MF, Gomes MJ. Espirito Intravenous immunoglobulin in lupus panniculitis. Clin Rev Allergy Immunol. 2010;38:307–18. p. 2-3 SRC - BaiduScholar.
56. Saeki Y, et al. Maintaining remission of lupus erythematosus profundus (LEP) with cyclosporin A. Lupus. 2000;9(5 SRC - BaiduScholar):390–2.
57. Ishiguro N, et al. Intractable ulceration in a patient with lupus erythematosus profundus successfully treated with cyclosporine. Int J Dermatol. 2012;51(9 SRC - BaiduScholar):1131–3.
58. Wozniacka A, et al. The dynamism of cutaneous lupus erythematosus: mild discoid lupus erythematosus evolving into SLE with SCLE and treatment-resistant lupus panniculitis. Clin Rheumatol. 2007;26(7 SRC - BaiduScholar):1176–9.
59. Guissa VR, et al. Lupus erythematosus panniculitis in children and adolescents. Acta Reumatol Port. 2012;37(1):82–5.
60. Eastham AB, et al. Lupus erythematosus panniculitis-induced facial atrophy: effective treatment with poly-L-lactic acid and hyaluronic acid dermal fillers. J Am Acad Dermatol. 2013;69(5 SRC - BaiduScholar):e260–2.
61. Costa IM, Salaro CP, Costa MC. Carvalho Polymethylmethacrylate facial implant: a successful personal experience in Brazil for more than 9 years. Dermatol Surg. 2009;35(8):1221–7.
62. Douvoyiannis M, et al. Panniculitis, infection, and dermatomyositis: case and literature review. Clin Rheumatol. 2009;1(28 Suppl SRC - BaiduScholar):S57–63.
63. Geddes MR, Sinnreich M, Chalk C. Minocycline-induced dermatomyositis. Muscle Nerve. 2010;41(4 SRC - BaiduScholar):547–9.
64. Nakamori A, et al. Vesiculobullous dermatomyositis with panniculitis without muscle disease. J Am Acad Dermatol. 2003;49(6 SRC - BaiduScholar):1136–9.
65. Romero-Aguilera G, Arpa M, Calle P, Rodríguez-Vázquez M, García-Martín-Dávila F, Cortina de la. Panniculitis associated with amyopathic dermatomyositis. Actas DermoSifiliogrficas. 2004;95(3 SRC - BaiduScholar):189–92.
66. Pau-Charles I, et al. Anti-MDA5 positive clinically amyopathic dermatomyositis presenting with severe cardiomyopathy. J Eur Acad Dermatol Venereol. 2014;28(8 SRC - BaiduScholar):1097–102.
67. Ciudad-Blanco C, et al. Dermatomyositis: assessment and follow-up of 20 patients. Actas Dermosifiliogr. 2011;102(6):448–55.
68. Janis JF, Winkelmann RK. Histopathology of the skin in dermatomyositis. A histopathologic study of 55 cases. Arch Dermatol. 1968;97(6 SRC - BaiduScholar):640–50.
69. Prendergast M, Hopkinson N. Breast calcinosis, panniculitis and fat hypertrophy in a 35-year-old woman with dermatomyositis. Rheumatology (Oxford). 2007;46(8 SRC - BaiduScholar):1378–9.
70. Kimura S, Fukuyama Y. Tubular cytoplasmic inclusions in a case of childhood dermatomyositis with migratory subcutaneous nodules. Eur J Pediatr. 1977;125(4 SRC - BaiduScholar):275–83.
71. Abdul-Wahab A, et al. Calcific panniculitis in adult-onset dermatomyositis. Clin Exp Dermatol. 2009;34(8 SRC - BaiduScholar):e854–6.
72. Commens C, et al. Dermatomyositis associated with multifocal lipoatrophy. J Am Acad Dermatol. 1990;22(5 Pt 2 SRC - BaiduScholar):966–9.
73. Bingham A, Mamyrova G, Rother KI. Predictors of acquired lipodystrophy in juvenile-onset dermatomyositis and a gradient of severity. Medicine (Baltimore). 2008;87(2 SRC - BaiduScholar):70–86.
74. Solans R, et al. Panniculitis: a cutaneous manifestation of dermatomyositis. J Am Acad Dermatol. 2002;46(5 Suppl SRC - BaiduScholar):S148–50.
75. Girouard SD, et al. Panniculitis associated with dermatomyositis and recurrent ovarian cancer. Arch Dermatol. 2012;148(6 SRC - BaiduScholar):740–4.
76. Ishikawa O, et al. Membranocystic changes in the panniculitis of dermatomyositis. Br J Dermatol. 1996;134(4 SRC - BaiduScholar):773–6.
77. Fusade T, et al. Subcutaneous changes in dermatomyositis. Br J Dermatol. 1993;128(4 SRC - BaiduScholar):451–3.
78. Spalding SJ, et al. Staphylococcus aureus panniculitis complicating juvenile dermatomyositis. Pediatrics. 2007;119(2):e528–30.
79. Leung YY, et al. Disseminated cutaneous infection with Mycobacterium chelonae mimicking pannicu-

litis in a patient with dermatomyositis. Hong Kong. 2005;11(6 SRC - BaiduScholar):515–9.
80. Kaieda S, et al. A subcutaneous panniculitis-like T-cell lymphoma mimicking dermatomyositis. Intern Med. 2014;53(13 SRC - BaiduScholar):1455.
81. Hemmi S, et al. Magnetic resonance imaging diagnosis of panniculitis in dermatomyositis. Muscle Nerve. 2010;41(1):151–3.
82. Molnar K, et al. Panniculitis in dermatomyositis: report of two cases. Br J Dermatol. 1998;139(1 SRC - BaiduScholar):161–3.
83. Kuriya N, Kinoshita N, Yokoyama N. Dermatomyositis with rhabdomyosarcoma and panniculitis. Report of an autopsy case. Nippon Naika Gakkai Zasshi. 1985;74(6 SRC - BaiduScholar):813–8.
84. Carrera E, et al. Dermatomyositis, lobar panniculitis and inflammatory myopathy with abundant macrophages. Neuromuscul Disord. 2006;16(7):468–71.
85. Femia AN, et al. Intravenous immunoglobulin for refractory cutaneous dermatomyositis: a retrospective analysis from an academic medical center. J Am Acad Dermatol. 2013;69(4 SRC - BaiduScholar):654–7.
86. Dalakas MC, et al. A controlled trial of high-dose intravenous immune globulin infusions as treatment for dermatomyositis. N Engl J Med. 1993;329(27 SRC - BaiduScholar):1993–2000.
87. Chao YY, Yang LJ. Dermatomyositis presenting as panniculitis. Int J Dermatol. 2000;39(2 SRC - BaiduScholar):141–4.
88. Sabroe RA, Wallington TB, Kennedy CT. Dermatomyositis treated with high-dose intravenous immunoglobulins and associated with panniculitis. Clin Exp Dermatol. 1995;20(2 SRC - BaiduScholar):164–7.
89. Su WP, Person JR. Morphea profunda. A new concept and a histopathologic study of 23 cases. Am J Dermatopathol. 1981;3(3 SRC - BaiduScholar):251–60.
90. Jinnin M, et al. Sclerosing panniculitis is associated with pulmonary hypertension in systemic sclerosis. Br J Dermatol. 2005;153(3 SRC - BaiduScholar):579–83.
91. Binesh VG, et al. Systemic sclerosis presenting as lobular panniculitis. Indian Dermatol Online J. 2012;3(3 SRC - BaiduScholar):222–4.
92. Almeida MS, et al. Panniculitis-an unusual cutaneous manifestation of systemic sclerosis. J Cutan Pathol. 2010;37(11 SRC - BaiduScholar):1170–3.
93. Zwischenberger BA, Jacobe HT. A systematic review of morphea treatments and therapeutic algorithm. J Am Acad Dermatol. 2011;65(5):925–41.
94. Fett N, Werth VP. Update on morphea: part II. Outcome measures and treatment. J Am Acad Dermatol. 2011;64(2 SRC - BaiduScholar):231–42; quiz 243–234.
95. Martini G, et al. Successful treatment of severe or methotrexate-resistant juvenile localized scleroderma with mycophenolate mofetil. Rheumatology (Oxford). 2009;48(11):1410–3.
96. Pérez Crespo M, Betlloch Mas I, Mataix Díaz J, Lucas Costa A, Ballester Nortes I, et al. Rapid response to cyclosporine and maintenance with methotrexate in linear scleroderma in a young girl. Pediatr Dermatol. 2009;26(1):118–20.
97. Strauss RM, et al. Good response of linear scleroderma in a child to ciclosporin. Br J Dermatol. 2004;150(4 SRC - BaiduScholar):790–2.
98. Peter RU, Ruzicka T, Eckert F. Low-dose cyclosporine A in the treatment of disabling morphea. Arch Dermatol. 1991;127(9 SRC - BaiduScholar):1420–1.
99. Worle B, et al. Cyclosporin in localized and systemic scleroderma-a clinical study. Dermatologica. 1990;181(3):215–20.
100. Cribier B, et al. Extracorporeal photochemotherapy in systemic sclerosis and severe morphea. Dermatology. 1995;191(1):25–31.
101. Neustadter JH, et al. Extracorporeal photochemotherapy for generalized deep morphea. Arch Dermatol. 2009;145(2 SRC - BaiduScholar):127–30.
102. Stausbol-Gron B, et al. Abatacept is a promising treatment for patients with disseminated morphea profunda: presentation of two cases. Acta Derm Venereol. 2011;91(6 SRC - BaiduScholar):686–8.
103. Roldan R, et al. Efficacy of bosentan in treatment of unresponsive cutaneous ulceration in disabling pansclerotic morphea in children. J Rheumatol. 2006;33(12 SRC - BaiduScholar):2538–40.
104. Song P, et al. Resolution of pansclerotic morphea after treatment with antithymocyte globulin. Nat Rev Rheumatol. 2009;5(9 SRC - BaiduScholar):513–6.
105. Choksi AN, Orringer JS. Linear morphea-induced atrophy treated with hyaluronic acid filler injections. Dermatol Surg. 2011;37(6 SRC - BaiduScholar):880–3.
106. Bennett ML, et al. Pyoderma gangrenosum. A comparison of typical and atypical forms with an emphasis on time to remission. Case review of 86 patients from 2 institutions. Medicine (Baltimore). 2000;79(1 SRC - BaiduScholar):37–46.
107. Powell FC, et al. Pyoderma gangrenosum: a review of 86 patients. Q J Med. 1985;55(217 SRC - BaiduScholar):173–86.
108. DeFilippis EM, et al. The genetics of pyoderma gangrenosum and implications for treatment: a systematic review. Br J Dermatol. 2015;172(6):1487–97.
109. Langan SM, et al. Incidence, mortality, and disease associations of pyoderma gangrenosum in the United Kingdom: a retrospective cohort study. J Invest Dermatol. 2012;132(9 SRC - BaiduScholar):2166–70.
110. Bernstein CN, et al. The prevalence of extraintestinal diseases in inflammatory bowel disease: a population-based study. Am J Gastroenterol. 2001;96(4 SRC - BaiduScholar):1116–22.
111. Binus AM, et al. Pyoderma gangrenosum: a retrospective review of patient characteristics, comor-

bidities and therapy in 103 patients. Br J Dermatol. 2011;165(6 SRC - BaiduScholar):1244–50.
112. Patel F, Fitzmaurice S, Duong C. Effective strategies for the management of pyoderma gangrenosum: a comprehensive review. Acta Derm Venereol. 2015;95(5):525–31.
113. Adachi Y, et al. Aberrant neutrophil trafficking and metabolic oscillations in severe pyoderma gangrenosum. J Invest Dermatol. 1998;111(2 SRC - BaiduScholar):259–68.
114. Oka M. Pyoderma gangrenosum and interleukin 8. Br J Dermatol. 2007;157(6 SRC - BaiduScholar):1279–81.
115. Oka M, Berking C, Nesbit M. Interleukin-8 overexpression is present in pyoderma gangrenosum ulcers and leads to ulcer formation in human skin xenografts. Lab Investig. 2000;80(4):595–604.
116. Saito S, et al. CD30+ anaplastic large cell lymphoma complicated by pyoderma gangrenosum with increased levels of serum cytokines. Eur J Haematol. 2006;77(3 SRC - BaiduScholar):251–4.
117. Ikeda K, et al. Beneficial effects of neutrophil-targeted therapy for pyoderma gangrenosum associated with ulcerative colitis. Eur J Haematol. 2011;21(5 SRC - BaiduScholar):804–5.
118. Larsen CG, et al. Production of interleukin-8 by human dermal fibroblasts and keratinocytes in response to interleukin-1 or tumour necrosis factor. Immunology. 1989;68(1):31–6.
119. Mielke V, et al. Detection of neutrophil-activating peptide NAP/IL-8 and NAP/IL-8 mRNA in human recombinant IL-1 alpha-and human recombinant tumor necrosis factor-alpha-stimulated human dermal fibroblasts. An immunocytochemical and fluorescent in situ hybridization study. J Immunol. 1990;144(1 SRC - BaiduScholar):153–61.
120. Huang W, Nath R, Zayed H. Results of an open-label, proof of concept study of gevokizumab in the treatment of the acute, inflammatory phase of pyoderma gangrenosum. Summer Academy Meeting of the American Academy of Dermatology August Chicago Illinois. 2014;7 SRC - BaiduScholar.
121. Brooklyn TN, Dunnill MGS, Shetty A. Infliximab for the treatment of pyoderma gangrenosum: a randomised, double blind, placebo controlled trial. Gut. 2006;55(4):505–9.
122. Brenner M, et al. Targeted treatment of pyoderma gangrenosum in PAPA (pyogenic arthritis, pyoderma gangrenosum and acne) syndrome with the recombinant human interleukin-1 receptor antagonist anakinra. Br J Dermatol. 2009;161(5 SRC - BaiduScholar):1199–201.
123. Brooklyn TN, et al. T-cell receptor repertoire in pyoderma gangrenosum: evidence for clonal expansions and trafficking. Br J Dermatol. 2007;157(5 SRC - BaiduScholar):960–6.
124. Reichrath J, et al. Treatment recommendations for pyoderma gangrenosum: an evidence-based review of the literature based on more than 350 patients. J Am Acad Dermatol. 2005;53(2 SRC - BaiduScholar):273–83.
125. Guenova E, Teske A, Fehrenbacher B. Interleukin 23 expression in pyoderma gangrenosum and targeted therapy with ustekinumab. Arch Dermatol. 2011;147(10 SRC - BaiduScholar):1203–5.
126. Fahmy M, et al. Ustekinumab for peristomal pyoderma gangrenosum. Am J Gastroenterol. 2012;107(5 SRC - BaiduScholar):794–5.
127. Goldminz AM, et al. Severely recalcitrant pyoderma gangrenosum successfully treated with ustekinumab. J Am Acad Dermatol. 2012;67(5 SRC - BaiduScholar):e237–8.
128. Cosgarea I, et al. Successful treatment of refractory pyoderma gangrenosum with ustekinumab only after excision of renal cell carcinoma. Int Wound J. 2016;13(5):1041–2.
129. Graham JA, et al. Pyoderma gangrenosum in infants and children. Pediatr Dermatol. 1994;11(1 SRC - BaiduScholar):10–7.
130. Shahi V, Wetter DA. Pyoderma gangrenosum associated with solid organ malignancies. Int J Dermatol. 2015;54(9):e351–7.
131. Madkaikar M, et al. Leukocyte adhesion deficiency-I with a novel intronic mutation presenting with pyoderma gangrenosum-like lesions. J Clin Immunol. 2015;35(4):431–4.
132. Sakiyama M, et al. Bullous pyoderma gangrenosum: a case report and review of the published work. J Dermatol. 2012;39:1010–5.
133. Langan SM, Powell FC. Vegetative pyoderma gangrenosum: a report of two new cases and a review of the literature. Int J Dermatol. 2005;44(8 SRC - BaiduScholar):623–9.
134. Callen JP, Jackson JM. Pyoderma gangrenosum: an update. Rheum Dis Clin North Am vi. 2007;33(4 SRC - BaiduScholar):787–802.
135. Ryu J, et al. Pyoderma gangrenosum presenting with leukemoid reaction: a report of 2 cases. Arch Dermatol. 2010;146(5 SRC - BaiduScholar):568–9.
136. Su WP, et al. Histopathologic and immunopathologic study of pyoderma gangrenosum. J Cutan Pathol. 1986;13(5 SRC - BaiduScholar):323–30.
137. Weenig RH, et al. Skin ulcers misdiagnosed as pyoderma gangrenosum. N Engl J Med. 2002;347(18 SRC - BaiduScholar):1412–8.
138. Su WPD, et al. Pyoderma gangrenosum: clinicopathologic correlation and proposed diagnostic criteria. Int J Dermatol. 2004;43(11 SRC - BaiduScholar):790–800.
139. Sheldon DG, et al. Twenty cases of peristomal pyoderma gangrenosum: diagnostic implications and management. Arch Surg. 2000;135(5):564–9.
140. Ahronowitz I, et al. Etiology and management of pyoderma gangrenosum: a comprehensive review. Am J Clin Dermatol. 2012;13(3 SRC - BaiduScholar):191–211.
141. Lyon CC, et al. Topical tacrolimus in the management of peristomal pyoderma gan-

grenosum. TreatmentUpdate. 2001;12(1 SRC - BaiduScholar):13–7.
142. Handler MZ, et al. Treatment of peristomal pyoderma gangrenosum with topical crushed dapsone. J Drugs Dermatol. 2011;10(9 SRC - BaiduScholar):1059–61.
143. Lynch WS, Bergfeld WF. Pyoderma gangrenosum responsive to minocycline hydrochloride. Cutis. 1978;21(4 SRC - BaiduScholar):535–8.
144. Cafardi J, Sami N. Intravenous immunoglobulin as salvage therapy in refractory pyoderma gangrenosum: report of a case and review of the literature. Case Rep Dermatol. 2014;6(3 SRC - BaiduScholar):239–44.
145. Hughes AP, Jackson JM, Callen JP. Clinical features and treatment of peristomal pyoderma gangrenosum. JAMA. 2000;284(12):1546–8.
146. Ormerod A, et al. Oral ciclosporin compared with prednisolone in pyoderma gangrenosum: a randomized controlled trial. Br J Dermatol. 2014;171 Suppl 1:2–8. SRC – BaiduScholar.
147. Miller J, et al. Pyoderma gangrenosum: a review and update on new therapies. J Am Acad Dermatol. 2010;62(4 SRC - BaiduScholar):646–54.
148. Budamakuntla L, et al. Autologous platelet rich plasma in pyoderma gangrenosum-two case reports. Indian Forester. 2015;60(2 SRC - BaiduScholar):204–5.
149. Schafer P. Apremilast mechanism of action and application to psoriasis and psoriatic arthritis. Biochem Pharmacol. 2012;83(12):1583–90.
150. Hatemi G, et al. Apremilast for Behcet's syndrome-a phase 2, placebo-controlled study. N Engl J Med. 2015;372(16 SRC - BaiduScholar):1510–8.
151. Borlu M, Utas S. Pyoderma gangrenosum after cholecystectomy. J Eur Acad Dermatol Venereol. 2001;15(2 SRC - BaiduScholar):185–6.
152. Harris AJ, Regan P, Burge S. Early diagnosis of pyoderma gangrenosum is important to prevent disfigurement. BMJ. 1998;316(7124):52–3.
153. Mahajan AL, et al. Could your case of necrotising fascitis be Pyoderma gangrenosum? Br J Plast Surg. 2005;58(3 SRC - BaiduScholar):409–12.
154. Kondo RN, Minelli L, Araújo FM. Pyoderma gangrenosum: skin grafting and hyperbaric oxygen as adjuvants in the treatment of a deep and extensive ulcer. An Bras Dermatol. 2013;88(6 Suppl 1 SRC - BaiduScholar):176–8.
155. Barańska-Rybak W, Kakol M, Naesstrom M, Komorowska O, Sokołowska Wojdyło M, et al. A retrospective study of 12 cases of pyoderma gangrenosum: why we should avoid surgical intervention and what therapy to apply. Am Surg. 2011;77(12):1644–9.
156. Tay YK, Friednash M, Aeling JL. Acute pyoderma gangrenosum does not require surgical therapy. Arch Fam Med. 1998;7(4):377–80.
157. Zakhireh M, Rockwell WB, Fryer RH. Stabilization of pyoderma gangrenosum ulcer with oral cyclosporine prior to skin grafting. Plast Reconstr Surg. 2004;113(5):1417–20.
158. de Imus G, et al. Accelerated healing of pyoderma gangrenosum treated with bioengineered skin and concomitant immunosuppression. J Am Acad Dermatol. 2001;44(1 SRC - BaiduScholar):61–6.
159. Toyozawa S, et al. Case report: a case of pyoderma gangrenosum with intractable leg ulcers treated by allogeneic cultured dermal substitutes. Dermatol Online J. 2008;14(11 SRC - BaiduScholar):17.
160. Wollina U, Karamfilov T. Treatment of recalcitrant ulcers in pyoderma gangrenosum with mycophenolate mofetil and autologous keratinocyte transplantation on a hyaluronic acid matrix. J Eur Acad Dermatol Venereol. 2000;14(3 SRC - BaiduScholar):187–90.
161. Cozzani E, et al. Pyoderma gangrenosum: a systematic review. Dermatol Venereol. 2014;149(5 SRC - BaiduScholar):587–600.
162. Venning VA, Ryan TJ. Subcorneal pustular dermatosis followed by pyoderma gangrenosum. Br J Dermatol. 1986;115(1 SRC - BaiduScholar):117–8.
163. Marsden JR, Millard LG. Pyoderma gangrenosum, subcorneal pustular dermatosis and IgA paraproteinaemia. Br J Dermatol. 1986;114(1 SRC - BaiduScholar):125–9.
164. Scerri L, et al. Pyoderma gangrenosum and subcorneal pustular dermatosis, without monoclonal gammopathy. Br J Dermatol. 1994;130(3 SRC - BaiduScholar):398–9.
165. Kohl PK, et al. Pyoderma gangrenosum followed by subcorneal pustular dermatosis in a patient with IgA paraproteinemia. J Am Acad Dermatol. 1991;24(2 Pt 2 SRC - BaiduScholar):325–8.
166. Davies MG, Hastings A. Sweet's syndrome progressing to pyoderma gangrenosum-a spectrum of neutrophilic skin disease in association with cryptogenic cirrhosis. Clin Exp Dermatol. 1991;16(4 SRC - BaiduScholar):279–82.
167. Chave TA, Hutchinson PE. Pyoderma gangrenosum, subcorneal pustular dermatosis, IgA paraproteinaemia and IgG antiepithelial antibodies. Br J Dermatol. 2001;145(5 SRC - BaiduScholar):852–4.
168. Puechguiral-Renaud I, et al. Subcorneal pustulosis and Pyoderma gangrenosum associated with a biclonal gammopathy. Eur J Dermatol. 2006;16(6 SRC - BaiduScholar):687–90.
169. Neoh CY, et al. Sweet's syndrome: a spectrum of unusual clinical presentations and associations. Br J Dermatol. 2007;156(3 SRC - BaiduScholar):480–5.
170. Castro-Fernandez M, et al. Coexistence of pyoderma gangrenosum and Sweet's syndrome in a patient with ulcerative colitis. Am J Gastroenterol. 2007;102(12 SRC - BaiduScholar):2865–6.
171. Ahmad K, Ramsay B. Pyoderma gangrenosum associated with subcorneal pustular dermatosis and IgA myeloma. Clin Exp Dermatol. 2009;34(1 SRC - BaiduScholar):46–8.
172. Caucanas M, et al. Associated pyoderma gangrenosum, erythema elevatum diutinum, and Sweet's syndrome: the concept of neutrophilic disease. Int J Dermatol. 2013;52(10 SRC - BaiduScholar):1185–8.

173. Rochet NM, et al. Sweet syndrome: clinical presentation, associations, and response to treatment in 77 patients. J Am Acad Dermatol. 2013;69(4 SRC - BaiduScholar):557–64.
174. Cohen PR. Sweet's syndrome-a comprehensive review of an acute febrile neutrophilic dermatosis. Orphanet J Rare Dis. 2007;2:34. SRC – BaiduScholar.
175. Halpern J, Salim A. Pediatric sweet syndrome: case report and literature review. Pediatr Dermatol. 2009;26(4 SRC - BaiduScholar):452–7.
176. Kawakami T, Ohashi S, Kawa Y. Elevated serum granulocyte colony-stimulating factor levels in patients with active phase of sweet syndrome and patients with active behcet disease: implication in neutrophil apoptosis dysfunction. Arch Dermatol. 2004;140(5 SRC - BaiduScholar):570–4.
177. Pauksen K, et al. Serum levels of granulocyte-colony stimulating factor (G-CSF) in bacterial and viral infections, and in atypical pneumonia. Br J Haematol. 1994;88(2 SRC - BaiduScholar):256–60.
178. Selig C, Nothdurft W. Cytokines and progenitor cells of granulocytopoiesis in peripheral blood of patients with bacterial infections. Infect Immun. 1995;63(1):104–9.
179. Umesaki N, et al. Plasma granulocyte colony stimulating factor concentrations in pregnant women. Gynecol Obstet Investig. 1995;40(1):5–7.
180. Matsubara K, et al. Concentrations of serum granulocyte-colony-stimulating factor in normal pregnancy and preeclampsia. Hypertens Pregnancy. 1999;18(1):95–106.
181. Soendergaard C, et al. Alpha-1 antitrypsin and granulocyte colony-stimulating factor as serum biomarkers of disease severity in ulcerative colitis. Inflamm Bowel Dis. 2015;21(5):1077–88.
182. Shinojima Y, et al. Sweet syndrome associated with intrahepatic cholangiocarcinoma producing granulocyte colony-stimulating factor. Br J Dermatol. 2006;155(5 SRC - BaiduScholar):1103–4.
183. Thompson DF, Montarella KE. Drug-induced Sweet's syndrome. Ann Pharmacother. 2007;41(5): 802–11.
184. Vanourny J, Swick BL. Sweet syndrome with systemic inflammatory response syndrome. Arch Dermatol. 2012;148(8 SRC - BaiduScholar):969–70.
185. Sawicki J, Morton RA, Ellis AK. Sweet syndrome with associated systemic inflammatory response syndrome: an ultimately fatal case. Ann Allergy Asthma Immunol. 2010;105(4):321–3.
186. Ratzinger G, et al. Acute febrile neutrophilic dermatosis: a histopathologic study of 31 cases with review of literature. Am J Dermatopathol. 2007;29(2 SRC - BaiduScholar):125–33.
187. Malone JC, Slone SP, Wills-Frank LA. Vascular inflammation (vasculitis) in sweet syndrome: a clinicopathologic study of 28 biopsy specimens from 21 patients. Arch Dermatol. 2002;138(3 SRC - BaiduScholar):345–9.
188. Requena L, Kutzner H, Palmedo G, Histiocytoid Sweet syndrome: a dermal infiltration of immature neutrophilic granulocytes. Arch Dermatol. 2005;141(7 SRC - BaiduScholar):834–42.
189. Chan MP, et al. Subcutaneous sweet syndrome in the setting of myeloid disorders: a case series and review of the literature. J Am Acad Dermatol. 2013;68(6 SRC - BaiduScholar):1006–15.
190. Kroshinsky D, et al. Necrotizing Sweet syndrome: a new variant of neutrophilic dermatosis mimicking necrotizing fasciitis. J Am Acad Dermatol. 2012;67(5 SRC - BaiduScholar):945–54.
191. Probert C, et al. Sweet's syndrome without granulocytosis. Int J Dermatol. 1998;37(2 SRC - BaiduScholar):108–12.
192. Su WP, Liu HN. Diagnostic criteria for Sweet's syndrome. Cutis. 1986;37(3 SRC - BaiduScholar):167–74.
193. von den Driesch P. Sweet's syndrome (acute febrile neutrophilic dermatosis). J Am Acad Dermatol. 1994;31(4 SRC - BaiduScholar):535–56; quiz 557560.
194. Rochael MC, Pantaleao L, Vilar EA. Sweet's syndrome: study of 73 cases, emphasizing histopathological findings. An Bras Dermatol. 2011;86(4 SRC - BaiduScholar):702–7.
195. Chavan RN, et al. Histiocytoid Sweet syndrome may indicate leukemia cutis: a novel application of fluorescence in situ hybridization. J Am Acad Dermatol. 2014;70(6 SRC - BaiduScholar):1021–7.
196. Tsuji H, et al. Sweet's syndrome associated with systemic lupus erythematosus: a case report and review of the literature. J Dermatol. 2013;40(8 SRC - BaiduScholar):641–8.
197. Cohen PR, Kurzrock R. Sweet's syndrome and cancer. Clin Dermatol. 1993;11(1):149–57.
198. Cohen PR, et al. Malignancy-associated Sweet's syndrome: review of the world literature. Oncologia. 1988;6(12 SRC - BaiduScholar):1887–97.
199. Krug B, et al. FDG PET utility in paraneoplastic sweet syndrome. Clin Nucl Med. 2004;29(2 SRC - BaiduScholar):91–2.
200. Dong A, et al. 18F-FDG PET/CT findings in a patient with Sweet syndrome associated with myelodysplastic syndrome. Clin Nucl Med. 2013;38(12):e454–7.
201. Larson AR, Granter SR. Systemic lupus erythematosus-associated neutrophilic dermatosis: a review and update. Adv Anat Pathol. 2014;21(4):248–53.
202. Maillard H, et al. Colchicine for Sweet's syndrome. A study of 20 cases. Br J Dermatol. 1999;140(3 SRC - BaiduScholar):565–6.
203. Horio T, et al. Potassium iodide in erythema nodosum and other erythematous dermatoses. J Am Acad Dermatol. 1983;9(1 SRC - BaiduScholar):77–81.
204. Jeanfils S, et al. Indomethacin treatment of eighteen patients with Sweet's syndrome. J Am Acad Dermatol. 1997;36(3 Pt 1 SRC - BaiduScholar):436–9.
205. Giovanna Brunasso AM, Massone C. Clinical images. Sweet syndrome during pregnancy. CMAJ. 2008;179(9 SRC - BaiduScholar):967.

206. Best J, et al. Pregnancy-associated Sweet's syndrome in an acute episode of ulcerative colitis. Z Gastroenterol. 2009;47(8 SRC - BaiduScholar):753–7.
207. Cohen PR. Pregnancy-associated Sweet's syndrome: world literature review. Obstet Gynecol Surv. 1993;48(8):584–7.
208. Truchuelo M, et al. Sweet-like lesions induced by bortezomib: a review of the literature and a report of 2 cases. Actas Dermosifiliogr. 2012;103(9 SRC - BaiduScholar):829–31.
209. Banuls J, et al. Interstitial granulomatous dermatitis with plaques and arthritis. Eur J Dermatol. 2003;13(3 SRC - BaiduScholar):308–10.
210. Altaykan A, et al. Interstitial granulomatous dermatitis with arthritis. Hum Pathol. 2004;35(7 SRC - BaiduScholar):892–4.
211. Verneuil L, et al. Interstitial granulomatous dermatitis with cutaneous cords and arthritis: a disorder associated with autoantibodies. J Am Acad Dermatol. 2001;45(2 SRC - BaiduScholar): 286–91.
212. Peroni A, et al. Interstitial granulomatous dermatitis: a distinct entity with characteristic histological and clinical pattern. Br J Dermatol. 2012;166(4 SRC - BaiduScholar):775–83.
213. Magro CM, et al. The interstitial granulomatous drug reaction: a distinctive clinical and pathological entity. J Cutan Pathol. 1998;25(2 SRC - BaiduScholar):72–8.
214. Hawryluk EB, et al. Non-infectious granulomatous diseases of the skin and their associated systemic diseases: an evidence-based update to important clinical questions. Am J Clin Dermatol. 2010;11(3 SRC - BaiduScholar):171–81.
215. Levine SD, et al. Interstitial granulomatous dermatitis in a patient with rheumatoid arthritis on etanercept. Cutis. 2009;83(1 SRC - BaiduScholar):50.
216. Szepetiuk G, Lesuisse M, Piérard GE, Quatresooz P, Piérard-Franchimont C. Autoimmunity-related granulomatous dermatitis in association with hepatitis. Case Rep Dermatol. 2012;4(1 SRC - BaiduScholar):80–4.
217. Chu P, Connolly MK, LeBoit PE. The histopathologic spectrum of palisaded neutrophilic and granulomatous dermatitis in patients with collagen vascular disease. Arch Dermatol. 1994;130(10 SRC - BaiduScholar):1278–83.
218. Ergun T, et al. Skin manifestations of rheumatoid arthritis: a study of 215 Turkish patients. Int J Dermatol. 2008;47(9 SRC - BaiduScholar):894–902.
219. Hantash BM, et al. Palisaded neutrophilic and granulomatous dermatitis associated with limited systemic sclerosis. J Am Acad Dermatol. 2008;58(4 SRC - BaiduScholar):661–4.
220. Finan MC, Winkelmann RK. The cutaneous extravascular necrotizing granuloma (Churg-Strauss granuloma) and systemic disease: a review of 27 cases. Medicine (Baltimore). 1983;62(3 SRC - BaiduScholar):142–58.
221. Higaki Y, et al. Rheumatoid papules: a report on four patients with histopathologic analysis. J Am Acad Dermatol. 1993;28(3 SRC - BaiduScholar):406–11.
222. Obermoser G, et al. Extravascular necrotizing palisaded granulomas as the presenting skin sign of systemic lupus erythematosus. Br J Dermatol. 2002;147(2 SRC - BaiduScholar):371–4.
223. Wilmoth GJ, Perniciaro C. Cutaneous extravascular necrotizing granuloma (Winkelmann granuloma): confirmation of the association with systemic disease. J Am Acad Dermatol. 1996;34(5 Pt 1 SRC - BaiduScholar):753–9.
224. Lee MW, Jang KA, Lim YS. Cutaneous extravascular necrotizing granuloma (Churg Strauss granuloma). Clin Exp Dermatol. 1999;24(3 SRC - BaiduScholar):193–5.
225. Bremner R, et al. Palisaded neutrophilic and granulomatous dermatitis: an unusual cutaneous manifestation of immune-mediated disorders. Semin Arthritis Rheum. 2004;34(3 SRC - BaiduScholar):610–6.
226. Hunt RD, et al. Palisaded neutrophilic and granulomatous dermatitis in an adolescent girl with perinuclear antineutrophil cytoplasmic antibody-positive pauci-immune glomerulonephritis and arthritis. J Am Acad Dermatol. 2012;67(4 SRC - BaiduScholar):e164–6.
227. Gutte R, Khopkar U. Isolated unilateral palisaded neutrophilic and granulomatous dermatitis. Indian J Dermatol Venereol Leprol. 2011;77(5 SRC - BaiduScholar):615–7.
228. Collaris EJ, et al. Cutaneous granulomas in rheumatoid arthritis. Int J Dermatol. 2007;46 Suppl 3 SRC - BaiduScholar:33–5.
229. Sangueza OP, et al. Palisaded neutrophilic granulomatous dermatitis in rheumatoid arthritis. J Am Acad Dermatol. 2002;47(2 SRC - BaiduScholar):251–7.
230. Germanas JP, et al. Palisaded neutrophilic granulomatous dermatitis in a 12-year-old girl with systemic lupus erythematosus. J Am Acad Dermatol. 2006;55(2 Suppl SRC - BaiduScholar):S60–2.
231. Umezawa Y, et al. Palisaded neutrophilic and granulomatous dermatitis in a rheumatoid arthritis patient after treatment with adalimumab. Eur J Dermatol. 2013;23(6 SRC - BaiduScholar):910–1.
232. Mahmoodi M, et al. Palisaded neutrophilic and granulomatous dermatitis in association with sarcoidosis. J Cutan Pathol. 2011;38(4 SRC - BaiduScholar):365–8.
233. Heidary N, et al. Palisaded neutrophilic and granulomatous dermatosis. Dermatol Online J. 2008;14(5 SRC - BaiduScholar):17.
234. Misago N, et al. Palisaded neutrophilic granulomatous dermatitis in systemic lupus erythematosus with a butterfly rash-like lesion. Eur J Dermatol. 2010;20(1 SRC - BaiduScholar):128–9.
235. Lee KJ, et al. Interstitial granulomatous dermatitis associated with autoimmune hepatitis. J Eur Acad Dermatol Venereol. 2007;21(5 SRC - BaiduScholar):684–5.
236. Gulati A, et al. Palisaded neutrophilic granulomatous dermatitis associated with systemic

lupus erythematosus presenting with the burning rope sign. J Am Acad Dermatol. 2009;61(4 SRC - BaiduScholar):711–4.

237. Kim SK, et al. Palisaded neutrophilic granulomatous dermatitis presenting as an unusual skin manifestation in a patient with Behcet's disease. Scand J Rheumatol. 2005;34(4 SRC - BaiduScholar):324–7.
238. Singh M, et al. Images in clinical medicine. Palisaded neutrophilic and granulomatous dermatitis. N Engl J Med. 2012;366(22 SRC - BaiduScholar):e33.
239. Asahina A, et al. Early lesion of palisaded neutrophilic granulomatous dermatitis in ulcerative colitis. Eur J Dermatol. 2007;17(3):234–7.
240. Newell EL, et al. A case of cutaneous extravascular necrotizing granuloma without systemic manifestations. Clin Exp Dermatol. 2007;32(5):509–12.
241. Fett N, Kovarik C, Bennett D. Palisaded neutrophilic granulomatous dermatitis without a definable underlying disorder treated with dapsone. J Am Acad Dermatol. 2011;65(3):e92–3.
242. Gordon K, et al. Allopurinol-induced palisaded neutrophilic and granulomatous dermatitis. Cutan Ocul Toxicol. 2012;31(4):338–40.
243. Stephenson SR, et al. Palisaded neutrophilic and granulomatous dermatitis presenting in a patient with rheumatoid arthritis on adalimumab. J Cutan Pathol. 2011;38(8):644–8.
244. de Unamuno Bustos B, et al. Palisaded neutrophilic and granulomatous dermatitis associated with ankylosing spondylitis. Am J Dermatopathol. 2013;35(8):847–50.
245. Al-Daraji WI, Coulson IH, Howat AJ. Palisaded neutrophilic and granulomatous dermatitis. Clin Exp Dermatol. 2005;30(5):578–9.
246. Paštar Z, et al. Palisaded neutrophilic and granulomatous dermatitis in association with subcutaneous nodular and systemic sarcoidosis. Acta Dermatovenerol Croat. 2013;21(4):245–9.
247. He Y, et al. Combination therapy with intralesional triamcinolone and oral dapsone for management of palisaded neutrophilic and granulomatous dermatitis. Dermatol Online J. 2013;19(2):17.
248. DiCaudo DJ, Connolly SM. Interstitial granulomatous dermatitis associated with pulmonary coccidioidomycosis. J Am Acad Dermatol. 2001;45(6):840–5.
249. Biswas A, et al. Palisaded neutrophilic and granulomatous dermatitis in a child with type I diabetes mellitus and coeliac disease. Br J Dermatol. 2008;159(2):488–9.
250. Brecher A. Palisaded neutrophilic and granulomatous dermatitis. Dermatol Online J. 2003;9(4):1.
251. Alghamdi R, et al. Intravenous immunoglobulins as a treatment of interstitial granulomatous dermatitis with arthritis. Br J Dermatol. 2012;167(1):218–20.
252. Kreuter A, et al. Infliximab therapy for interstitial granulomatous dermatitis. J Eur Acad Dermatol Venereol. 2007;21(2 SRC - BaiduScholar):251–2.
253. Antunes J, et al. Autoimmune thyroiditis presenting as interstitial granulomatous dermatitis. An Bras Dermatol. 2012;87(5):748–51.
254. Balin SJ, et al. Myelodysplastic syndrome presenting as generalized granulomatous dermatitis. Arch Dermatol. 2011;147(3 SRC - BaiduScholar):331–5.
255. Busquets-Perez N, et al. Interstitial granulomatous dermatitis with arthritis (Ackerman syndrome). J Rheumatol. 2006;33(6 SRC - BaiduScholar):1207–9.
256. Chen DL, et al. A novel case of polyfibromatosis and interstitial granulomatous dermatitis with arthritis. J Am Acad Dermatol. 2006;55(2 Suppl SRC - BaiduScholar):S32–7.
257. Tomasini C, Pippione M. Interstitial granulomatous dermatitis with plaques. J Am Acad Dermatol. 2002;46(6 SRC - BaiduScholar):892–9.
258. Martin G, et al. Interstitial granulomatous dermatitis with arthritis associated with trastuzumab. J Eur Acad Dermatol Venereol. 2010;24(4 SRC - BaiduScholar):493–4.
259. Martinez-Moran C, Najera L, Ruiz-Casado AI. Interstitial granulomatous drug reaction to sorafenib. Arch Dermatol. 2011;147(9 SRC - BaiduScholar):1118–9.
260. Marcollo Pini A, et al. Interstitial granulomatous drug reaction following intravenous ganciclovir. Br J Dermatol. 2008;158(6 SRC - BaiduScholar):1391–3.
261. Fujita Y, et al. A case of interstitial granulomatous drug reaction due to sennoside. Br J Dermatol. 2004;150(5 SRC - BaiduScholar):1035–7.
262. Yazganoglu KD, et al. Interstitial granulomatous drug reaction due to thalidomide. J Eur Acad Dermatol Venereol. 2009;23(4 SRC - BaiduScholar):490–3.
263. Mason HR, et al. Interstitial granulomatous dermatitis associated with darifenacin. J Drugs Dermatol. 2008;7(9 SRC - BaiduScholar):895–7.
264. Chen YC, et al. Interstitial granulomatous drug reaction presenting as erythroderma: remission after discontinuation of enalapril maleate. Br J Dermatol. 2008;158(5 SRC - BaiduScholar):1143–5.
265. Deng A, Harvey V, Sina B. Interstitial granulomatous dermatitis associated with the use of tumor necrosis factor alpha inhibitors. Arch Dermatol. 2006;142(2 SRC BaiduScholar):198–202.
266. Martorell-Calatayud A, et al. Interstitial granulomatous drug reaction to adalimumab. Am J Dermatopathol. 2010;32(4 SRC - BaiduScholar):408–9.
267. Hu S, et al. Interstitial granulomatous dermatitis in a patient with rheumatoid arthritis on etanercept. Cutis. 2008;81(4):336–8.
268. Du XF, et al. Interstitial granulomatous drug reaction to a Chinese herb extract. Eur J Dermatol. 2012;22(3 SRC - BaiduScholar):419–20.
269. Laura A, et al. Interstitial granulomatous drug reaction due to febuxostat. Indian J Dermatol Venereol Leprol. 2014;80(2 SRC - BaiduScholar):182–4.
270. Hernandez N, et al. Generalized erythematous-violaceous plaques in a patient with a history of dyslipidemia. Interstitial granulomatous drug reaction IGDR. Int J Dermatol. 2013;52(4 SRC - BaiduScholar):393–4.

271. Groves C, et al. Interstitial granulomatous reaction to strontium ranelate. Arch Dermatol. 2008;144(2 SRC - BaiduScholar):268–9.
272. Fernando SL, et al. Drug-induced hypersensitivity syndrome with superficial granulomatous dermatitis-a novel finding. Am J Dermatopathol. 2009;31(6 SRC - BaiduScholar):611–3.
273. Kim MS, et al. Allopurinol-induced DRESS syndrome with a histologic pattern consistent with interstitial granulomatous drug reaction. Am J Dermatopathol. 2014;36(2 SRC - BaiduScholar):193–6.
274. Sakaizawa K, et al. Interstitial granulomatous dermatitis with plaques. Eur J Dermatol. 2008;18(5 SRC - BaiduScholar):600–1.
275. Garcia-Rabasco A, et al. Interstitial granulomatous dermatitis in a patient with lupus erythematosus. Am J Dermatopathol. 2011;33(8 SRC - BaiduScholar):871–2.
276. Wong HK, et al. A palpable erythematous cord over the trunk in a patient with systemic lupus erythematosus. Interstitial granulomatous dermatitis IGD. JAMA Dermatol. 2013;149(5 SRC - BaiduScholar):609–14.
277. Blaise S, Salameire D, Carpentier PH. Interstitial granulomatous dermatitis: a misdiagnosed cutaneous form of systemic lupus erythematosus? Clin Exp Dermatol. 2008;33(6 SRC - BaiduScholar):712–4.
278. Marmon S, et al. Lupus-erythematous-associated interstitial granulomatous dermatitis. Dermatol Online J. 2012;18(12 SRC - BaiduScholar):31.
279. Felcht M, et al. Interstitial granulomatous dermatitis (Ackerman's Syndrome). Eur J Dermatol. 2010;20(5 SRC - BaiduScholar):661–2.
280. Lee HW, et al. Interstitial granulomatous dermatitis with plaques associated with antiphospholipid syndrome. Br J Dermatol. 2005;152(4 SRC - BaiduScholar):814–6.
281. Swing DC Jr, et al. Interstitial granulomatous dermatitis secondary to acute promyelocytic leukemia. Am J Dermatopathol. 2008;30(2 SRC - BaiduScholar):197–9.
282. Schreckenberg C, Asch PH, Sibilia J. [Interstitial granulomatous dermatitis and paraneoplastic rheumatoid polyarthritis disclosing cancer of the lung]. Ann Dermatol Venereol. 1998;125(9 SRC - BaiduScholar):585–8.
283. Lucas A, Banuls J, Mataix J. Localized acquired cutis laxa secondary to interstitial granulomatous dermatitis. Clin Exp Dermatol. 2009;34(5):e102–5.
284. Long D, et al. Interstitial granulomatous dermatitis with arthritis. J Am Acad Dermatol. 1996;34(6 SRC - BaiduScholar):957–61.
285. Patsatsi A, et al. Interstitial granulomatous dermatitis: another clinical variant. Case Rep Dermatol. 2011;3(3 SRC - BaiduScholar):195–200.
286. Dubey S, Merry P. Clinical vignette. Interstitial granulomatous dermatitis Ackermans syndrome in SLE presenting with the rope sign. Rheumatology (Oxford). 2007;46(1 SRC - BaiduScholar):80.
287. Jabbari A, et al. Interstitial granulomatous dermatitis with arthritis. Dermatol Online J. 2009;15(8 SRC - BaiduScholar):22.
288. Schanz S, Schmalzing M, Guenova E. Interstitial granulomatous dermatitis with arthritis responding to tocilizumab. Arch Dermatol. 2012;148(1):17–20.
289. Wollina U, et al. Interstitial granulomatous dermatitis with plaques and arthritis. Clin Rheumatol. 2003;22:347–9. p. 4–5 SRC - BaiduScholar.
290. Zoli A, et al. Interstitial granulomatous dermatitis in rheumatoid arthritis responsive to etanercept. Clin Rheumatol. 2010;29(1):99–101.
291. Johnson H, et al. Interstitial granulomatous dermatitis. Dermatol Online J. 2008;14(5 SRC - BaiduScholar):18.
292. Warycha MA, et al. Interstitial granulomatous dermatitis in a child with chronic uveitis. J Am Acad Dermatol. 2008;58(5 Suppl 1 SRC - BaiduScholar):S100–2.

11 Iatrogenic Disease and Drug Induced Toxicities Related to Anti-Inflammatory and Immunomodulatory Agents

Shelly Rivas and Allireza Alloo

Key Points

- DMARDs and other anti-inflammatory medications are associated with unique cutaneous and extracutaneous toxicities.
- In addition to cutaneous hypersensitivity reactions, patients on such medications are potentially at higher risk for infections, hematologic abnormalities, and malignancy.
- Medication reconciliation is important in recognizing drug-induced connective tissue disease.

Interdisciplinary Introduction

This chapter focuses on medication reactions relevant to treating patients with inflammatory dermatoses and connective tissue diseases. It is divided into two sections. The first reviews adverse drug reactions to immunomodulatory agents used to manage inflammatory dermatologic conditions. The second section highlights medications that can cause drug-induced lupus erythematosus and drug-induced dermatomyositis.

S. Rivas · A. Alloo (✉)
Department of Dermatology, Donald and Barbara Zucker School of Medicine at Hofstra Northwell, Hempstead, NY, USA
e-mail: aalloo@northwell.edu

Toxicities of Anti-Inflammatory and Immunomodulatory Agents

Improvements in existing disease-modifying anti-rheumatic drugs and the development of novel immunomodulatory agents have significantly augmented the potential for disease control in patients with connective tissue diseases. However, these medications are not without risk. In this section, we will review the side effects of various immunomodulatory agents, with particular attention to toxicities that affect the skin, hair, and nails.

Antimalarials

Antimalarial agents have been used to treat dermatologic conditions since the late nineteenth century. Chloroquine and hydroxychloroquine, the antimalarials most commonly used today, are indicated for a variety of cutaneous and systemic conditions including discoid lupus, subacute cutaneous lupus erythematosus (SCLE), systemic lupus erythematosus, dermatomyositis, sarcoidosis, granuloma annulare, lichen planus, porphyria cutanea tarda, and polymorphous light eruption [1].

Mechanism of Action

The mechanism of action of antimalarial agents is not fully understood. They are believed to have

A. Garg et al. (eds.), *Interdisciplinary Approaches to Overlap Disorders in Dermatology & Rheumatology*,
https://doi.org/10.1007/978-3-319-18446-3_11

a role in suppressing T-lymphocyte proliferation and leukocyte chemotaxis, as well as stabilizing lysosomal enzymes [2]. Antimalarial agents have an affinity for pigment-containing tissues, including the skin and the melanin-rich iris and choroid of the eye [2].

Cutaneous Side Effects

Cutaneous adverse effects of hydroxychloroquine and chloroquine include dyspigmentation, likely secondary to the binding of hydroxychloriquine or chloroquine to melanin [3]. Classically, patients present with blue-gray to black macules, most commonly involving the anterior legs, arms, face, oral mucosa and nails (Fig. 11.1) [4, 5]. Reversible hypopigmentation or bleaching of hair roots has also been noted with chloroquine [6, 7]. Quinacrine, which is used less frequently, can cause yellowing of the skin, similar to the skin findings of jaundice [8, 9]. Pigmentary changes are usually reversible with cessation of the drug. While the exact incidence and time course of anti-malarial dyspigmentation is unknown, estimates are as high as 25%, with dyspigmentation occurring months to years after initiation of medication [10].

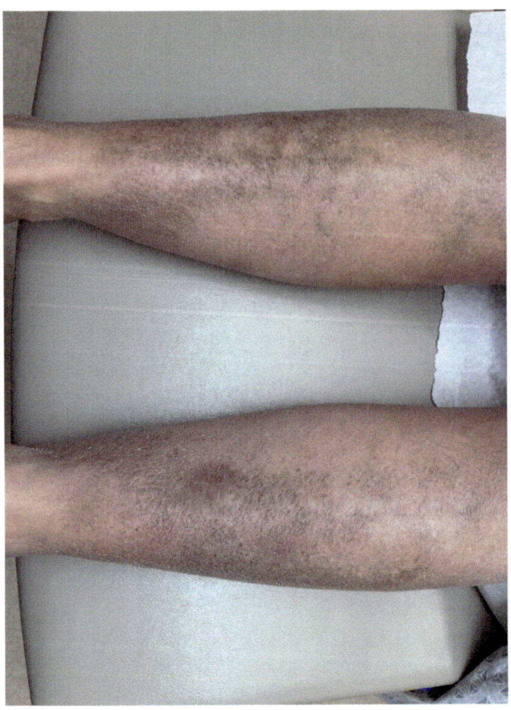

Fig. 11.1 Hydroxycholoroquine Dyspigmentation on the Anterior Shins. (Image Courtesy of Joseph F. Merola, MD MMSC)

Idiosyncratic cutaneous adverse drug reactions have also been noted with antimalarials. These are often lichenoid eruptions [11, 12]; in addition, more serious drug reactions, including acute generalized exanthematous pustulosis (AGEP), drug-induced hypersensitivity syndrome (DIHS), and toxic epidermal necrolysis (TEN), have been observed [13–15]. Of note, recent cases of AGEP induced by hydroxychloroquine have been found to be recalcitrant to drug cessation alone, often requiring systemic treatment [16, 17]. Interestingly, when hydroxychloroquine is used to treat dermatomyositis, evidence suggests that patients are more prone to drug hypersensitivity reactions than when the same agent is used for other indications [18]. Lastly, as antimalarials are well-known photosensitizing agents, phototoxic and photoallergic eruptions can also occur [19].

Extracutaneous and Systemic Side Effects

The most widely reported adverse effect of antimalarial drugs is retinal toxicity. This sequela appears to be agent-specific and dose-dependent: ocular toxicity rarely occurs at dosages greater than 250 mg/d for chloroquine or greater than 6.4 mg/kg/d for hydroxychloroquine, with chloroquine carrying a greater risk for retinal toxicity overall [2]. Concomitant use of hydroxychloroquine and chloroquine confers an additive risk of retinal toxicity. To manage this risk, in patients without a history of maculopathy, a baseline fundus exam is recommended with annual screenings commencing after five years of treatment [20].

Antimalarials may less often cause systemic toxicities, including agranulocytosis, hemolysis in patients with G6-deficiency, gastrointestinal distress, and neuromuscular and neuropsychiatric effects such as irritability, hyperexcitability, and seizures [1]. Cardiac risks including but not limited to QTc prolongation have been reported. While no formal guidelines exist at present, consider baseline ECG in patients with multiple risk factors as well as follow-up ECG and screening for cardiac symptoms in patients with prolonged QTc or those receiving antimalarials in combination with other QTc-prolonging therapies. Hydroxychloroquine-induced cardiomyopathy has also been reported.

Azathioprine

Azathioprine, a derivative of 6-mercaptopurine, is a potent immunosuppressive and anti-inflammatory agent used in dermatology for the treatment of immunobullous diseases, vasculitides, dermatomyositis, scleroderma, and Behcet's disease [21, 22].

Mechanism of Action

Azathioprine's active metabolite, 6-thioguanine, is a purine analog whose structure is similar to that of adenine and guanine. Its incorporation into nucleic acid synthesis halts purine metabolism. This leads to decreased cell division and inhibition of B and T cell function [2].

Cutaneous Side Effects

Azathioprine increases patients' risk of non-melanoma skin cancer (NMSC) [23]. It has also been associated with a severe hypersensitivity syndrome, in which patients present with a morbilliform eruption, fever, leukocytosis, transaminitis, gastrointestinal distress, and in severe cases, cardiogenic shock [24, 25]. Such reactions are typically seen within a month of initiating therapy. In the context of this hypersensitivity reaction, several cases of reactive inflammatory dermatoses, such as Sweet's syndrome and erythema nodosum, have been reported [26–29]. Both the azathioprine-associated drug hypersensitivity syndrome and the associated reactive dermatoses typically remit with drug discontinuation. Therapy, as for all other hypersensitivity reactions, is primarily supportive.

Extracutaneous and Systemic Side Effects

The extracutaneous adverse effects most commonly associated with azathioprine are infection, bone marrow suppression, and increased malignancy risk. Specifically, evidence suggests a two to five-fold increased risk of B and T-cell lymphoma [23].

Cyclosporine

Cyclosporine was first used by rheumatologists more than 40 years ago for the treatment of arthritis [30]. Dermatologists have used it for the past two decades to treat inflammatory skin diseases, including atopic dermatitis, immunobullous disorders and pyoderma gangrenosum. Cyclosporine is also now FDA-approved for the treatment of severe, recalcitrant and disabling psoriasis [31].

Mechanism of Action

Cyclosporine works by counteracting the upregulation of pro-inflammatory cytokines, including IL-2, which are required for T-cell activation. This in turn leads to decreased B and T cell function [31]. For the treatment of recalcitrant dermatoses, cyclosporine is used primarily as a short-term temporizing therapy to control flares, acting as a bridge while an alternative immunosuppresive medication takes effect.

Cutaneous Side Effects

The cutaneous adverse effects most commonly attributed to cyclosporine are gingival hyperplasia and hypertrichosis; the latter has been shown to occur in up to 60% patients [32, 33]. Diffuse sebaceous hyperplasia has been reported in transplant patients on long-term cyclosporine [34, 35]. Cutaneous pseudolymphoma secondary to cyclosporine has also been described [36]. While the increased risk of NMSC in patients on long-term cyclosporine therapy has been well described [30], it has not been shown to be increased in patients on low-dose or short term treatments except in those previously treated with PUVA [37].

Extracutaneous and Systemic Side Effects

Extracutaneous toxicities of cyclosporine most commonly include hypertension and kidney injury secondary to the vasoconstrictive effect of cyclosporine on afferent glomerular arterioles [30, 37]. Both hypertension and acute kidney injury are dose-dependent. Patients who develop hypertension can be managed either by reducing the cyclosporine dose by 25–50% or adding an antihypertensive agent, preferably a calcium channel blocker of the dihydropyridine class, such as amlodipine or nifedipine [31]. While kidney injury is usually reversible during short-term therapy and may be managed with dose reduction or treatment cessation, irreversible damage to the kidney has been observed in patients on long-term cyclosporine therapy (>2 years) even without previous abnormal blood pressure or kidney function tests [38].

Less frequently, hyperlipidemia, gastrointestinal distress, and neurological symptoms such as headaches, tremor and psychosis have also been reported in patients on cyclosporine [37].

Dapsone

Dapsone is a sulfone drug used for its anti-inflammatory and anti-parasitic properties [39]. It was adopted in the early twentieth century for treatment of infections including those caused by atypical mycobacteria [39]. Prior to the introduction of isotretinoin, dapsone was the drug of choice for the treatment of nodulocystic acne [40]. Today, dapsone is employed primarily in the treatment of neutrophilic and eosinophilic dermatoses [39]. It is also used to treat leprosy, dermatitis herpetiformis, linear IgA dermatosis, IgA pemphigus, subcorneal pustular dermatosis, and erythema elevatum diutinum [41].

Mechanism of Action

Dapsone works by inhibiting neutrophil myeloperoxidase, eosinophil peroxidase and neutrophil chemotaxis [39].

Cutaneous Side Effects

A potentially fatal hypersensitivity reaction consisting of morbilliform eruption associated with fever and hepatitis has been observed in 0.5–3.6% of patients within four to six weeks of dapsone initiation [42, 43]. AGEP has also been reported [43]. When used to treat leprosy, dapsone may also precipitate the development of erythema nodosum leprosum, which can be controlled with thalidomide [2].

Extracutaneous and Systemic Side Effects

Dapsone is metabolized by cytochrome P450 in the liver to form hydroxylamines, metabolites which can lead to methemoglobinemia and promote hemolysis, particularly in patients with a glucose-6-phosphate dehydrogenase (G6PD) deficiency [39]. For this reason, G6PD levels should be checked prior to initiating therapy. In rare circumstances, dapsone has also been associated with other hematologic toxicities, such as agranulocytosis [44]. Other observed toxicities include peripheral neuropathy and hepatoxicity, which appear to be dose-dependent [41].

Mycophenolate Mofetil

Mycophenolate mofetil (MMF), a synthetic derivative of mycophenolic acid (MPA) with greater bioavailability, was originally used as an immunosuppressant in patients who received solid organ transplants. In dermatology, MPA was initially adopted for the treatment of psoriasis. Since the 1990s, MMF has been used as a steroid-sparing agent in the treatment of recalcitrant immunobullous diseases, pyoderma gangrenosum, bullous lichen planus, connective tissue diseases and vasculitides, among other dermatoses [45].

Mechanism of Action

MMF is hydrolyzed to MPA after ingestion. MPA works by selectively inhibiting the enzyme inosine monophosphate dehydrogenase, blocking production of guanosine-5-phosphate [2]. Depletion of the guanosine pool in the cell prevents de novo purine synthesis, leading to a subsequent decrease in B and T lymphocytes. Additionally, MPA suppresses immunoglobulin production by B lymphocytes and plays a role in decreasing intercellular adhesion and leukocyte recruitment [2].

Cutaneous Side Effects

Cutaneous side effects of MMF have not been widely reported.

Extracutaneous and Systemic Side Effects

Given its role as an immunosuppressant, MMF renders patients to higher risk of infections. Overall, however, it has a limited side-effect profile. The most commonly reported side effects are gastrointestinal disturbances including nausea, vomiting, diarrhea and abdominal pain [2]. Mycopenolic acid may be considered in cases of MMF gastrointestinal intolerance. Hematologic abnormalities and hepatotoxicity can occur but are uncommon [46]. Other toxicities reported include neuropsychiatric effects such as headache and insomnia [47].

Methotrexate

Originally used in oncology as a chemotherapeutic agent, low-dose methotrexate (MTX) has been FDA-approved for the treatment of severe, debilitating and recalcitrant psoriasis for nearly half a century [48]. It is also used by dermatologists for the treatment of other inflammatory skin conditions, including pityriasis rubra pilaris, atopic dermatitis and lichen planus [49].

Mechanism of Action

MTX works by inhibiting dihydrofolate reductase, thereby blocking purine production necessary for DNA synthesis [50]. MTX exerts anti-inflammatory effects secondarily, by suppressing neutrophil and macrophage chemotaxis, stimulating apoptosis of T and B lymphocytes, and inhibiting proliferation of proinflammatory cytokines [2].

Cutaneous Side Effects

MTX may rarely cause erosions or ulcerations within psoriatic plaques [51, 52]. Erosions have also been reported in non-psoriatic skin of patients treated with MTX for arthritis and are considered a possible portent of ensuing pancytopenia [53, 54]. MTX therapy also commonly causes increased photosensitivity [54]. Radiation recall has also been reported [55–57]. Rheumatoid nodules have been found to develop at an accelerated rate in rheumatoid arthritis patients treated with MTX [58]. Lastly, MTX may cause non-scarring alopecia [2].

Extracutaneous and Systemic Side Effects

Among the most common side effects of MTX is gastrointestinal upset. Increasing doses of folic acid typically help abate this symptom [59]. More serious potential side effects include infection, pancytopenia and hepatotoxicity [49]. Pancytopenia can occur within days to weeks of initiating the medication and is reversible with drug cessation. Severe hepatoxicity in the form of fibrosis or cirrhosis, by contrast, typically develops over years and is irreversible. The risk of hepatotoxicity rises directly with cumulative MTX dose and is compounded by a history of liver disease, alcoholic liver damage, or obesity [49]. Assessment for hepatic fibrosis has traditionally included periodic liver biopsies; more recent investigations have focused on potential serologic markers such as procollagen 3 aminopeptide, alpha-2 macroglobulin, tissue inhibitor of metalloproteinase-1 (TIMP-1) and hyaluronic acid [50, 60]. Patients on long-term MTX therapy should be referred to hepatology for evaluation.

Studies have suggested an increased risk of lymphoproliferative disorders during therapy with MTX [61]. Specifically, methotrexate-induced lymphoproliferative disease (MTX-LPD) has been observed more often in patients with rheumatoid arthritis treated with MTX than in any other patient cohort [62, 63]. However, there is limited evidence linking patients treated with MTX for psoriasis, or any other chronic cutaneous disease, with an increased risk for lymphoproliferative disorders.

Tumor Necrosis Factor Inhibitors

Tumor necrosis factor (TNF)-alpha inhibitors are widely utilized in dermatology for management of psoriasis, with three agents (etanercept, infliximab and adalimumab) FDA-approved for this indication. TNF-alpha inhibitors have also been employed to treat other inflammatory dermatoses, including hidradenitis suppurativa, dermatomyositis, immunobullous disease, neutrophilic dermatoses, and others.

Mechanism of Action

All TNF inhibitors block activation of TNF-alpha, a pro-inflammatory cytokine. Four TNF alpha inhibitors are monoclonal antibodies: infliximab, adalimumab, golimumab, and certolizumab pegol. Etanercept is a dimeric fusion protein.

Cutaneous Side Effects

The incidence of cutaneous toxicities secondary to TNF-alpha inhibitors is low. Most commonly, local injection/infusion site reactions are observed [64]. Other reported cutaneous adverse reactions to TNF-alpha inhibitors include cutaneous small-vessel vasculitis, cutaneous infections, interstitial granulomatous dermatitis and palisaded neutrophilic and granulomatous dermatitis, generalized eczematous and lichenoid reactions, psoriasis and psoriasiform lesions (Table 11.1) [64–67]. Up to one third of patients presenting with psoriatic lesions after starting TNF-alpha inhibitor therapy will present with a palmoplantar pustulosis, a pustular, pruritic eruption on the palms and soles (Figs. 11.2 and 11.3) [64, 68]. Patients may also develop typical psoriatic lesions on the trunk, extremities and scalp. Lastly,

Table 11.1 Summary of Cutaneous Toxicities of Anti-Rheumatic Agents

Medication	Mechanism of Action	Reported adverse cutaneous side effects
Antimalarials	Exact mechanism is unclear; possibly suppress T-lymphocyte proliferation and leukocyte chemotaxis, and stabilize lysosomal enzymes	Blue-gray dyspigmentation of legs, arms, face, oral mucosa and nails Bleaching of hair roots Yellowing of skin (quinacrine) Lichenoid drug eruption, AGEP, TEN, phototoxic and photoallergic eruptions
Azathioprine	Inhibits B and T cells via blockade of purine synthesis	Hypersensitivity reaction Sweet's syndrome Erythema nodosum
Cyclosporine	Downregulates IL-2, B and T cell function	Gingival hyperplasia Hypertrichosis Sebaceous hyperplasia Cutaneous pseudolymphoma
Dapsone	Inhibits neutrophil myeloperoxidase and eosinophil peroxidase, disrupts neutrophil chemotaxis	Hypersensitivity syndrome AGEP Erythema nodosum leprosum
Mycophenolate mofetil (MMF)	Selectively inhibits inosine monophosphate dehydrogenase, preventing de novo purine production and subsequent suppression of B and T lymphocytes	Rarely reported
Methotrexate (MTX)	Inhibits dihydrofolate reductase, thereby blocking purine production and subsequent B and T cell production	Photosensitivity Radiation recall Rheumatoid nodules Alopecia Mucosal erosions Ulceration of psoriatic plaques
TNF-alpha inhibitors	Blocks activation of TNF-alpha, a pro-inflammatory cytokine	Local injection site reactions Psoriasis and psoriasiform dermatitis SCLE-like eruption CCLE-like eruption Vasculitis PNGD Generalized lichenoid and eczematous eruptions

AGEP Acute and Generalized Exanthematous Pustulosis, *DIHS* Drug-Induced Hypersensitivity Syndrome, *TEN* Toxic Epidermal Necrolysis, *SCLE* Subacute Cutaneous Lupus Erythematosus, *CCLE* Chronic Cutaneous Lupus Erythematosus, *PNGD* Palisaded and Neutrophilic Granulomatous Dermatitis

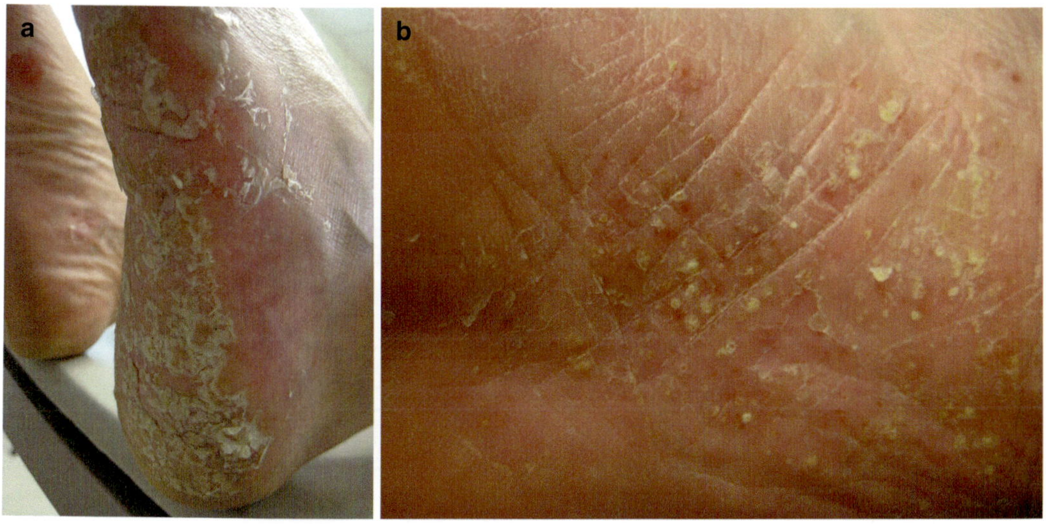

Fig. 11.2 (**a**, **b**) Anti-TNF Induced Plantar Pustulosis. (Image Courtesy of Joseph F. Merola, MD MMSC)

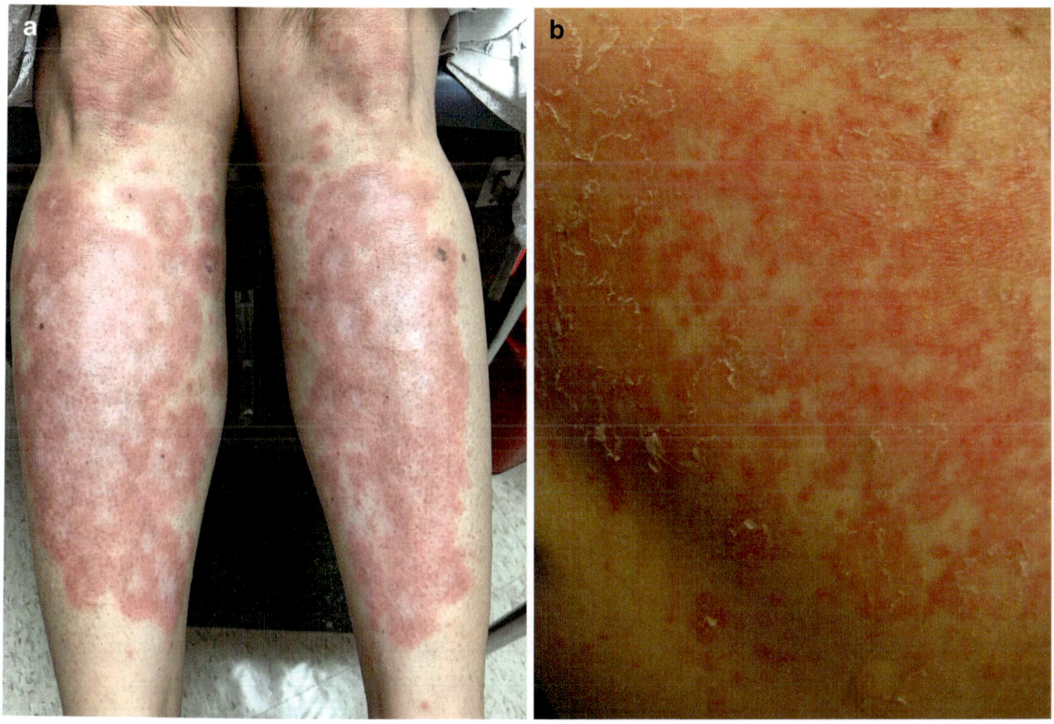

Fig. 11.3 (**a**, **b**) Drug-Induced Subacute Cutaneous Lupus. (Image Courtesy of Joseph F. Merola, MD MMSC)

TNF-alpha inhibitors can also induce subacute cutaneous and discoid lupus erythematosus, which are reversible within weeks of drug discontinuation [64].

Extracutaneous and Systemic Side Effects

TNF-alpha inhibitors will often lead to the development of antinuclear antibodies (ANA) and antibodies against double-stranded DNA (dsDNA) [69]. They can also induce a reversible syndrome mimicking systemic lupus erythematosus that subsides within weeks of drug cessation [64]. Despite concern to the contrary, patients with psoriasis and/or psoriatic arthritis treated with TNF-alpha inhibitors have not been found to have an increased risk of lymphoma or internal malignancy [70–72].

Drug-Induced Lupus Erythematosus and Drug-Induced Dermatomyositis

Though immunomodulatory agents are most often used in dermatology to manage inflammatory and connective tissue diseases, it is important to appreciate that these same agents, along with other common medications, can themselves paradoxically trigger the development of rheumatologic syndromes. Conscientious medication reconciliation is therefore of vital importance when considering a new diagnosis of connective tissue disease. In this section, we will review the important features of drug-induced lupus and drug-induced dermatomyositis, including commonly implicated medications.

Drug-Induced Lupus Erythematosus

The incidence of drug-induced lupus erythematosus, both systemic and cutaneous, has grown in recent years. In drug-induced SCLE, patients develop annular, papulosquamous plaques typically in a photodistribution, which may be clinically indistinguishable from native SCLE (Fig. 11.4) [72]. Additionally, patients typically will have antibodies against SSA/Ro. Evidence suggests that up to 20% of cases of SCLE are drug-induced, necessitating a thorough consideration of medication history when encountering a new diagnosis of SCLE [73].

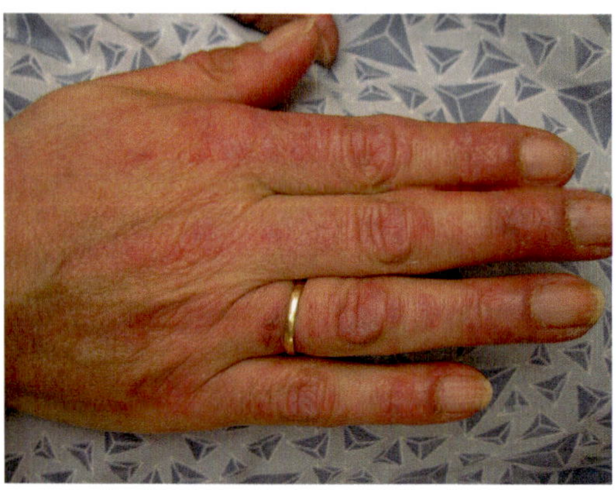

Fig. 11.4 Drug-induced Dermatomyositis. (Image Courtesy of Joseph F. Merola, MD MMSC)

In drug-induced systemic lupus, cutaneous findings may be absent or may include malar erythema or a photodistributed erythematous eruption [72]. Systemic features often predominate: patients may experience fatigue, fever, weight loss, arthritis, myalgias and serositis [72]. These cases of drug-induced systemic lupus are often associated with positive antinuclear antibody titers, specifically anti-histone antibodies.

The medication profile specific to each entity has been listed in Table 11.2.

Drug-Induced Dermatomyositis

Drug-induced dermatomyositis presents with characteristic skin findings identical to that of idiopathic dermatomyositis. The pathophysiology has not yet been elucidated; the cutaneous findings usually develop after long-term therapy of a potential causative agent, typically at least two years [76].

Drug-induced dermatomyositis has been linked to a variety of medications, including hydroxyurea, penicillamine, statins, cyclophosphamide, BCG vaccine administration, zolendronic acid, TNF-alpha inhibitors, and ipilimumab [76–80]. As with most cases of drug hypersensitivity, identification and cessation of such offending drugs often leads to resolution of symptoms.

Summary

Disease-modifying anti-rheumatic drugs and steroid-sparing agents serve as powerful tools in the management of cutaneous inflammatory and

Table 11.2 Key distinguishing features of Drug-Induced SLE vs. Drug-induced SCLE. (Adapted from Callen JP. Drug-induced subacute cutaneous lupus erythematosus. Lupus. 2010 Aug;19 (9):1107–11)

	Drug-induced SLE	Drug-induced SCLE
Morphology of Skin lesions	Rare	Annular, gyrate, papulosquamous plaques
Serologies	Anti-histone antibodies	Anti-Ro/SSA antibodies, rarely anti-histone antibodies
Serositis	Common	Occasional
Implicated drugs	Procainamide, hydralazine, isoniazid, minocycline, ticlodipine, TNF-alpha inhibitors [71]	Hydrochlorothiazide, proton pump inhibitors, calcium-channel blockers, terbinafine, ACE-inhibitors, TNF-alpha inhibitors, antifungals, diuretics, beta blockers, antiepileptics, lipid-lowering agents, antimalarials and sulfonylureas, docetaxel, paclitaxel, tamoxifen, fluorouracil, capecitabine, doxorubicin and cyclophosphamide [72, 74, 75]

TNF tumor necrosis factor, *ACE* angiotensin-converting-enzyme

connective tissue disease. However, in addition to their efficacy, such agents are also associated with distinct cutaneous and extracutaneous toxicities. Clinicians who aim to use such medications should have a detailed understanding of such reactions as early recognition and timely intervention could prevent life-threatening sequelae.

References

1. Kali S, Dutz JP. New concepts in antimalarial use and mode of action in dermatology. Dermatol Ther. 2007;20:160–74.
2. Katzung BG, Masters SB, Trevor AJ. Basic & clinical pharmacology. New York: Lange Medical Books/McGraw-Hill; 2015.
3. Puri PK, Lountzis NI, Tyler W, Ferringer T. Hydroxychloroquine-induced hyperpigmentation: the staining pattern. J Cutan Pathol. 2008;35(12):1134–7.
4. Kleinegger CL, Hammond HL, Finkelstein MW. Oral mucosal hyperpigmentation secondary to antimalarial drug therapy. Oral Surg Oral Med Oral Pathol Oral Radiol Endod. 2000;90:189–94.
5. Rosen T, Aponte C. Cutaneous hyperpigmentation due to chronic quinine ingestion. Cutis. 2005;75(2):114–6.
6. Asch PH, Caussade P, Marquart-Elbaz C, Boehm N, Grosshans E. Chloroquine-induced achromotrichia: an ultrastructural study. Ann Dermatol Venereol. 1997;124:552–6.
7. Donovan JC, Price VH. Images in clinical medicine. Chloroquine-induced hair hypopigmentation. N Engl J Med. 2010;363(4):372.
8. Vidal D, Altés J, Smandia JA. Yellow skin discoloration induced by quinacrine in a patient with cutaneous lupus erythematosus. Actas Dermosifiliogr. 2013;104(1):89–90.
9. Sokol RJ, Lichtenstein PK, Farrell MK. Quinacrine hydrochloride induced yellow discoloration of the skin in children. Pediatrics. 1982;69:232–3.
10. Dereure O. Drug-induced skin pigmentation. Am J Clin Dermatol. 2001;2(4):253–62.
11. Halevy S, Shai A. Lichenoid drug eruptions. J Am Acad Dermatol. 1993;29:249–55.
12. Bauer F. Quinacrine hydrochloride drug eruption (tropical lichenoid dermatitis). Its early and late sequelae and its malignant potential: a review. J Am Acad Dermatol. 1981;4(2):239–48.
13. Paradisi A, Bugatti L, Sisto T, Filosa G, Amerio PL, Capizzi R. Acute generalized exanthematous pustulosis induced by hydroxychloroquine: three cases and a review of the literature. Clin Ther. 2008;30(5):930–40.
14. Volpe A, Marchetta A, Caramaschi P, Biasi D, Bambara LM, Arcaro G. Hydroxychloroquine-induced DRESS syndrome. Clin Rheumatol. 2008;27(4):537–9.
15. Callaly EL, FitzGerald O, Rogers S. Hydroxychloroquine-associated, photo-induced toxic epidermal necrolysis. Clin Exp Dermatol. 2008;33(5):572–4.
16. Pearson KC, Morrell DS, Runge SR, Jolly P. Prolonged pustular eruption from hydroxychloroquine: an unusual case of acute generalized exanthematous pustulosis. Cutis. 2016;97(3):212–6.
17. Yalçın B, Çakmak S, Yıldırım B. Successful treatment of hydroxychloroquine-induced recalcitrant acute generalized exanthematous pustulosis with cyclosporine: case report and literature review. Ann Dermatol. 2015;4:431–4.
18. Pelle MT, Callen JP. Adverse cutaneous reactions to hydroxychloroquine are more common in patients with dermatomyositis than in patients with cutaneous lupus erythematosus. Arch Dermatol. 2002;138(9):1231–3.
19. Lisi P, Assalve D, Hansel K. Phototoxic and photoallergic dermatitis caused by hydroxychloroquine. Contact Dermatitis. 2004;50(4):255–6.
20. Marmor MF, Kellner U, Lai TY, Melles RB, Mieler WF, American Academy of Ophthalmology. Recommendations on screening for chloroquine and

hydroxychloroquine retinopathy (2016 Revision). Ophthalmology. 2016;123:1386–94.
21. Patel AA, Swerlick RA, McCall CO. Azathioprine in dermatology: the past, the present, and the future. J Am Acad Dermatol. 2006;55:369–89.
22. Wise M, Callen JP. Azathioprine: a guide for the management of dermatology patients. Dermatol Ther. 2007;20:206–15.
23. Feldman M, Friedman LS, Brandt LJ. Sleisenger and Fordtran's gastrointestinal and liver disease: pathophysiology, diagnosis, management, expert consult premium edition-enhanced online features. Elsevier Health Sciences; 2010 May 3.
24. Jeurissen ME, Boerbooms AM, Van de Putte LB, Kruijsen MW. Azathioprine induced fever, chills, rash, and hepatotoxicity in rheumatoid arthritis. Ann Rheum Dis. 1990;49(1):25–7.
25. Rosenthal E. Azathioprine shock. Postgrad Med J. 1986;62(729):677–8.
26. Biswas SN, Chakraborty PP, Gantait K, Bar C. Azathioprine-induced bullous Sweet's syndrome: a rare association. BMJ Case Rep. 2016;2016. https://doi.org/10.1136/bcr-2016-215192. PMID 27090551.
27. Choonhakarn C, Chaowattanapanit S. Azathioprine-induced Sweet's syndrome and published work review. J Dermatol. 2013;40(4):267–71.
28. Turow A, Yong TY, Fok JS, Li JY. Azathioprine hypersensitivity presenting as cardiogenic shock and Sweet's syndrome in a patient with microscopic polyangiitis. Intern Med. 2012;51(14):1889–92.
29. De Fonclare AL, Khosrotehrani K, Aractingi S, Duriez P, Cosnes J, Beaugerie L. Erythema nodosum–like eruption as a manifestation of azathioprine hypersensitivity in patients with inflammatory bowel disease. Arch Dermatol. 2007;143(6):744–8.
30. Bhutani T, Lee CS, Koo JY. Cyclosporine. In: Wolverton SE, editor. Comprehensive dermatologic drug therapy. 3rd ed. Edinburgh: Elsevier; 2013. 1991-211.
31. Amor KT, Ryan C, Menter A. The use of cyclosporine in dermatology: part I. J Am Acad Dermatol. 2010;63(6):925–46.
32. Doufexi A, Mina M, Ioannidou E. Gingival overgrowth in children: epidemiology, pathogenesis, and complications. A literature review. J Periodontol. 2005;76(1):3–10.
33. Bencini PL, Montagnino G, Sala F, De Vecchi A, Crosti C, Tarantino A. Cutaneous lesions in 67 cyclosporin-treated renal transplant recipients. Dermatology. 1986;172(1):24–30.
34. de Berker DA, Taylor AE, Quinn AG, Simpson NB. Sebaceous hyperplasia in organ transplant recipients: shared aspects of hyperplastic and dysplastic processes? J Am Acad Dermatol. 1996;35(5):696–9.
35. Wilken R, Fung MA, Shi VY, Cheng MY, Sultani H, Maverakis E. Cyclosporine-induced sebaceous hyperplasia in a hematopoetic stem cell transplant patient: delayed onset of a common adverse event. Dermatol Online J. 2016;22(1):13030/qt4865202s.
36. Foley C, Leonard N, Wynne B. Cutaneous pseudolymphoma: A rare side effect of cyclosporine. J Am Acad Dermatol. 2015;72(3):e85–6.
37. Ryan C, Amor KT, Menter A. The use of cyclosporine in dermatology: part II. J Am Acad Dermatol. 2010;63(6):949–72.
38. Zachariae H. Renal toxicity of long-term cyclosporine. Scand J Rheumatol. 1999;28(2):65–8.
39. Wozel G, Blasum C. Dapsone in dermatology and beyond. Arch Dermatol Res. 2014;306(2):103–24.
40. Stotland M, Shalita AR, Kissling RF. Dapsone 5% gel. Am J Clin Dermatol. 2009;10(4):221–7.
41. Edhegard K, Hall RP. Dapsone. In: Wolverton SE, editor. Comprehensive dermatologic drug therapy. 3rd ed. Edinburgh: Elsevier; 2013. p. 228–40.
42. Hoogeveen RM, van der Bom T, de Boer HH, Thurlings RM, Wind BS, de Vries HJ, van Lent AU, Beuers U, van der Wal AC, Nellen FJ. A lethal case of the dapsone hypersensitivity syndrome involving the myocardium. Neth J Med. 2016;74(2):89–92.
43. Schulkes KJ, Tervaert JC, Rijken F, Haas LE. Dapsone hypersensitivity syndrome not related to G6PD deficiency. BMJ Case Rep. 2015;2015:bcr2015212742.
44. Jollow DJ, Bradshaw TP, Mcmillan DC. Dapsone-induced hemolytic anemia. Drug Metab Rev. 1995;27(1–2):107–24.
45. Narasimharao P, Pratap DV, Suneetha S. Acute generalized exanthematous pustulosis (AGEP) due to dapsone in a patient with leprosy. Lepr Rev. 2009;80(1):81.
46. Zwerner J, Fiorentino D. Mycophenolate mofetil. Dermatol Ther. 2007;20:229–38.
47. Liu V, Mackool BT. Mycophenolate in dermatology. J Dermatolog Treat. 2003;14:203–11.
48. Weinstein GD. Methotrexate. Ann Intern Med. 1977;86(2):199–204.
49. Callen JP, Kulp-Shorten CL. Methotrexate. In: Wolverton SE, editor. Comprehensive dermatologic drug therapy. 3rd ed. Edinburgh: Elsevier; 2013. p. 169–81.
50. Poordad FF. FIBROSpect II: a potential noninvasive test to assess hepatic fibrosis. Expert Rev Mol Diagn. 2004;4(5):593–7.
51. Souza CF, Suarez OM, Silva TF, Gorenstein AC, Quintella LP, Avelleira JC. Ulcerations due to methotrexate toxicity in a psoriasis patient. An Bras Dermatol. 2016;91(3):375–7.
52. Koçak AY, Koçak O, Aslan F, Tektaş M. Methotrexate toxicity presenting as cutaneous ulcerations on psoriatic plaques. Cutan Ocul Toxicol. 2013;32(4):333–5.
53. Shiver MB, Hall LA, Conner KB, Brown GE, Cheung WL, Wirges ML. Cutaneous erosions: a herald for impending pancytopenia in methotrexate toxicity. Dermatol Online J. 2014;20(7):13030/qt46k975h8.
54. Ben-Amitai D, Hodak E, David M. Cutaneous ulceration: an unusual sign of methotrexate toxic-

ity—first report in a patient without psoriasis. Ann Pharmacother. 1998;32(6):651–3.
55. Mallory SB, Berry DH. Severe reactivation of sunburn following methotrexate use. Pediatrics. 1986;78(3):514–5.
56. Guzzo C, Kaidby K. Recurrent recall of sunburn by methotrexate. Photodermatol Photoimmunol Photomed. 1995;11(2):55–6.
57. Devore KJ. Solar burn reactivation induced by methrotrexate. Pharmacotherapy. 2010;30(4):123e–6e.
58. Tilstra JS, Lienesch DW. Rheumatoid nodules. Dermatol Clin. 2015;33(3):361–71.
59. Shea B, Swinden MV, Tanjong Ghogomu E, Ortiz Z, Katchamart W, Rader T, Bombardier C, Wells GA, Tugwell P. Folic acid and folinic acid for reducing side effects in patients receiving methotrexate for rheumatoid arthritis. Cochrane Database Syst Rev. 2013;5.
60. Chalmers RJ, Kirby B, Smith A, Burrows P, Little R, Horan M, Hextall JM, Smith CH, Klaber M, Rogers S. Replacement of routine liver biopsy by procollagen III aminopeptide for monitoring patients with psoriasis receiving long-term methotrexate: a multicentre audit and health economic analysis. Br J Dermatol. 2005;152(3):444–50.
61. Patel RV, Clark LN, Lebwohl M, Weinberg JM. Treatments for psoriasis and the risk of malignancy. J Am Acad Dermatol. 2009;60:1001–17.
62. Hoshida Y, Xu JX, Fujita S, Nakamichi I, Ikeda JI, Tomita Y, Nakatsuka SI, Tamaru JI, Iizuka A, Takeuchi T, Aozasa K. Lymphoproliferative disorders in rheumatoid arthritis: clinicopathological analysis of 76 cases in relation to methotrexate medication. J Rheumatol. 2007;34(2):322–31.
63. Clarke LE, Junkins-Hopkins J, Seykora JT, Adler DJ, Elenitsas R. Methotrexate-associated lymphoproliferative disorder in a patient with rheumatoid arthritis presenting in the skin. J Am Acad Dermatol. 2007;56(4):686–90.
64. Moustou AE, Matekovits A, Dessinioti C, Antoniou C, Sfikakis PP, Stratigos AJ. Cutaneous side effects of anti–tumor necrosis factor biologic therapy: a clinical review. J Am Acad Dermatol. 2009;61(3):486–504.
65. Sokumbi O, Wetter DA, Makol A, Warrington KJ. Vasculitis associated with tumor necrosis factor-α inhibitors. Mayo Clin Proc. Elsevier. 2012;87(8):739–45.
66. Stephenson SR, Campbell SM, Drew GS, Magro CM. Palisaded neutrophlic and granulomatous dermatitis presenting in a patient with rheumatoid arthritis on adalimumab. J Cutan Pathol. 2011;38(8):644–8.
67. Jayasekera PS, Walsh ML, Hurrell D, Parslew RG. Case report of lichen planopilaris occurring in a pediatric patient receiving a tumor necrosis factor α inhibitor and a review of the literature. Pediatr Dermatol. 2016;33:e143–6.
68. Shmidt E, Wetter DA, Ferguson SB, Pittelkow MR. Psoriasis and palmoplantar pustulosis associated with tumor necrosis factor-α inhibitors: the Mayo Clinic experience, 1998 to 2010. J Am Acad Dermatol. 2012;67(5):e179–85.
69. Eriksson C, Engstrand S, Sundqvist KG, Rantapaa-Dahlqvist S. Autoantibody formation in patients with rheumatoid arthritis treated with anti-TNF alpha. Ann Rheum Dis. 2005;64:403–7.
70. Dommasch ED, Abuabara K, Shin DB, Nguyen J, Troxel AB, Gelfand JM. The risk of infection and malignancy with tumor necrosis factor antagonists in adults with psoriatic disease: a systematic review and meta-analysis of randomized controlled trials. J Am Acad Dermatol. 2011;64(6):1035–50.
71. Costa L, et al. Incidence of malignancies in a cohort of psoriatic arthritis patients taking traditional disease modifying antirheumatic drug and tumor necrosis factor inhibitor therapy: an observational study. J Rheumatol. 2016;43:2149–54.
72. Callen JP. Drug-induced subacute cutaneous lupus erythematosus. Lupus. 2010;19(9):1107–11.
73. Laurinaviciene R, Sandholdt LH, Bygum A. Drug-induced cutaneous lupus erythematosus: 88 new cases. Eur J Dermatol. 2017;27(1):28–33.
74. Lowe GC, Henderson CL, Hansen CB, Sontheimer RD. A systematic review of drug-induced subacute cutaneous lupus erythematosus. Br J Dermatol. 2011;164(3):465–72.
75. Wiznia LE, Subtil A, Choi JN. Subacute cutaneous lupus induced by chemotherapy: gemcitabine as a causative agent. JAMA Dermatol. 2013;149(9):1071–5.
76. Seidler AM, Gottlieb AB. Dermatomyositis induced by drug therapy: a review of case reports. J Am Acad Dermatol. 2008;59(5):872–80.
77. Liu SW, Velez NF, Lam C, Femia A, Granter SR, Townsend HB, Vleugels RA. Dermatomyositis induced by anti–tumor necrosis factor in a patient with juvenile idiopathic arthritis. JAMA Dermatol. 2013;149(10):1204–8.
78. Succaria F, Collier M, Mahalingam M. Zoledronic acid–induced interface dermatitis. Am J Dermatopathol. 2015;37(12):933–5.
79. Tong PL, Yu LL, Chan JJ. Drug-induced dermatomyositis after zoledronic acid. Australas J Dermatol. 2012;53(4):e73–5.
80. Ali SS, Goddard AL, Luke JJ, Donahue H, Todd DJ, Werchniak A, Vleugels RA. Drug-associated dermatomyositis following ipilimumab therapy: a novel immune-mediated adverse event associated with cytotoxic T-lymphocyte antigen 4 blockade. JAMA Dermatol. 2015;151(2):195–9.

Index

A. Garg et al. (eds.), *Interdisciplinary Approaches to Overlap Disorders in Dermatology & Rheumatology*,
https://doi.org/10.1007/978-3-319-18446-3

Printed by Printforce, the Netherlands